OPHTHALMOLOGY CLINICS-2

for Postgraduates

Basic Sciences, Instruments, Investigations, Imaging, Interpretation and Viva Voice

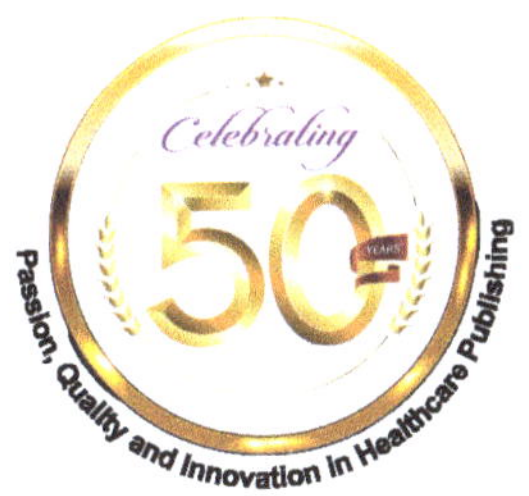

OPHTHALMOLOGY CLINICS-2

for Postgraduates

Basic Sciences, Instruments, Investigations, Imaging, Interpretation and Viva Voice

Editors

Prafulla Kumar Maharana
MD DNB
Assistant Professor
Dr Rajendra Prasad Centre for Ophthalmic Sciences
All India Institute of Medical Sciences
New Delhi, India

Namrata Sharma
MD
Professor
Dr Rajendra Prasad Centre for Ophthalmic Sciences
All India Institute of Medical Sciences
New Delhi, India

Atul Kumar
MD FAMS
Professor and Chief
Dr Rajendra Prasad Centre for Ophthalmic Sciences
All India Institute of Medical Sciences
New Delhi, India

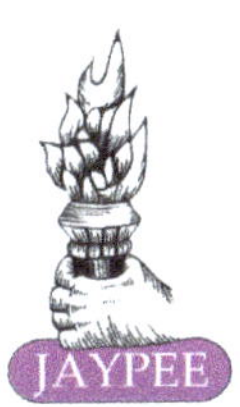

JAYPEE BROTHERS MEDICAL PUBLISHERS
The Health Sciences Publisher
New Delhi | London

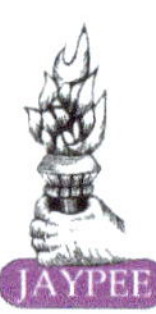

Jaypee Brothers Medical Publishers (P) Ltd.

Headquarters
Jaypee Brothers Medical Publishers (P) Ltd.
4838/24, Ansari Road, Daryaganj
New Delhi 110 002, India
Phone: +91-11-43574357
Fax: +91-11-43574314
Email: jaypee@jaypeebrothers.com

Overseas Office
JP Medical Ltd.
83, Victoria Street, London
SW1H 0HW (UK)
Phone: +44 20 3170 8910
Fax: +44 (0)20 3008 6180
E-mail: info@jpmedpub.com

Website: www.jaypeebrothers.com
Website: www.jaypeedigital.com

Inquiries for bulk sales may be solicited at: jaypee@jaypeebrothers.com

Ophthalmology Clinics-2 for Postgraduates: Basic Sciences, Instruments, Investigations, Imaging, Interpretation and Viva Voice

First Edition: **2020**

ISBN: 978-93-89188-60-8

Dedicated to

My parents, Mr Devendra Maharana and
Mrs Binadini Maharana, and My Students.

—Prafulla Kumar Maharana

My parents, Dr Ramesh C Sharma and Mrs Maitreyi Pushpa,
my husband, Dr Subhash Chandra, and daughter, Vasavdatta

—Namrata Sharma

My late parents, Mr Sanat Kumar and Mrs Swarna Kumar,
my wife, Mrs Parul Kumar, and children, Aman and Arshi

—Atul Kumar

CONTRIBUTORS

Abhipsa Sharma MBBS
Junior Resident
Dr Rajendra Prasad Centre for Ophthalmic Sciences
All India Institute of Medical Sciences
New Delhi, India

Aditi Dubey MS
Assistant Professor
Department of Ophthalmology
Gandhi Medical College (GMC)
Bhopal, Madhya Pradesh, India

Alisha Kishore MD
Senior Resident
Dr Rajendra Prasad Centre for Ophthalmic Sciences
All India Institute of Medical Sciences
New Delhi, India

Amber Bhayana MD
Senior Resident
Dr Rajendra Prasad Centre for Ophthalmic Sciences
All India Institute of Medical Sciences
New Delhi, India

Anin Sethi MD
Senior Resident
Dr Rajendra Prasad Centre for Ophthalmic Sciences
All India Institute of Medical Sciences
New Delhi, India

Ankit Singh Tomar MD
Oculoplastics Fellow
Centre for Sight Superspeciality Eye Hospital
Hyderabad, Telangana, India

Anusha Sachan MD
Senior Resident
Dr Rajendra Prasad Centre for Ophthalmic Sciences
All India Institute of Medical Sciences
New Delhi, India

Arpit Sharma MBBS
Junior Resident
Dr Rajendra Prasad Centre for Ophthalmic Sciences
All India Institute of Medical Sciences
New Delhi, India

Asha Samdani MD
Senior Resident
Dr Rajendra Prasad Centre for Ophthalmic Sciences
All India Institute of Medical Sciences
New Delhi, India

Atul Kumar MD FAMS
Professor and Chief
Dr Rajendra Prasad Centre for Ophthalmic Sciences
All India Institute of Medical Sciences
New Delhi, India

Brijesh Takkar MD
Assistant Professor
Department of Ophthalmology
All India Institute of Medical Sciences
Bhopal, Madhya Pradesh, India

Deepali Singhal MD
Senior Resident
Dr Rajendra Prasad Centre for Ophthalmic Sciences
All India Institute of Medical Sciences
New Delhi, India

Devesh Kumawat MD
Assistant professor
Department of Ophthalmology
All India Institute of Medical Sciences
Rishikesh, Uttarakhand, India

Divya Agarwal MD
Senior Resident
Dr Rajendra Prasad Centre for Ophthalmic Sciences
All India Institute of Medical Sciences
New Delhi, India

Gaurav Garg MD
Oculoplastics Fellow
Centre for Sight Superspeciality Eye Hospital
Hyderabad, Telangana, India

Geeta Satpathy MD
Professor
Department of Microbiology
Dr Rajendra Prasad Centre for Ophthalmic Sciences
All India Institute of Medical Sciences
New Delhi, India

Gunjan Saluja MD
Senior Resident
Dr Rajendra Prasad Centre for Ophthalmic Sciences
All India Institute of Medical Sciences
New Delhi, India

Hannah Shiny R MBBS
Junior Resident
Dr Rajendra Prasad Centre for Ophthalmic Sciences
All India Institute of Medical Sciences
New Delhi, India

Harika Regani MBBS
Junior Resident
Dr Rajendra Prasad Centre for Ophthalmic Sciences
All India Institute of Medical Sciences
New Delhi, India

Jeewan Singh Titiyal MD
Professor
Dr Rajendra Prasad Centre for Ophthalmic Sciences
All India Institute of Medical Sciences
New Delhi, India

Jyoti Shakrawal MD
Senior Resident
Dr Rajendra Prasad Centre for Ophthalmic Sciences
All India Institute of Medical Sciences
New Delhi, India

Karthika Bhaskaran MD
Senior Resident
Dr Rajendra Prasad Centre for Ophthalmic Sciences
All India Institute of Medical Sciences
New Delhi, India

Lohith Rambarki MD
Senior Resident
Dr Rajendra Prasad Centre for Ophthalmic Sciences
All India Institute of Medical Sciences
New Delhi, India

Meenakshi Wadhwani MS DNB
Assistant Professor
Department of Ophthalmology
Chacha Nehru Bal Chikitsalaya
New Delhi, India

Mohamed Ibrahime Asif MD
Senior Resident
Dr Rajendra Prasad Centre for Ophthalmic Sciences
All India Institute of Medical Sciences
New Delhi, India

Mousumi Bannerjee MBBS
Junior Resident
Dr Rajendra Prasad Centre for Ophthalmic Sciences
All India Institute of Medical Sciences
New Delhi, India

Namrata Sharma MD
Professor
Dr Rajendra Prasad Centre for Ophthalmic Sciences
All India Institute of Medical Sciences
New Delhi, India

Nasiq Hasan MD
Senior Resident
Dr Rajendra Prasad Centre for Ophthalmic Sciences
All India Institute of Medical Sciences
New Delhi, India

Nawazish Shaikh MBBS
Junior Resident
Dr Rajendra Prasad Centre for Ophthalmic Sciences
All India Institute of Medical Sciences
New Delhi, India

Nikita Gupta MD
Resident
Dr Rajendra Prasad Centre for Ophthalmic Sciences
All India Institute of Medical Sciences
New Delhi, India

Nishat Hussain Ahmed MD
Assistant Professor
Department of Microbiology
Dr Rajendra Prasad Centre for Ophthalmic Sciences
All India Institute of Medical Sciences
New Delhi, India

Pallavi Shukla MD
Scientist B
Department of Community Ophthalmology
Dr Rajendra Prasad Centre for Ophthalmic Sciences
All India Institute of Medical Sciences
New Delhi, India

Pallavi Singh MD
Senior Resident
Dr Rajendra Prasad Centre for Ophthalmic Sciences
All India Institute of Medical Sciences
New Delhi, India

Prafulla Kumar Maharana MD DNB
Assistant Professor
Dr Rajendra Prasad Centre for Ophthalmic Sciences
All India Institute of Medical Sciences
New Delhi, India

Pranita Sahay MD
Scientist
Dr Rajendra Prasad Centre for Ophthalmic Sciences
All India Institute of Medical Sciences
New Delhi, India

Praveen Vashist MD MSc (CEH)
Professor
Department of Community Ophthalmology
Dr Rajendra Prasad Centre for Ophthalmic Sciences
All India Institute of Medical Sciences
New Delhi, India

Priyanka MS
Senior Resident
Department of Ophthalmology
All India Institute of Medical Sciences
Bhopal, Madhya Pradesh, India

Priyanka Ramesh MD
Senior Resident
Dr Rajendra Prasad Centre for Ophthalmic Sciences
All India Institute of Medical Sciences
New Delhi, India

Rinky Agarwal MD
Senior Resident
Dr Rajendra Prasad Centre for Ophthalmic Sciences
All India Institute of Medical Sciences
New Delhi, India

Ritu Nagpal MD
Senior Research Associate
Dr Rajendra Prasad Centre for Ophthalmic Sciences
All India Institute of Medical Sciences
New Delhi, India

Rohan Chawla MD
Assistant Professor
Dr Rajendra Prasad Centre for Ophthalmic Sciences
All India Institute of Medical Sciences
New Delhi, India

Sahil Agrawal MD
Senior Resident
Dr Rajendra Prasad Centre for Ophthalmic Sciences
All India Institute of Medical Sciences
New Delhi, India

Saloni Gupta MS
Divisional Medical Officer
Department of Ophthalmology
Northern Railway Central Hospital (NRCH)
New Delhi, India

Sanjay Sharma MD
Professor
Department of Radiodiagnosis
Dr Rajendra Prasad Centre for Ophthalmic Sciences
All India Institute of Medical Sciences
New Delhi, India

Saurabh Verma MD
Senior Resident
Dr Rajendra Prasad Centre for Ophthalmic Sciences
All India Institute of Medical Sciences
New Delhi, India

Savinay Kapur MD
Senior Resident
Department of Radiodiagnosis
Dr Rajendra Prasad Centre for Ophthalmic Sciences
All India Institute of Medical Sciences
New Delhi, India

Seema Kashyap MD
Professor
Department of Pathology
Dr Rajendra Prasad Centre for Ophthalmic Sciences
All India Institute of Medical Sciences
New Delhi, India

Shahnaz Anjum MBBS
Junior Resident
Dr Rajendra Prasad Centre for Ophthalmic Sciences
All India Institute of Medical Sciences
New Delhi, India

Shipra Singhi MD
Consultant
Department of Ophthalmology
Medipulse Hospital
Jodhpur, Rajasthan, India

Shreya Nayak MBBS
Junior Resident
Dr Rajendra Prasad Centre for Ophthalmic Sciences
All India Institute of Medical Sciences
New Delhi, India

Siddhi Goel MD
Senior Resident
Dr Rajendra Prasad Centre for Ophthalmic Sciences
All India Institute of Medical Sciences
New Delhi, India

Sitesh Kumar Bergaal MD
Senior Resident
Dr Rajendra Prasad Centre for Ophthalmic Sciences
All India Institute of Medical Sciences
New Delhi, India

Sourabh Verma MD
Senior Resident
Dr Rajendra Prasad Centre for Ophthalmic Sciences
All India Institute of Medical Sciences
New Delhi, India

Suman Dhanda MD
Senior Resident
Dr Rajendra Prasad Centre for Ophthalmic Sciences
All India Institute of Medical Sciences
New Delhi, India

Suman Meena MBBS
Junior Resident
Dr Rajendra Prasad Centre for Ophthalmic Sciences
All India Institute of Medical Sciences
New Delhi, India

Suraj S Senjam MD
Associate Professor
Department of Community Ophthalmology
Dr Rajendra Prasad Centre for Ophthalmic Sciences
All India Institute of Medical Sciences
New Delhi, India

Surg Cdr Srujana D MS
Associate Professor
Department of Ophthalmology
Armed Forces Medical College
Pune, Maharashtra, India

Talvir Sidhu MD
Assistant Professor
Department of Ophthalmology
Government Medical College
Patiala, Punjab, India

Tanuj Dada MD
Professor
Dr Rajendra Prasad Centre for Ophthalmic Sciences
All India Institute of Medical Sciences
New Delhi, India

Vatika Jain MBBS
Junior Resident
Dr Rajendra Prasad Centre for Ophthalmic Sciences
All India Institute of Medical Sciences
New Delhi, India

Vatsalya Venkatraman MBBS
Junior Resident
Dr Rajendra Prasad Centre for Ophthalmic Sciences
All India Institute of Medical Sciences
New Delhi, India

Vivek Gupta MD
Assistant Professor
Department of Community Ophthalmology
Dr Rajendra Prasad Centre for Ophthalmic Sciences
All India Institute of Medical Sciences
New Delhi, India

Yogita Gupta MD
Senior Resident
Dr Rajendra Prasad Centre for Ophthalmic Sciences
All India Institute of Medical Sciences
New Delhi, India

PREFACE

First of all, we thank the readers for the tremendous positive response to our earlier book "Ophthalmology Clinics for Postgraduates". Just to reiterate "Postgraduate examination is one of the most difficult and stressful milestones in the medical profession. It entails a tremendous amount of stress on the candidates who appear for the examination." Our previous book was primarily targeted at the discussion on cases that are often given as long and short cases. However, any examination is not complete without going through the much difficult phase of viva based on the various investigations, their result and interpretation. Besides, investigations and their interpretation are an invaluable tool for diagnosis of common clinical problems seen in day-to-day practice.

Imaging in ophthalmology has dramatically advanced over the last decade. It is often difficult for a student to get information about all the investigation tools at one place. Similarly, a general practitioner often finds it difficult to interpret the outputs of so many investigating tools. This book attempts to present the important investigative tools in a format that is exactly the same as required in the practical examinations and day-to-day practice for an ophthalmologist.

The primary focus is on principles of different investigative tools, and the clinical interpretation of their outputs. Special emphasis has been given to present the outputs in different clinical cases that are often encountered in day-to-day practice and postgraduate examinations. Every possible effort has been made to include photographs of all-important cases seen in outpatient department (OPD), and given as cases in examinations.

A section on Basic Sciences such as Ocular Pathology, Ocular Microbiology, and Community Ophthalmology have been included. This will help the students to appear in viva examinations. A section on Orbital Imaging will help the students and practitioners to be able to diagnose the common clinical situations seen in day-to-day practice. In addition, a chapter on instruments has been included with every section, which is invariably a part of all postgraduate practical examinations. The editors and all the contributors have made sincere efforts to make things simple and concise to facilitate quick and thorough revision. Each chapter ends with a section on viva questions that will help the candidates to mentally prepare for the viva before the final examination.

Lastly, we remind the postgraduate students that the book is not a replacement for the standard textbooks, but it will make their understanding and application easier whenever there is some doubt or confusion.

The editors wish best of luck to the students for their examinations!

Prafulla Kumar Maharana
Namrata Sharma
Atul Kumar

CONTENTS

SECTION 1 Appliances and Instruments

SECTION 2 Basic Sciences

SECTION 3 Interpretation of Images and Reports

1

SECTION

APPLIANCES AND INSTRUMENTS

1 CHAPTER

Oculoplasty and Orbital Imaging

1.1 EXOPHTHALMOMETRY

Pallavi Singh, Siddhi Goel

INTRODUCTION

Disorders of the orbit are quite commonly seen in ophthalmic practice. These are often associated with displacement of the globe from its normal position in the orbit. Exophthalmometer is an instrument used for measuring the degree of displacement of the globe. It is used for measurement of both exophthalmos as well as enophthalmos.

PRINCIPLE

Exophthalmometry is the science of quantitatively assessing the position of the globe in the orbit, by measuring the distance of the anterior corneal apex from the lateral margins. There are three different types of clinical exophthalmometry:

1. *Absolute*: Comparison with the normal values seen in the general population.
2. *Relative*: Comparison of one eye with the other.
3. *Comparative*: Comparison of measurements of one eye over a period.

TYPES OF EXOPHTHALMOMETER

Various types of exophthalmometer have been described over the years. The first such device, called ophthalmoprostatometer was developed by Cohn in 1865.[1] Perpendicular globe position was obtained by Zehender, by placing a mirror medial to the cornea and parallel to his ruler. A sighting device was placed lateral to the ruler and exactly opposite to the marked center of the mirror, to ensure perpendicular position of the globe. The Hertel exophthalmometer was introduced in 1905 and till date remains, the most popular device used for clinical exophthalmometry. Luedde invented a pocket-sized device in 1938, which was an inexpensive and useful alternative to the previous devices. In 1970, Davanger sought to eliminate the error caused in measurement by parallax by introducing a prism, which moves forward and back. Naugle and Couvillion described their exophthalmometer in 1992, which uses superior and inferior orbital rims as reference points, thus enabling measurements in cases of lateral orbital wall fractures. Hertel's exophthalmometer has been variously modified to use the external auditory meatus as the point of reference (Yeatts) and with a fixation adapter to fixate on the forehead and nose (Kratky and Hurwitz). Computed tomography scans can be used to document the degree of proptosis accurately, however, they are expensive, time consuming and cause radiation exposure.[1]

TECHNIQUE

To use the Hertel's exophthalmometer, the examiner sits opposite the patient at eye level. The instrument is then placed at both the lateral orbital rims and the base distance between the two is noted. The examiner asks the patient to look straight ahead with eyelids wide open. Each eye is measured separately for proptosis by looking into the mirror (which has a millimeter scale marked on it) with one eye and moving the head side to side until the red fixation lines match up, thus eliminating any parallax. The examiner can now determine the position of the corneal apex of the patient from the millimeter reading.

NORMAL VALUES

The normal values in exophthalmometry are taken as 10–23 mm (average 16 mm) in whites, and 12–23 mm (average 18 mm) in blacks. On an average, in the Indian population, a value of greater than 21 mm or a difference of 2 mm or greater between two eyes is considered significant.[2,3]

VIVA QUESTIONS

1. What are the different types of exophthalmometry?

Ans. There are three different types of exophthalmometry:

i. *Absolute*: Comparison with the normal values seen in the general population.

ii. *Relative*:
- Comparison of one eye with the other
- Normal values are ≤2 mm.

iii. *Comparative*:
- Serial exophthalmometry readings of the same eye are compared over time
- It is better to use the same instrument
- Useful in Graves' disease
- Hertel preferred over Luedde.

2. Name different types of exophthalmometer.

Ans. Hertel, Naugle, Luedde, Zehender, Davanger, and Gormaz are a few different types of exophthalmometers.

Hertel's (Figs. 1.1.1 and 1.1.2)

- It has a Foot-plates (or yokes) "grooved arc" to fit over bony temporal margin of lateral orbital rim; a crossbar to establish baseline and to allow for binocular reading.
- It uses prisms (Marco's) or mirrors (B&L's or Lombart's) incline at 45° from sagittal plane.
- Overall dimensions are 25 × 7 × 2 cm. Weight is 117 g (4.1 oz)/light weight or 216 g (7.6 oz)/heavy duty.
- Scale for orbital wall goes from 75 mm to 121 mm.
- The scale to measure the proptosis ranges from 0 mm to 35 mm.

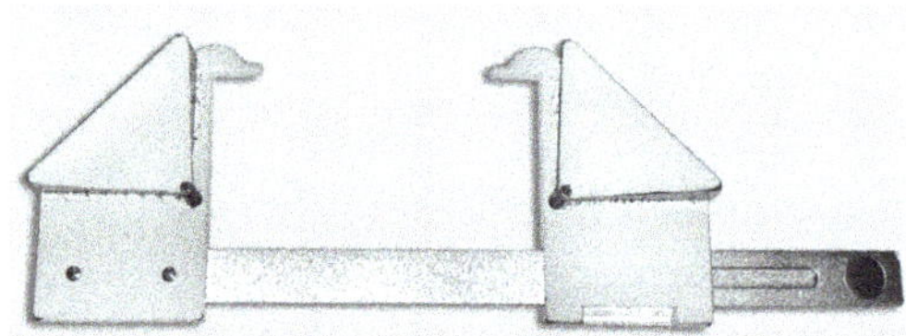

Fig. 1.1.1: Hertel's exophthalmometer.

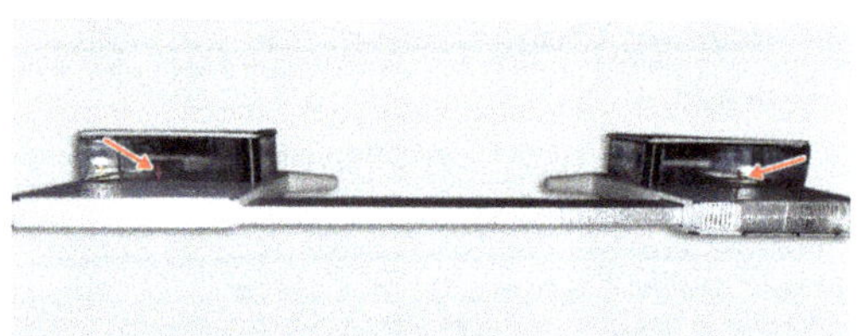

Fig. 1.1.2: Hertel's exophthalmometer with the redline used for parallax.

Luedde (Fig. 1.1.3)

- It is a transparent plastic mm ruler. It has a notch that conforms to angle of lateral orbital rim
- *Scale readings*: 0 mm (end of notch) to 40 mm
- Parallax is minimized by using scale on both sides of the rod (advantages of using Luedde over a standard ophthalmic millimeter ruler).

Naugle's Exophthalmometer (Fig. 1.1.4)

This is an inferior and superior rim-based instrument. It may be used when the lateral orbital rim is not intact.

3. What are the advantages of Hertel's exophthalmometer?

Ans. The advantages are:

- *Binocular reading*: It provides the ability to measure both eyes simultaneously and the measurement of the distance between lateral orbital rims.
- *Baseline for sequential readings*: It is also useful for serial follow-ups of the same patient.
- Best for comparative exophthalmometry.

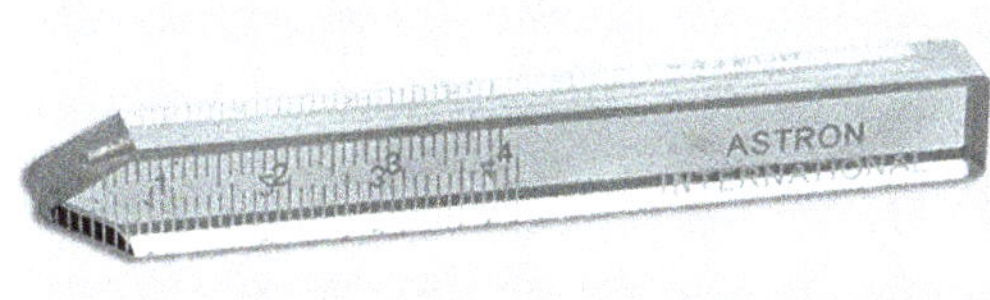

Fig. 1.1.3: Luedde Exophthalmometer.

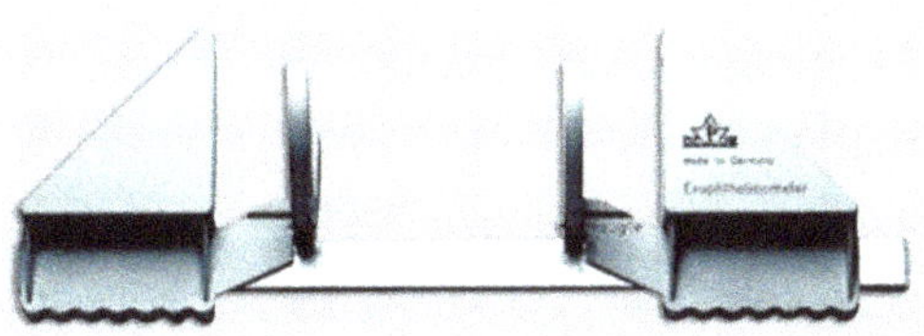

Fig. 1.1.4: Naugle's exophthalmometer.

4. What are the disadvantages of Hertel's exophthalmometer?

Ans. The disadvantages are:

- Parallax error while performing measurements—tilting of instrument leading to minor deviations in position result in gross variations in reading.
- Difficulty of visualizing the scale under conditions of low illumination, which may result in inaccurate readings.
- Variations in the distance between the two halves of the instruments lead to displacement of the footplate which considerably affects the measurement.
- It is also a relatively expensive instrument.
- Induced error may occur when measuring globes that are not horizontally at the same level.
- Narrow base on Hertel—difficult setting up.
- Facial bone deformity—may cause unreliable measurements due to unparalleled placement of device while measuring globes that are not horizontally at the same level.
- Poor fixation or convergence can lead to unreliable measurement.

5. What are the advantages of Luedde's exophthalmometer over Hertel's?

Ans. The advantages are:

- Luedde's exophthalmometer measures degree of proptosis of each eye separately, thus is useful in cases of *facial asymmetry*.
- It is pocket-sized, portable, and easily stored.
- It is easier to clean and sterilize.
- It is cheaper as compared to the Hertel's exophthalmometer.
- It can be used in presence of *strabismus*.

6. What are the advantages of Naugle's exophthalmometer over Hertel's?

Ans. Advantages are:

- Naugle's exophthalmometer uses a prism that can move backward and forward, which *eliminates parallax*.

- It utilizes superior and inferior orbital rims for measurement, thus can be used in cases of *lateral orbital rim fractures.*
- It also has the advantage of measuring hyperophthalmos and hypo-ophthalmos with a vertical gradient scale.

7. What is the definition of exophthalmos/ enophthalmos?

Ans. Exophthalmos is a protrusion of the eyeball due to an increase in orbital contents in a normal bony orbit. Protrusion of the eyeball more than 21 mm or a difference of 2 mm between both the eyes is defined as proptosis/exophthalmos. Enophthalmos is abnormal posterior displacement of globe (sinking of eyeball into orbit).

8. What are the causes of pseudoproptosis?

Ans. Causes are:

- Facial asymmetry
- Unilateral high myopia
- Buphthalmic eye
- Lid retraction
- Enophthalmos of the other eye.

9. What is exorbitism?

Ans. Exorbitism is a protrusion of the eyeball due to a decrease in capacity of the orbital container, with a normal orbital content volume, as seen in Crouzon's syndrome.

10. How is proptosis measured on CT scan?

Ans. The method described by Hilal and Trokel is most commonly used.[4] In a mid-axial CT scan, a line is drawn connecting the tips of the orbital rims. The perpendicular distance from this line to each corneal apex is measured. Proptosis is present if either line measures greater than 21 mm or the difference between the two eyes is more than 2 mm.

11. What are clinical ways to assess exophthalmos?

Ans. The various examination techniques are:

- *Worm's eye view*: Looking at the patient from down below, when the head is tilted backward to look for protrusion of the eyeball.
- *Naffziger's view*: Looking at patient from above, with the head tilted backward, to look for eyeball protrusion. Alternatively, asking the patient to close eyes and then open them, with the head tilted backward, to see which cornea is seen first on eye opening.
- *Ruler method*: Placing a ruler parallel to the coronal plane, touching the superior and inferior orbital rims, and looking for the relative position of the corneal apex to the ruler.

12. What are the factors influencing exophthalmometry reading?

Ans. Several factors can influence exophthalmometry reading such as:[3]

- *Age*: Lower readings are recorded for children (average 14 mm). In children and teenagers mean exophthalmometric measurements increase with age.[5]
    - <4 years old (13.2 mm)
    - 5–8 years old (14.4 mm)
    - 9–12 years old (15.2 mm)
    - 13–17 years old (16.2 mm)
- *Sex*: Males have higher readings (~1 mm)
- *Posture*: In supine position normal eyes sink back 1–3 mm in Graves' disease, eyes are not affected by this phenomena.
- *Ethnicity*: Blacks have higher reading. Asians have smaller ranges.
- *Spherical equivalent*: Negatively correlated.[3]
- *Axial length*: Positively correlated.[3]

REFERENCES

1. Genders SW, Mourits DL, Jasem M, et al. Parallax-free Exophthalmometry: a comprehensive review of the literature on clinical Exophthalmometry and the introduction of the first parallax-free exophthalmometer. Orbit Amst Neth. 2015;34(1):23-9.

2. Karti O, Selver OB, Karahan E, et al. The Effect of Age, Gender, Refractive Status and Axial Length on the Measurements of Hertel Exophthalmometry. Open Ophthalmol J. 2015;9:113-5.
3. Ramli N, Kala S, Samsudin A, et al. Proptosis—Correlation and Agreement between Hertel Exophthalmometry and Computed Tomography. Orbit Amst Neth. 2015;34(5):257-62.
4. Hilal SK, Trokel SL. Computerized tomography of the orbit using thin sections. Semin Roentgenol. 1977;12(2):137-47.
5. Dijkstal JM, Bothun ED, Harrison AR, et al. Normal Exophthalmometry measurements in a United States pediatric population. Ophthal Plast Reconstr Surg. 2012;28(1): 54-6.

1.2 ORBITAL IMAGING TECHNIQUES

Sanjay Sharma, Savinay Kapur

ORBITAL RADIOGRAPHS

Standard projections for the bony orbit include posteroanterior (PA) (Fig. 1.2.1A), lateral (Fig. 1.2.1B), and optic foramen view (Fig. 1.2.1C). The patient can either be seated, standing or semiprone. The PA projection also called the occipitofrontal view is done with a 20° caudal tilt, with the central beam exiting at the nasion. On the radiographs, the innominate line (Fig. 1.2.1A, black arrows) should cross the greater wing of sphenoid on

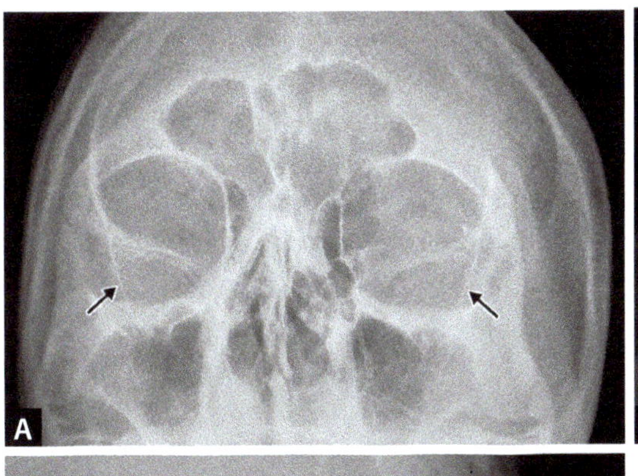

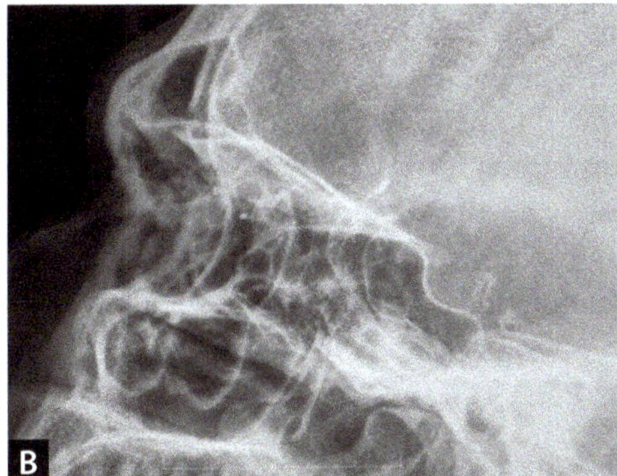

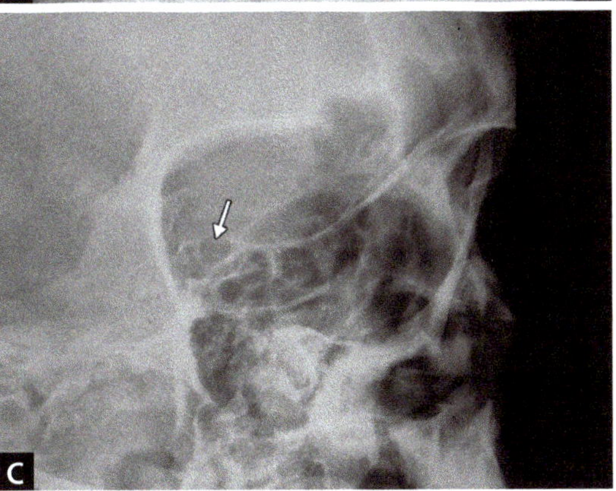

Figs. 1.2.1A to C: Different commonly done normal orbital radiographs views. (A) Anteroposterior (AP) view; (B) Lateral view; and (C) Optic foramen view (marked by a white arrow). Black arrows mark the innominate line.

the temporal side of the orbit. For the lateral view, the patient is positioned with the mid sagittal plane of the skull placed parallel to the image receptor. The beam is centered at a point 2.5 cm posterior to the outer canthus. To evaluate whether a radiograph is true lateral or not, look at the superimposition of the floor of the anterior cranial fossa on both sides. For visualizing the optic foramen, Rhese projection is used. Here the head is placed on the detector face first such that cheek, nose, and chin touch the detector, with orbit in center. The head is tilted in a manner such that the orbitomeatal line is perpendicular to the detector, keeping the mid sagittal plane at an angle of 53° to the image receptor. Beam is centered 2.5 cm superior and 2.5 cm posterior to the upper external auditory meatus. The superior orbital fissure and optic foramen are well seen on this view as are the margins of the orbit. With the increasing use of modern cross-sectional imaging this view is not commonly requested. The current use of orbital radiographs are limited to patients with trauma or suspected intraorbital foreign body. In many centers, it is now restricted only to exclude foreign body prior to a magnetic resonance imaging (MRI) examination.

ULTRASOUND

Nowadays, ultrasound is considered as an extension of physical examination due to its easy availability and noninvasive nature. It is the first line of investigation for evaluation of ocular and orbital pathology. Its main utility lies in evaluation of intraocular lesions, especially when the media is opaque. It also acts as a problem solving tool after computed tomography (CT)/ MRI as it allows for differentiation of cystic from solid lesions. Also, being a dynamic modality, it can be used to assess intraorbital pathologies and extraocular muscles (EOMs) in various stages of contraction. However, an inherent limitation of ultrasound is the trade-off between image resolution and depth of evaluation. High frequency probes permit high resolution imaging, but allow only limited depth of evaluation. Hence, its utility for evaluation of deep seated orbital pathologies is limited. Both A (amplitude) and B (brightness) (Fig. 1.2.2A) mode scans are used. The A-mode scan is mainly used by ophthalmologists where spikes are produced by the returning echoes from different interfaces within the eye. B-mode scan of the eyeball is done with a linear high resolution array transducer with frequency between 7.5 MHz and 10 MHz. For evaluation of the orbit, a lower frequency probe with 5–7.5 MHz bandwidth is used. To maintain an air free interface, coupling gel is applied over closed eyelids. In a normal individual, the anterior and posterior chambers are cystic (no echoes seen within anechoic) with an echogenic lens present between the two. Posterior to the globe, echogenic fat (Fig. 1.2.2A) is seen with a central hypoechoic linear structure representing the optic nerve sheath complex (Fig. 1.2.2A). A color Doppler evaluation may be done to evaluate the blood

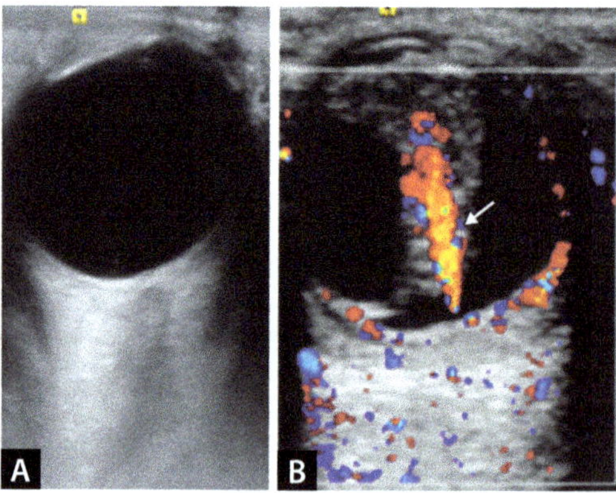

Figs. 1.2.2A and B: (A) Normal orbital ultrasound; and (B) Doppler in a child with persistent hyperplastic primary vitreous (PHPV) showing embryonic vascular channel marked by a white arrow.

flow in suspected persistent hyperplastic primary vitreous (PHPV) (Fig. 1.2.2B, shown by a white arrow) tumors and vascular malformations. In vascular lesions such as arteriovenous malformation (AVMs) and caroticocavernous fistula, spectral trace can be obtained to confirm the arterial or venous nature of flow. This information has an important therapeutic implication. Another new tool which can add to the evaluation of intraocular masses is contrast-enhanced ultrasound. Microbubble-based ultrasound contrast agents stay within the intravascular compartment and hence differentiate masses from pseudomasses (like retinal detachment/hemorrhage) as well as can potentially help to characterize masses as these tend to have different contrast kinetics. Ultrasound elastography is a yet another tool that evaluates the elasticity of a tissue that may find applications in times to come. Ultrasound biomicroscopy (UBM) is another exciting application for the evaluation of anterior chamber. It uses a high more than 30 MHz transducer to produce high resolution two-dimensional grayscale images of the anterior chamber.

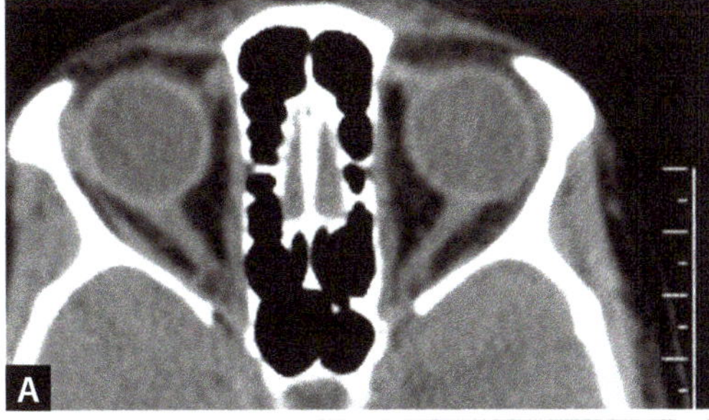

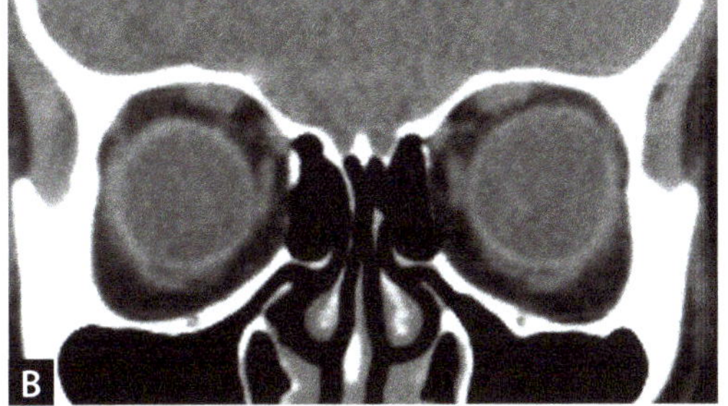

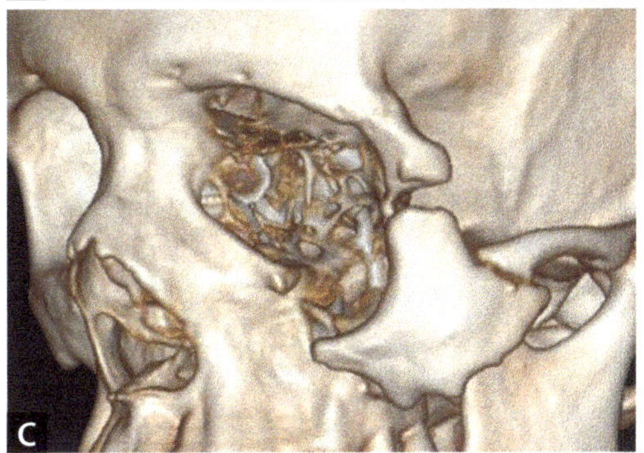

Figs. 1.2.3A to C: Normal orbital computed tomography (CT) sections; (A) Axial; and (B) Coronal; (C) A 3D volume rendered view in an adult with left tripod fracture.

COMPUTED TOMOGRAPHY

Computed tomography is a main orbital imaging modality which utilizes X-rays to generate cross-sectional images (slices). This volumetric cross-sectional information is used by software techniques to provide multiplanar images [along axial (Fig. 1.2.3A)/ coronal (Fig. 1.2.3B)/sagittal/curved planes] as well as volume rendered imaging (3D dataset, Fig. 1.2.3C).

CT scanning is based on the following principles:

- The images are acquired by a 360° rapid rotation of the X-ray tube around the patient. In modern CT scanners, the table moves horizontally through the gantry which houses the X-ray source and the detectors to generate helical (spiral) dataset.
- As the X-rays pass through the patient, they are attenuated depending on the radiographic density (attenuation coefficient) of tissues through which they pass. The scattered and transmitted radiation is then measured by a ring of sensitive detectors located in the gantry around the patient.

- Hence, each point in the body is imaged by a number of X-ray beams at different angles which allows for depth assessment (third dimension). The final image is reconstructed from multiple X-ray projections depending on the attenuation coefficients of the tissues through which beam passes.
- Filtered back projection is the most commonly used method by which attenuation data is converted to an image.
- The attenuation value of tissues is expressed on a scale named *Hounsfield units (HU)* with a range of 3,000 HU. Cortex of bones generally has an attenuation value of around +800 to +1,000 HU (white on the CT image), air has an attenuation value in the range of –800 to –1,000 HU (black on the CT image), muscles and soft tissues have an attenuation value of +40 to +80 HU while fat has an attenuation of –40 to –80 HU. Water is defined by having zero attenuation as a standard reference.

CONTRAST-ENHANCED COMPUTED TOMOGRAPHY IMAGING

Contrast-enhanced CT (CECT) imaging of the orbit and brain is obtained following intravenous injection of an iodinated contrast medium. Enhancement of various tissues following contrast administration depends on their blood flow and vascular permeability. Iso-osmolar iodinated contrast media like iohexol (Omnipaque) and iodixanol (Visipaque) are used routinely with iodine concentration between 300 mgI/mL and 350 mgI/mL. Orbital fat provides an intrinsic background contrast against which some orbital pathologies can be visualized without requiring a contrast medium.

Q. When to order a contrast-enhanced CT scan?

Ans. The following clinical situations require an additional injection of a contrast medium:
- *Mass lesions*: Benign/malignant tumors
- *Vascular lesions*: Caroticocavernous fistula (CT angiogram)/cavernous sinus pathology
- *Inflammatory conditions*: Optic neuritis, cysticercosis, panophthalmitis/orbital cellulitis, especially if suspecting an abscess.

Q. (More importantly) when to order a noncontrast enhanced CT scan?

Ans.
- Where the clinical indication is for detection and localization of foreign bodies or trauma where assessment of bony fractures/extraocular muscle entrapment is of primary concern.
- To differentiate between acute hemorrhage and mass lesions as both would be bright on contrast-enhanced images [blood is hyperdense on noncontrast computed tomography scan (NCCT), most mass lesions are not).
- As a complimentary tool for detection of calcification/bony destruction in masses already being evaluated by MRI.
- When there is a contraindication to iodinated contrast media—renal function derangement/known contrast allergy.
- Thyroid ophthalmopathy to evaluate anatomy of EOMs and crowding at orbital apex.

ACQUISITION AND INTERPRETATION OF COMPUTED TOMOGRAPHY

The first step in acquisition of CT scans is obtaining a scout image/scannogram/localizer. For orbital CT, a lateral scout view is obtained which is a low dose X-ray projection where there is no gantry rotation around the patient but taken with a fixed position of the X-ray source and detectors. The use of a scannogram is to plan the acquisition and specify the craniocaudal extent of the scan. Volumetric data is now obtained with overlap between slices of the helix so that 3D reconstruction can be obtained.

Contrast can be given hand injected or by a pressure injector. For routine CECT, a hand injection is a safer, cheaper, and acceptable technique. Generally 50 mL of contrast in adults (2 mL/kg for children) would suffice for most indications. However, in cases where CT angiogram is required a pressure injector must be used. Angiograms are arterial phase images to evaluate arterial anatomy/supply (like in suspected AVMs and sometimes caroticocavernous fistula).

On hard copy CT films, the scannogram is usually displayed as the first image on the CT film, preceding the series of axial images. The scout view not only gives an overview, but also allows confirmation of the fact that the entire region of interest has been included in the scanned area

MAGNETIC RESONANCE IMAGING

Principle

Hydrogen is the most abundant element in human body. It has unpaired protons in their nuclei and therefore behaves as tiny magnet. These protons precess about their axis and as a result have a very small associated magnetic field. However, as they precess in different directions and are randomly oriented inside the body, the net magnetization vector is nullified. However, it changes when the human body is placed in a strong external magnetic field. The protons inside the hydrogen atoms act like tiny dipoles and get aligned along the direction of magnetic field, being either parallel or antiparallel to the field (longitudinal magnetization). They also rotate around their axes following the strength of the magnetic field. When a radiofrequency pulse is applied, these tiny dipoles are tilted off the equilibrium and start to precess in phase with one another in a direction perpendicular to the axis of the main magnetic field (transverse magnetization). When external pulse is switched off, the longitudinal magnetization is regained with time (T1 relaxation). There is also a loss of the transverse magnetization (T2 relaxation). T1 and T2 relaxation times (time needed to regain 66% of longitudinal magnetization and lose 66% of transverse magnetization, respectively) depend upon the composition of the tissue and also the environment in which the tissue is situated. Hence, different magnetic resonance sequences can be designed to make use of this difference in T1 and T2 relaxation times to display difference in composition of different tissues. These sequences can have different T1 and T2 weighting to display contrast between tissues which have different T1 and T2 relaxation times.

Magnetic Resonance Imaging Contrast Media

Most commonly used compounds for contrast enhancement are gadolinium-based. These are also extracellular agents like CT contrast media and are distributed in the intravascular and interstitial tissues depending on the blood flow and permeability. They shorten the T1 relaxation times and hence are bright on T1-weighted (T1W) images. Because fat is also bright on T1W images it needs to be suppressed so that enhancement is not masked due to bright signal of fat. Hence, postcontrast images are generally fat suppressed.

When to Choose MRI over CT?

- Higher contrast resolution needed—characterization of masses and soft tissue lesions

- To assess intracranial pathologies including cranial nerves and cavernous sinus pathologies
- To see intracranial extent/spread of extracranial pathologies like fungal sinusitis
- Children.

Basic Image Sequences in MRI

T1-weighted Images (Figs. 1.2.4A and 1.2.5A)

Tissues with shorter T1 relaxation times such as fat appear brighter than those with longer T1 relaxation times such as water, vitreous, and cerebrospinal fluid (CSF).

It is the best sequence for studying anatomy.

> *Substances bright on T1 images:*
> - *Fat*
> - *Melanin*
> - *Gadolinium*
> - *Soft calcium*
> - Methemoglobin (subacute hemorrhage)
> - High protein/exudative fluid like in craniopharyngiomas/posterior pituitary

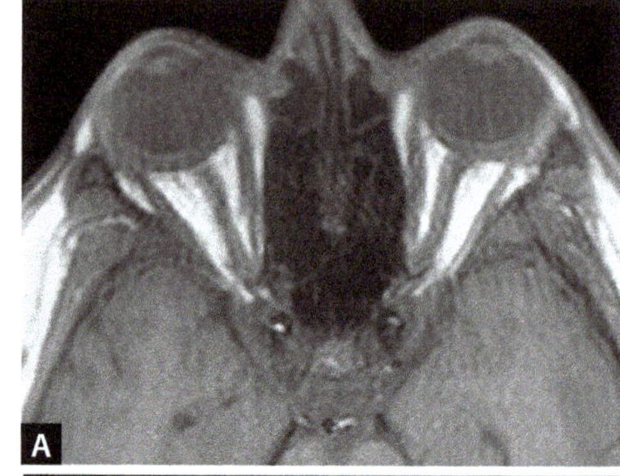

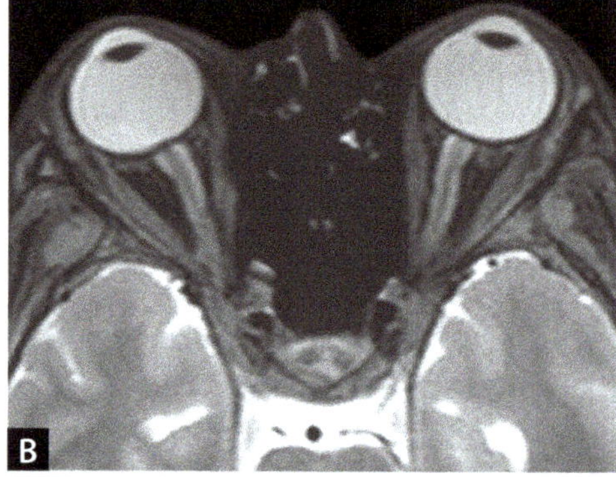

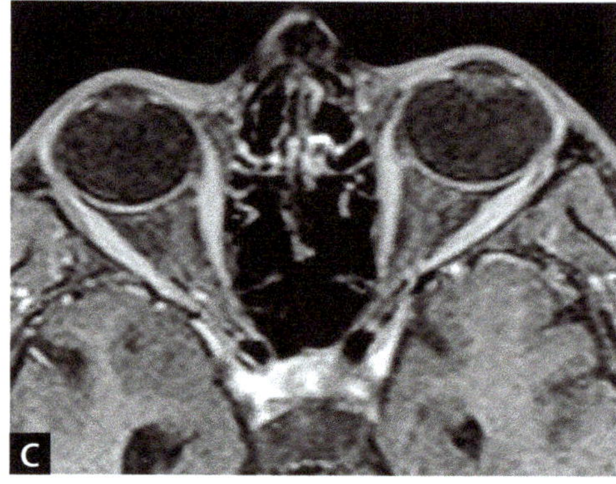

Figs. 1.2.4A to C: Routine normal magnetic resonance imaging (MRI) sequences of orbit in axial plane. (A) T1-weighted; (B) T2-weighted fat suppressed; and (C) T1-weighted postcontrast images.

T2-weighted Images (Figs. 1.2.4B and 1.2.5B)

Tissues with longer T2-relaxation like water, vitreous, and CSF appear brighter than tissues with shorter T2-relaxation such as blood products.

Fluid Attenuation Inversion Recovery (Fig. 1.2.5C)

Signals from free fluid can be suppressed using the fluid attenuation inversion recovery (FLAIR) sequence. FLAIR is especially useful in demyelinating conditions where white matter hyperintensities on T2W images are better appreciated when the bright signal from the adjacent CSF in the ventricles is nulled.

It is the best sequence for studying in brain pathology.

Fat-suppressed Images (Figs. 1.2.4B and C)

Bright signals from intraorbital fat can mask the signal and enhancing pathologies. This problem can be overcome by suppressing the signal of fat by unique fat suppression sequences. It is an ideal sequence for identifying intraorbital pathology along with postcontrast T1W images.

Postcontrast Images (Figs. 1.2.4C and 1.2.5D)

Gadolinium does not cross the blood-brain barrier (BBB) and hence does not cause enhancement in the brain when BBB is intact. When the BBB is disrupted, gadolinium diffuses into the interstitial spaces resulting in their enhancement.

> *Normally enhancing structures in orbit:*
> - *Lacrimal glands, EOMs, and uveal tract*
>   - *Structure which never enhances normally:*
> - *Optic nerve*

Diffusion-weighted Images

Primary application of diffusion-weighted images (DWI) in the brain is to look for acute infarcts. When there is cytotoxic edema, the cells swell and there is a restriction of diffusion in the extracellular space. This is reflected as a bright signal on DWI and low signal on apparent diffusion coefficient (ADC) maps. Always look at ADC maps to differentiate true diffusion restriction from "T2 shine through" (T2 bright areas may appear bright on DWI images without having diffusion restriction, however these are bright on ADC images as well).

Susceptibility-weighted Images

Magnetic resonance imaging sequences can either be spin echo or gradient echo

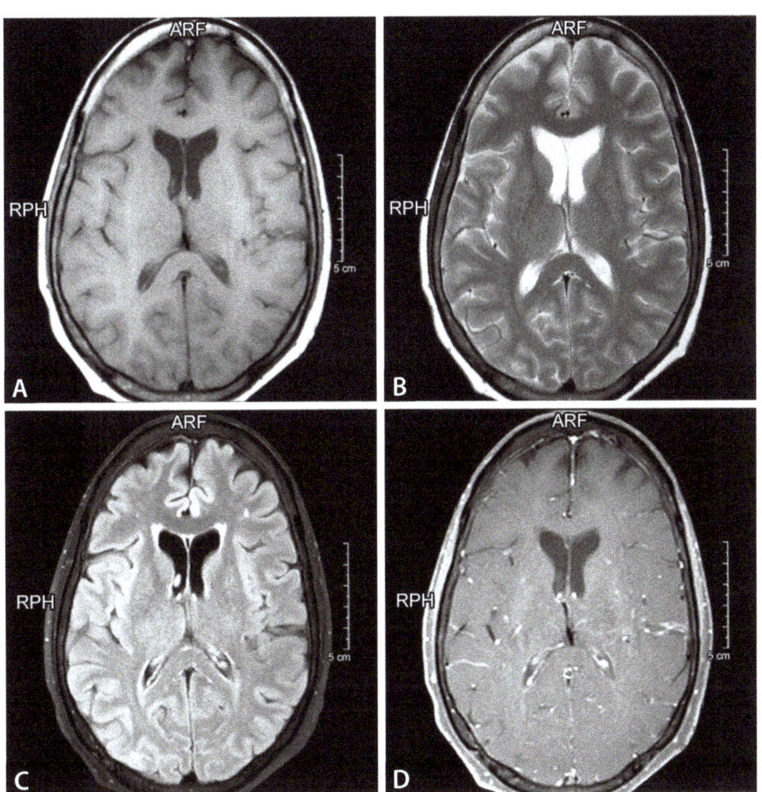

Figs. 1.2.5A to D: Routine normal magnetic resonance imaging (MRI) sequences of brain in axial plane. (A) T1-weighted; (B) T2-weighted; (C) Fluid attenuation inversion recovery (FLAIR); and (D) T1-weighted postcontrast images.

Table 1.2.1: Appearances (signal) of various tissues on standard MRI sequence.

Tissues	*T1WI*	*T2WI*	*FLAIR/Fat saturation*
Free water (like in cysts/CSF)	Dark	Bright	Suppressed (dark)
Fat	Bright	Bright	Suppressed (dark)
Interstitial fluid secondary to increased vascular permeability in inflammatory/neoplastic pathology	Dark	Bright	Bright

(CSF: cerebrospinal fluid; CT: computed tomography; FLAIR: fluid attenuation inversion recovery; MRI: magnetic resonance imaging; T1WI: T1-weighted image; T2WI: T2-weighted image)
Note: The terminology used to describe images is as follows:
Dark = hypointense
Bright = hyperintense
(On CT; dark = hypodense, bright = hyperdense)

sequences. The technique of gradient echo images is beyond the scope of this book. However, it is important to know the utility of these images (Table 1.2.1). Susceptibility-weighted images (SWIs) are very sensitive to local field inhomogeneities and hence are therefore best to look for calcification and deoxyhemoglobin (hemorrhage).

Standard brain protocol—routine sections are taken at 5 mm

1. Axial T2
2. Sagittal T2
3. Axial T1
4. Axial FLAIR

} Basic protocol

5. SWI
6. DWI
7. Post-Gd—axial/sagittal/coronal images

} Extended protocol

Orbit protocol:

1. Thin (3 mm sections) T2 axial
2. Thin T1 axial
3. Thin T2 fat saturation axial, coronal (oblique sagittal on the side of pathology)
4. Thin T1 fat saturation postcontrast images in all three planes.

For brain lesions, intensity is defined with respect to grey matter. Any lesion with signal intensity higher than the cortex (brighter) is said to be hyperintense and lesions darker than grey matter are hypointense by definition.

EMISSION COMPUTED TOMOGRAPHY

Emission computed tomography is a form of scintigraphy wherein a radioactive tracer substance is injected intravenously. The tracer substance acts as a source of radiation for imaging. However, the spatial resolution is lower compared to CT as well as MRI. With single-photon emission computed tomography (SPECT), the radionuclides emit gamma and X-rays, and the images are obtained using a rotating gamma camera. This technique allows detection of disturbances of BBB as well as abnormalities of cerebral blood flow. *Positron emission tomography (PET)* on the other hand utilizes a β+ emitting nuclide (^{11}carbon and ^{18}fluorine) and is based on the concept of positron annihilation. It is frequently employed when there is suspicion of a systemic disease coexisting with orbital disease.

1.3 A PATTERN-BASED APPROACH TO RADIOLOGIC DIAGNOSIS IN OPHTHALMOLOGY: PART I

Sanjay Sharma, Savinay Kapur

Most orbital pathologies can be divided into six basic imaging patterns:

1. *Intraocular*: Retinoblastoma (RB), melanoma, metastasis, and endophthalmitis.
2. *Intraconal*: Cavernous malformation, venous varix, lymphoproliferative disease and metastasis, and venolymphatic malformation.
3. *Extraconal*: Dermoid, lacrimal gland masses, bone lesions, venolymphatic malformation, schwannoma, hemangiopericytoma, capillary hemangioma, sinonasal masses with orbital extension, postseptal infection, and lymphoproliferative lesions *(Subperiosteal space is separate from extraconal compartment).*
4. *Optic nerve sheath complex (ONSC) lesions*: Meningioma, glioma, sarcoidosis, optic neuritis, idiopathic orbital inflammation, and lymphoproliferative disease *(These are intraconal lesions).*
5. Conal *[extraocular muscle (EOM) enlargement of various etiologies)*: Thyroid-associated orbitopathy, idiopathic orbital inflammation, carotid cavernous fistula (CCF), sarcoidosis, lymphoproliferative disease and metastasis, myocysticercus, and traumatic contusion.
6. *Infiltrative diseases*: Metastasis, idiopathic orbital inflammation, lymphoproliferative disease, cellulitis, sarcoidosis, plexiform neurofibroma, and rhabdomyosarcoma.

Pearl:

- Three most common intraorbital pathologies—thyroid orbitopathy, lymphoproliferative disorders, and idiopathic orbital inflammation.
- Three most common transcompartmental orbital lesions—idiopathic orbital inflammation, capillary hemangioma, and venolymphatic malformation.

INTRACONAL LESIONS

Cavernous Hemangioma (A Slow Flow Venous Malformation)

Typical presentation: Painless, progressive proptosis in a middle-aged woman.

Imaging findings: They appear as well-defined (pathologically encapsulated), oval to round, and homogeneous masses with a density somewhat greater than that of the muscle. They are typically located within the intraconal space (especially laterally), but larger lesions may extend outside the muscle cone. Bone remodeling is seen with large and longstanding lesions. Small foci of calcification are sometimes present which represent phleboliths. Enhancement is generally moderate owing to the low vascular flow. The lesion enhances progressively with homogeneous enhancement on delayed images (Fig. 1.3.1). On magnetic resonance imaging (MRI), the lesion is hypointense on T1, hyperintense on T2-weighted images (T2WIs). Intralesional hemorrhage is uncommon (cf. cerebral cavernous malformation and lymphatic malformation).

Lymphangioma (Venolymphatic Malformation)

Typical presentation: Gradual, painless progressive proptosis in a child, often painful when sudden in onset.

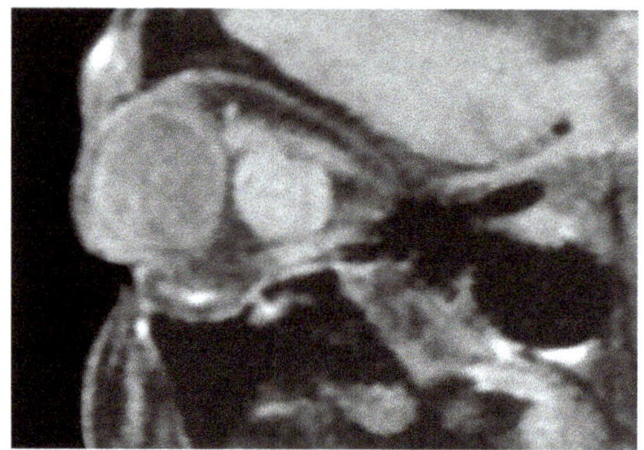

Fig. 1.3.1: Oblique parasagittal T1-weighted (T1W) fat suppressed postcontrast magnetic resonance imaging (MRI), with *cavernous hemangioma*, showing an ovoid enhancing soft tissue intraconal mass separate from the optic nerve.

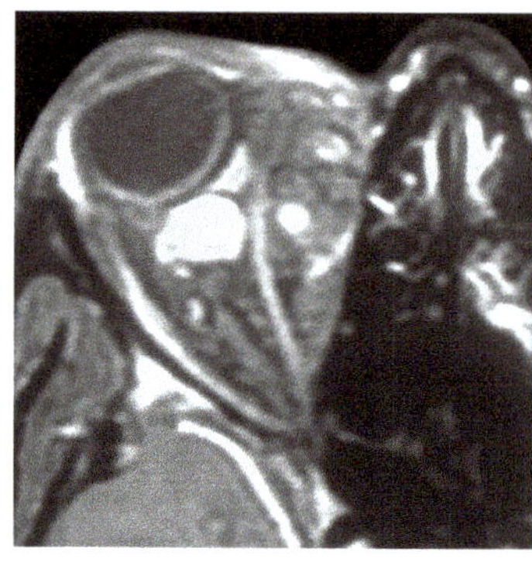

Fig. 1.3.2: Axial T1-weighted (T1W) fat suppressed postcontrast magnetic resonance imaging (MRI), with *lymphangioma (synonyms. venolymphatic malformation)* showing a transcompartmental ill circumscribed mass lesion with foci of hemorrhage and fluid–fluid levels.

Imaging findings: They appear as irregular heterogeneous masses, which are poorly defined (pathologically unencapsulated) and insinuate along normal orbital structures. They are known to cross anatomic boundaries such as the orbital septum and fascial layers. They can be macrocystic or microcystic. The macrocystic variant has multiple low-density cystic areas while in the microcystic variants the cysts are too small (to be seen on imaging) and hence look like a soft tissue mass. There is mild or no contrast enhancement. The wall and septae may show patchy enhancement, typically less than capillary hemangioma. Larger lesions may cause bone remodeling with extension into preseptal or infratemporal fossa through the inferior orbital fissure. Magnetic resonance (MR) is the investigation of choice for evaluating the extent of lesion. Signal characteristics depend on the presence or absence of proteinaceous contents/blood products within the lesion. In the absence of these, the cystic areas are hypointense on T1 and hyperintense on T2. Blood-fluid levels are characteristically seen in the setting of recent intralesional hemorrhage (Fig. 1.3.2).

Venous Varix

Typical presentation: Painless, progressive proptosis that increases on stooping forward/ Valsalva.

Imaging findings: Orbital varix represents a form of hamartoma, with thin-walled distensible venous channels that communicate with the normal orbital venous vasculature. Ultrasound is a highly useful modality for their diagnosis as it allows for dynamic assessment. The dilated venous channels collapse in the upright posture or at rest, but on straining, the increased blood flow with dilation of channels becomes obvious. On computed tomography (CT) the varices appear as an irregular or smooth variably enhancing lesion located at the orbital apex, which significantly increases in size with straining. However, as the study requires dynamicity and straining CT and MRI are seldom used for diagnosis. Once it is thrombosed, patients may present with acute onset retro-orbital pain and proptosis. CT at this time shows no change on straining and absence of enhancement. The lesion may appear hyperdense on noncontrast computed tomography (NCCT) due to hemorrhagic contents. MRI done at this time will show a well-defined T1/T2 heterogeneously hyperintense lesion due to hemorrhagic contents.

Pearl

Orbital varices can be a difficult radiologic diagnosis (on CT/MRI), as the discrete venous channels are seldom visualized.

Lymphoproliferative Disease and Intraconal Metastasis

Difficult to differentiate from other intraconal masses. Need evidence of a primary elsewhere to make this diagnosis. Rapid increase in size may be a pointer. Systemic work is warranted.

EXTRACONAL LESIONS

Dermoid Cyst

Typical presentation: Child or young adult with a mass near the frontozygomatic/frontoethmoid suture often with globe dystopia.

Imaging findings: It typically appears as a round to oval, well-defined lesion, located in the anterior superotemporal orbit. It is almost always extraconal and has a cystic center with areas of fat within (Fig. 1.3.3). A fat-fluid level may be present. Denser foci within the lesion represent flecks of keratin and sebum. The cyst is surrounded by a thin rim of tissue that may be partially calcified. Adjacent bone commonly shows remodeling/sutural widening. Occasionally the cystic cavity extends into the temporal fossa or the intracranial space. Contrast administration may produce mild enhancement of cyst rim, but not its center. On MRI, the lesion tends to be heterogeneously hyperintense on T2WI and hypointense on T1WI, however, areas of T1 hyperintensity are seen within the mass which show signal dropout on fat suppressed images.

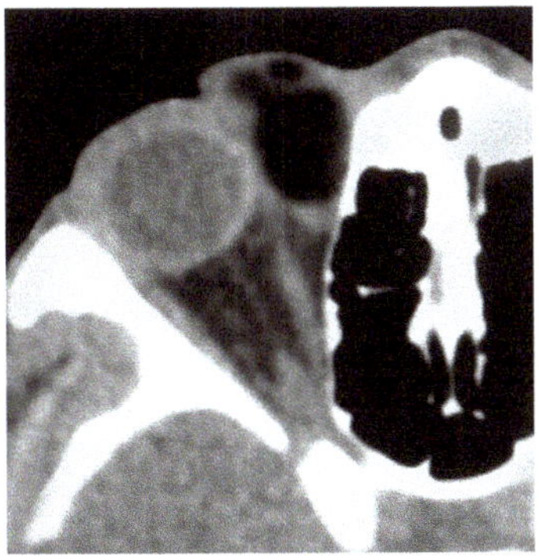

Fig. 1.3.3: Axial noncontrast computed tomography (CT), with right medial angular *dermoid*, showing a well-defined mass of fat attenuation.

Orbital Schwannoma

Typical presentation: Painless, progressive proptosis along with symptoms due to mass effect on surrounding structures. May be present acutely with painful proptosis in cases of hemorrhage into the lesion.

Imaging findings: They are typically extraconal though they can be intraconal or extraconal or both. Commonly involves the frontal branches of the ophthalmic division of the trigeminal nerve. Schwannomas have a heterogeneous T2 signal (Fig. 1.3.4) and variable patterns of enhancement with homogeneous or ring enhancement being most common.

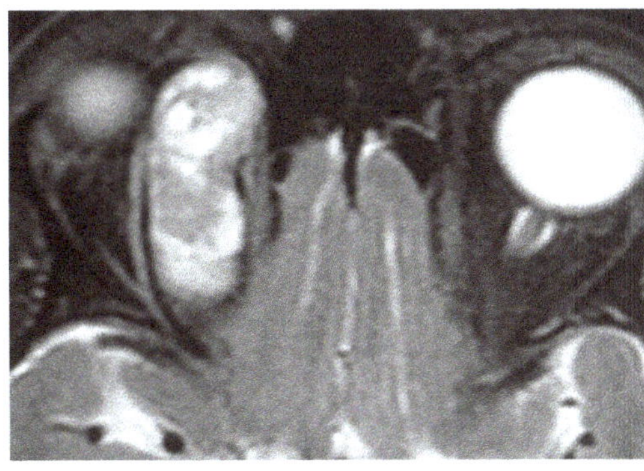

Fig. 1.3.4: Axial T2-weighted (T2W) fat suppressed magnetic resonance imaging (MRI), with right *intraorbital schwannoma* showing an elongated extraconal heterogeneous well-defined mass lesion with foci of necrosis and hemorrhage.

> *Orbital schwannomas can show delayed homogeneous enhancement like cavernous malformations, but do not follow the centripetal enhancement pattern of the latter.*

Hemangiopericytoma (Solitary Fibrous Tumor of Orbit)

These appear as homogeneous to heterogeneous, rounded or elongated masses of moderate density in an extraconal location most commonly along the paranasal sinuses. The borders are smooth and well circumscribed, similar to cavernous hemangioma. Calcification may be seen in up to one-fourth of cases. Bone erosion is unusual, but some degree of cortical disruption is sometimes seen along with rare periosteal reaction. Following contrast administration, enhancement is moderate to mark. Dynamic CT may show prominent early enhancement with rapid washout. The MRI image shows a round to oval tumor with well-defined borders. On the T1WI, the signal is isointense to cortical gray matter and muscle, and hypointense to fat. On the T2WI, the lesion is hyperintense to fat. Low-intensity signal voids represent large vessels with rapid blood flow. Moderate, diffuse, and homogeneous enhancement is seen with gadolinium.

Capillary Hemangioma

Typical history: Cutaneous discoloration or leash of vessels on the lids, periocular soft tissues; present at birth during infancy, grows with the child say up to 5-7 years age, and disappear by 10 years.

Imaging findings: They appear as ill-defined to irregularly marginated, lobulated, infiltrating masses most commonly located anterior to the globe in the eyelid. They show moderate to marked contrast enhancement.

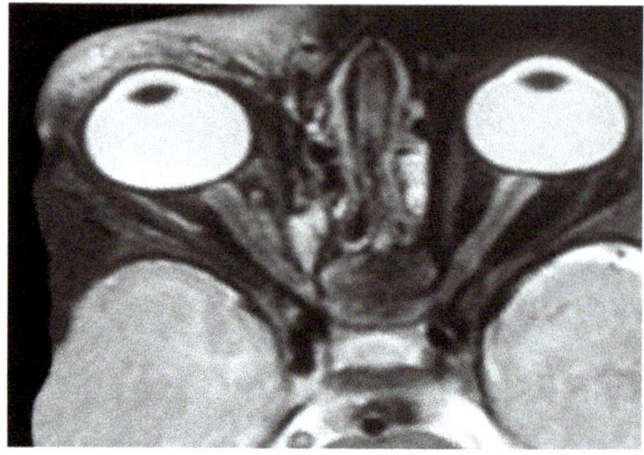

Fig. 1.3.5: Axial T2-weighted (T2W) fat suppressed magnetic resonance imaging (MRI), with right *orbital capillary hemangioma*, showing an ill-defined transcompartmental mass with areas of flow void. It showed marked contrast enhancement (in another section not shown).

Longstanding lesions in young children may cause expansion of bony orbital volume. Rarely occur as intraosseous lesions forming expansile masses with intact tables. In its proliferative phase, the mass shows intense and early enhancement (in arterial phase) with multiple flow voids on T1W/T2W images. However, in its involuting phase or if it does not involute completely, they tend to have heterogeneous high signal intensity on T1W and T2W (Fig. 1.3.5) with heterogeneous enhancement on contrast images.

Rhabdomyosarcoma

These lesions appear as irregular, moderate to well-defined soft tissue masses, mostly occupying the extraconal space, with about half extending into the intraconal space. Two-thirds of tumors arise in the superonasal quadrant of orbit. The density is similar to that of the EOMs, but may be heterogeneous due to intervening focal areas of hemorrhage. The tumor may conform to adjacent bony walls and orbital structures such as the globe. Bony erosion or destruction is unusual, but with larger lesions can be seen in up to 40% of cases. With contrast administration, mild to moderate uniform enhancement is observed.

Pearl

Most common malignancy of the orbit (head and neck region) in a child.

Lacrimal Gland Lesions

Benign neoplasms like pleomorphic adenoma present as indolent painless enlargement of the gland. Malignant and inflammatory lesions present with a shorter history and pain. They are broadly divided into epithelial and nonepithelial lesions. Epithelial lesions arise from the acini and tend to be neoplastic while nonepithelial lesions are predominantly inflammatory or infiltrative in nature. Adenoid cystic carcinoma is the most common malignancy of the lacrimal gland with propensity for perineural spread. CT scan of these lesions shows a heterogeneous mass in the lacrimal gland fossa area (Fig. 1.3.6). They can be irregular in shape with poorly demarcated margins or be round to oval in shape with well-defined borders. Larger tumors may extend along the lateral orbital wall to reach up to the orbital apex. Foci of calcification are frequently present within the lesion. Destruction or sclerosis of adjacent bone is a common phenomenon, especially with large tumors. Contrast administration shows areas of marked and focal enhancement.

On MR, pleomorphic adenoma is typically isointense to muscle with bright enhancement. Lymphomas on the other hand have a homogeneous T2 hypointense signal higher than muscle. Lacrimal glands are the second most common location for idiopathic orbital inflammation.

Pearl

Idiopathic inflammatory inflammation and lymphomas are the two most common masses of lacrimal gland.

Bony Orbital Lesions

Orbital bone lesions are malignant or benign. Metastatic lesions are more common than primary malignancy. In children, the common causes are Ewing's and neuroblastoma (Fig. 1.3.7) while in adults metastases are common from lung, breast, and prostate. Meningiomas of the greater wing of sphenoid cause intraosseous growth, which may cause

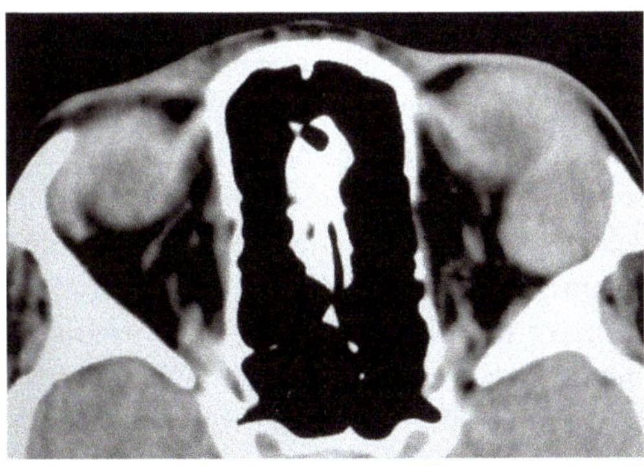

Fig. 1.3.6: Axial contrast computed tomography (CT), with a left *lacrimal gland mass* (pleomorphic adenoma), showing heterogeneous enhancement, remodeling of the adjacent bone, and abaxial proptosis.

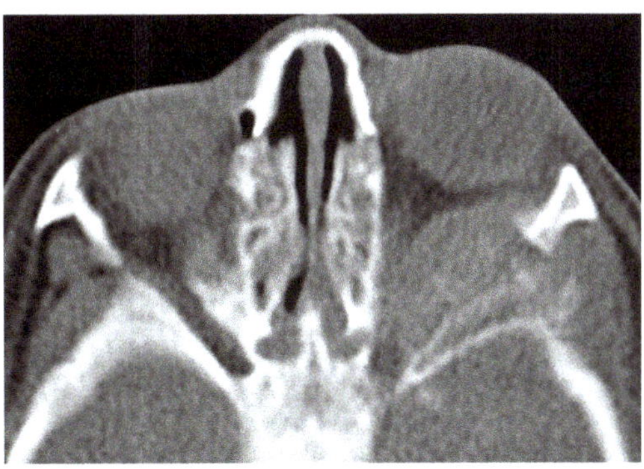

Fig. 1.3.7: Axial computed tomography (CT) (bone window), in a 2-year-old child with *metastatic neuroblastoma*, showing a destructive left sphenoid bone lesion with spiculated periosteal reaction and abaxial proptosis.

narrowing of intraorbital foramina. This sclerosis can be more easily seen on the CT images while on MR there is increase in the dark signal of the bone. Non-neoplastic benign fibro-osseous lesions include fibrous dysplasia (FD) and ossifying fibroma. FD is seen in patients less than 30 years of age. On CT, characteristic ground glass density is seen, with T1/T2 hypointensity on MR. Sagittal and oblique planes are helpful for evaluating the orbital apex and optic canal.

Ossifying fibromas may have internal mineralization, which can mimic that of FD on CT. However, ossifying fibroma usually has borders that are better defined than those of FD, which tends to have a poorly defined transition zone.

Mucocele

Longstanding lesions appear as masses opacifying one or more paranasal sinuses, extending into the orbit. The most common sinuses to get involved are frontal and ethmoid. The intervening bone may be expanded or remodeled or dehiscent around the cyst. This is best evaluated in bone window settings. Orbital structures are displaced, usually laterally or inferiorly. The cystic cavity is usually filled with a homogeneous, low-density mucoid material. The lesion lacks contrast enhancement unless contains pus. Longstanding inspissated secretions and proteinaceous contents appear T1 hyperintense and hyperdense on NCCT (Fig. 1.3.8) despite their cystic character.

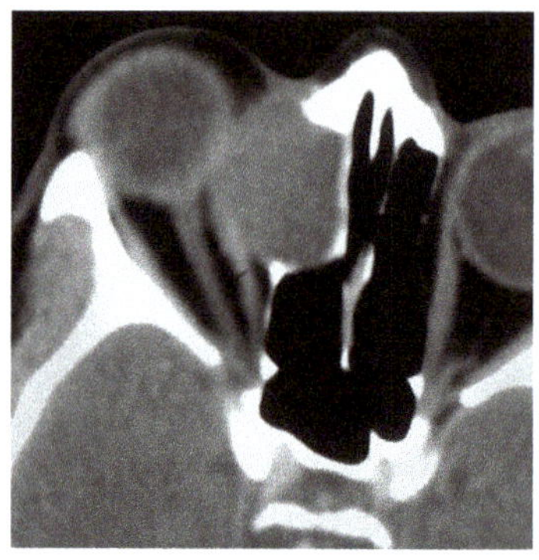

Fig. 1.3.8: Axial contrast computed tomography (CT), with right *ethmoid mucocele*, showing an expansile hyperattenuating lesion centered in the right anterior ethmoid sinus seen breaking into the orbit through the dehiscent lamina papyracea and causing abaxial proptosis.

INTRAOCULAR MASS

Metastases

In half of these cases, the intraocular metastases are asymptomatic, but in the other, they may present with vision loss or scotoma.

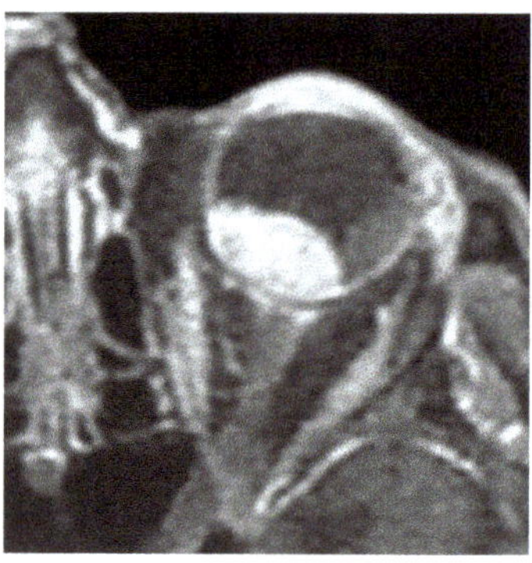

Fig. 1.3.9: Axial T1-weighted (T1W) fat suppressed magnetic resonance imaging (MRI), with left intraocular *metastatic lung cancer* showing bright homogeneous enhancement and retinal detachment.

Uvea is the most common site for intraocular metastasis, mostly localized to the choroid. These tend to occur as flatter/broad based lesions (posterior to the equator) (Fig. 1.3.9), compared to melanoma which tend to mushroom shaped. The most common primary tumors responsible for intraocular metastases are lung for men and breast for women. The prevalence of orbital metastases ranges from 2% to 5%. Few tumors have a propensity to metastasize to particular tissues (prostate to bone, melanoma to EOMs, breast to fatty tissue, and EOMs). The overall distribution of orbital metastases is in a ratio of 2:2:1, bone:fat:muscle.

Retinal Detachment

Retinal detachment (RD) typically begins with posterior vitreous detachment and is typically a clinical diagnosis based on history and examination. On imaging, there is a characteristic V-shaped area of abnormal density in the posterior globe which is limited by the anterior attachment of the retina, in contradistinction to suprachoroidal collections, which extend anteriorly to the level of the ciliary body.

Pearl

Ultrasound is the best radiologic modality for its detection. A CT may completely miss the RD.

Uveal Melanoma

Uveal melanoma is the most common primary intraocular malignancy in adults, constituting 5–6% of melanoma diagnoses with up to 50% of patients developing distant metastases. It may arise in any part of the uvea, including the ciliary body, iris, or choroid (most common). Cross-sectional imaging is of use when ocular opacities limit assessment. MRI is the investigation of choice with characteristic findings of melanoma being marked hyperintensity on T1WIs and hypointensity on T2WIs (Figs. 1.3.10A and B) which makes this a unique tumor. It enhances brightly on contrast-enhanced CT and MR, however subtraction MR imaging may be needed to demonstrate enhancement as the tumor is bright on T1 images as well. MR is also useful for distinguishing the tumor from associated hemorrhage.

Pearl

Ultrasound should be the first-line radiologic modality for the evaluation of suspected intraocular masses, and MRI later, if required. Systemic workup is necessary for staging.

Retinoblastoma

Child typically presents with white reflex or strabismus. It is the most common intraocular malignancy in childhood. It is considered a clinical diagnosis supported by ultrasound.

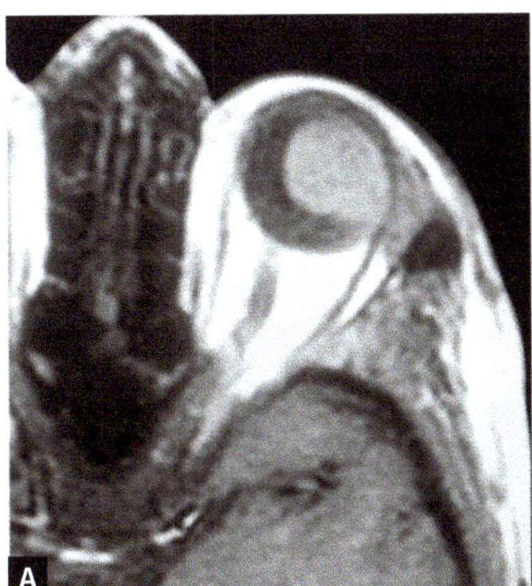

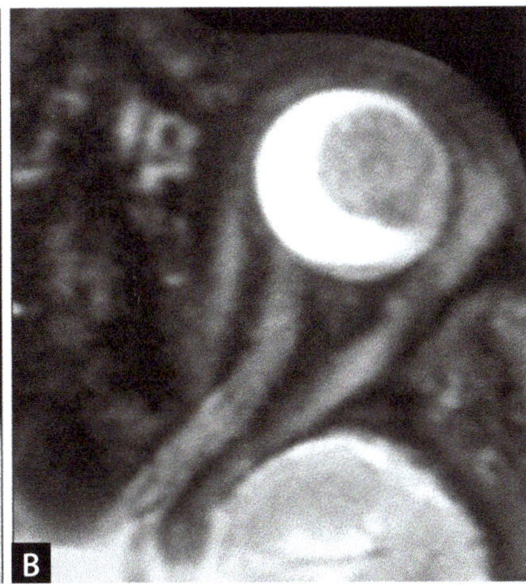

Figs. 1.3.10A and B: Axial T1-weighted (T1W) (A) and T2-weighted (T2W) (B) fat suppressed magnetic resonance imaging (MRI), in an elderly man, with a polypoidal left intraocular mass, a *uveal melanoma*, which is bight on T1W and dark on T2W images.

MRI is required for the larger tumors for local staging. Ultrasonography and MRI can both be useful to distinguish RB from other differential diagnoses, viz. Coats' disease, persistent hyperplastic primary vitreous, retinopathy of prematurity (Fig. 1.3.11) or toxocariasis. CT is only considered a problem solving tool due to the radiation risk, CT is an excellent modality to detect small calcifications which may be diagnostic in doubtful cases (Fig. 1.3.12A).

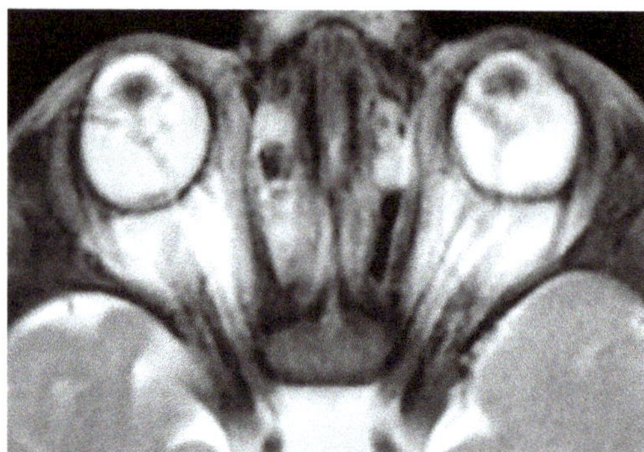

Fig. 1.3.11: Axial T2-weighted (T2W) magnetic resonance imaging (MRI), in a premature child who received oxygen in neonatal care for 2 weeks, having *retinopathy of prematurity*, showing bilateral microphthalmia, retinal detachment, and bilateral intraocular hemorrhage but no mass.

However, an A-mode ultrasound is a popular modality to evaluate calcification in the tumors. MRI is the preferred imaging modality for delineating the morphology and extent of the tumor, especially extraocular spread and optic nerve involvement (Fig. 1.3.12B). RB has characteristic low T2 signal, because of its high cellular density and variable postcontrast MR enhancement.

Pearl

Evaluation of white reflex in a child is a common and difficult clinical problem. The diagnosis is often not apparent even after thorough clinically evaluation and radiology.

Endophthalmitis

Endophthalmitis occurs either following surgery or trauma due to local inoculation or even secondary to hematogenous spread of infection from a distant anatomic site. Although usually a clinical diagnosis, the role of imaging remains detection of complications like formation of intraorbital abscess, RD, cavernous sinus involvement,

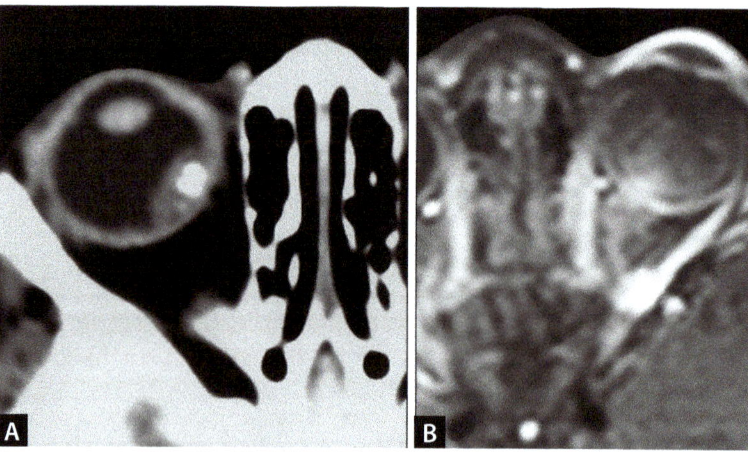

Figs. 1.3.12A and B: Axial noncontrast computed tomography (CT) (A) and T1-weighted (T1W) fat suppressed contrast-enhanced (CE) magnetic resonance imaging (MRI) (B) in another child with *retinoblastoma*, showing calcified right intraocular mass (A) and enhancing left intraocular mass with optic nerve involvement up to the apex.

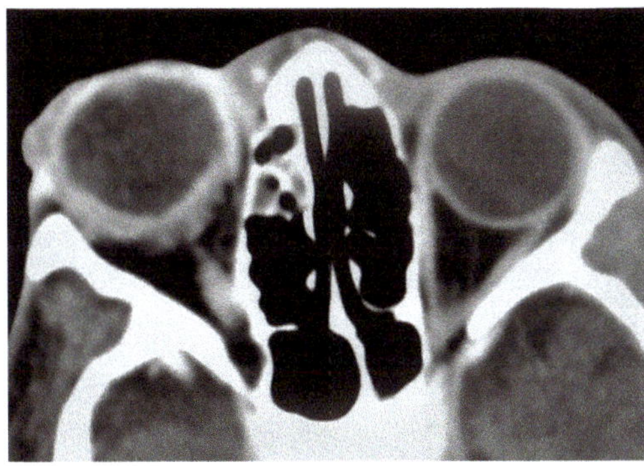

Fig. 1.3.13: Axial contrast computed tomography (CT), with right metastatic *endophthalmitis*, showing diffuse thickening of right ocular coats but no fluid collection or abscess. An active abdominal sepsis was presumed to be the cause of his disease.

and development of phthisis bulbi. The ocular coats are seen to be diffusely thickened (Fig. 1.3.13). Abscesses can also occur in both the suprachoroidal space and the subretinal space. On CT and MR, abscesses are peripherally enhancing layers of predominantly fluid attenuation. On T2WI, the high signal of vitreous may obscure pathology; however, the inflamed uveal tract can be clearly seen separately from the vitreous on fluid-attenuated inversion recovery (FLAIR) imaging. Contrast MRI assisted may be useful in demonstrating abscesses.

1.4 A PATTERN-BASED APPROACH TO RADIOLOGIC DIAGNOSIS IN OPHTHALMOLOGY: PART II

Sanjay Sharma, Savinay Kapur

OPTIC NERVE SHEATH COMPLEX LESIONS

Optic Glioma

Typical presentation: Decreased visual activity, visual field defect, proptosis, and relative afferent pupillary defect (RAPD).

Imaging findings: These are glial tumors which in the brain arise from the parenchyma of white matter, but often also involve the adjacent gray matter. The Dodge classification divides these tumors into just three groups based on anatomical localization:

1. *Stage 1*: Optic nerves only
2. *Stage 2*: Chiasm involved (with or without optic nerve involvement)
3. *Stage 3*: Hypothalamic involvement and/ or other adjacent structures.

> *Neurofibromatosis type 1 (NF1) associated—more likely to involve the optic nerve. Sporadic—more likely to involve the chiasm.*

In patients of neurofibromatosis (NF), these lesions appear on computed tomography (CT) as hypodense and poorly-defined masses. The optic nerve cannot be seen separate from the mass; hence, the nerve appears tubular, tortuous, and kinked. Minimal or no enhancement is seen in the lesion. Sporadic gliomas tend to have solid cystic appearance similar to pilocytic astrocytomas. The solid areas are generally T2 hyperintense and show contrast enhancement (Fig. 1.4.1).

Pearls

If unilateral, NF1 in 20% patients; if bilateral—pathognomonic of NF1.

Optic Nerve Sheath Meningioma

Typical presentation: Insidious vision loss over months to years.

Imaging findings: The typically appear as smooth tubular enlargement of the optic

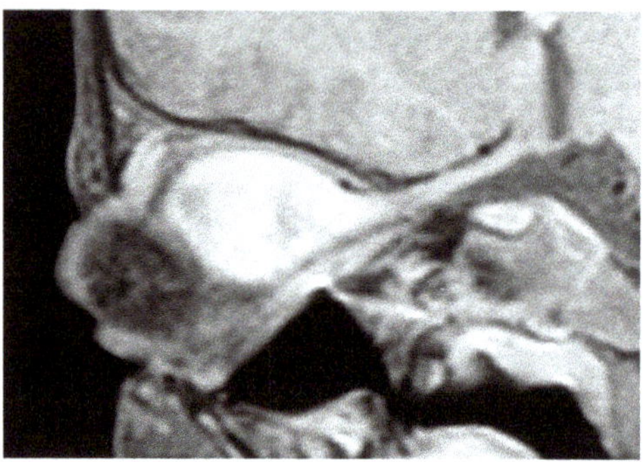

Fig. 1.4.1: Oblique sagittal T1-weight (T1W) postcontrast magnetic resonance imaging (MRI) of *optic nerve glioma*, showing a fusiform enhancing tumor not separate from the optic nerve.

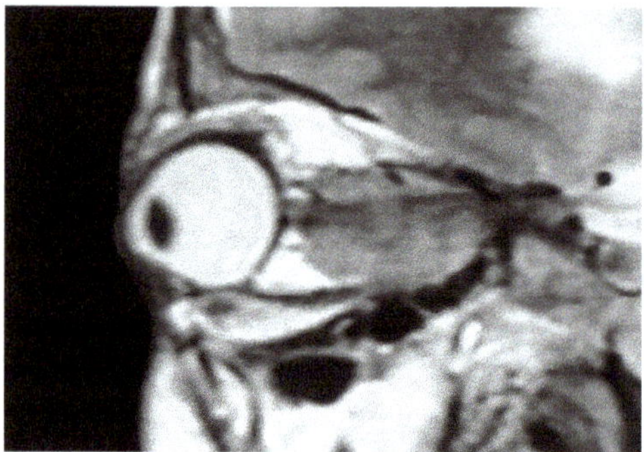

Fig. 1.4.2: Oblique sagittal T2-weight (T2W) magnetic resonance imaging (MRI) with *optic sheath meningioma*, showing a fusiform intermediate signal intensity neoplasm encasing the optic nerve. Note that the neoplasm is seen distinct from the optic nerve.

nerve. Less commonly, they may be fusiform or globular in appearance in case the dura is breached. The lesion appears iso to hyperdense on CT and may show foci of calcification in 20–50% of cases. There is marked and homogeneous contrast enhancement of the mass, often with a linear central zone of reduced density representing the normal optic nerve (tram-tracking sign). Expansion of bony orbital walls is seen in case the tumor is longstanding. Meningiomas generally produce isointense signals on T1-weighted (T1W) images with respect to normal optic nerve and cortical gray matter. The T2-weighted (T2W) image is heterogeneous and varies from being slightly hypointense to slightly hyperintense (Fig. 1.4.2) with respect to the gray matter. The fibroblastic stromal elements give meningiomas their characteristic hypointense signal. The postgadolinium T1W image shows marked enhancement of the tumor surrounding an optic nerve of lower signal intensity with a dural tail. This is best distinguished on fat suppression sequences. A subtle intracranial extension may only be visible on the contrast image.

Pearl

Think of NF2, if multiple or associated with other neoplasms like schwannomas or ependymomas.

Optic Neuritis

Typical presentation: Unilateral rapid onset of vision loss; eye pain worsened with eye movements.

Imaging findings: Optic neuritis is a magnetic resonance imaging (MRI) diagnosis; CT has no role. Key imaging sequences—axial, coronal T2 FS, and T1 FS postcontrast are required. Optic nerve involvement may be segmental or diffuse. Optic neuritis manifests as increased T2 signal and bulk of the nerve which may be associated with abnormal enhancement.

Pearls

1st pearl: Always image the brain if optic neuritis presents as there is 25% risk of multiple sclerosis. Can also be seen with neuromyelitis optica (NMO).

2nd pearl: Hence screening of cervical spine with STIR sequence may be done.

3rd pearl: If bilateral (Fig. 1.4.3), then think of infectious causes, such as viral prodrome in children.

Idiopathic Orbital Inflammation

Typical presentation: Unilateral more common than bilateral, rapid onset pain ± diplopia ± vision loss and redness.

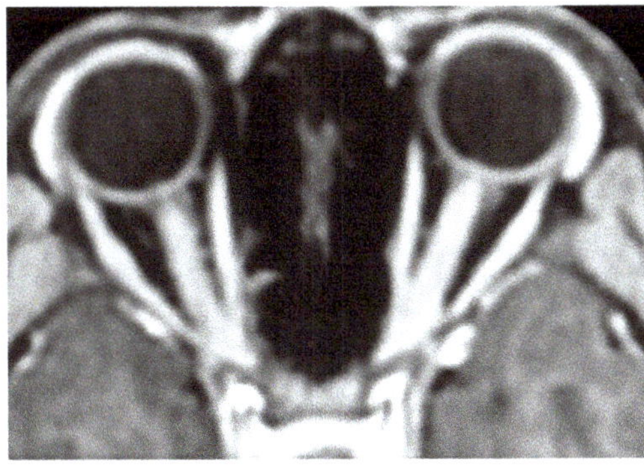

Fig. 1.4.3: Axial postcontrast fat suppressed T1-weight (T1W) magnetic resonance imaging (MRI) with *bilateral optic neuritis* showing a marked enhancement of both optic nerves. Note that the normal optic nerves never enhance as brightly as the extraocular muscles (EOMs), as in this case.

Imaging findings: Orbital inflammation may be seen in a variety of orbital conditions, however, about 5–15% have no discernible cause and hence classified as idiopathic. Also called orbital pseudotumor, idiopathic orbital pseudotumor or nonspecific orbital inflammation. Many patients would have underlying systemic vasculitis as a cause. It may be related to immunoglobulin G4 (IgG4) disease. Here the optic nerve sheath is involved instead of the optic nerve itself. There is frequent involvement of retrobulbar fat, EOMs, lacrimal glands, and optic nerve. The masses are ill defined on CT. On MRI they are T1 intermediate, T2 dark, and show variable enhancement.

Radiological differential diagnosis—lymphoproliferative disease/sarcoidosis (neither has a similar clinical presentation), systemic vasculitis, and IgG4-related orbital disease.

Lymphoproliferative Disease

Includes lymphoma (most common), lymphoid hyperplasia and atypical lymphoid hyperplasia, and ocular adnexal lymphoma. Around a quarter of all masses in patients older than 60 years are lymphomas. Non-Hodgkin's lymphoma, specifically the mucosa-associated lymphoid tissue (MALT) form is the most common primary orbital lymphoma.

Sarcoidosis

Presentation is similar to inflammatory pseudotumor. Most common site of involvement is the uvea or lacrimal gland. On MRI, involvement of the optic nerve sheath may show linear tram-track enhancement. On imaging, if there is isolated optic nerve involvement, it may be indistinguishable from the above two conditions. Laboratory investigations [serum calcium and angiotensin-converting enzyme (ACE) levels] are supportive, besides the systemic workup for the evidence of the disease elsewhere in the body to help make the diagnosis.

CONAL (EXTRAOCULAR MUSCLE ENLARGEMENT)

Thyroid-associated Orbitopathy

Typical presentation: Bilateral painless axial proptosis.

Imaging findings: Most common extra-thyroidal manifestation of Graves disease (25–50% patients). Caused by accumulation of glycosaminoglycans in the orbital soft tissues and increased fat volume. On CT, enlargement of EOMs is the imaging hallmark of the disease and is best appreciated on axial and coronal scans (Figs. 1.4.4A and B). The enlarged muscles are sharply defined, sometimes demonstrating increased density. There may be focal areas of low density, reflecting fatty infiltration. Typically, only the muscle bellies are involved, with relatively normal tendinous insertion referred to as the "coca-cola" sign seen on axial images (cf. pseudotumor). The inferior and the medial rectus muscles are the most frequently involved ones. The superior ophthalmic vein may be enlarged as a result of apical compression. The bulky EOMs are isointense on T1, slightly hyperintense on T2W images. The thickened tensor intermuscularis appears as a prominent curved band between the superior and lateral rectus muscles. Contrast administration is not necessary for imaging to make a diagnosis. Up to 8% of patients with thromboangiitis obliterans (TAO) develop dystrophic optic neuropathy (DON) likely secondary to optic nerve compression by the enlarged EOMs. The presentation may sometimes be asymmetric (unilateral) or even antedate the clinical disease.

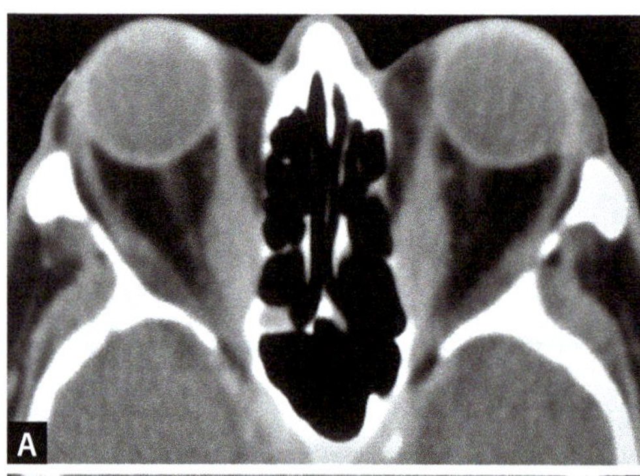

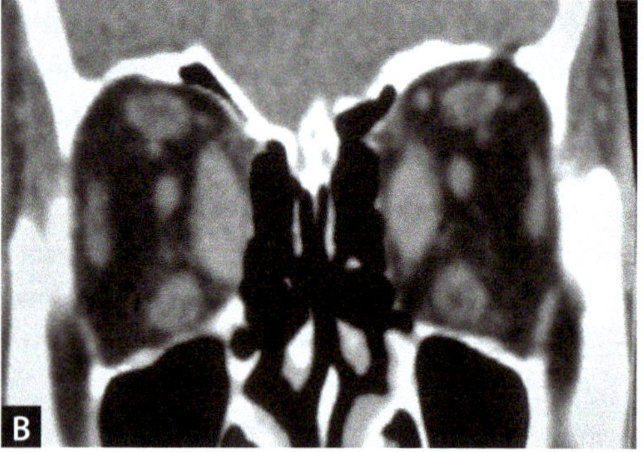

Figs. 1.4.4A and B: Axial (A) and coronal (B) contrast-enhanced computed tomography (CECT) scan in *thyroid-associated orbitopathy*, shows bulky bellies of bilateral extraocular muscles (EOMs) especially inferior and medial recti. Note the typical tendinous sparing.

Idiopathic Orbital Inflammation

Typical presentation: Pain, ocular dysmotility, and redness.

Imaging findings: Myositis is one of the most common orbital manifestations of IOI. In contradistinction to TAO, IOI of the EOMs is typically unilateral, painful, and rapid in onset (hours to days). However, some patients may have an atypical presentation, with a relatively painless manifestation, or bilateral disease (25% of patients, common in children). On imaging, the differentiation is based on involvement of tendinous insertion with inflammation in the adjacent fat.

Carotid-cavernous Fistula

They have been variously classified by their hemodynamics (high or low flow), cause (spontaneous or posttraumatic), or vascular anatomy (direct or indirect) or vascular anatomy (direct or indirect, Table 1.4.1).

Computed tomography scan in these cases demonstrates proptosis with the prominence of the orbital vasculature. The superior ophthalmic vein is dilated in most cases. Low density, nonenhancing areas within the vessel or the cavernous sinus represent thrombosis. Symmetrical enlargement of EOMs from vascular engorgement is commonly seen.

Table 1.4.1: Direct and indirect carotid-cavernous fistula (CCF).

Direct CCF	*Indirect CCF*
Frequently associated with trauma (spontaneous may be to aneurysm rupture) and direct flow from CCA to cavernous sinus	Dural shunting of arterial flow from branches of ICA/ECA/ both into the cavernous sinus
Progresses rapidly	Insidious onset
High flow	Low flow

(CCA: cavernous carotid artery; ECA: external carotid artery; ICA: internal carotid artery)

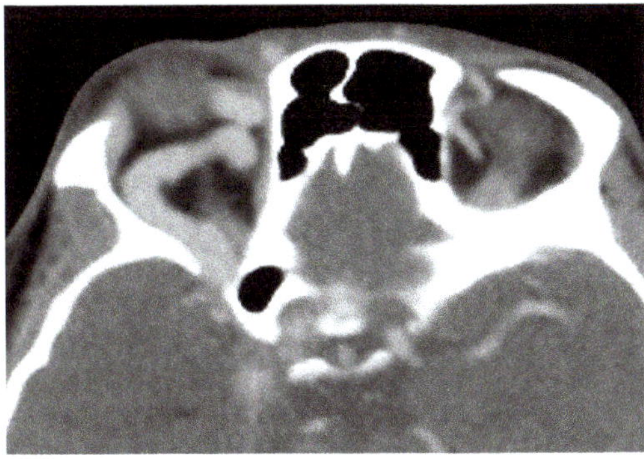

Fig. 1.4.5: Axial contrast-enhanced computed tomography (CECT) in a young male with *carotico-cavernous fistula*, showing engorged right superior ophthalmic vein. The swelling of left extraocular muscles is not seen in this section.

Enlargement of cavernous sinus may be appreciated, and in longstanding cases, the superior orbital fissure can be widened. Contrast CT is generally diagnostic in most cases (Fig. 1.4.5). However, invasive digital subtraction angiography (DSA) may be necessary some occasionally times, especially to demonstrate an indirect fistula or for interventional radiological treatment of CCF. On magnetic resonance (MR), vessels with fast flowing blood show a signal void on both T1W and T2W images and these can be demonstrated on gadolinium-enhanced magnetic resonance angiography (MRA) images.

Sarcoidosis

Involvement of the EOMs by sarcoidosis is unusual and can have a variety of presentations. There may be involvement of multiple muscles on one side or bilateral, painful or indolent, with or without involvement of other orbital soft tissues such as the lacrimal gland. It may spare or involve the tendinous insertions, and hence is difficult to differentiate from TAO or IOI by physical examination and imaging, especially if there is no evidence of systemic sarcoidosis.

Lymphoproliferative Disease and Metastases

Intramuscular metastases and lymphoma are rare. Metastases and lymphoma or other lymphoproliferative diseases occurring in the EOMs have been reported only sporadically in the literature. Carcinoma (predominantly breast), melanoma, non-Hodgkin lymphoma, and neuroendocrine tumors such as carcinoid are better known primaries. Breast carcinoma may sometimes involve the EOMs in a bilateral symmetric pattern with sparing of the tendons, which may be difficult to distinguish from TAO on imaging.

INFILTRATIVE DISEASES

Metastasis

Most common primary malignancy to metastasize to the orbits is breast carcinoma. Diffuse intraconal disease is one of many imaging patterns that may be seen in breast cancer, in addition to intramuscular or osseous masses. Infiltrative scirrhous breast carcinoma may cause enophthalmos, because fibrous tissue replaces the normal orbital fat.

Idiopathic Orbital Inflammation

Diffuse involvement of the orbital fat is less common than involvement of other orbital structures such as the lacrimal gland or EOMs (Fig. 1.4.6). The eponym "Tolosa-Hunt syndrome" applies when there is predominantly involvement of the orbital apex or cavernous sinus.

Lymphoproliferative Disease

Similar to IOI, lymphoproliferative disease such as lymphoma may present with an infiltrative pattern, involving any orbital structure. However, in contrast to IOI, lymphoproliferative disease presents with

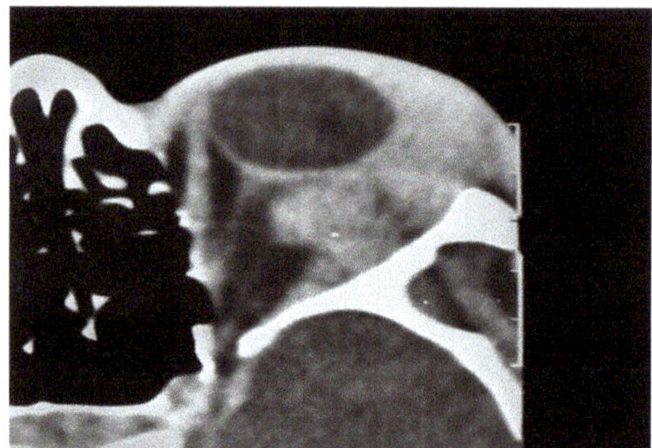

Fig. 1.4.6: Axial contrast-enhanced computed tomography (CECT) in a middle-aged woman with *idiopathic orbital inflammation*, showing the infiltrating multicompartmental soft tissue mass involving left lateral rectus, lacrimal gland, retrobulbar fat, and preseptal soft tissues.

minimal or no pain and with gradual progression. In some series, diffuse ill-defined orbital disease was found to be commoner than a well-circumscribed round or oblong mass. On MRI, T2W signal isointense or hypointense to muscle is typical of lymphoproliferative disease and restricted diffusion may also be seen.

Orbital Cellulitis

Involvement of the soft tissues posterior to the orbital septum is the imaging hallmark of orbital cellulitis (cf. preseptal cellulitis). It is important to make this distinction as orbital cellulitis has a higher complication rate and may be associated with optic neuropathy, encephalomeningitis, cavernous sinus thrombosis, sepsis, and intracranial abscess. Orbital cellulitis in early stages is characterized by eyelid edema and sinusitis on CT images. Postcontrast scans show marked increased in enhancement. More typically inflammation is seen in the medial or superomedial orbit adjacent to the opacified sinus, associated with fat stranding, i.e. heterogeneity in the retrobulbar fat (Fig. 1.4.7). An orbital abscess appears as a well-defined mass with a low density necrotic center, and an enhancing rim. On MRI,

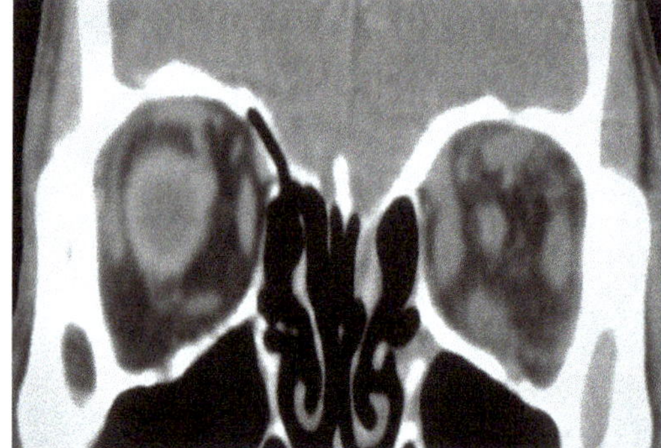

Fig. 1.4.7: Coronal contrast-enhanced computed tomography (CECT) in left *orbital cellulitis*, showing swollen left extraocular muscles and fat stranding.

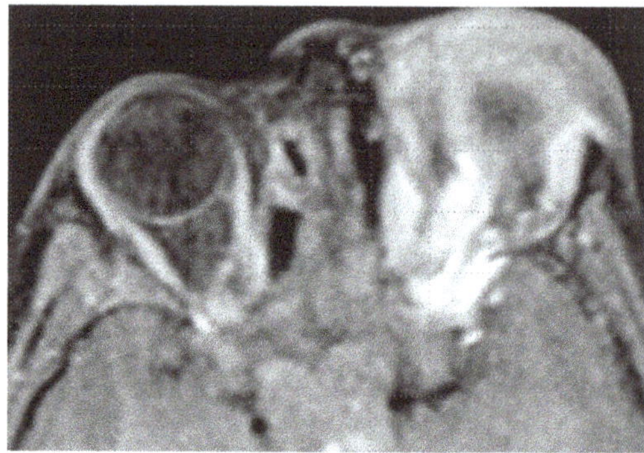

Fig. 1.4.8: Axial postcontrast fat suppressed T1-weighted (T1W) magnetic resonance imaging (MRI) with left orbital *plexiform neurofibroma* showing an infiltrating enhancing soft tissue mass in a patient with neurofibromatosis type 1 (NF1).

orbital inflammation and edema produce a diffuse signal that is isointense to muscle. On the T2W image, a fluid level may be visible as a layered hyperintense signal in an abscess or sinus. The inflammatory exudate remains hypointense. The necrotic abscess center remains dark, but there is an enhancement of the peripheral rim.

Plexiform Neurofibroma

It occurs in about one-third of patients with NF1 (Fig. 1.4.8). It commonly affects the trigeminal nerve, especially the ophthalmic and maxillary divisions. PNF has a multispatial growth pattern, similar to venous and lymphatic malformations that follow vessels. The patient's age and relevant history are the key to the correct diagnosis. On imaging, PNF follows the distribution of the involved nerves through fascial boundaries with a characteristic targetoid appearance on T2W images.

Rhabdomyosarcoma

Rhabdomyosarcoma is the most common soft tissue sarcoma of the head and neck in childhood (mean age is 8 years), with 10% of all cases involving in the orbit. Proptosis and blepharoptosis are common presenting symptoms of orbital RMS. Pain is uncommon and may indicate an advanced tumor. Typically, it presents as an extraconal well-defined mass without osseous destruction, however more advanced cases can be both extra- and intraconal and infiltrative with destroy bone. It can involve any part of the orbit, including the EOMs. On noncontrast CT (NCCT), the mass is isodense to muscle. On MR imaging, RMS is typically T2 hyperintense with areas of high T1 signal secondary to hemorrhage, with some contrast enhancement.

MISCELLANEOUS PATHOLOGIES

Intraocular/Intraorbital Foreign Body

Noncontrast CT scan is the imaging modality of choice for evaluation of suspected intraorbital foreign bodies. It has an advantage over the plain radiographs owing to its superior spatial resolution; it can often identify nonmetallic foreign bodies like wood also. Helical CT scans allow precise localization of the foreign body and delineation of its relationship with the surrounding structures (Fig. 1.4.9). MRI is contraindicated for evaluating metallic intraorbital foreign bodies.

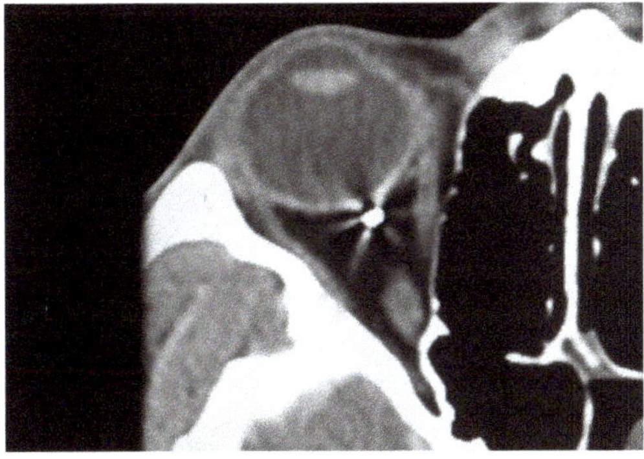

Fig. 1.4.9: Axial noncontrast computed tomography (NCCT) shows a tiny *metallic foreign body* just behind the right globe, adjacent to the optic disc. It clearly shows that it is lying in extraocular location.

Cysticercosis

Ultrasound is often the first-line imaging modality for evaluating suspected cysticercus (Figs. 1.4.10A and B), especially if intraocular. MRI is preferred over CT for identification of myocysticercosis. Orbital cysticercosis on MRI scans appears as a T2 hyperintense cystic lesion often with an eccentric hypointense scolex within the EOM. The muscle itself may be bulky with perilesional T2 hyperintensity suggestive of edema (Figs. 1.4.10A and B). Contrast-enhanced CT (CECT) may show a ring enhancing lesion in one of the EOMs with an eccentric focus of enhancement or calcification representing the scolex.

Orbital Trauma

Computed tomography is the preferred imaging modality for evaluation of orbital and cranial fractures because of its ability to provide detailed bony images in high spatial resolution. A NCCT with bone and soft tissue windows with multiplanar reconstruction is employed (Figs. 1.4.11A and B). Diffuse hyperdense areas suggest acute intraorbital bleed while air pockets represent orbital emphysema. A "blowout" orbital fracture involving the medial wall and floor is a frequent injury. In a pure blowout fracture of the orbital floor, it is displaced downward into the maxillary sinus (Figs. 1.4.11A and B). In children, due to resilient bones, there is often a minimal bony displacement and herniation of orbital contents

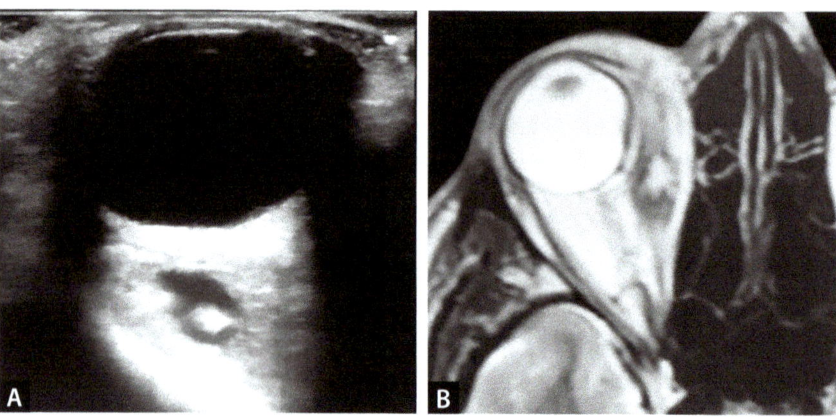

Figs. 1.4.10A and B: Ultrasound (A) and axial T2-weighted (T2W) magnetic resonance imaging (MRI) (B) in *myocysticercus* showing a cystic intraorbital lesion in the lateral rectus with a hyperechoic center suggesting a scolex (A); another patient showing a swollen medial rectus with a cyst and nodule.

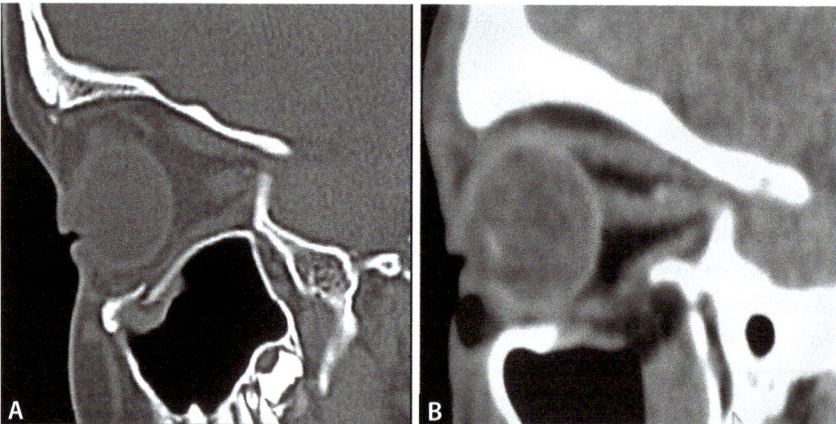

Figs. 1.4.11A and B: Oblique sagittal computed tomography (CT) reconstruction, bone window (A) soft tissue window (B), in two different patients of *blowout fracture* of the orbit. Note clearly the orbital floor fractures with normal inferior rectus (IR) and tear drop shaped hemorrhage pouting in the maxillary sinus in (A) and entrapped swollen IR in (B).

but inferior rectus may still get entrapped, referred to as "trapdoor fracture". The muscle may be bulky, heterogeneous with a rounded contour suggesting hematoma or contusion. Medial wall fractures show displacement of the lamina papyracea into the ethmoid air cells often with opacification of the sinus. The medial rectus muscle with intraorbital fat may also be displaced into the fracture site.

Axial images are best for the evaluation of the maxillary antrum, pterygoid plates, zygomatic arches, and the medial and lateral orbital walls. Coronal images are more useful for evaluation of orbital rims, the orbital floor and roof, the cribriform plate, and the skull base. Reformatted images in the orthogonal sagittal and oblique planes are helpful for evaluating subtle orbital apex and optic canal fractures.

Pearl

Magnetic resonance imaging may miss fractures as the bony structures are not quite conspicuous.

1.5 ULTRASONOGRAPHY

Asha Samdani, Aditi Dubey

INTRODUCTION

Ultrasonography (USG) has broad application in ophthalmology. In 1793, Lazzaro Spallanzani (Italy) discovered that bats orient themselves with the help of sound whistles while flying in darkness. This was the basis of modern ultrasound application. Two types of devices, are used diagnostically, i.e. A-scan and B-scan. *A-scan* is a one-dimensional amplitude modulation scan commonly used for measurement of axial length (AL) and pachymetry.

Along with B-scan, it is used to determine the ultrasonic properties such as internal reflectivity, and dimensions of posterior segment masses. *B-scan* is a two-dimensional, cross-section brightness scan. Its use is primarily to evaluate posterior segment and orbital pathology when the ocular media are cloudy, and a direct view is not possible. High-resolution B-scan or *ultrasound biomicroscopy (UBM)* uses higher frequency probes (20–50 MHz vs the standard 10 MHz) to provide detailed images of anterior segment structures such as the angle, iris, and ciliary body. This chapter deals with B-scan USG primarily.

For sound to be considered ultrasound, it must have a frequency of greater than 20,000 oscillations per second, or 20 KHz, rendering it inaudible to human ears. Ultrasonography of the eye is an indispensable noninvasive tool in the diagnosis and management of various ocular orbital diseases. It was first used in ophthalmology in 1956 by Mundt and Hughes as A-scan. Baum and Greenwood introduced the first B-scan in 1958. Coleman in the 70s developed the first commercially available B-scan.

PRINCIPLE

Ophthalmic ultrasound (Figs. 1.5.1 and 1.5.2) uses high-frequency ultrasound waves, which are transmitted from probe to eye. Tissue penetration is directly proportional to resolution and inversely to frequency. That is why; USG probes used for Ocular USG are of higher frequency (10 MHz) as it needs much less tissue penetration. As the sound waves strike intraocular structures, they are reflected back to the probe and converted into an electric signal. These signals are subsequently reconstructed as an image on a monitor.

The ophthalmic B-scan probe has high frequencies of 10 MHz and contains piezoelectric crystal. Marker on probe helps in the understanding orientation of the image on the screen (Fig. 1.5.2). The orientation of

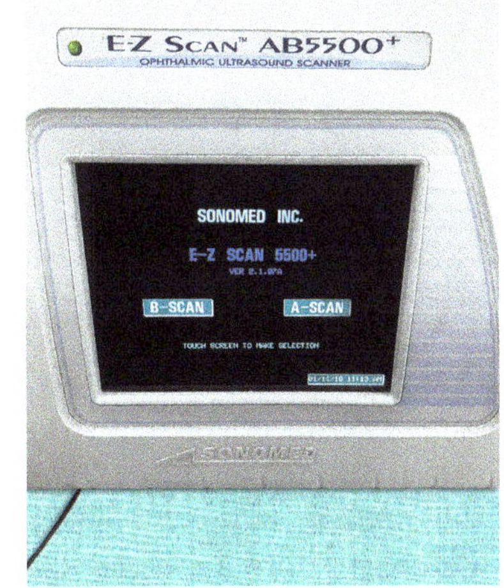

Fig. 1.5.1: Ultrasonography display.

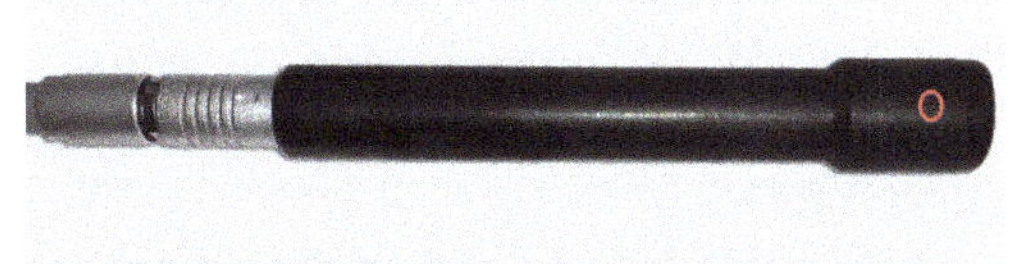

Fig. 1.5.2: Ultrasonography probe.

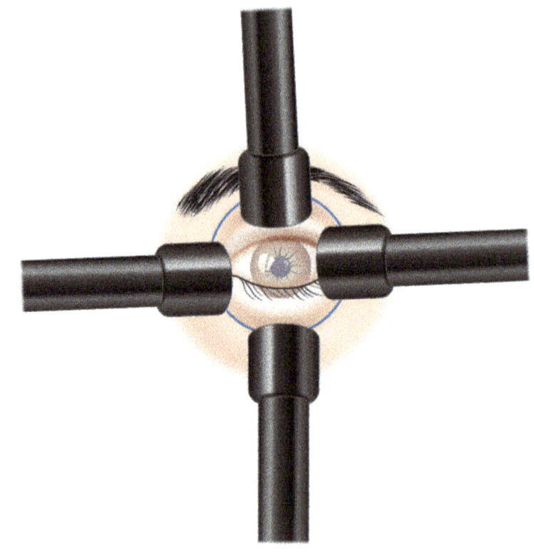
Fig. 1.5.3: Orientation of USG probe while performing scanning.

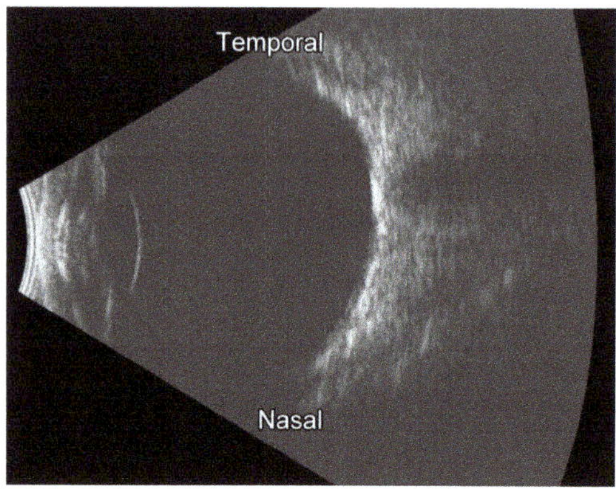

Fig. 1.5.4: Orientation.

the marker (Fig. 1.5.3) is directly correlated to the sound beam orientation. Wherever the marker is directed on the eye *represents the upper portion* of the echogram (Fig. 1.5.4) and, in most instances, the probe is placed opposite the area of the eye to be examined.

Velocity depends on the density of the medium. Sound travels faster through solids than liquids in aqueous and vitreous = 1,532 m/s, and in cornea and lens = 1,641 m/s (Table 1.5.1).

Reflectivity is higher when the echoes are stronger and thus producing brighter dots.

Table 1.5.1: Velocity of sound in various media.

980	Silicone IOL
986	Silicone oil
1480	Fresh water
1532	Aqueous, vitreous
1550	Solid tissue: Intraocular and orbital soft tissue blood
1640	Clear crystalline lens

(IOL: intraocular lens)

The angle of incidence of the probe is critical. When the probe is held perpendicular to the area of interest, more of the echo is reflected directly back into the probe tip and sent to the display screen. When held oblique to the area imaged, part of the echo is reflected away from the probe tip, and less is sent to the display screen the higher the perpendicularity.

Absorption: The density of the solid lid structure results in absorption of part of the sound wave when B-scan is performed through the closed eye, thereby compromising the image of the posterior segment.

Shadowing reduction in echo amplitude posterior to a strongly reflecting or attenuating surface can also lead to poor quality of the image.

Gain: The amplification of the display can be altered by adjusting the gain, which is measured in decibels (dB). When the gain is high, weaker signals are displayed, such as vitreous opacities and posterior vitreous detachments (PVDs). When the gain is low, the weaker signals disappear, and only the stronger echoes, such as the retina, remain on the screen.

BASIC SCREENING TECHNIQUE

Probe positions: The probe can be used in the following positions:

- *Transverse position*: Most commonly used. The probe is positioned parallel to limbus (on opposite scleral surface). It demonstrates the lateral extent of pathology (approximately 6 o'clock hours) (Fig. 1.5.4).

- *Longitudinal position*: The probe is perpendicular to the limbus. It represents the radial extent of pathology and proximity to the optic nerve and demonstrates only 1 o'clock hour that represents optic nerve to the periphery.
- *Axial position*: Patient is fixating in primary gaze, probe face centered on the cornea. Displays the lens and the optic nerve. Horizontal axial scan-marker is toward the patient's nose. Vertical axial scan-marker toward the 12 o'clock position.
- *Oblique position*: The patient is asked to look at various gazes and probe is placed at the oblique axis.

An examination performed when there is no view into the eye because of opaque media, and the determination of the status of the posterior segment is required. The highest gain setting must be used to visualize any weak signals, such as vitreous opacities and posterior vitreous detachments, or to gauge the extent of vitreous hemorrhages. If any pathology such as retinal or choroidal detachments (CDs) is found, then the gain may be reduced for better resolution of the stronger signals from these structures. The entire globe must be examined, from the posterior pole out to the far periphery.

Using a limbus-to-fornix approach, the four major quadrants include the 12-o'clock, 3-o'clock, 6-o'clock, and 9-o'clock positions, and each centered on the right side of the echogram in transverse approaches are evaluated. The posterior pole with a horizontal axial scan is evaluated, which incorporates both the optic nerve and the macula in one echogram. If no additional pathology is detected, these five echograms complete the examination.

In case of any posterior pathology is detected during basic screening, it should be centered on the right side of the echogram to achieve the highest resolution. This is accomplished by determining the clock hour represented in the transverse scan where it was discovered. Once determined, the patient should be instructed to redirect his or her gaze to that meridian, with the probe then placed on the opposite scleral surface. The gain is now reduced until the highest resolution is achieved, and photographic documentation is produced.

Macular localizing: The four methods of localizing and centering of the macula are horizontal, vertical, transverse, and longitudinal. In the horizontal and vertical method, the probe is on the corneal vertex and should be aimed straight ahead to center the macula with marker directed nasally in horizontal while the marker is in the 12-o'clock position in the vertical method. In the transverse and longitudinal method, patient fixating slightly temporally and the probe is placed onto the nasal sclera with the marker at the 12-o'clock position in transverse method while toward the limbus or temporally toward the macula in the longitudinal method. These scan bypasses the lens, thereby preventing absorption or reverberation artifacts from an intraocular lens

Indications for B-scan

- *Opaque ocular media*:
  - *Anterior segment*: For example, corneal opacification, hyphema or hypopyon, miosis, cataract, pupillary or retrolenticular membrane
  - *Posterior segment*: For example, vitreous hemorrhage or inflammation
- *Clear ocular media*:
  - *Anterior segment*: For example, iris lesions, ciliary body lesions

- *Posterior segment*: Tumors, choroidal detachment (CD), retinal detachment (RD), optic disc abnormalities
- *Intraocular foreign bodies*: For detection and localization.

VIVA QUESTIONS

1. Different examination modes of ultrasonography (USG).

Ans. Various examination modes in ophthalmic ultrasonography are:

- *A-scan*: Amplitude modulation scan
- *B-scan*: Brightness modulation scan
- Vector A-scan
- Doppler ultrasonography
- UBM (high-frequency ultrasound).

A-scan: Amplitude modulation scan—salient features are:

- Axial length
- Time-amplitude scan
- Pressure, falsely low AL
- It can also be used for pachymetry
- The frequency of the probe is around 8 MHz
- Quantitative USG:
  - Helps to determine the texture of lesion
  - Based on reflectivity
- It is semiquantitative (Table 1.5.2).

B-scan (brightness modulation scan):

- Multiple A-scans
- As internal emitter is rapidly swept back and forth
- Two-dimensional (2D)

Table 1.5.2: A-scan amplitude.

Category	*Spike height (%)*
Extremely low	0–5
Low	5–40
Medium	40–60
Medium to high	60–80
High	80–100

- Topographic examination for shape, border, location, and extent
- *Kinetic USG*: Mobility, after movements, vascularity (Valsalva).
- It can assess:
  - Vitreoretinal status
  - Macula
  - ONH
  - Anterior two-thirds of orbit
  - Extraocular muscle (EOM)

Doppler ultrasound:

- Using frequency shifts from acoustic reflections to measure movements, flow conditions within vessels is detected
- Presentation as false color based on the frequency
- Three-dimensional reconstructions.

2. Differences between retinal detachment (RD), choroidal detachment (CD), and posterior vitreous detachment (PVD).

Ans. See Table 1.5.3. Other important points include:

- *Retinal detachment*: It appears as a highly reflective, attached to the ora serrata anteriorly and the optic nerve (Fig. 1.5.5). It has moderate mobility and translucent subretinal space. Maintains 100% reflectivity even on low gain.
  - There is a gradual separation of the membrane from the ocular wall unlike in CD
  - Attachment at disc is broad and at the periphery of the disc
  - Persists at low gain
  - Thickness corresponds to PVR
  - Configuration—convex RRD, concave TRD, double layer sign in GRT.
  - The configuration of funnel (Figs. 1.5.6 and 1.5.7), retinoschisis
  - Coexisting findings can be peripheral retinal looping, cyst formation in long-standing RD (Fig. 1.5.8)
  - Tractional RD common finding in vascular retinopathies caused strong

Table 1.5.3: Differences between RD, CD, and PVD.

	CD	*RD*	*PVD*
Topography	Dome shaped	Linear, V	V, U
Location	Periphery (pre-equator)	Variable	Variable
Attachment to optic disc	No	Yes	Variable
Others	Kissing choroids, vortex vein	Folds, breaks	Inferior, thicker
Quantitative (A)			
Spike height	90–100%	80–100%	40–90%
Spike peak	Double	Single	Single
Kinetic (A and B)			
Mobility	Minimal	Moderate	Marked
After movement	Absent	Minimal to moderate	Marked

(CD: choroidal detachment; PVD: posterior vitreous detachment; RD: retinal detachment)

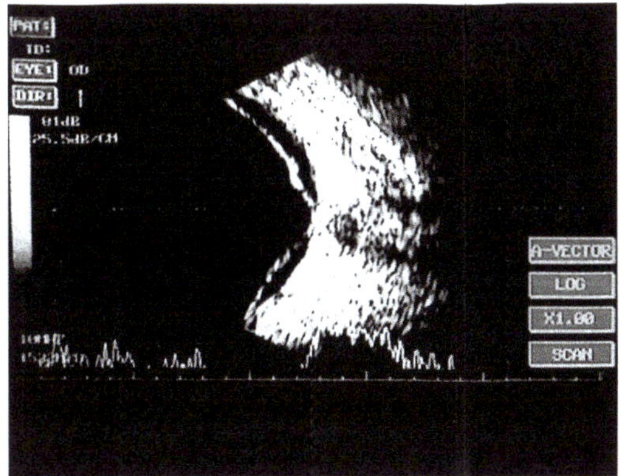

Fig. 1.5.5: Retinal detachment.

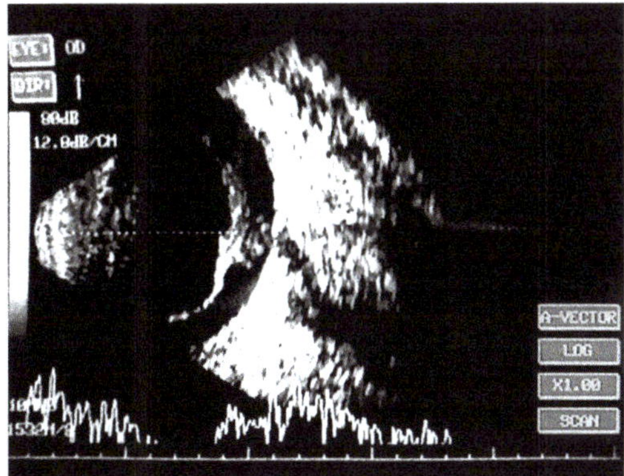

Fig. 1.5.6: Open funnel retinal detachment (RD).

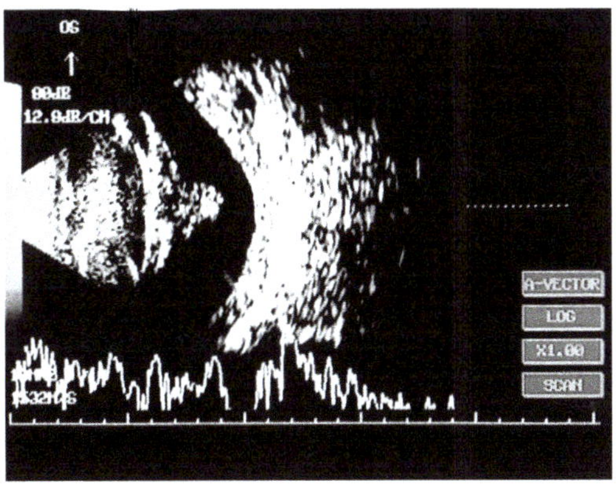

Fig. 1.5.7: Closed funnel retinal detachment (RD).

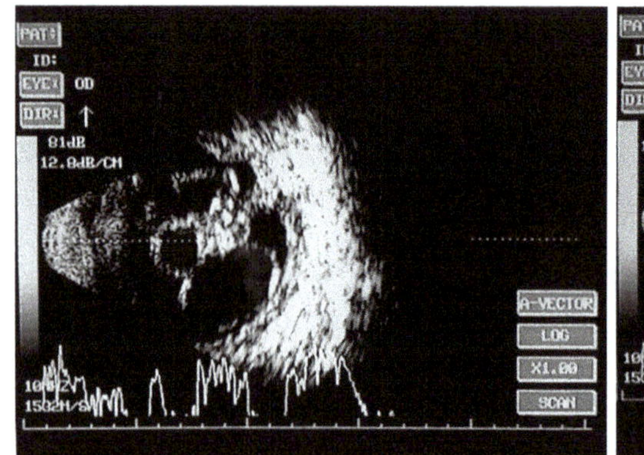

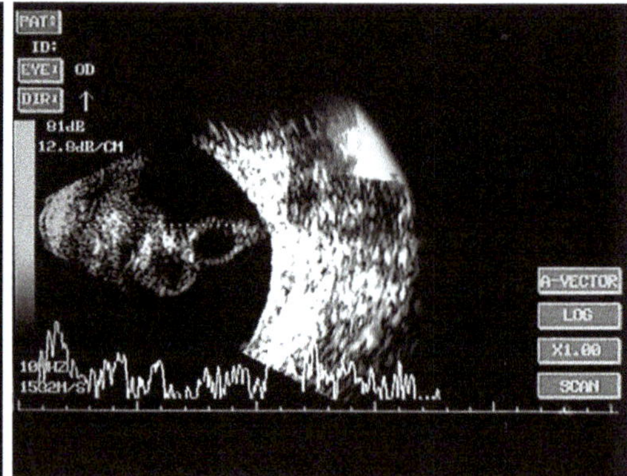

Fig. 1.5.8: Retinal cyst in old retinal detachment (RD).

adhesion (Fig. 1.5.9) and subsequent traction detached retina—concave appearance
- Giant retinal tears appear as large tears with rolled out tissue and clear breach

- *Posterior vitreous detachment*: In PVD with the normal eye, the reflectivity is very low, high gain (90 dB) setting is required (Fig. 1.5.10). The reflectivity disappears on lowering the gain under 70 dB. Kinetic echography typically shows a very undulating movement that continues after the eye movements' stop.
  - Attachment at disc narrow or none
  - About 40–90% spike height decreasing anteriorly
  - The height of PVD generally more superiorly
  - Thick PVD spike may persist at low gain
  - How to differentiate from RD? Measure the difference in decibels between the 50% spike height of membrane and sclera
- *Choroidal detachment*: Choroidal detachment is smooth, dome-shaped and thick, no movement seen with eye movement (Fig. 1.5.11). When extensive, one can see multiple dome-shaped detachments, which may "kiss" in the central vitreous cavity.

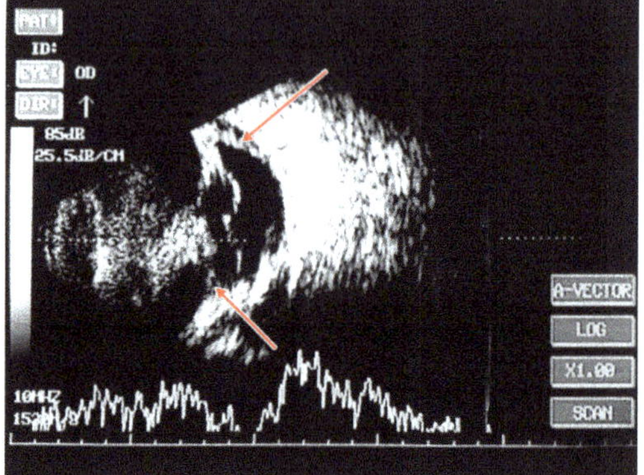

Fig. 1.5.9: Tractional retinal detachment (RD).

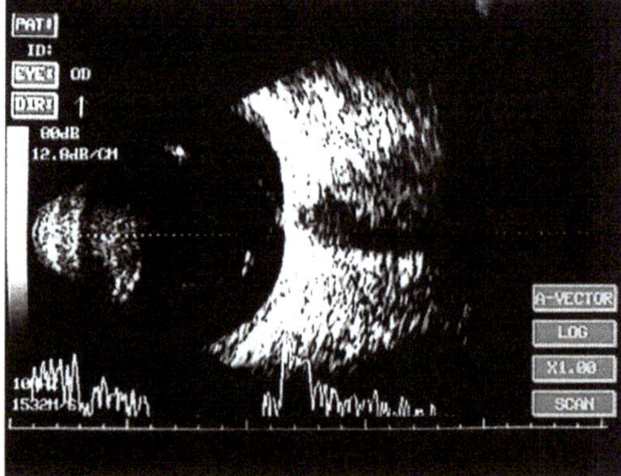

Fig. 1.5.10: Posterior vitreous detachment.

  - *Serous* CD has anechoic suprachoroidal space
  - *Hemorrhagic* CD has dispersed opacities (Fig. 1.5.12)

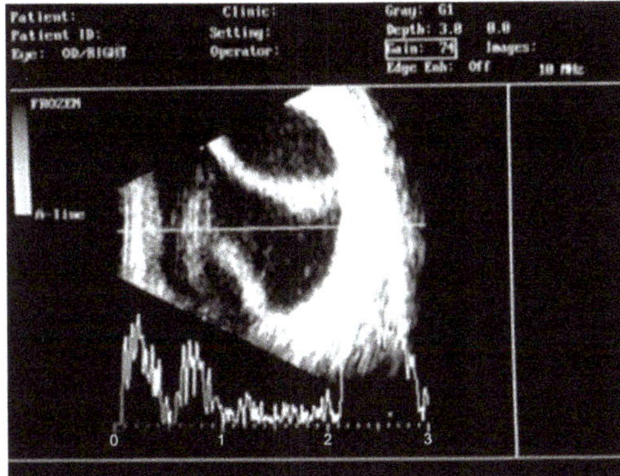

Fig. 1.5.11: Choroidal detachment.

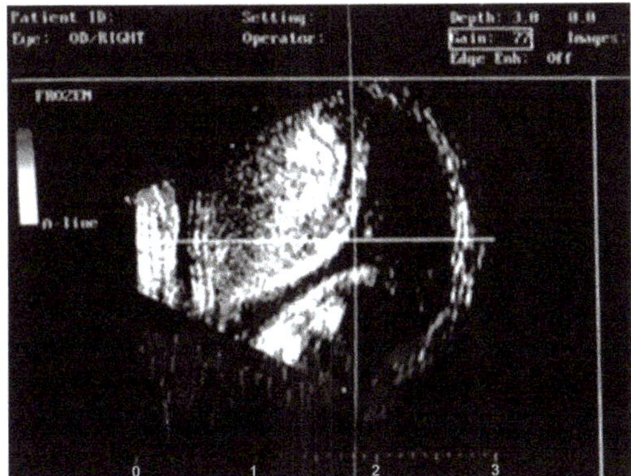

Fig. 1.5.12: Hemorrhagic choroidal detachment (CD) with kissing choroids.

- Seen as thick bright opacity even at low gain
- Sometimes thin stretched cord-like opacity extending between the wall and detached choroidal layer presumed to be vortex vein.

3. Vitreous hemorrhage.

Ans. A fresh mild hemorrhage appears as small dots or linear areas of low reflective mobile vitreous opacities (Fig. 1.5.13). Old vitreous hemorrhage appears vitreous filled with multiple large opacities that are higher in their reflectively and membranes as the blood organizes.

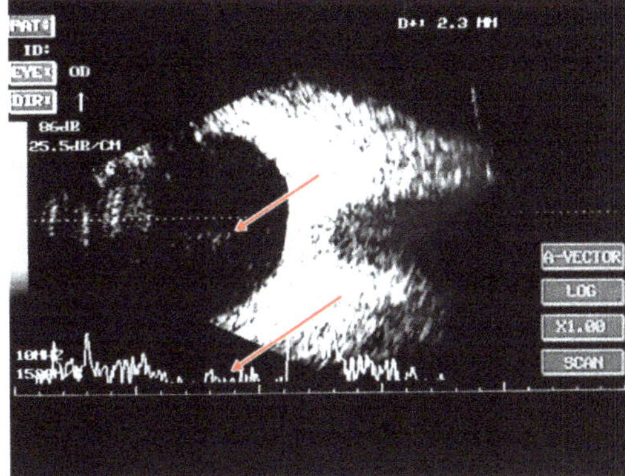

Fig. 1.5.13: Vitreous hemorrhage.

Differentiation between vitreous hemorrhage and asteroid hyalosis: Asteroid hyalosis is calcium deposits in vitreous cavity and appear as bright round signals on B scan with echo-free space in front of the retina.

- Asteroid hyalosis is highly echogenic, and they are still visible when the gain setting is reduced up to 60 dB whereas vitreous hemorrhage which usually disappears by 60 dB.

4. USG appearance of endophthalmitis.

Ans. It depends on the degree and severity of infection and extent of vitreous involvement.

- Low to moderate cases—hyper-reflective opacities noted
- Severe cases—moderate or coarse opacities with membrane formation (Fig. 1.5.14).

5. USG appearance of persistent fetal vasculature:

Ans. It is a congenital abnormality when the fetal hyaloid artery does not resorb. Very thin persistent hyaloidal vessel coursing from the disc to the lens can be seen. Globe size is usually small (Fig. 1.5.15).

6. USG appearance of intraocular foreign body.

Ans:

- *A-scan*:
  - Steeply rising wide echo spike along the baseline between the initial spike and ocular wall spike.

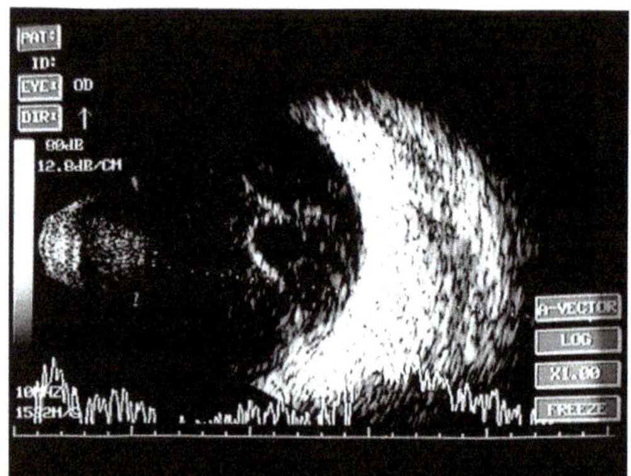

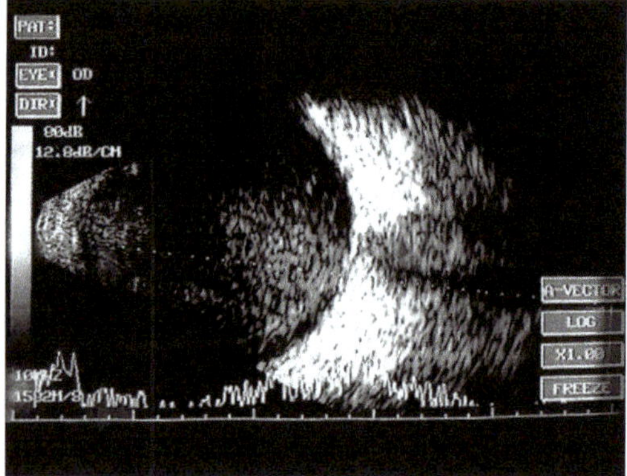

Fig. 1.5.14: Endophthalmitis.

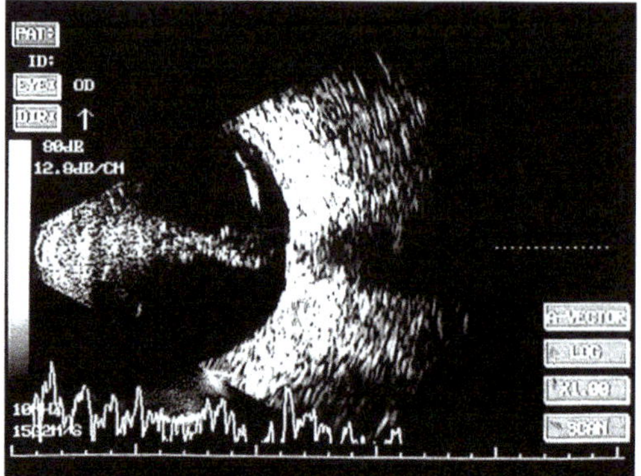

Fig. 1.5.15: Persistent fetal vasculature.

- Extremely high reflectivity (100% spike), which persists on low gain (Fig. 1.5.16).
- The distance between the intraocular foreign body and the adjacent sclera is accurately measured at lower system sensitivity.
- Sound attenuation is very strong.

- *B-scan*:
  - Acoustically opaque contrasting with the acoustically clear vitreous.
  - Persists even when the system sensitivity is decreased by 20–30 db.
  - Topographic and kinetic echography will show if the foreign body is adherent to the retina or if it is floating in the vitreous.

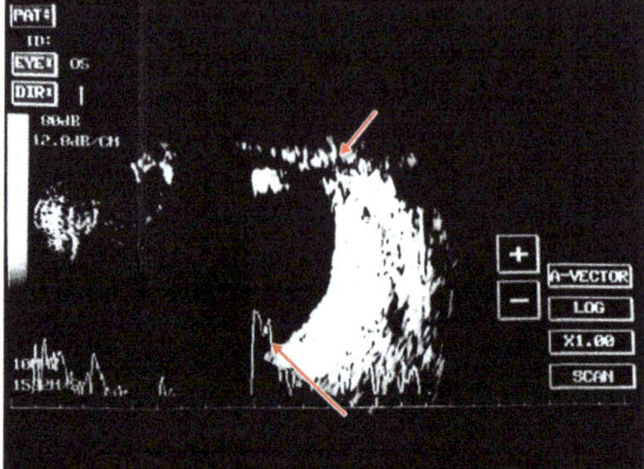

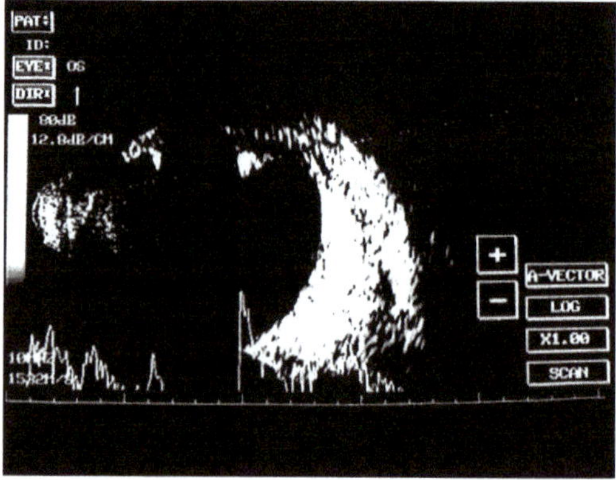

Fig. 1.5.16: Intraocular foreign body.

  - Sound attenuation is very strong.
  - Shadowing of the ocular and orbital tissues behind it as it totally reflects the sound beams preventing its propagation within tissues behind it (Fig. 1.5.16).

- Associated findings like vitreous hemorrhage, vitreous bands, fibrosis, RD, CD, and even scleral entry wounds can be assessed.

7. USG appearance of posterior staphyloma.

Ans. Appears as a shallow excavation of posterior pole with smooth edges in highly myopic eyes (focal area of thinned sclera) (Fig. 1.5.17).

8. USG appearance of posterior scleritis.

Ans. The degree of scleral thickening can vary from mild to severe. It is commonly, associated edema adjacent to the sclera. This manifests itself as an echolucent area in the tenon space, it forms a "T-sign" USG is the best modality for diagnosis (Figs. 1.5.18A and B).

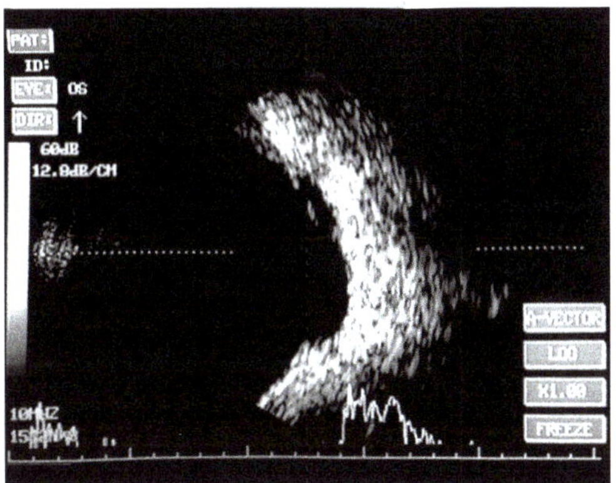

Fig. 1.5.17: Posterior staphyloma.

9. USG appearance of optic nerve pathologies.

Ans.

- Optic disc drusen—appears as an echogenic focus within or on the surface of the optic nerve head (Fig. 1.5.19). Posterior acoustic shadowing may be present with larger lesions. Astrocytic hamartomas may confuse with drusen and can be differentiated by following points:
  - Seen in patients with tuberous sclerosis or neurofibromatosis
  - Usually unilateral
  - Usually larger
  - Associated with RD
- Optic nerve head cupping—appears as an excavation of the disc (Figs. 1.5.20 and 1.5.21). It is important to note that USG can detect cupping reliably only in advanced cases.

10. USG appearance of intraocular tumors.

Ans. Ultrasonographic appearance of intraocular tumors has been summarized in Table 1.5.4.

- *Choroidal melanoma*:
  - Mushroom shaped is caused by tumor growth through a break in Bruch's membrane)
  - Choroidal excavation (produced by dome-shaped fundus lesions in ultrasound beam path)

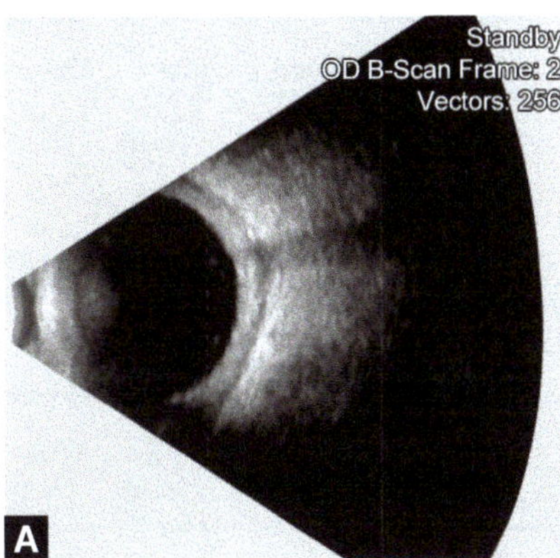

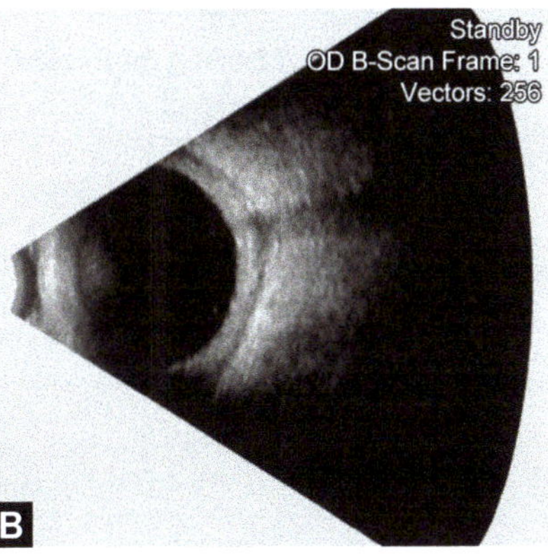

Figs. 1.5.18A and B: Posterior scleritis. (A) "T" sign in the right eye; and (B) Left eye.

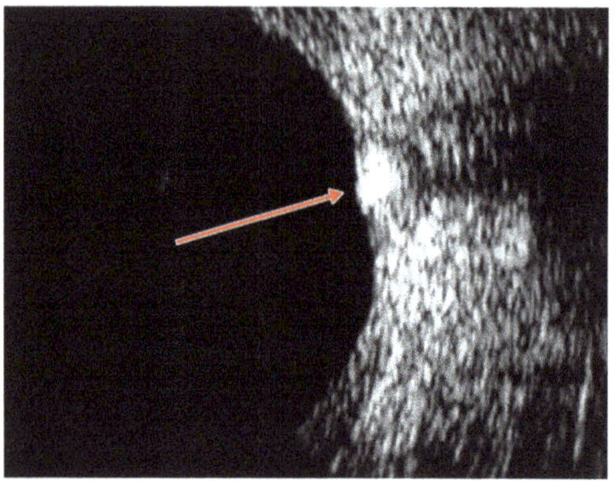

Fig. 1.5.19: Optic disc drusen.

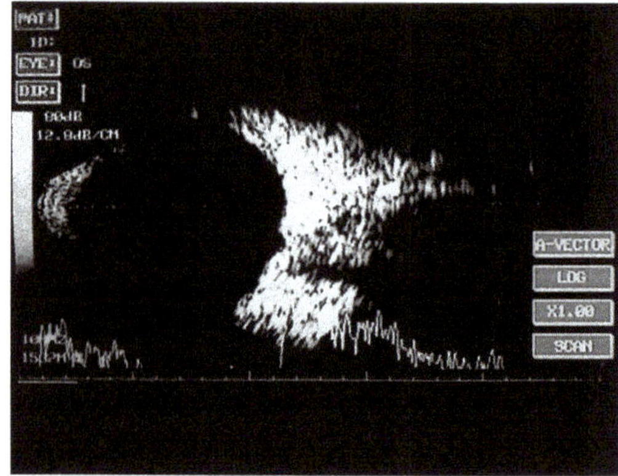

Fig. 1.5.20: Early optic nerve head cupping.

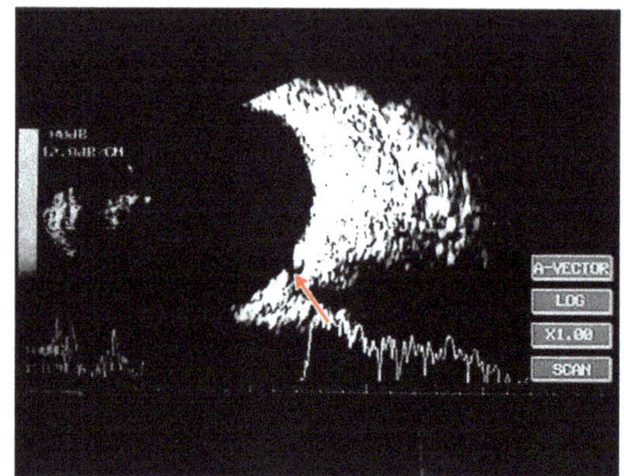

Fig. 1.5.21: Advanced optic nerve head cupping.

Table 1.5.4: Common intraocular tumors in ultrasonography (USG).

	Melanoma	*Metastasis*	*Hemangioma*
Shape	Domed, mushroom	Domed/bi-domed, irregular	Domed
Location	Variable	Near macula	Near disc
Associated RD	Variable	Common	Rare
Growth	Variable	Rapid	Slow
Quantitative (A)			
Reflectivity	Low/medium	Variable	High
Internal structure	Regular	Irregular	Regular
Sound attenuation	Strong	Variable	Weak
Kinetic (A)			
Vascularity	Present	Absent	Absent

(RD: retinal detachment)

- ◆ Solid mass with shadowing (Fig. 1.5.22)
- ◆ The scleral extension should be watched for
- *Choroidal metastasis*: The tumor has an irregular outline and heterogeneous internal structure.
- *Hemangioma*: A scan honeycomb spikes, spikes do not touch baseline.

11. USG appearance of cysticercosis extraocular muscle.

Ans. Extraocular muscle (EOM) cysticercosis manifests as a well-demarcated cyst in relation to the right recti muscle with a central echodense, highly reflective structure within the sonolucent cyst, corresponding to the scolex (Fig. 1.5.23). EOM involvement is the most common variety of orbital cysticercosis. The subconjunctival space is the next common site, followed by the eyelid, optic nerve, retro-orbital space, and lacrimal gland. All the extraocular muscles are involved in myocysticercosis. However, the lateral rectus, medial rectus, and the superior oblique muscles have been found to be affected to a greater extent.

12. USG appearance retinopathy of prematurity (ROP).

Ans.

- Multiple membranes in the periphery
- Retinal detachment (RD)
- Focal fibrovascular fonds
- Open funnel RD
- Closed funnel RD.

13. USG appearance coats.

Ans.

- Unilateral
- RD, turbid SRF.

14. RB (Retinoblastoma)

Ans.

- Solid tumor
- Calcification
- Moderate internal reflectivity
- *If necrosis, calcification*: High reflectivity (Fig. 1.5.24).
- Sound attenuation moderate to high
- If glaucoma: Globe enlarged.

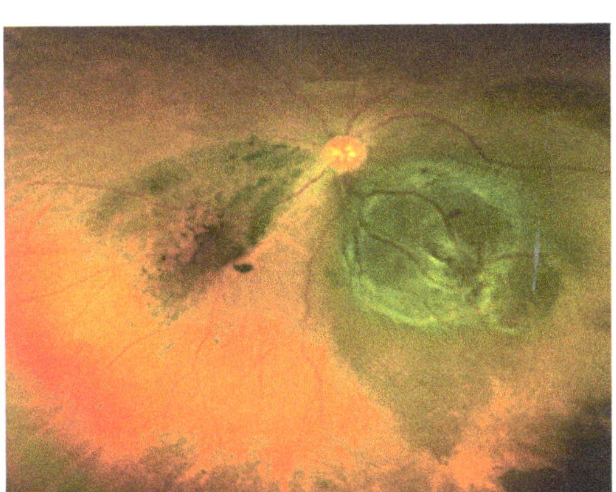

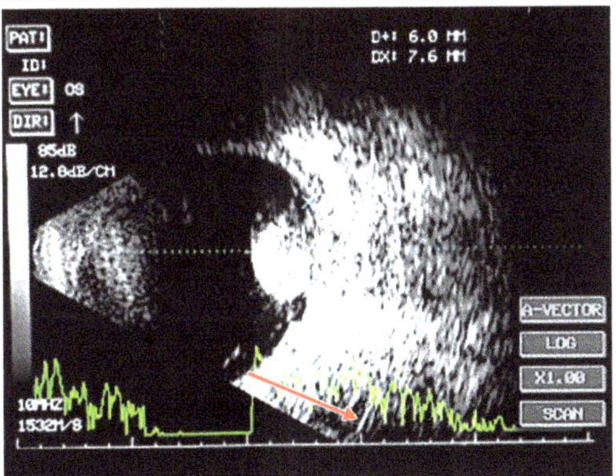

Fig. 1.5.22: Choroidal melanoma.

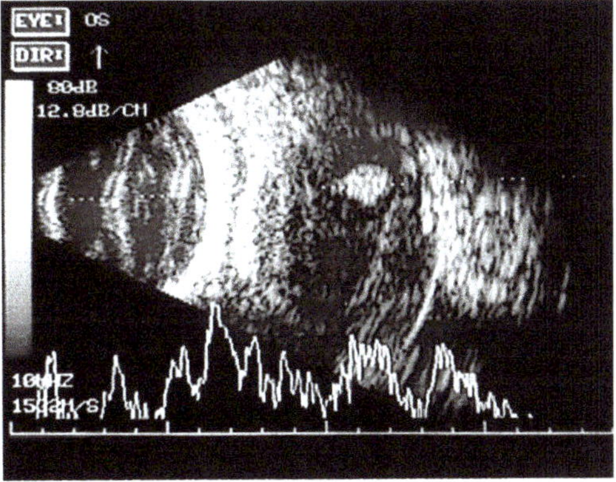

Fig. 1.5.23: Cysticercosis extraocular muscle.

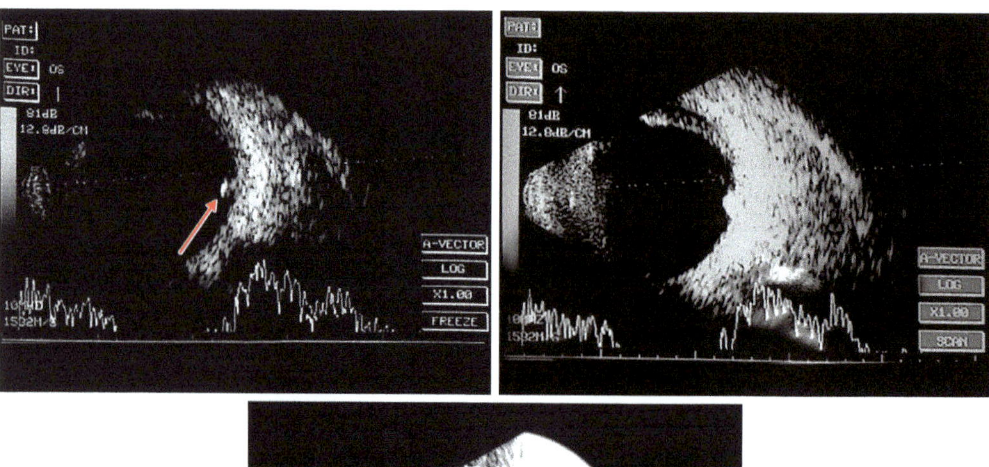

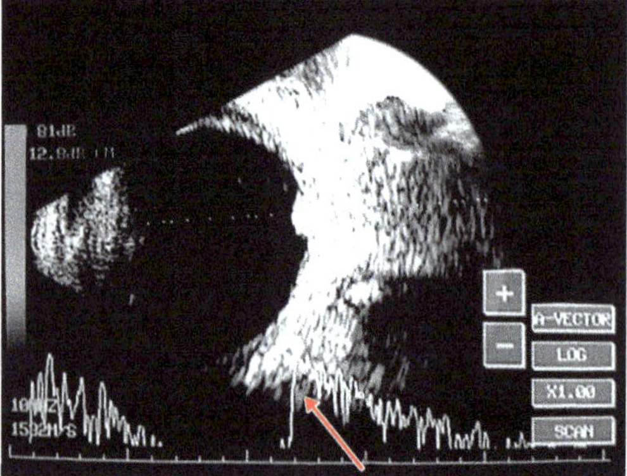

Fig. 1.5.24: Retinoblastoma.

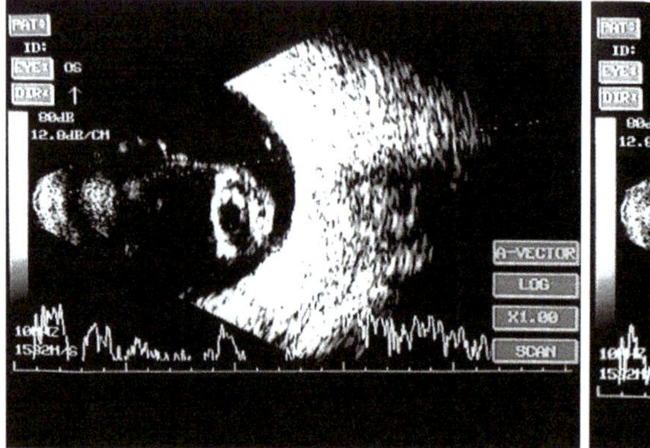

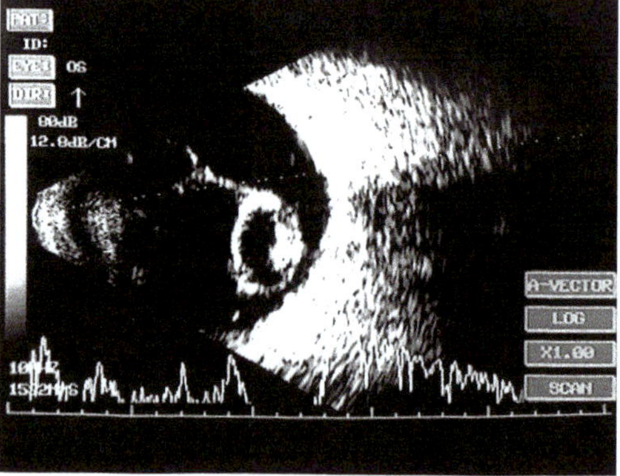

Fig. 1.5.25: Nucleus drop.

15. Nucleus drop.

Ans.

- Biconvex-shaped structure (Fig. 1.5.25)
- Surrounding mild to moderate spikes suggesting vitritis.

16. Choroidal coloboma.

Ans.

- Following findings can be there:
  - Excavation of posterior layer (Fig. 1.5.26)
  - Cyst

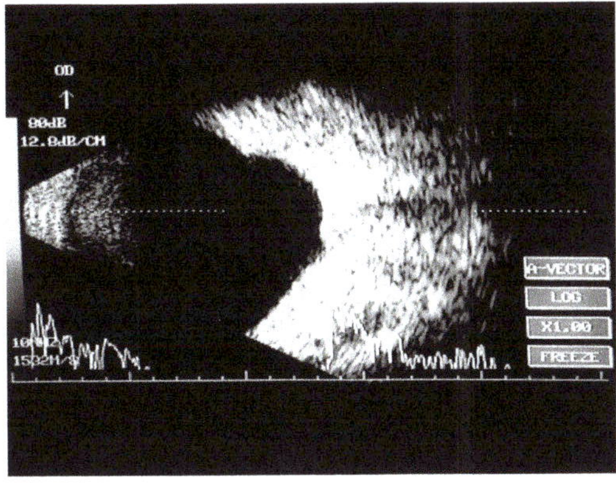

Fig. 1.5.26: Choroidal coloboma.

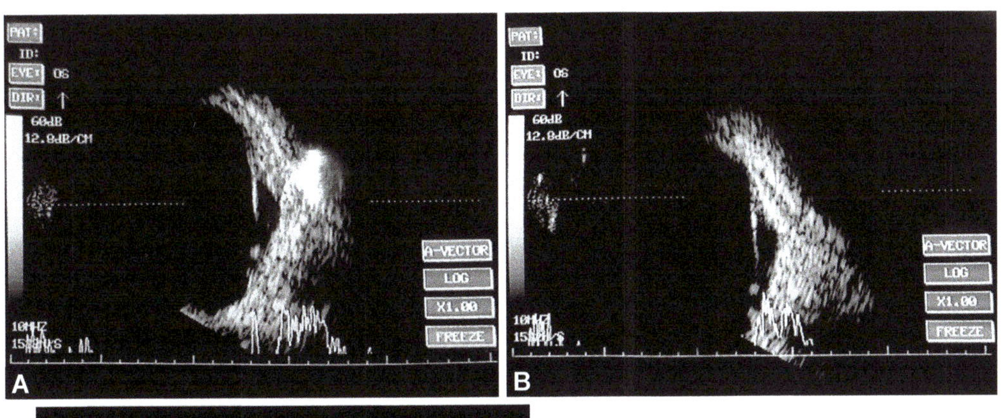

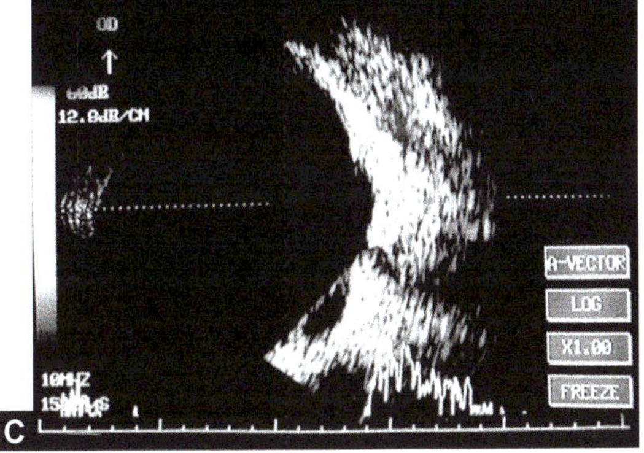

Figs. 1.5.27A to C: Choroidal coloboma with RD.

- RD (Figs. 1.5.27A to C)
- Small eyeball.

BIBLIOGRAPHY

1. Aironi VD, Gandage SG. Pictorial essay: B-scan ultrasonography in ocular abnormalities. Indian J Radiol Imaging. 2009;19(2): 109-15.
2. Coleman JD, Silverman RH, Lizzi FL, et al. Ultrasonography of eye and orbit, 2nd edition. Lippincott Williams and Wilkins; 2005. pp. 47-122.
3. Pushker N, Bajaj MS, Chandra M, et al. Ocular and orbital cysticercosis. Acta Ophthalmol Scand. 2001;79(4):408-13.

1.6 APPLIANCES AND INSTRUMENTS IN OCULOPLASTY

Saloni Gupta, Sahil Agrawal, Pranita Sahay

The commonly used instruments in oculoplasty surgery include the following:

1. Lid clamp or Snellen's entropion clamp (Fig. 1.6.1)
2. Jaeger's lid spatula (Fig. 1.6.2)
3. Epilation forceps (Fig. 1.6.3)
4. Plain forceps (Fig. 1.6.4)
5. Artery (hemostatic) forceps (Fig. 1.6.5)
6. Arruga's needle holder (Fig. 1.6.6)
7. Stevens tenotomy scissors (Fig. 1.6.7)
8. Berke's ptosis clamp (Fig. 1.6.8)
9. Well's enucleation spoon (Fig. 1.6.9)
10. Enucleation scissors (Fig. 1.6.10)
11. Mule's evisceration spatula (Fig. 1.6.11)
12. Evisceration curette (Fig. 1.6.12)
13. Chalazion clamp (Fig. 1.6.13)
14. Chalazion scoop (Fig. 1.6.14)
15. Nettleship's punctum dilator (Fig. 1.6.15)
16. Bowman lacrimal probe (Fig. 1.6.16)
17. Freer periosteal elevator (Fig. 1.6.17)

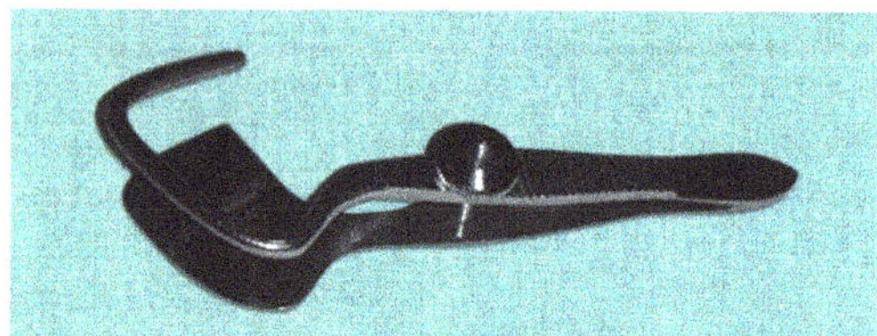

Fig. 1.6.1: Lid clamp or Snellen's entropion clamp.

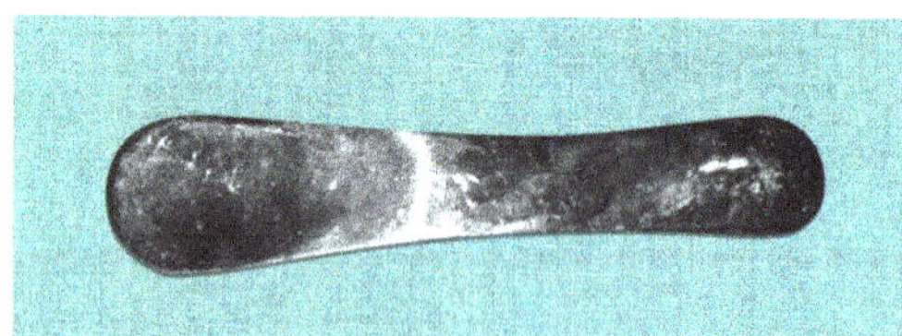

Fig. 1.6.2: Jaeger's lid spatula.

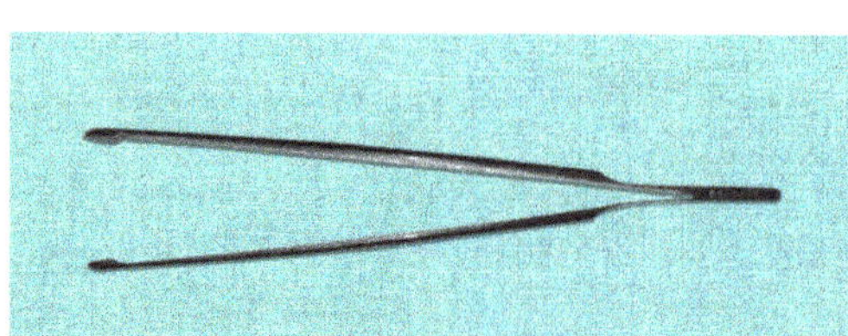

Fig. 1.6.3: Epilation forceps.

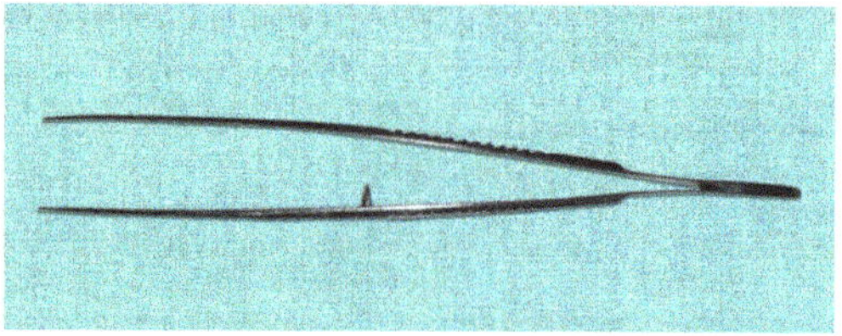

Fig. 1.6.4: Plain forceps.

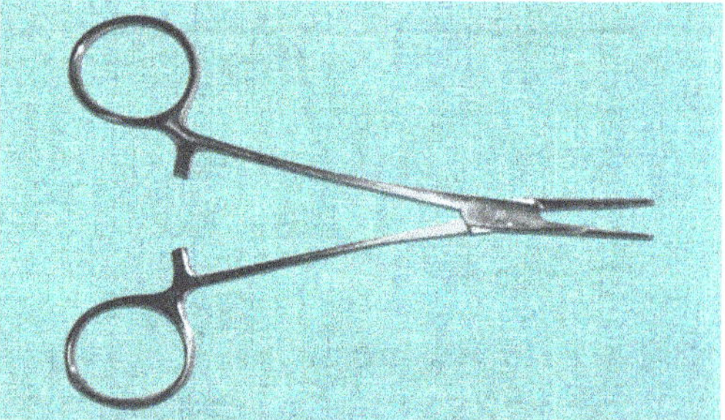

Fig. 1.6.5: Artery (hemostatic) forceps.

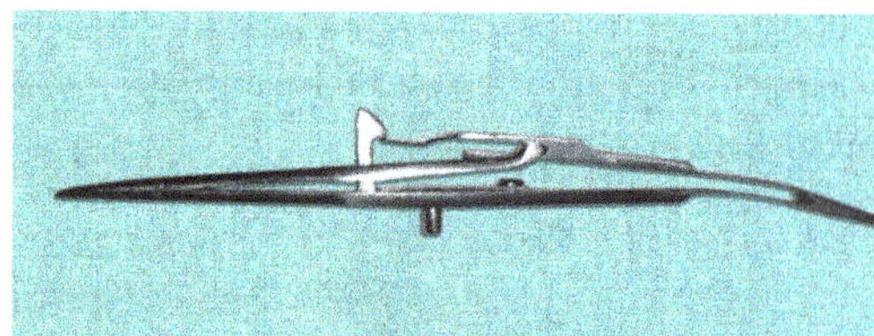

Fig. 1.6.6: Arruga's needle holder.

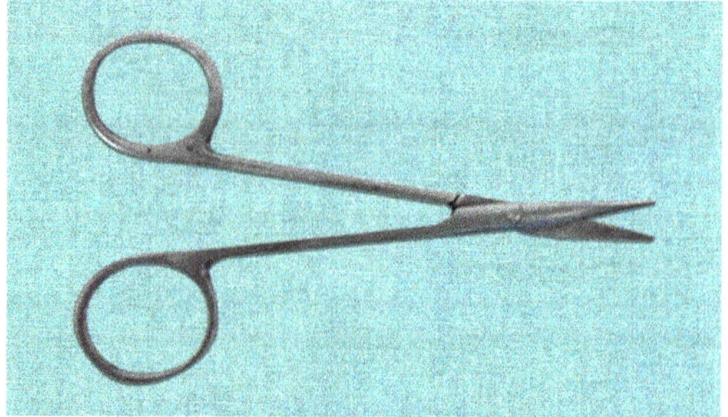

Fig. 1.6.7: Stevens tenotomy scissors.

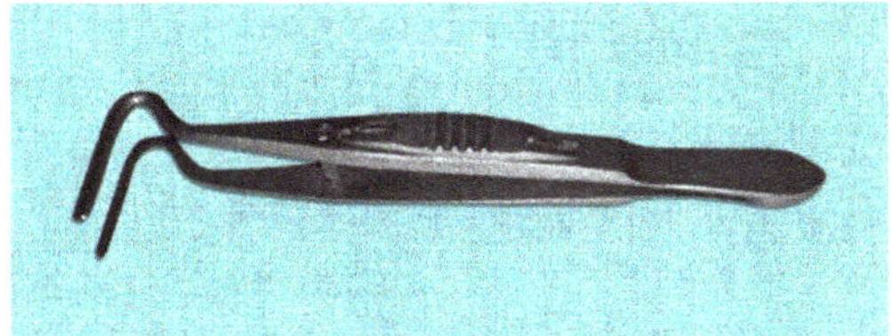

Fig. 1.6.8: Berke's ptosis clamp.

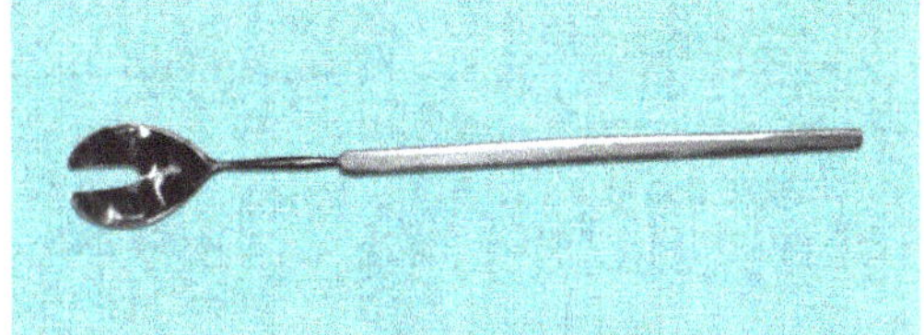

Fig. 1.6.9: Well's enucleation spoon.

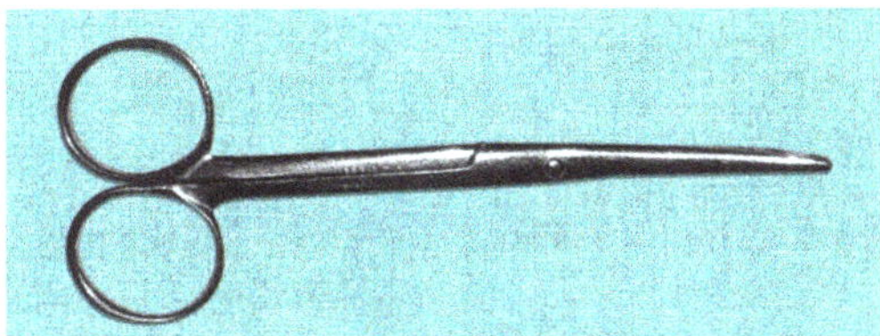

Fig. 1.6.10: Enucleation scissors.

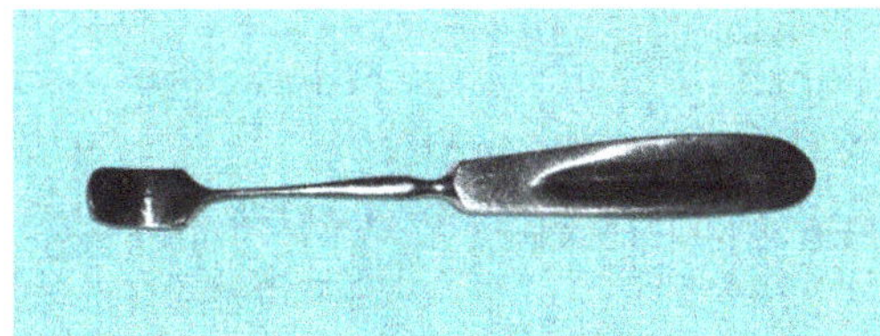

Fig. 1.6.11: Mule's evisceration spatula.

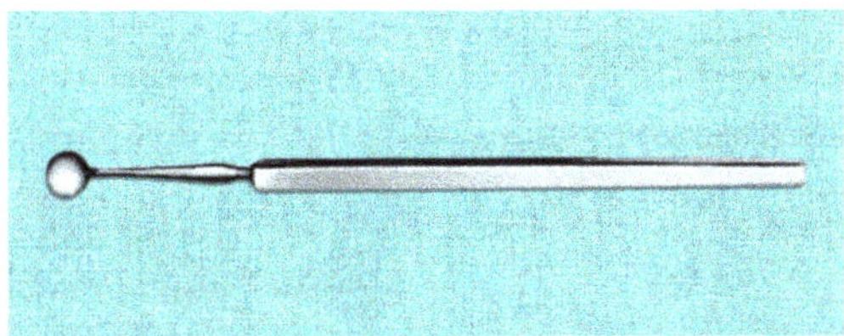

Fig. 1.6.12: Evisceration curette.

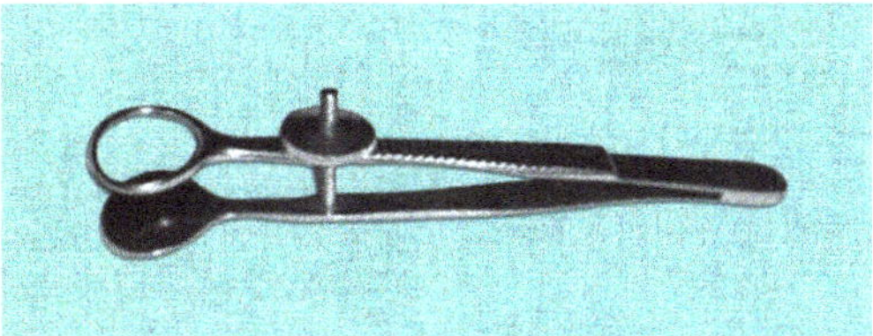

Fig. 1.6.13: Chalazion clamp.

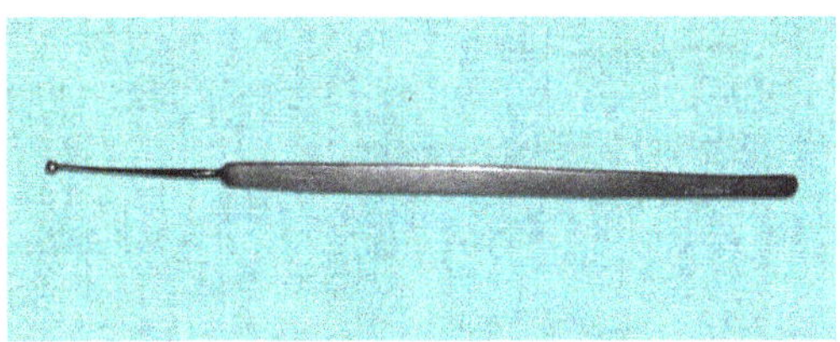

Fig. 1.6.14: Chalazion scoop.

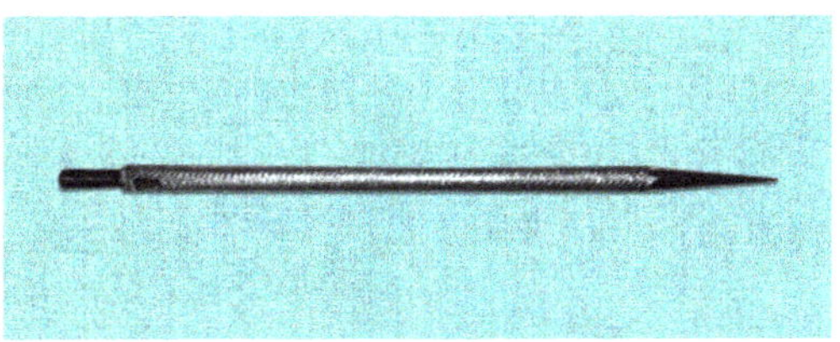

Fig. 1.6.15: Nettleship's punctum dilator.

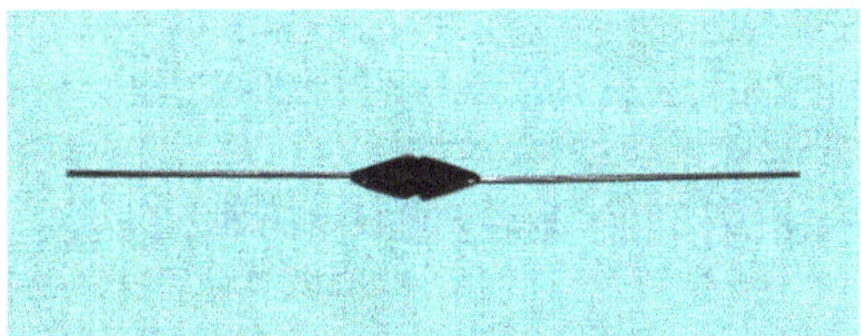

Fig. 1.6.16: Bowman lacrimal probe.

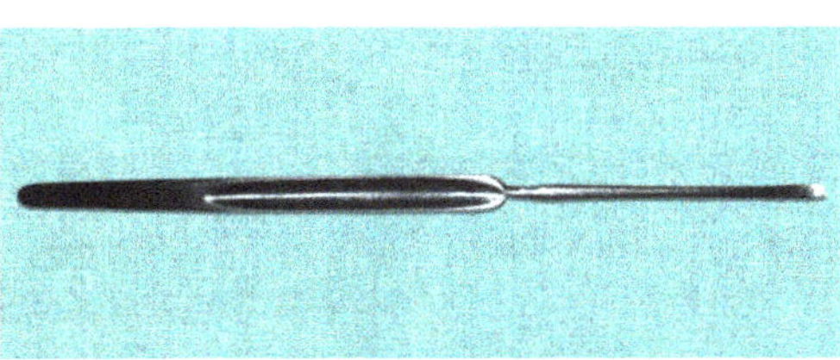

Fig. 1.6.17: Freer periosteal elevator.

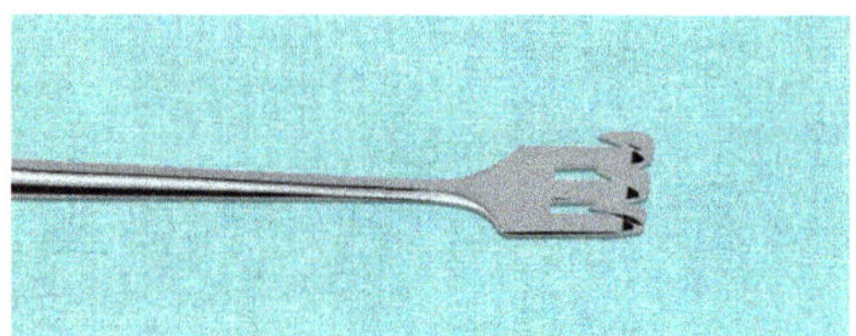

Fig. 1.6.18: Cat's paw lacrimal wound retractor.

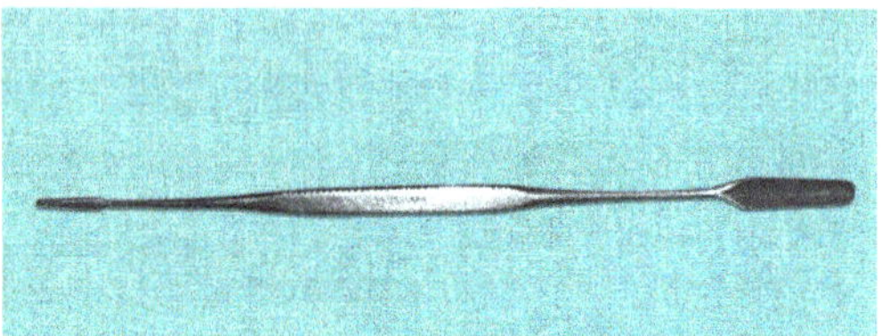

Fig. 1.6.19: Lacrimal sac dissector and currete

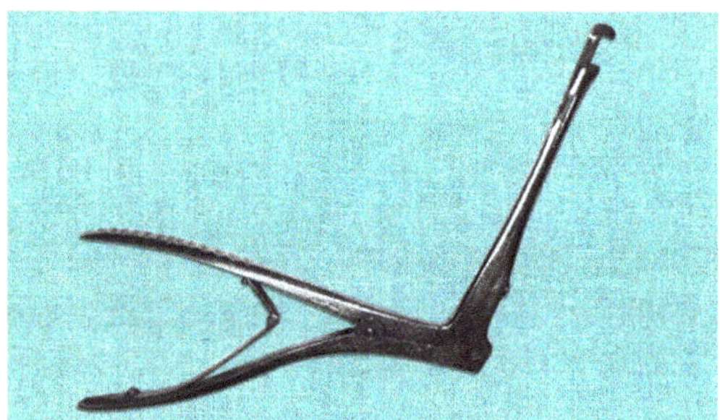

Fig. 1.6.20: Kerrison bone punch.

18. Cat's paw lacrimal wound retractor (Fig. 1.6.18)
19. Lacrimal sac dissector and currete (Fig. 1.6.19)
20. Kerrison bone punch (Fig. 1.6.20)

The details of the above-mentioned instruments have discussed in Ophthalmology Clinics for Postgraduates 2016.

PTOSIS

The three categories of surgical procedures most commonly used in ptosis are:

1. *External approach*: Transcutaneous levator advancement
2. *Internal approach*: Levator/tarsus/Müller muscle resection (*Putterman müllerectomy, Fasanella-Servat procedure)*
3. Frontalis muscle suspension using sling.

The most common determining factors in the choice of the surgical procedure for ptosis repair are:

- The amount and type of ptosis
- Levator function
- Surgeon's comfort level and experience with various procedures.

Surgical correction of the levator aponeurosis is preferred in cases with good levator function.

- *External (transcutaneous)* levator advancement surgery is most commonly used when levator function is normal and the upper eyelid crease is high. In this setting, the levator muscle itself is normal, but the levator aponeurosis (its tendinous attachment to the tarsal plate) is stretched or disinserted, thus requiring advancement. It also allows the surgeon to simultaneously remove excess eyelid skin.
- For repair of minimal ptosis (2 mm)—Putterman müllerectomy if 2.5% phenylephrine test is positive or *Fasanella-Servat procedure* (requires removal of the superior tarsus).
- Frontalis muscle suspension techniques done in cases where levator function is poor or absent.

Amount of Resection

Berke's Rule

Levator function	*Intraoperative lid height*
2–3 mm	At upper limbus
4–5 mm	1–2 mm overlap
6–7 mm	2 mm overlap
8–9 mm	3–4 mm
10–11 mm	5 mm overlap

Beard's Rule

Preoperative margin to reflex distance	*Amount of resection*
10–13 mm	3–4 mm
14–17 mm	2–3 mm
18–22 mm	1–2 mm
>23 mm	0–1 mm

Complications of Ptosis Surgery

- Overcorrection
- Undercorrection
- Lid contour abnormalities
- Lid lag and lagophthalmos
- Lid crease and fold asymmetry
- Keratopathy
- Infection and/or inflammation
- Hemorrhage.

Complications of Ptosis Clamp

- Oculocardiac reflex (Aschner phenomenon or Aschner-Dagnini reflex) is a known complication. Compression, traction or any manipulation of the extraocular muscles can lead to a sudden decrease in pulse rate/bradycardia.
- Afferent pathway is ophthalmic branch of the Vth cranial nerve via the ciliary ganglion.
- Efferent pathway is the vagus nerve.
- The reflex is mediated by visceral motor nucleus of the vagus nerve in the brain stem, stimulation of which leads to decreased output of the sinoatrial (SA) node of heart causing bradycardia, junctional rhythm, and asystole. Most commonly seen in neonates and children during strabismus correction surgery. However, it can occur with other ocular surgeries and adults.

Management

- Immediate removal of the stimulus can results in the restoration of normal sinus rhythm.
- If not, the use of atropine or glycopyrrolate can revert the attack.
- In severe cases, such as asystole, cardiopulmonary resuscitation (CPR) is required.
- Surgery can be continued if the attack can be reversed successfully.

Materials for Sling Surgery

- Autologous tissue:
    - Fascia Lata (both autologous and preserved)
    - Palmaris longus tendon
    - Temporalis fascia
- Synthetic material:
    - Silicone nonabsorbable sutures, Gore-Tex strips (polytetrafluoroethylene), polypropylene (Prolene), polyester mesh, monofilament nylon, and Supramid Extra (polyfilament and nylon).

Management of Residual Ptosis

- The moderate to severe cases of residual ptosis were tackled by levator resection by skin approach which has all the advantages like ease of the proper exposure of levator and its dissection, availability of adequate amount of levator muscle for resection after cutting the horns, and proper lid fold formation is possible.
- The cases of mild ptosis with faint lid folds were managed by proper lid fold formation.

Nonsurgical Management of Ptosis

A dropped eyelid can be managed nonsurgically by:

- External mechanical devices (skin-taping, adhesives, or spectacle-based lid crutches) to retract the upper lid
- Stimulating Müller's muscle (topical eye drops)
- Weakening orbicularis muscle tone (injectable botulinum toxin).

ENUCLEATION

1. Current indications of enucleation:
    - Intraocular malignancy (uveal melanoma and retinoblastoma)
    - Trauma
    - Painful blind eye

- Sympathetic ophthalmitis
- Microphthalmos.

2. Evisceration versus enucleation: Table 1.6.1 shows difference between evisceration and enucleation.
3. Causes of bleeding during enucleation:
   - Bleeding from central retinal vessels following optic nerve transection.
   - Bleeding from anterior ciliary arteries during muscle transection.
4. Hemostasis during enucleation:
   - Retrobulbar injection of lignocaine and adrenaline preoperatively can help in intraoperative hemostasis.
   - Small amount of bleeding can be controlled by firm digital pressure.
   - Use of cautery is rarely required and should be used with caution near the orbital apex to prevent damage to extraocular muscles and oculomotor nerves.
   - Postoperatively a pressure patch for the first 48 hours helps in maintain hemostasis.
5. Types of enucleation:
   - Based on technique:
     - Conventional (imbrication) technique of enucleation
     - Myoconjunctival technique of enucleation—where extraocular muscles are attached to the respective fornices instead of imbricating over the implant.
     - Modifications of conventional:
       - 4-petal technique
       - Double petal technique
       - Scleral patch/orbital fat over porous implants.
   - Based on primary or secondary implant.
6. Best approach to achieve optimal optic nerve length in retinoblastoma:
   - Gentle traction is applied to cause subluxation of globe out of rim.
   - Use of blunt 15° curved tenotomy scissors from the *lateral* aspect to transect the nerve.
7. Complications of enucleation:
   - *Intraoperative*:
     - Damage to or loss of extraocular muscles
     - Hemorrhage
     - Extensive dissection and mishandling of conjunctiva and tenons, leading to poor closure.
     - Improper implant sizing.

Table 1.6.1: Differences between evisceration and enucleation.

	Evisceration	*Enucleation*
Definition	Surgical technique of removing the intraocular contents, at the same time preserving the remaining scleral shell, extraocular muscle attachments, and surrounding orbital adnexa	Surgical procedure of removal of the entire globe and its intraocular contents, while preserving all other periorbital and orbital structures
Indications	• Endophthalmitis • Penetrating ocular trauma • Painful blind eye	• Intraocular malignancy (uveal melanoma and retinoblastoma) • Trauma • Painful blind eye • Sympathetic ophthalmitis • Microphthalmos
Advantages	Shorter duration of surgery • Less complex procedure • Less disruption of orbital tissues • Improved postoperative prosthesis motility and better orbital volume • In cases of infection, less chance of spread to central nervous system (CNS) • Less painful more cost-efficient	• Lesser risk of sympathetic ophthalmitis • Lesser risk of intraocular tumor dissemination

Table 1.6.2: Types of exenteration.

Types	*Contents removed*
Anterior exenteration/extended enucleation	Globe, posterior lamella of eyelid, and conjunctival sac
Lid sparing exenteration/subtotal exenteration	Orbital contents including periosteum of orbital walls
Total exenteration/eyelid sacrificing	Orbital contents, periorbita and lids
Radical/extended exenteration	Dissection involves paranasal sinuses, face, jaw, palate, and skull base

- *Postoperative:*
  - Infection
  - Hemorrhage
  - Wound dehiscence
  - Extrusion of the conformer
  - Contraction of the fornices
  - Exposure, extrusion or migration of the implant
  - Ptosis
  - Hollow or deep superior sulcus
  - Poorly fitting prosthesis
  - Enophthalmos
  - Socket contracture
  - Postenucleation socket syndrome
  - Orbital cellulitis.

8. Calculate the size of implant:
   - Formula for enucleation implant size: Implant diameter = Axial length-2 mm
   - Subtract 1mm from the above implant diameter for evisceration or hyperopia.
   - With a proper sized implant, almost no chances of superior sulcus deformity or enophthalmos.
   - The implant replaces the volume, leaving space for prosthesis 1.5–2.5 mL.
9. Types of implant:
   - Nonintegrated [silicone, acrylic, and semi-integrated implants (Universal and Iowa) polymethyl methacrylate (PMMA)] and integrated (hydroxyapatite, porous polyethylene, and bioceramic).
   - Buried and exposed implants.
10. *Exenteration*: Exenteration is a surgical procedure involving removal of the entire globe and its adnexa (including muscles, fat, nerves, and eyelids). Types of exenteration are shown in Table 1.6.2.

EVISCERATION

1. Current indications of evisceration:
   - Blind painful eye
   - Endophthalmitis
   - Phthisis bulbi
   - Staphylomatous globe
   - Severe traumatic injury
   - End-stage glaucoma.
2. Difference between enucleation and evisceration: As answered above in Table 1.6.1.
3. Causes of bleeding during evisceration: From retained uveal tissue.
4. Hemostasis during evisceration:
   - Subconjunctival injection of lignocaine and adrenaline preoperatively can help in intraoperative hemostasis.
   - Complete removal of uveal tissue adherent to scleral shell.
   - Inner side of empty scleral cup should be cleaned with sponge soaked in absolute alcohol aids in removing residual uveal tissue.
   - Small amount of bleeding can be controlled by firm digital pressure.
   - In case of excessive bleeding, cautery can be used.
5. *Types of evisceration*: Two-flap technique and four-flap technique.
6. What is anophthalmic socket?
   - Anophthalmic socket is defined as the absence of the globe and ocular tissue from the orbit.
   - The majority of cases of anophthalmos are seen following evisceration or enucleation. Congenital anophthal-

mos, although seen rarely, happens due to the arrest of embryogenesis during formation of the optic vesicle.

7. *Types of implant*: See enucleation.

CHALAZION

1. Nonsurgical management of chalazion:
   - Warm compresses and lid hygiene.
   - Tetracycline class of antibiotics [non-antimicrobial effects—inhibiting polymorph degranulation, reducing meibomian secretion viscosity, decreasing collagenase production, and inhibiting matrix metalloproteinase-9 (MMP-9) activity].
   - Topical steroids—to prevent the chronic inflammatory response.
   - Local intralesional injection of a steroid (triamcinolone or methylprednisolone)—reduces inflammation and cause regression of the chalazion.

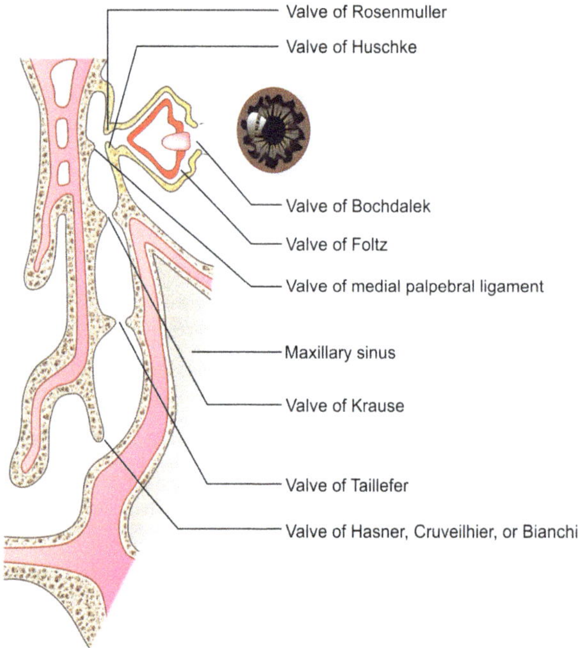

2. Intralesional steroid: agents, dose, technique, indication, and complication:
   - Local intralesional injection of a steroid (triamcinolone or methylprednisolone) 0.2 mL of 40 mg/mL into the chalazion's center.
   - *Indications*:
     - As an alternative first-line treatment when biopsy is not required
     - When the lesion is located near the lacrimal drainage system
     - Where an incision could cause complications involving tear flow.
   - *Complications*: Hypopigmentation and atrophy of the area, a visible depot of medication, corneal perforation, traumatic cataract, elevated intraocular pressure, and bacterial or viral infections.
3. How to prevent recurrence following chalazion excision?

- Adequate curettage and drainage may prevent recurrences.
- Cauterization of the meibomian gland with a hyfrecator, phenol or trichloroacetic acid, and helps in preventing recurrences.
- Long-term low-dose tetracycline class therapy frequently has also been shown to prevent recurrence.

4. Approaches for excision:
   - Transconjunctival vertical incision—to avoid damage to nearby glands.
   - External (skin) horizontal incision—if a chalazion threatens to break through the skin or has drained through.

DACRYOCYSTORHINOSTOMY

1. Valves in nasolacrimal duct (NLD) system and their clinical importance?
   - *Valves in NLD system*: The mucous membrane folds in the lacrimal pathways form a type of valve and serve to block the backward tear outflow.
   - *Valve of Rosenmüller*: It is a fold of mucosa at the junction between common canaliculi and lacrimal sac. It prevents reflux of tear from sac back into canaliculi.
   - *Valve of Hasner*: It is located at the junction of the opening of duct into inferior meatus of nose. It prevents sudden blast of air entering the lacrimal sac while blowing the nose.
   - *Other valves*: Valve of Huschke, Bochdalek, Folta, Krause, Hyrtl, Taillefer.
2. Lengths/distance of surgically important landmarks in NLD system:
   - The NLD is located, on average, 24.6 ± 3.56 mm posterior to the anterior nasal spine.
   - The marginal vessels lie medial to medial canthus while angular vein lies 8 mm medial to medial canthus. Thus, it is important to plan the skin incision and dissect tissues carefully.
   - The uncinate process is attached just posterior to the NLD, which is only 4 mm anterior to the maxillary sinus ostium.
   - Maxillary sinus ostium is also an important landmark to determine the location of the NLD.
3. What is false passage in probing?
   At the time of probing, lacrimal probe may pierce through and go into a different track instead of NLD system creating a false passage.
4. What is the size of probes preferred in congenital nasolacrimal duct obstruction?
   Size: 0–00
5. Lacrimal sac dimensions and parts:
   - *Lacrimal sac*:
     - Length 15 mm
     - Breadth 5–6 mm
     - Volume 20 mm^3
   - *Parts*:
     - Fundus (3–5 mm)—portion above the opening of canaliculi
     - Body (10–12 mm)—middle part
     - Neck—lower small part
6. What is lacrimal pump?
   - Lacrimal pump is a system helping in tear drainage.
   - In the relaxed state, the puncta lie in the tear lake.
   - With eyelid closure, the orbicularis oculi muscle contracts. The pretarsal orbicularis squeezes and closes the puncta and canaliculi. The preseptal orbicularis, which inserts into the lacrimal sac, pulls the lacrimal sac open and draws the tears into the sac by creating a negative pressure within sac.
   - With eyelid opening, the orbicularis relaxes, the puncta open, and the lacrimal sac collapses, propelling tears down the duct. Simultaneously, with the puncta opened, the canaliculi refill, completing the cycle.

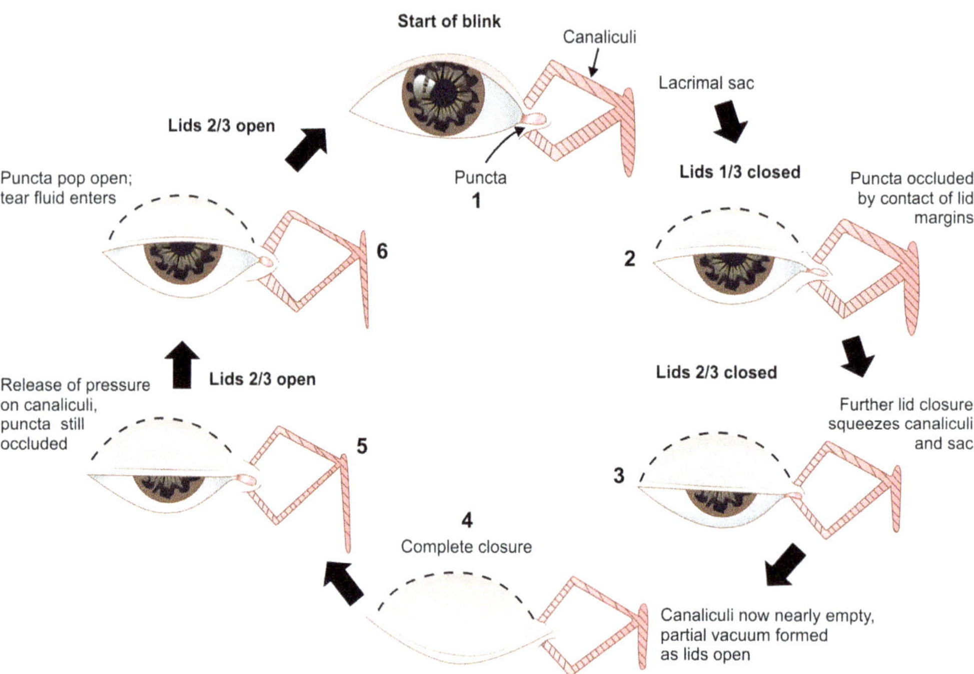

Table 1.6.3: Advantages and disadvantages of endoscopic dacryocystorhinostomy (DCR).

Advantages	*Disadvantages*
No external scar	Requires extensive knowledge of endonasal anatomy
Endonasal anatomy is directly visualized	Requires skills
In cases of primary failure, scar tissue under direct visualization can be easily mended	Increased operative time
If indicated concomitant sinus surgery performed	Expensive equipment

7. Muscles of lacrimal pump mechanism:
   - *Horner's muscle (pars lacrimalis)*: Fibers of pretarsal portion arising from lacrimal fascia and upper part of post lacrimal crest. They help in draining tears by lacrimal sac
   - *Muscle of Riolan (pars ciliaris)*: Fibers of pretarsal portion which run along lid margins behind ciliary follicles. They keep lid in close opposition to globe.
8. What is percentage of tear drainage through upper and lower puncta?

   70% tear enter the lower canaliculus while 30% enter the upper.
9. Types of dacryocystorhinostomy (DCR):
   - External DCR
   - Endonasal DCR
   - Transcanalicular endoscopic DCR
   - Conjunctival DCR
   - Canalicular DCR.
10. Advantage and disadvantage of endoscopic dacryocystorhinostomy.

    Advantage and disadvantage of endoscopic DCR are shown in Table 1.6.3.

11. Site of ostium in DCR:
    - The bony ostium is initiated at the junction of lacrimal bone and lamina papyracea.
    - Extension:
        - *Superiorly*: About 2 mm above the medial canthal tendon (MCT)
        - *Inferiorly*: Till the upper edge of NLD
        - *Posteriorly*: Including the lamina papyracea
        - *Anteriorly*: Till 3-4 mm above the level of anterior crest.
12. What is sump syndrome?
    - Lacrimal sump syndrome occurs as result of incomplete opening of inferior portion of the lacrimal sac, or the bone adjacent to the inferior sac, such that dependent fluid continues to collect in the sac. It can also result when mucosal healing leads to reapproximation of cut surfaces.
    - It is an uncommon cause of failed DCR.
13. Describe indications of intubation DCR.
    Not indicated in uncomplicated DCR as tube induced granulation tissue formation can itself cause closure of anastomosis.
    Indications of intubation DCR are as follows:
    - Canalicular stenosis
    - Fibrosed sac with inadequate mucosal flaps
    - Repeat DCR
    - Loss of mucosal flaps during surgery
14. Different types of intubation tubes (stents).
    Two main types of stents are bicanalicular and monocanalicular.
    1. *Bicanalicular stent*: Pass through both the upper and lower canaliculus. For example Crawford stent, Ritleng stent, Pigtail/Donut stent, and Kaneka Lacriflow stent.
    2. *Monocanalicular stents*: Do not provide a closed loop system, only intubating either the upper or lower canaliculus. Types—Mini-Monoka stent and Jones tube.
15. Cerebrospinal fluid rhinorrhea in DCR:
    - Cerebrospinal fluid (CSF) leakage or rhinorrhea is a very rare complication of DCR
    - The cause of CSF leak after external DCR can either be the direct or indirect mode of bone injury. Inadvertent extension of the osteotomy to the anterior part of the base of the skull can produce direct injury
    - With the development of new surgical procedures such as endoscopic DCR the incidence of iatrogenic CSF rhinorrhea has increased
    - It is more likely to occur during a pediatric DCR as children have low lying cribriform plate as compared to adults.
    - Most of the iatrogenic CSF leaks resolve within 7-10 days with conservative management. The main goal of management of CSF rhinorrhea is to prevent ascending meningitis.
16. *Rate of failed DCR*: The failure of DCR in most series is less than 10% of cases.
17. Difference between DCR and dacryocystectomy (DCT)

- Dacryocystectomy is a surgical procedure of complete extirpation of the lacrimal sac.
    - It was the standard of care for management of dacryocystitis and lacrimal fistulas before the advent of DCR.
    - Indications for DCT include fibrotic sac, lacrimal sac tumor, tuberculosis (TB) of lacrimal sac, and nasolacrimal duct obstruction (NLDO) associated with atrophic rhinitis.

18. Appropriate age for massage, probing, and DCR in congenital NLDO?
    - Conservative management (Crigglers' sac massage) of congenital NLDO up to 6–12 months of age
    - Nasolacrimal duct probing (therapeutic):
        - 12–18 months if conservative treatment fails
        - Before 1 year in special cases (mucocele, prior to intraocular surgery, and repeated episodes of dacryocystitis)
    - Dacryocystorhinostomy—after at least three trial of failed probing.
19. How to confirm that regurgitated fluid is from sac not canaliculus?
    - Regurgitated fluid from canaliculus is clear fluid whereas from sac is mucoid/pus.
    - It can be confirmed by dacryocystography.

2 CHAPTER

Cornea

2.1 SLIT-LAMP BIOMICROSCOPY

Rinky Agarwal, Sitesh Kumar Bergaal, Ritu Nagpal, Namrata Sharma

INTRODUCTION

Ocular diseases can involve any part of the eye starting from adnexa to optic nerve and numerous instruments can aid in their diagnosis. Naked eye examination with a bright light projected from a torch forms the most basic part of ocular examination. However, this being limited by lack of magnification leads to overlooking of minute but extremely important details required for diagnosis of several ocular pathologies. Gullstrand combined principles of microscope and illumination in a single instrument and introduced slit lamp in early 20th century to aid enthusiastic ophthalmologists obtain a magnified as well as detailed view of various ocular parts.[1] Mawas later on introduced the word *biomicroscopy* and defined it as examination of living eye by means of corneal microscope and a slit lamp.

Modern day slit-lamp biomicroscopy (SLB) with its auxiliary devices forms an indispensable tool for complete examination of the eye. It not only provides a magnified view of every part of the eye from adnexa to cornea to retina, but also allows clinical photography for documentation. In addition to qualitative assessment, quantitative measurement of intraocular pressure, pupil size, corneal thickness, endothelial cell morphology, and anterior chamber depth can also be obtained with modern day SLB.

PARTS OF SLIT LAMP

Slit lamp, in a simplified language is a horizontally mounted microscope with provision for bright light especially designed for ophthalmic use (Fig. 2.1.1).

Observation System (Microscope)

The observation system, essentially composed of two optical elements, an objective lens (providing a power of +22 D

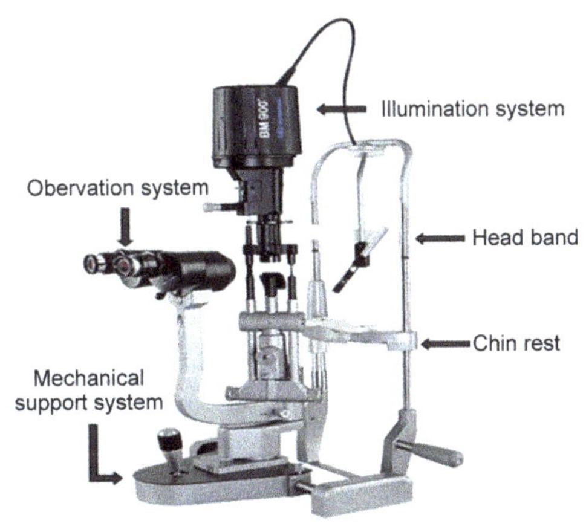

Fig. 2.1.1: Parts of a slit lamp (Haag-Streit).

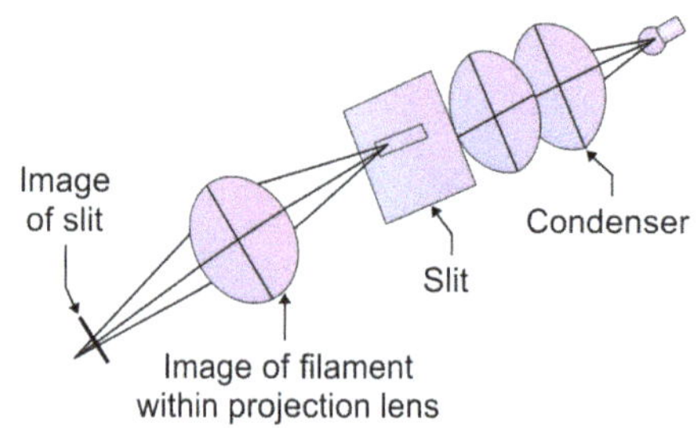

Fig. 2.1.2: Optical principle of slit lamp.

by two plano-convex lenses) and an eyepiece (power of +10 D), presents an enlarged but inverted image of near object to the observer, a problem overcome by use of prisms between objective and eyepiece. Two eyepieces are independently adjustable to match observer's interpupillary distance and refractive error (Fig. 2.1.2).

Modern day slit lamps provide a range of magnification from 6X to 40X. Three types of magnification systems used in different models of slit lamps comprise:

1. Czapskiscope with rotating objectives (different objectives placed in a turret type of arrangement)
2. Littmann-Galilean telescope principle of magnification
3. Zoom system.

Nowadays, observation arm has a high quality digital camera, connected to a computer, incorporated for real-time photographic and videographic documentation of ocular details permitting future references and teaching.[2]

Illumination System

The Gullstand's illumination system is designed to provide a bright, evenly illuminated, finely focused, and highly malleable slit of light. It is composed of a light source which provides an illumination of 2×10^5 to 4×10^5 lux and a condenser lens system with a couple of plano-convex lenses with their convex lenses in apposition to focus light on the desired object. A projection lens provided in the system ensures a high-quality image of slit at the eye by decreasing aberrations and increasing its depth of focus. A mirror or prism placed perpendicular to the projection system allows latter to pass easily from one side of the microscope to the other. Whenever required for examination of fundus, illumination system can be made to coincide with the viewing axis without obstructing the field of view by use of a narrow prism or mirror.

Adjustment of height and width of the slit and its rotation in both vertical and horizontal meridian is facilitated by use of different knobs specifically provided for this purpose. Various filters like cobalt blue filter and red-free filter attached to the illumination system provide enhanced view of iron lines and corneal epithelial defects and blood vessels, respectively.

Mechanical Support System

Thorough ocular examination requires a confident clinician, a comfortable patient, and a long working distance between observer and patient's eye. The former is an art learnt with time, patience, and perseverance while the latter two are supplemented by an ergonomically supportive mechanical system, which has changed little over years.

Mechanical coupling of microscope and illumination system allows them to rotate along a common axis that coincides with their focal planes. This safeguards parfocality between slit beam and microscope for adequate illumination of patient's eye while examination. Slight decentration may, however, be required while performing added procedures like gonioscopy and fundoscopy with accessory lenses.

Back and forth, side-by-side, and up-down movement of microscope and illumination system is facilitated by joystick provided in the slit lamp. Movement of the instrument relative to chinrest (to accommodate individuals of all sizes and age) and movement of chinrest relative to patient's face are aided by a screw device fitted in the mechanical system. A movable fixation target in accordance with clinician's requirement and a black mark on the chinrest coinciding with the eyebrow of the patient allow an unimpeded ocular examination.

BASIC PRINCIPLES OF SLIT-LAMP ILLUMINATION

Three specific types of illumination provided by slit lamp enhance examiner's ability to see details of ocular structure examined.

1. *Focal illumination*, achieved by narrowing the slit beam horizontally or vertically permits examination of specific areas without any extraneous light outside area of examination.
2. *Oblique illumination*, obtained by projecting light oblique to the tissue examined is essential for examining different layers of ocular structures.
3. *Optical slit section*, which makes the instrument unique, is used to examine internal details of all layers of ocular structure examined. Importance of slit beam of light cannot be overemphasized in revolutionizing ophthalmologic expansions. Incorporation of this simple idea in intraoperative microscope has reformed clinician's ability to objectively judge intraoperative depth of a lesion tremendously.[3] Newer devices like Orbscan also utilize slit scanning technology for assessment of corneal topography.

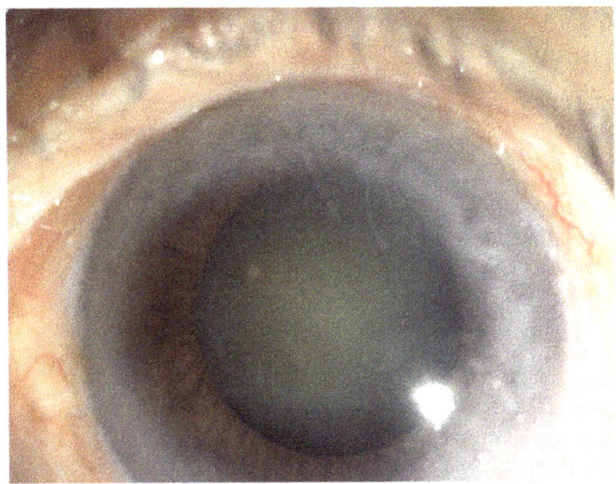

Fig. 2.1.3: Target sign seen on diffuse illumination in pseudoexfoliation syndrome.

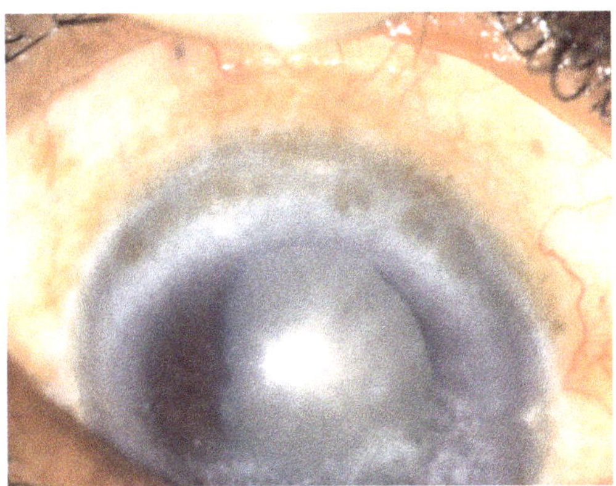

Fig. 2.1.4: Herbert's pits seen superiorly diffuse illumination in healed trachoma.

TECHNIQUE OF BIOMICROSCOPY

Methods of Illumination

1. *Diffuse illumination*: Diffuse illumination is facilitated by use of widest slit beam (medium-to-high illumination and medium-to-high magnification), the intensity of which can made more endurable to the patient with the aid of a neutral density diffuse filter and shortest examination time possible to avoid phototoxicity of retina. The maximum beam height ranges from 8 mm to 14 mm depending on the model of slit lamp. This height is still less for examination of adnexa in entirety, therefore beam has to be moved up-down and side-to-side to overcome omission of any additional details (Figs. 2.1.3 and 2.1.4).
2. *Direct focal slit illumination*: Direct focal examination of ocular structure is enabled by projecting a narrow slit beam

at an angle to coincide with exact focus of the microscope (Figs. 2.1.5 and 2.1.6). This can be done as an optical section, as parallelepiped beam or conical beam. Narrowing the slit beam, although reduces the amount of illumination available for examination, helps clinician acquire comprehensive information about various layers of cornea. The problem of low illumination can be overcome by maintaining dim background lights. This makes examiner's eyes more sensitive to low illumination of light.

A special form of direct focal illumination called *broad tangential illumination*, attained by reflecting light at an extremely oblique illumination angle, helps in diagnosing surface abnormalities of cornea and in corneal photography.

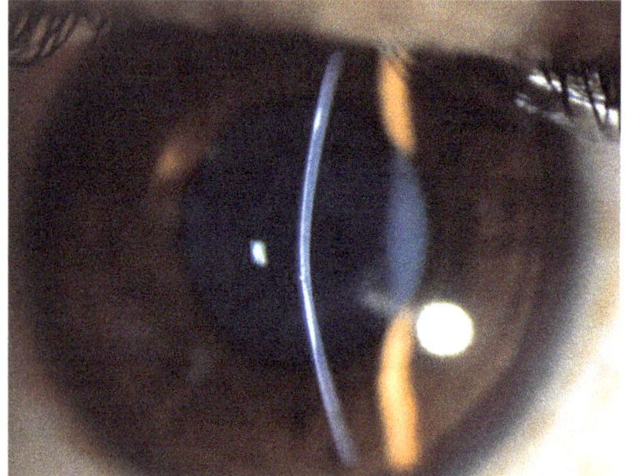

Fig. 2.1.5: Central steepening and thinning of cornea in keratoconus as seen on direct slit illumination.

3. *Sclerotic scatter*: Examination of faintest corneal opacities can be heightened by technique of scleral scatter, where light beam focused at one side of scleral limbus emerges from entire circumference of limbus by utilizing principle of *total internal reflection* (provided cornea is transparent) (Fig. 2.1.7). Complete loss of parfocality between illumination and microscope for this technique is ensured by focusing broad beam of light at 3 or 9 o'clock scleral limbus (till halo of light appears around entire limbus) and examining cornea independently by microscope.
4. *Retroillumination*: Retroillumination, as the name implies, means inspection of any pathological area with aid of light reflected from structure posterior to it. A corneal or lenticular abnormality can be assessed by broad illuminating light reflected by iris (Fig. 2.1.8) or fundus (red reflex emerging from retinal pigmented epithelium and choroid) (Fig. 2.1.9) under either direct illumination (pathology is

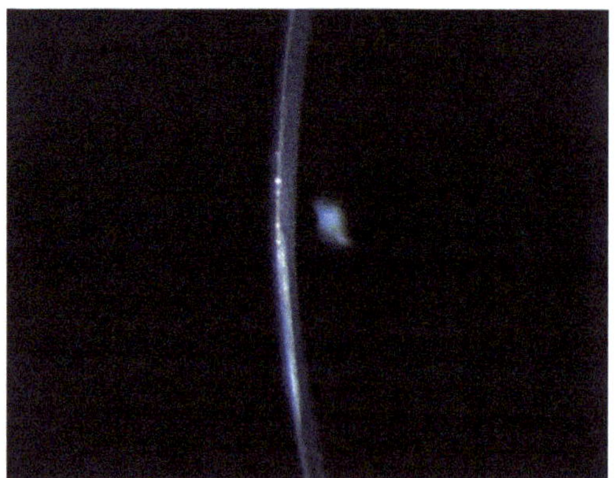

Fig. 2.1.6: Magnified slit view of Figure 2.1.5 also showing anterior stromal scarring.

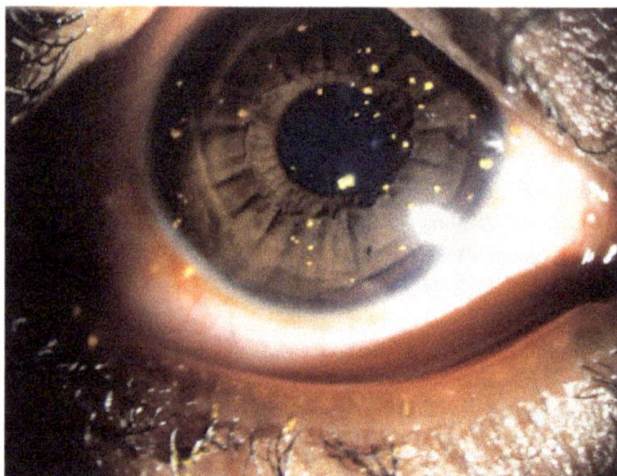

Fig. 2.1.7: Multiple corneal foreign bodies seen on scleral scatter.

seen against illuminated background) or indirect illumination (as light is at right angle to observed pathology, it is seen against dark background).

5. *Proximal (indirect) illumination*: Proximal illumination, a technique which syndicates sclerotic scatter and retroillumination, can be employed to assess any pathological area by directing light adjacent to the area under examination. Indirect illumination permits visualization of additional details of any abnormality by preventing dazzling light from masking underlying structures (Fig. 2.1.10). When a moderately wide beam of light is directed adjacent to a particular area, transparency of that area causes light to travel effortlessly within it whereas any opacity reflects it back to the observer, permitting its enhanced identification.

6. *Specular reflection*: Specular reflection, based on principle of *Snell's law*, is a method used to examine planar surfaces by means of total internal reflection. Clinically, this principle is largely used to scrutinize corneal endothelial cells (Fig. 2.1.11). When light is incident on endothelial layer, dazzling reflex of light reflected from zone of discontinuity leads to specular reflection. For this patient

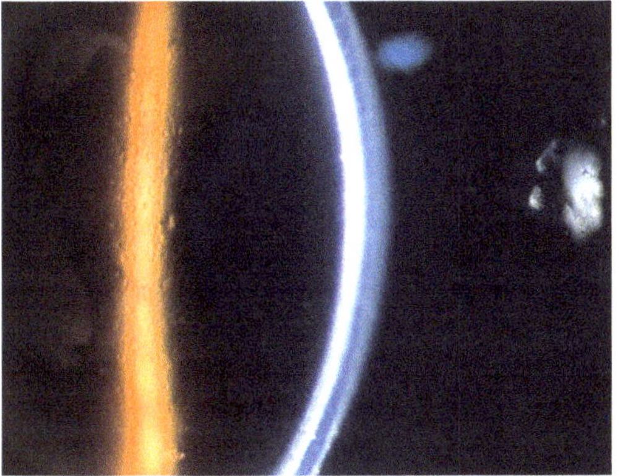

Fig. 2.1.8: Recurrence of spheroidal degeneration at interface post lamellar keratoplasty appreciated on retroillumination from iris.

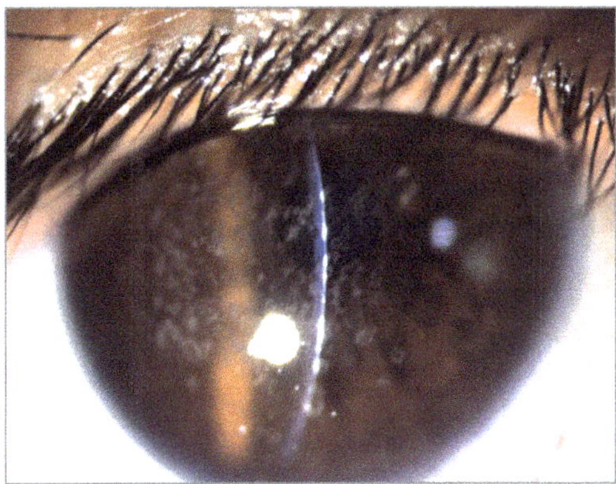

Fig. 2.1.10: Hyaline deposits of granular dystrophy seen on proximal illumination.

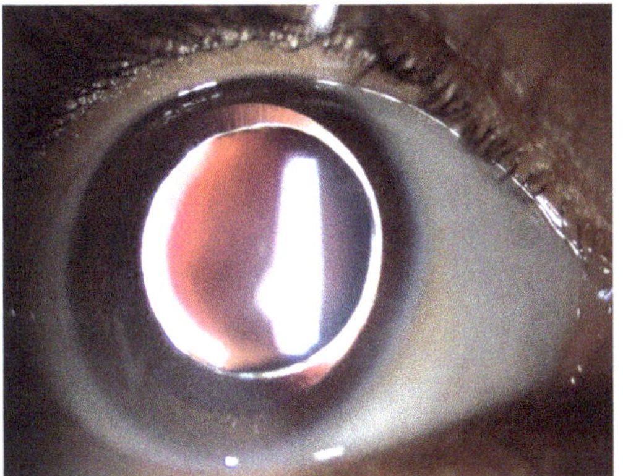

Fig. 2.1.9: Crystalline lens in microspherophakia best appreciated on retroillumination from fundus.

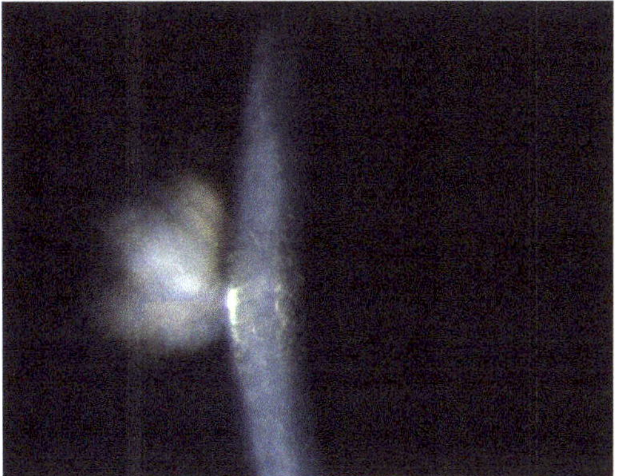

Fig. 2.1.11: Specular endothelium at endothelium shows presence of guttae.

is instructed to look 30° temporally and light is incident from opposite side such that angle between microscope and light is 60°. A parallelepiped beam under high illumination and high magnification is required for this purpose.[4]

All these techniques are mentioned comprehensively in Table 2.1.1.[5]

Table 2.1.1: Different techniques of slit-lamp examination.[5]

Method of slit-lamp examination		*Angle between microscope and illumination*	*Slit beam*	*Structures/lesions seen*
Diffuse illumination		30–45°	Diffuse	Generalized view of adnexa, lids, ocular surface, and anterior segment
Direct focal illumination	Optical section	30–45°	Narrow slit beam	• Cornea • Epithelial layer (dark), Bowman's membrane (bright), stroma (gray), Descemet's membrane (brightest) • Crystalline lens • Anterior capsule, anterior cortical layer, nucleus, cortical layer, posterior capsule • Anterior one-third of vitreous
	Parallelopiped section	30–45°	2–3 mm wide slit beam	Corneal scars and infiltrates (appear brighter than surroundings because of more density)
	Conical beam	45–60°	Semi-circular pattern	• Flare—gray or milky haze in anterior chamber • Cells—white dots
	Broad tangential illumination	70–80°	Wide beam	• Anterior surface irregularities of cornea like band-shaped keratopathy (BSK), punctate keratopathy • Posterior corneal surface irregularities like Descemet's folds
Retroillumination	Iris (undilated pupil)	60° slightly rotated off-axis	Moderately broad beam	Epithelial microcysts, refractile materials like Salzmann's nodules and amyloid deposits, stromal infiltrates, blood vessels, pigmented deposits and Descemet's excrescences
	Fundus (dilated pupil)	Slit beam is coaxial to microscope and centered in the pupil	Moderately broad beam	• Corneal scars, epithelial basement membrane and lattice corneal dystrophy, guttae, ridges in Descemet's membrane, oil droplet reflex in keratoconus • Lenticular opacities like blue dot cataract, posterior subcapsular cataract

Contd...

Contd...

Method of slit-lamp examination	*Angle between microscope and illumination*	*Slit beam*	*Structures/lesions seen*
Sclerotic scatter	15° slightly decentered	Maximum slit height, moderate width	Faintest of corneal opacities like subepithelial infiltrates, epithelial edema, stromal edema
Indirect illumination	>45°	2–3 mm height, 0.2 mm broad, decentered beam	Corneal infiltrates, microcysts and vacuoles
Specular reflection	60°	40X magnification, 3–4 mm height, 0.5 mm wide beam	Tear film abnormalities, corneal endothelial cells

DYNAMIC SLIT-LAMP BIOMICROSCOPY

Slit-lamp biomicroscopy is a dynamic process in which examiner constantly integrates various types of illumination techniques to obtain an accurate, three-dimensional, fully detailed, and complete mental image of ocular structures examined. Every clinician must establish an individualized protocol for a systematic, multidirectional, and unbiased examination to gather every possible data within single, if required repeated, examination (Fig. 2.1.12).

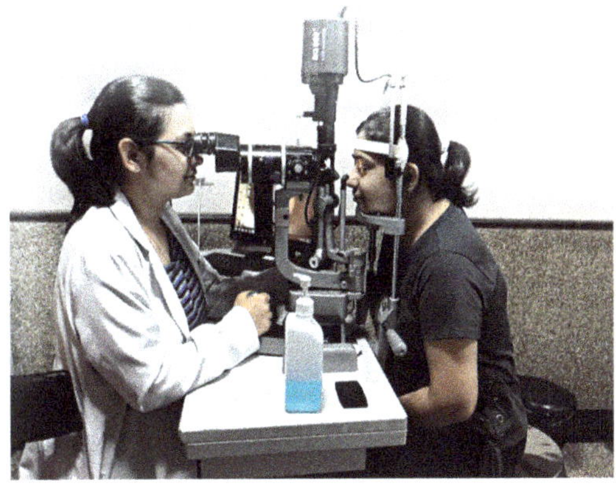

Fig. 2.1.12: Dynamic slit-lamp biomicroscopy.

- A semi-dark room ensures adaptation of examiner to low sensitivities of light for a comprehensive examination of fine details.
- Key step for an unhindered examination is adjustment of instrument according to comfort of both patient and the clinician. Clinician should adapt to an erect posture owing to ill-effects of bad ergonomics on clinician's spine and muscles in the long-run.
- Slit-lamp examination begins with diffuse examination of both eyes at lowest magnification with filtered slit beam to locate any gross abnormalities. This is followed by detailed examination of each eye under high magnification.
- Sclerotic scatter from temporal limbus is used to identify faintest of corneal opacities. Direct focal and indirect illumination of affected area is followed by visualization of internal details of abnormality against retroillumination of iris and fundus. Two or three scans across cornea with light beam projected from nasal, temporal, superior, and

inferior directions guarantee complete impression of extent and severity of any abnormality if present.

- Examination of lens and anterior vitreous against red reflex of fundus, direct and indirect illumination methods follows evaluation of cornea.
- Clinician should make it a habit to constantly move the instrument from anterior to posterior part of eye to encompass every single detail piecemeal and later on reconstruct the mental image in toto on a drawing using color coding for repeated interpretation of details (Table 2.1.2).[6]

Table 2.1.2: Color coding of corneal disorders.

Color	*Corneal disorder*	*Representation*
Black	• Nebular opacity • Macular opacity • Leucomatous opacity	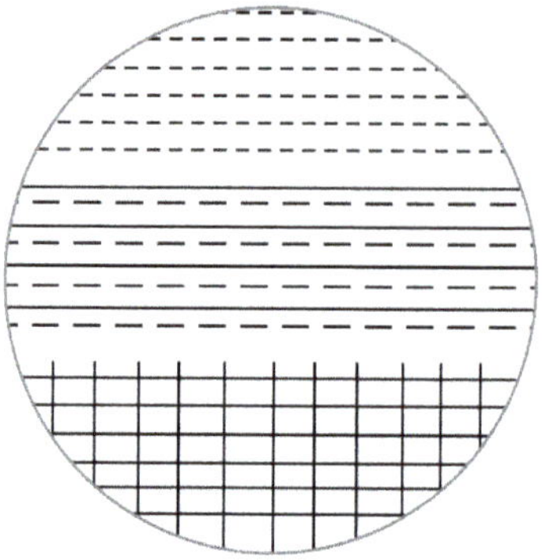
Blue	• Descemet's folds • Epithelial edema • Stromal edema	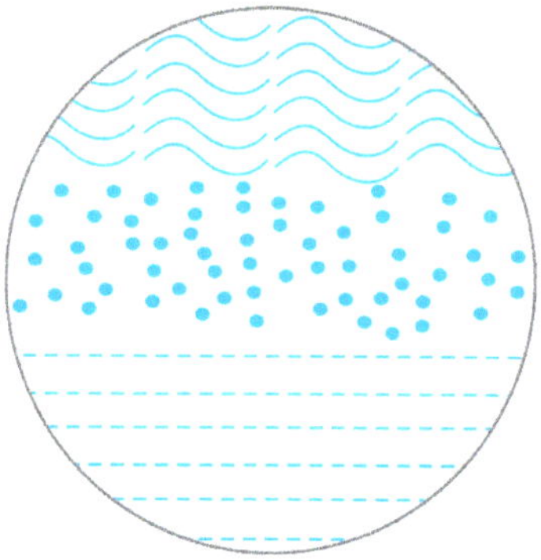
Red brown	• Iron pigmentation • Deep intrastromal blood vessel—straight lines extending till limbus • Superficial conjunctival blood vessels—dotted lines extending • beyond limbus • Intracorneal blood	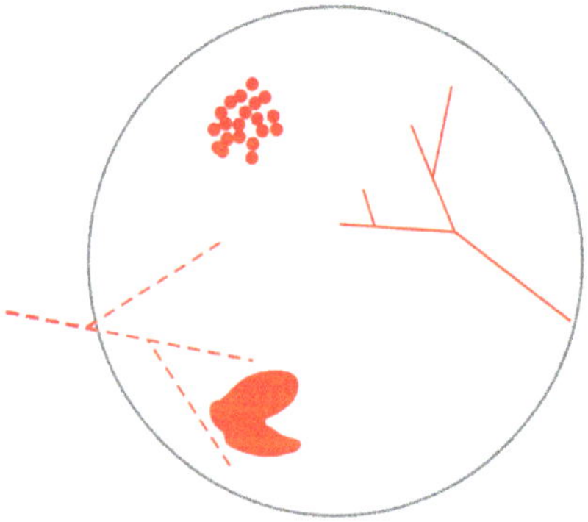

Contd...

Contd...

Color	*Corneal disorder*	*Representation*
Yellow	• Keratic precipitates • Hypopyon • Infiltrate	
Green	• Filaments • Punctate staining • Epithelial defect	

- Application of any vital dyes, medications or accessory procedures are performed after an unhindered primary examination described above.

ACCESSORY DEVICES

The addition of accessory devices to slit lamp allows performance of various specialized examinations necessary to substantiate clinical findings.

- Various types of staining to diagnose, measure, and monitor treatment success (Fig. 2.1.13)
- One of the most commonly performed accessory examinations; applanation tonometry with a prism particularly designed for this purpose is presently the gold standard for estimation the intraocular pressure.

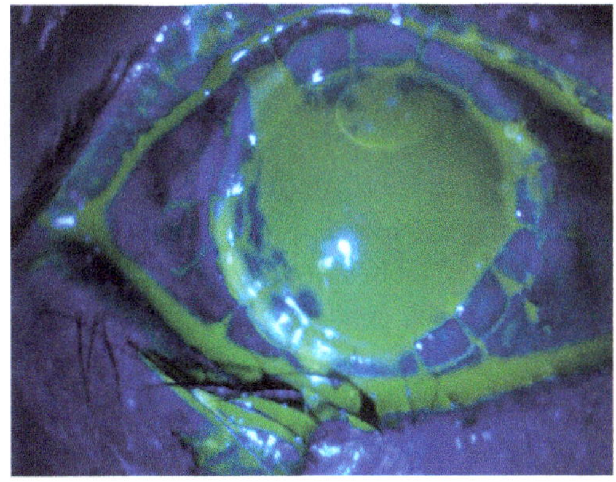

Fig. 2.1.13: Epithelial defect as seen under cobalt blue light after fluorescein staining.

- Gonioscopy utilizes the principle of total internal reflection to examine angle recess by means of an accessory convex lens (Figs. 2.1.14A and B). Fundoscopy with highly convex (90 D) or concave

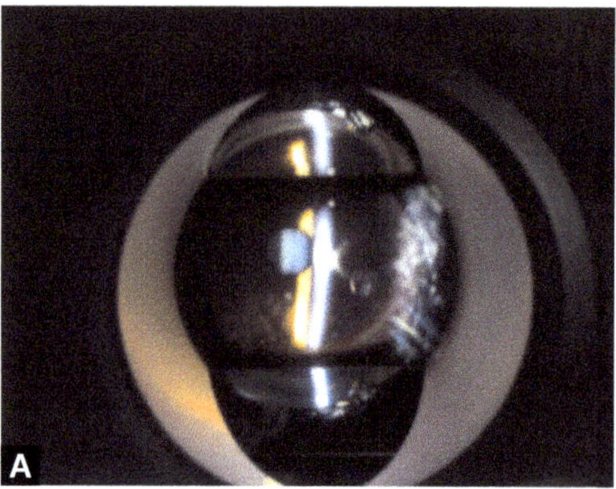

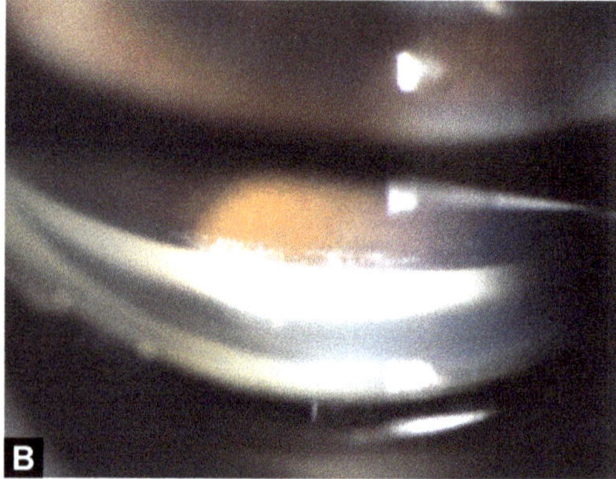

Figs. 2.1.14A and B: (A) Gonioscopy procedure being performed with Goldmann two mirror lens; (B) Widened ciliary body band seen on gonioscopy in angle recession.

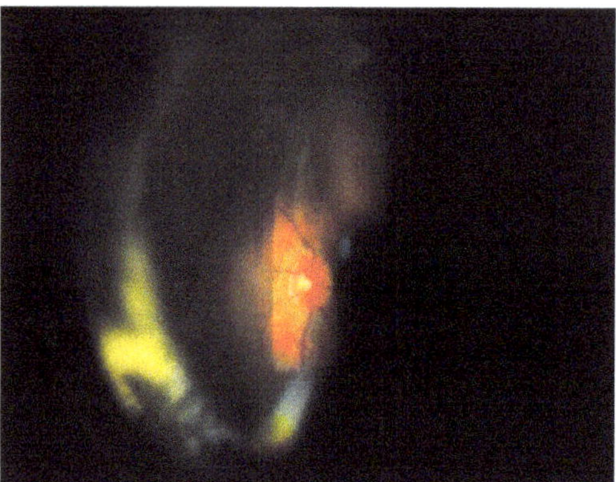

Fig. 2.1.15: Magnified disc details appreciated on slit-lamp biomicroscopy examination with 90 D.

(Hruby lens) lens provides magnified slit view of macula and disc (Fig. 2.1.15).

- In contact lens users, SLB plays a paramount role in assessment of contact lens fitting, centration, and movement (by means of tear film formation between contact lens and cornea after fluorescein staining) along with inspection of any secondary effects and aftercare at every follow-up.
- Accessory laser delivery devices attached to slit lamp can be used to perform laser capsulotomy, iridotomy, trabeculoplasty, and retinal photocoagulation as outpatient procedures.
- Laser interferometry and potential acuity meter also exploit slit lamp for gauging visual potential of a patient.

VIVA QUESTIONS

1. What are the different filters in a slit lamp? Enumerate their clinical uses?

Ans. Refer to Table 2.1.3.

2. Dyes used for corneal staining; specific uses, staining property, advantages, and disadvantages.

Ans. Refer to Table 2.1.4.

3. How to mark the axis, preoperatively for toric intraocular lens (IOL) on slit lamp?

Ans.

- There are various markers available for preoperative toric axis marking such as Gimble marker (ASICO) and the Nuits/Lane Pre-op Toric Reference Marker (bubble), Neuhann-Nuijts One-Step Toric Marker, AXsys™ One Step Electronic Toric Marking Device, and pendulum-attached marker.
- Manual marking can also be done accurately. The eye should be marked while the patient is sitting upright and fixing with the other eye at a distant target to avoid cyclotorsion. Make slit lamp's illuminating column coaxial with viewing

Table 2.1.3: Different filters in a slit lamp.	
Filter	*Use*
Cobalt blue filter	• Fluorescein staining • Goldmann applanation tonometry • Fleischer ring
Yellow filter	Increases contrast enhancement when using cobalt blue filter
Red free/green filter	• Rose bengal staining • Blood vessels • Hemorrhages
Diffuser and white filter	Generalized examination of eye and adnexa
Neutral density filter and gray filter	Decrease brightness for photophobic patients
Heat absorbing	Decreases patient discomfort

Table 2.1.4: Dyes used for corneal staining.			
Dye	*Staining property*	*Advantages*	*Disadvantages*
Sodium fluorescein	• Yellow color water-soluble dye • Stains epithelium bright green as seen under cobalt blue filter, diffuses into intercellular spaces, does not stain devitalized tissue	Can be used for assessment of ocular surface integrity and function, tear film breakup time (TBUT), corneal epithelial defects, rigid contact lens fitting, applanation tonometry, Seidel's test, Jones dye test, fluorescein dye disappearance test (FDDT)	Can exhibit pseudoflare, stain soft contact lens and promote growth of *Pseudomonas aeruginosa* in solution
Rose bengal	Red color under red-free/green filter, stains dead or degenerated cells and mucus strands	For staining of conjunctiva and evaluation of herpetic keratouveitis, true dendrites, superficial punctate keratitis	Intrinsic cellular toxicity to corneal epithelial cells, patient discomfort, particularly stinging upon instillation
Lissamine green	• Green color under white light • Preferentially stains dead and devitalized cells, does not stain normal ocular surface	• Detects dead or degenerate conjunctival cells • Minimal effect on corneal epithelial cells and minimal stinging on application	

column. For 0–180° reference marking, a narrow slit beam can be focused on the cornea and the axis can be marked. Maintain steady fixation of the patient by closing contralateral eye and asking patient to look straight ahead into the slit lamp. Mark axis on peripheral cornea using gentian violet marker pen or a 26 G sterile needle on a 2 mL syringe at the point where slit beam cuts limbus. This type of marking uses the first Purkinje image principle.

4. How to calculate magnification in SLB with 90 D?

Ans. Image magnification factor for emmetropic eye = 60/90 D X magnification of slit lamp.

5. Color coding in corneal ulcer.

Ans. Refer to Table 2.1.2.

6. How to perform specular microscopy?

Ans.

- Instruct the patient to look straight ahead
- Project slit beam from onto the central cornea from temporal side
- Shorten the size of the beam (3–4 mm height and 0.5 mm width) and increase magnification (25X or 40X)
- Coincide slit beam with light reflected from nasal iris and first catoptric/Purkinje image (it has rectangular shape of the slit-lamp mirror)
- Paving stone pattern consisting of hexagonal endothelial cells with dark center and bright borders can be appreciated.

7. Method for grading cells and flare.

Ans. Refer to Tables 2.1.5 and 2.1.6. Laser flare/cell photometry is based on measurement of light [incoming laser (helium-neon/diode) beam] scattered in anterior chamber. ASOCT-based measurements like aqueous-to-air relative intensity (ARI) index method to examine retrolental cells have also been described.

Table 2.1.5: Clinical grading on aqueous cells on slit lamp.

Standardization of Uveitis Nomenclature (SUN) classification of cells grading		
Grade	*Cells**	*Flare*
0	<1	None
0.5+	1–5	
1+	6–15	Faint (barely detectable)
2+	16–25	Moderate (iris/lens details clear)
3+	26–50	Marked (iris/lens details hazy)
4+	>50	Intense (fibrin/plastic aqueous)

*Slit-lamp beam field size is 1 × 1 mm^2, preferably 16X magnification.

Table 2.1.6: Grading of flare on slit lamp.

Grade	*Description*	*Findings*
0	None	
1+	Faint	Mild anterior chamber turbidity
2+	Moderate	Iris and lens details clear
3+	Marked	Iris and lens details hazy
4+	Intense	Fibrin or plastic aqueous

REFERENCES

1. Timoney PJ, Breathnach CS. Allvar Gullstrand and the slit lamp 1911. Ir J Med Sci. 2013;182(2):301-5.
2. Martin R. Cornea and anterior eye assessment with slit lamp biomicroscopy, specular microscopy, confocal microscopy, and ultrasound biomicroscopy. Indian J Ophthalmol. 2018;66(2):195.
3. KA. Biomicroscopie du Cristallin. Arch Ophthalmol. 1931;5(1):154.
4. Bourne WM, Kaufman HE. Specular microscopy of human corneal endothelium in vivo. Am J Ophthalmol. 1976;81(3):319-23.
5. Krachmer JH, Mannis MJ, Holland EJ. Cornea. St. Louis Missouri: Mosby/Elsevier; 2011. p. 1967.
6. Waring GO, Laibson PR. A systematic method of drawing corneal pathologic conditions. Arch Ophthalmol. 1977;95(9):1540-2.

2.2 KERATOMETER

Ritu Nagpal, Siddhi Goel, Shipra Singhi, Prafulla Kumar Maharana

INTRODUCTION

Keratometer (Fig. 2.2.1) is a device used to measure the anterior curvature of the central 3 mm of cornea. It is an essential tool for biometry of cases undergoing cataract surgery. Besides, it is useful for contact lens (CL) trial and diagnosis of irregular astigmatism. Although new generation videokeratography devices have superseded its role, it is still considered as the gold standard for calculation of keratometry before cataract surgery.

PRINCIPLES

The keratometer assumes that the cornea is a perfect, thin, dry and inelastic sphere and calculates the corneal power using the following principles:[1-3]

- The cornea is a convex refracting surface.
- In order to find the refracting power of the cornea, we need to reflect an object of a known size at a known distance to the corneal surface.
- Keeping the distance between the eye and keratometer fixed, the corneal radius is directly proportional to the size of the reflected image which is nothing but the 1st Purkinje image and indirectly proportional to the size of the object.
- The anterior corneal curvature is then calculated using the convex mirror formula. The size of the reflecting image is determined with a measuring telescope, and the refractive power of the cornea is calculated based on the refractive index of n = 1.3375 (this may vary depending upon the type of instrument).
- The corneal power is calculated based on Snell's law of refraction:

  Surface power formula: $D = n_2 - n_1 / R$

  D = The dioptric power of the cornea

  n_1 = Refractive index of the first medium (air-cornea)

  n_2 = Refractive index of the second medium (cornea-aqueous)

  R = The radius of curvature of the cornea in meters.
- The keratometer does not take into account the power of posterior corneal curvature, instead adjusts the index of refraction (1.3375 vs 1.376) to account for the posterior corneal power.
- *Doubling principle*: Due to involuntary eye movements of the eye the image formed on cornea will not be stable. To overcome this Ramsden developed the doubling technique where a prism is introduced into the optical system so that two images are formed and the prism is moved until the images touch each other.

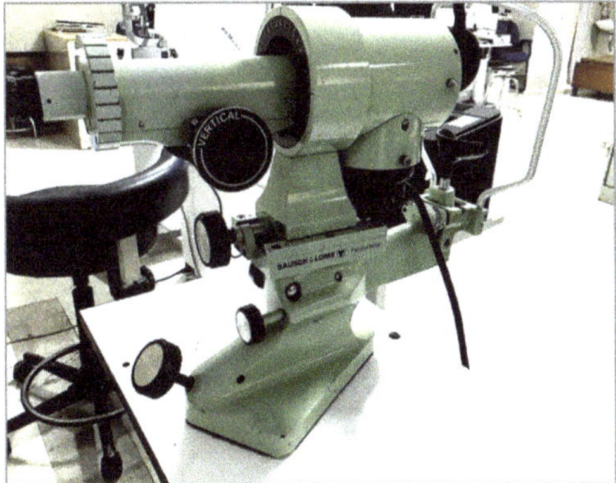

Fig. 2.2.1: Bausch and Lomb keratometer.

TYPES OF KERATOMETER

Keratometer can be classified based on:

1. Principles of keratometer:[4]
   i. *Javal-Schiotz keratometer*: Fixed image size with variable object size (fixed

doubling). Here, Wollaston prisms are used.

ii. *Bausch and Lomb keratometer*: Fixed object size with variable image size (variable doubling). There are two prisms, one prism in the horizontal direction and the other in the vertical direction. There are two apertures through which whatever the rays are passing; they are undeviated.

Other keratometers described includes:

- *Helmholtz Doubling Principle Keratometer*: It consists of two rotating prisms that create an angle with each other
- *Original American Optical Keratometer*: Here, bi-prisms are used.

2. Depending upon the need to rotate the prism:
   - *One position keratometer*: Horizontal and vertical meridian can be assessed without rotation because it consists of horizontal and vertical direction prism. Examples include Bausch and Lomb keratometer and Appa Swamy keratometer.[4]
   - *Two position keratometer*: In this type horizontal meridian is assessed first following which the keratometer is rotated 90° apart to assess another meridian. Here, Wollaston prism is used, e.g. Javal-Schiotz keratometer.[4]
3. Depending upon working:
   - Automated
   - Manual.

PARTS OF KERATOMETER

- Telescope
- Eyepiece at one end (near to examiner)
- Objective (near to the patient)
- Knobs for adjustment of vertical and horizontal curvature on the telescope
- Knobs adjusting the height of telescope
- Chin rest-adjusting knobs
- Bulb for illumination
- Knob for focusing of mires
- Model cornea with the occluder.

Performing Keratometry

- Looking through the eyepiece of the keratometer, use the eyepiece to focus the crosshair.
- The patient can comfortably put the chin and forehead on the appropriate rests.
- Use the occluder attached to the keratometer to cover the eye not being measured.
- Then use the height adjustment knob of the keratometer to position the light reflections at the level of the cornea (Figs. 2.2.2 and 2.2.3).

INTERPRETATION

Measurement Range

- 36–52 D
- Its lower limit can be extended up to 30 D by interposing –1.0 D in front of the objective of the telescope

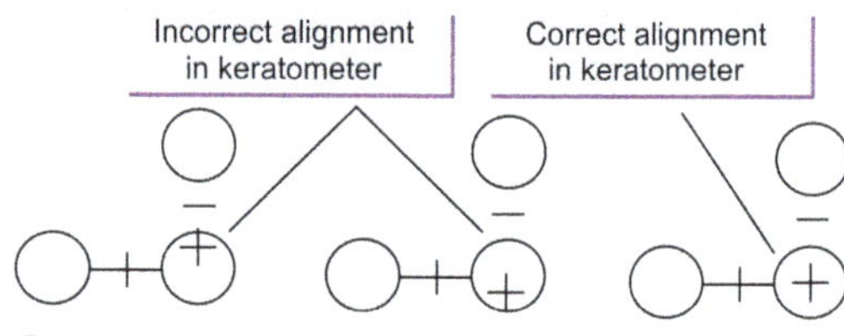

Fig. 2.2.2: Correct and incorrect alignment in keratometer.

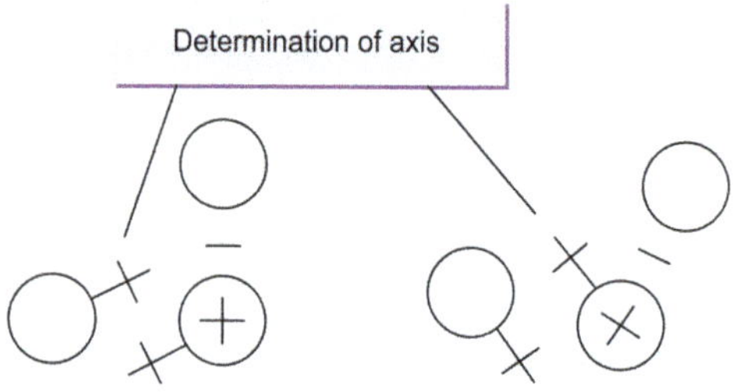

Fig. 2.2.3: Determination of steep and flat axis.

- Its upper limit can be extended up to 61 D by interposing a lens of +1.25 D in front of the objective of the telescope
- *Normal keratometry*:
  - The cornea contributes for two-thirds of the refractive power of the eye
  - Around 98% of the population has a corneal power between 40–48 D.[2]
  - Around 68% have a cornea power between 42 D and 45 D.[2]

Limitations

- Measures only two points at the 3–4 mm zone, does not provide information about the cornea central or peripheral to these points.
- It assumes that the cornea is spherocylindrical and symmetric with a major and minor axis separated by 90°, which is not always true thus it ignores spherical aberration.
- Focusing and misalignment errors.
- Cannot accurately measure irregular corneas.
- It does not measure the posterior corneal surface that contributes approximately 0.4 D of against-the-rule astigmatism to the total corneal power. This is important when calculating the amount of total corneal astigmatism for toric intraocular lens (IOL) implantation and refractive lens exchange with multifocal IOL implantation.

SOURCES OF ERRORS IN KERATOMETRY

There are many factors that can lead to inaccuracies in measurement, as follows:[2,3]

- *Diurnal variations in corneal physiology*: The refractive index of the cornea shows diurnal fluctuations due to variations in corneal hydration. Although not that significant, repeated measurements should be done at the same time of the day when some research is planned.
- *Contact lens wearers*: Contact lens can cause temporary alterations in the curvature of the cornea. Patients must discontinue CL wear for 2 weeks for soft CLs, and 4 weeks for rigid CLs before measurement of keratometry.
- *Nonsphericity of the cornea*: A keratometer assumes that the cornea is thin, inelastic, and a perfect sphere. On the contrary, the normal cornea has some thickness, is spherocylindrical, and elastic.
- *Improper calibration*: Steel balls are used to calibrate manual keratometers. Routine calibration is a must to avoid any error.
- *Failure to focus eyepieces*: To achieve focus, first, the eye-pieces are turned anticlockwise and then slowly turned clockwise until the mires are in sharp focus. The observer's refractive error must be neutralized to avoid any erroneous measurements.
- *Tear film breakup*: Disruptions of the corneal surface, either due to dry eye, corneal scarring or due to insufficiencies in the tear film can lead to errors. One drop of artificial tear drop before the examination can abolish this error.
- *Previous refractive surgery*: Keratometers assume that the Gullstrand ratio, i.e. relation between the front and back surface of the cornea is similar in corneas of different patients. However, corneal laser surgery results in changes in the relationship between the curvature of the anterior and posterior surfaces of the cornea and thus the posterior corneal power cannot be ignored in such cases.
- Drooping eyelids.
- *Irregular cornea*: Inaccuracies can be avoided by repeat keratometry, if:
  - Corneal curvature more than 47 D or less than 40 D
  - The difference in the corneal cylinder is more than 1 D between eyes.

VIVA QUESTIONS

1. What are the types of keratometry?
Ans. Refer to text.

2. How to calibrate keratometer?
Ans. The keratometer is callibrated using steel balls. A steel ball of known radius of curvature is placed before the keratometer and its value is set on the dial. The mires are focused by rotating the eye piece by trial and error method. When the mires are focused, calibration is said to be complete.

3. What is the principle of keratometer?
Ans. Refer to text.

4. Disadvantages of keratometer.
Ans. Refer to text, limitations of keratometer.

5. Can you measure the central K in keratometer?
Ans. No.

6. What is the normal range of keratometer?
Ans. 36–52 D.

7. How can the range of measurement be increased?
Ans. Refer to text.

8. Which equipment can give you an accurate estimation of posterior corneal surface power?
Ans. Pentacam.

9. Which equipment can give you total astigmatism?
Ans. Cassini (based on ray tracing principle) and Pentacam (total power map).

10. Conditions where posterior corneal power cannot be ignored.
Ans. Postrefractive surgery and postradial keratotomy.

REFERENCES

1. Friedman NJ, Kaiser PK. Optics/Refraction. Case Reviews in Ophthalmology, 2nd edition. New York, United States: Elsevier;2017. pp. 1-46.
2. Elliott DB. Determination of the refractive correction. Clinical Procedures in Primary Eye Care, 3rd edition. Edinburgh: Butterworth-Heinemann; 2007. pp. 83-150.
3. Embleton SJ. Pre-operative biometry and intra-ocular lens calculation. Cataract. Edinburgh: Butterworth-Heinemann; 2008. pp. 33-72.
4. Chowdhury PH, Shah BH, Tiwari N. Keratometer: Easy to Understand. J Ophthalmol. 2018;3(S1):000S1-016.

2.3 PENTACAM

Siddhi Goel, Pranita Sahay, Anin Sethi, Prafulla Kumar Maharana, Jeewan Singh Titiyal

INTRODUCTION

Cornea is the principal refractive element of the human eye. Out of around 58–60 D, cornea contributes around 42–45 D or almost two-thirds of the total power of the eye. The anterior surface of cornea accounts for the maximum refraction that occurs in the eye. The considerable difference in the refractive index of air and cornea accounts for this (air $\mu = 1$; corneal $\mu = 1.37$). Thus, evaluation and characterization of the corneal surface is an essential component for the diagnosis, planning, treatment, and postoperative

Table 2.3.1: Various corneal topographers/ tomographers.	
Principle	*Device*
Placido based	• Placido disc • Videokeratoscope
Slit scanning system	Orbscan
Slit scanning system + Placido	Orbscan II
Scheimpflug	• Pentacam • Sirius • Galilei
Ray tracing	Cassini

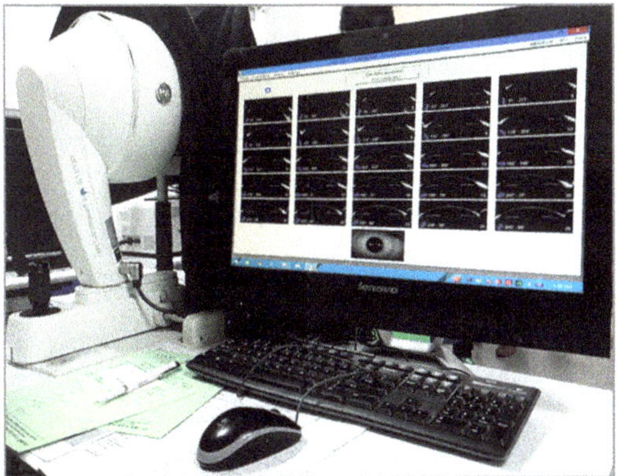

Fig. 2.3.1: Pentacam.

follow-up of many corneal disorders such as keratoconus (KC) and other ectatic disorders, refractive surgery, and contact lens fitting.

Corneal topography refers to the graphic representation of the geometrical properties of the cornea whereas corneal tomography includes three-dimensional (3D) characterization of the cornea. Nowadays, various corneal topographic and tomographic systems are available which are noninvasive and easy to operate and interpret (Table 2.3.1). Further discussion in this chapter would be on the Pentacam system (Fig. 2.3.1).

PRINCIPLE

The Pentacam is based on the Scheimpflug principle, introduced by Theodore Scheimpflug,[1] a cartographer of the Austrian naval forces. This was initially used for topographic imaging for military purposes with cameras attached to the gliders or hot air balloons with the prototype devices. The Scheimpflug law states that "In order to get a higher depth of focus, the picture plane, the objective plane, and the film plane should be moved in such a way that they cut each other in one line or one point of intersection, known as the Scheimpflug intersection" (Fig. 2.3.2). Typically, in a camera, the lens plane, the image plane, and the plane of focus are parallel to each other, resulting in a decreased depth of focus. Scheimpflug based imaging system provides a high depth-of-focus, sharp images of the anterior as well as posterior corneal surface, iris, and lens. The depth of penetration though depends upon the media transparency and pupillary diameter.[2]

EXAMINATION METHODS

The Pentacam uses a combination of a rotating Scheimpflug camera and a static camera. It uses a monochromatic slit-light, ultraviolet (UV) free blue light-emitting diode (LED), of wavelength 475 nm. The camera takes a total of 50 images in maximum 2 seconds, from 0° to 180°, with each of the photographs is an image of the cornea at a specific angle. The software combines all these images and provides a 360° image of the anterior segment consisting of as many as 25,000 (in case of Pentacam HR it is 138,000) true elevation points.

The addition of the second camera improves the reproducibility of Pentacam significantly when compared to other corneal topography systems. It detects any eye movement of the fixating eye and corrects the position accordingly. This significantly increases the reliability and repeatability of Pentacam.

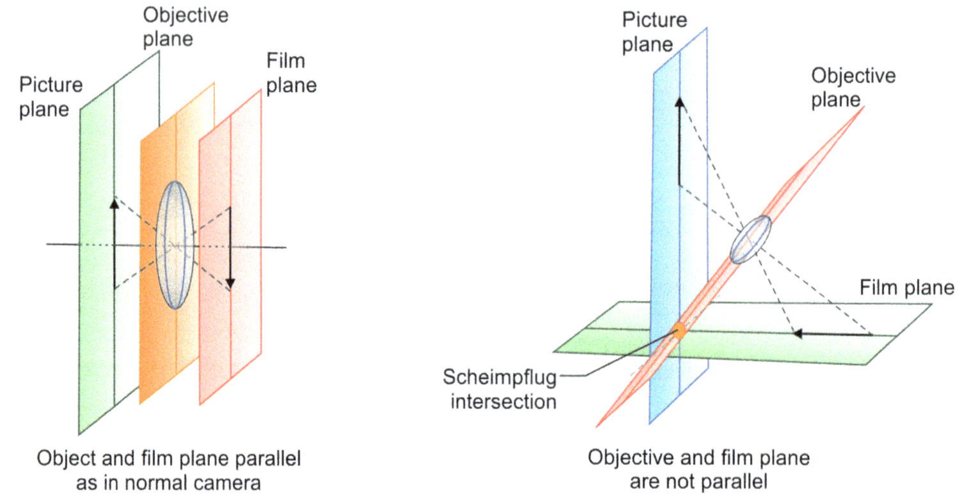

Fig. 2.3.2: Image formation in a normal camera versus Scheimpflug principle.

INTERPRETATION

As shown in Figure 2.3.3, the Pentacam output consists of corneal, anterior chamber (AC) parameters on the left side, and the "quad map" on the right side. The quad map consists of the anterior curvature sagittal map, the anterior and posterior elevation maps, and the pachymetry map. However, the display can be modified as per the need of the investigator.

Curvature Maps

They give information about pattern, symmetry, and skewing of the axis of the anterior surface of the cornea. The usual pattern is the symmetric bowtie (SB), where the two segments are equal in size and their axes are aligned (Fig. 2.3.3). The SB represents regular astigmatism. This can be with-the-rule, against-the-rule (ATR) or oblique depending upon the orientation of the bowties. Various other patterns include (Figs. 2.3.4 and 2.3.5):

- Round—steepest part of the cornea is round but decentered.
- Oval—steepest part is oval and it can be centered or decentered.
- Superior steep—steepest part is located in the superior quadrant.
- Inferior steep—steepest part is located in the inferior quadrant.
- Irregular—no particular shape.
- *Abnormal SB*:
  - *Symmetric bowtie with skewed radial axis (SB/SRAX)*: The angle between the axes of the two lobes is > 22°.
  - *Asymmetric bowtie with inferior steepening (AB/IS)*: The IS difference is > 1.5D
  - *Asymmetric bowtie with superior steepening (AB/SS)*: The SI difference is > 2.5D
  - *Asymmetric bowtie with skewed radial axis (AB/SRAX)*: The angle between the axes of the two lobes is > 22°.
- Butterfly.
- Claw pattern or "kissing birds"—seen in pellucid marginal degeneration (PMD).
- Junctional (vertical D)—circular shape, where two segments are connected laterally.

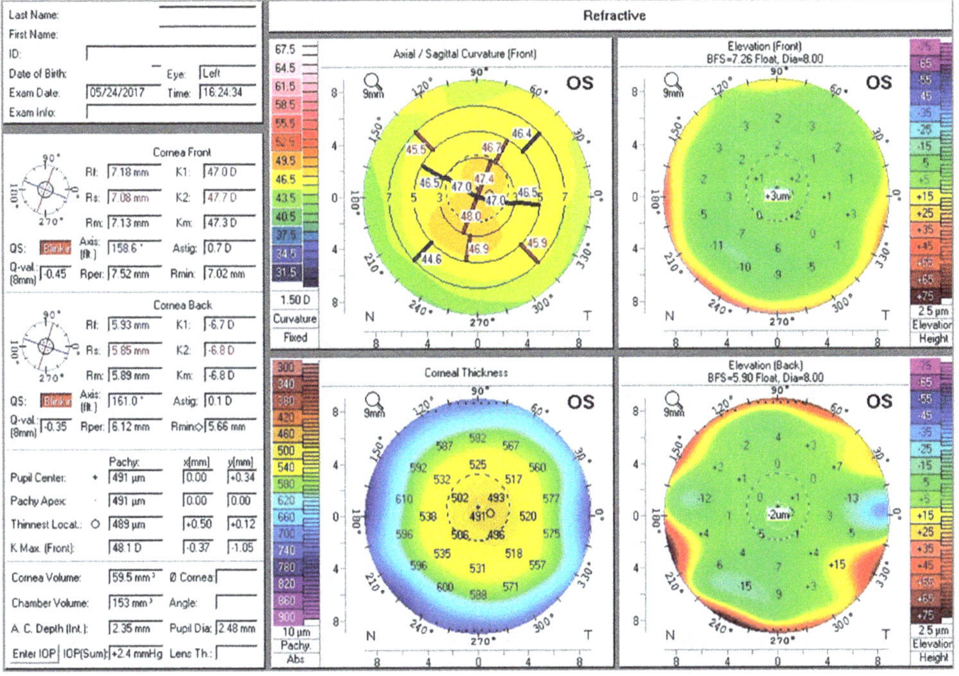

Fig. 2.3.3: Corneal tomography. On the left is the table of corneal parameters and on the right is the four-view refractive composite map.

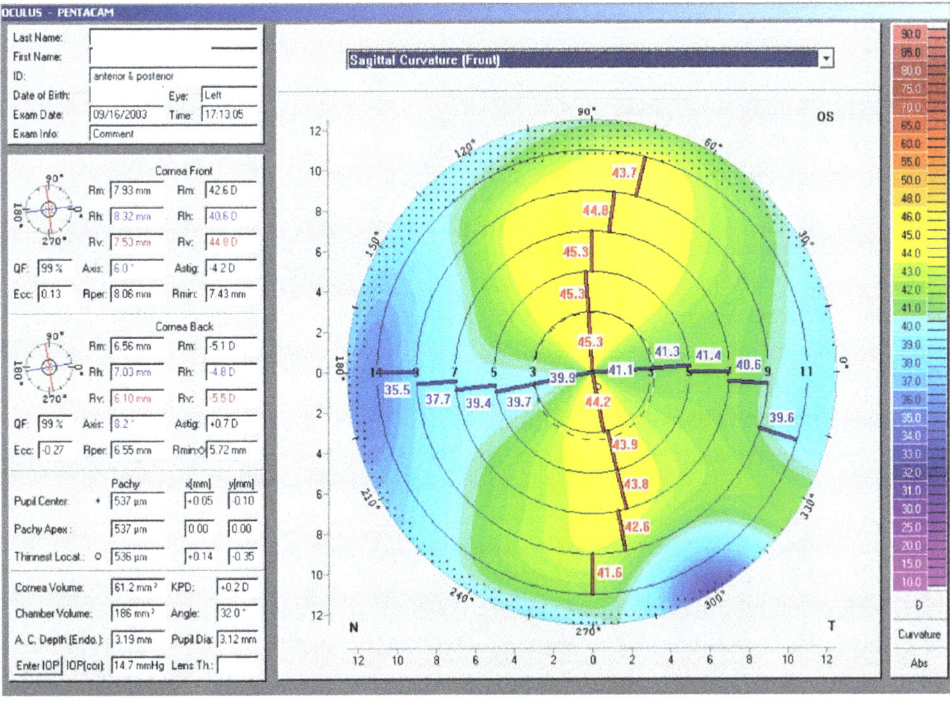

Fig. 2.3.4: Anterior sagittal map showing symmetric bowtie pattern.

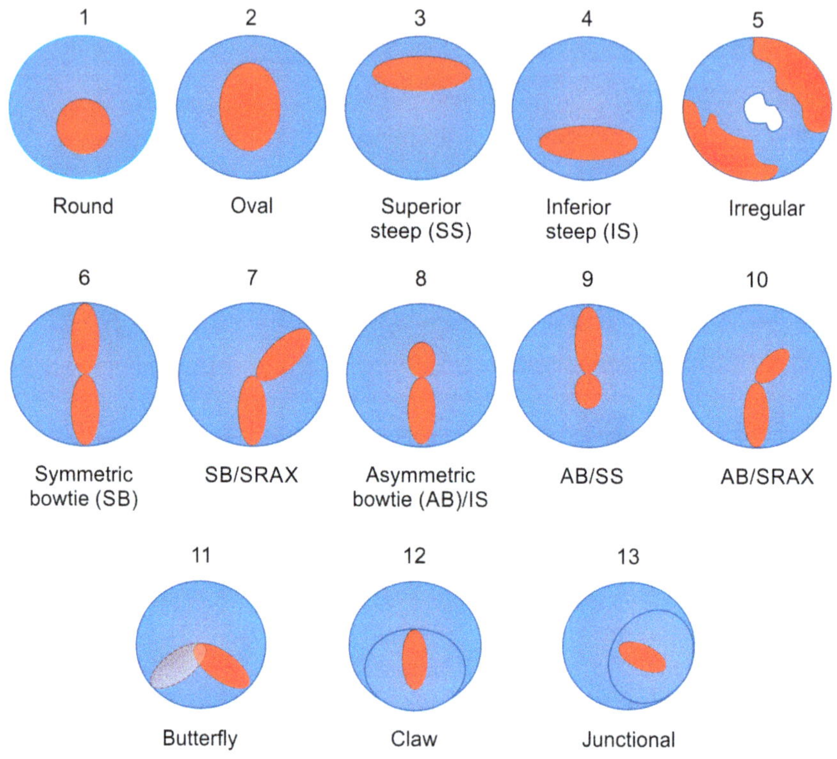

Fig. 2.3.5: Various patterns of the anterior sagittal map. (SRAX: skewed radial axis)

- Smiling face—may be an indicator of KC and postoperative ectasia.
- Vortex—the steep and flat segments are distributed in a vortex pattern. It is an indicator of corneal instability.

A phenomenon occasionally exists in some individuals; the sagittal map in one eye appears as a mirror shape of that in the other eye, this is known as "enantiomorphism". When this phenomenon is seen, borderline irregularities can be considered normal.

Elevation Maps

The normal cornea is prolate; it rises centrally above the reference sphere resulting in a central hill. This hill is surrounded by an annular sea as the cornea dips below the reference surface. As we move to the periphery, the cornea rises above the reference surface resulting in peripheral highlands (Fig. 2.3.6).

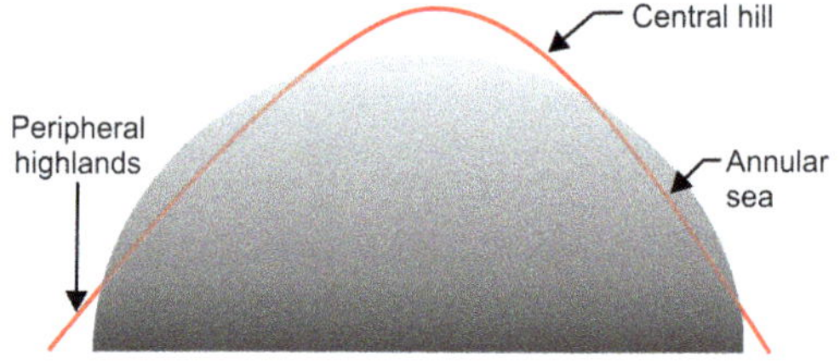

Fig. 2.3.6: Illustration demonstrating normal cornea against a best-fit sphere.

Reference Plane

Various points on the corneal surface are compared against a reference plane and any point higher than the reference plane is represented with warm colors and points lower than reference are represented with cooler colors. Three selectable reference bodies are available:

1. *Best-fit toric ellipsoid (BFTE)*—matches perfectly to astigmatic corneas (most frequently used).
2. *Ellipsoid*—matches optimal to the actual shape of the cornea.
3. *Best-fit sphere (BFS)*—comparable to Orbscan.

The Pentacam displays both the front and back elevation maps (Fig. 2.3.7).

- *Elevation on the front surface*: While interpreting, we look at the values within the central 5 mm circle on the map in BFTE mode. Clinical interpretation is as follows:
  - Normal < +12 μ
  - +13 to +15 μ—suspected
  - More than +15 μ is a risk factor

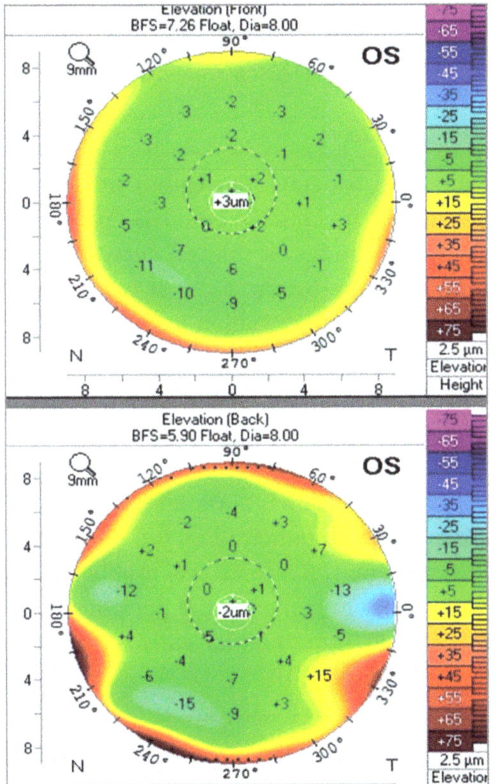

Fig. 2.3.7: Front and back elevation maps.

- *Elevation at the back surface*: Clinical interpretation is as follows:
  - Normal—< +17 μ
  - +18 to +20 μ—suspected
  - More than 20 μ is a risk factor.

The difference between front and back surfaces should be < +5 μ. Any isolated island on either the anterior or posterior surface is suspicious even in the presence of normal values.

Thickness/Pachymetry Maps

The true thickness of the cornea is the difference between the anterior and posterior elevations (Fig. 2.3.8). The Pentacam generates 25,000 data points to describe the true thickness whereas a standard ultrasound pachymetry can only image one single data point. Pachymetry is important for the diagnosis of ectatic disorders and preoperative planning of various corneal procedures like laser in situ keratomileusis (LASIK), small incision lenticule extraction (SMILE), Intacs, and collagen cross-linking. Clinical interpretation is as follows:

- Inferior steepening ratio compares the superior and inferior values at 5 mm circle. A difference of > 30 μ is suspicious.

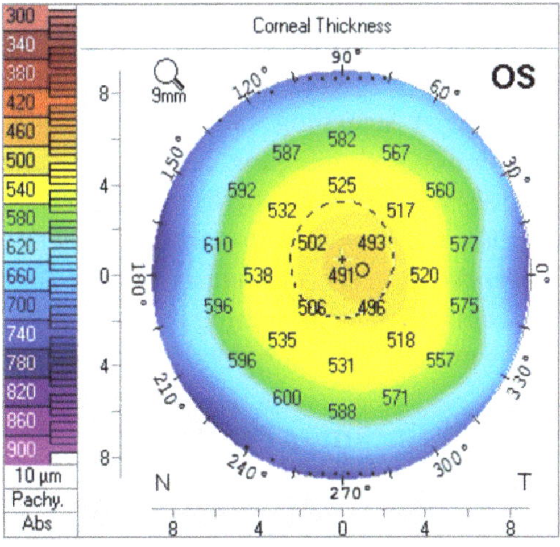

Fig. 2.3.8: Corneal pachymetry map.

- Difference between thinnest pachy and pachy at apex should be < 10 μ
- The difference of thinnest pachy between the two eyes should be < 30 μ
- If the thinnest point is decentered from apex by > 500 μ, suspect KC.

Asphericity of Cornea

If the rays passing through the corneal periphery are refracted more than the rays passing through the central part, then it will give rise to spherical aberration. Therefore, in the case of an oblate cornea where the radius of curvature becomes smaller towards the periphery, stronger spherical aberrations are encountered.

On the contrary, in case of a prolate cornea, the radius of curvature increases towards the periphery and thus spherical aberration decreases.

The corneal asphericity is described in terms of Q value. Q value of normal cornea is –0.26 to 0.35. Q value is negative when the cornea is prolate as the rays from corneal periphery would fall behind the central rays. On the contrary, Q value is positive in the oblate cornea as the peripheral rays would fall ahead of the central rays.

Belin/Ambrosio Enhanced Ectasia Display

Belin/Ambrosio Enhanced Ectasia Display (BAD) is a screening tool that combines elevation based mapping and progression analysis of corneal pachymetry (Fig. 2.3.9). This is an extremely important tool for early diagnosis of corneal ectasia and hence frequently used for screening of cases for KC before any refractive surgery.

Corneal Thickness Progression Analysis

The corneal thickness progression analysis (CTPA) is measured by taking the thickness of cornea at multiple concentric rings, starting from the thinnest point and 2, 4, 6, 8, and 10 mm. corneal-thickness spatial profile (CTSP) is calculated by measuring the corneal thickness at the thinnest location and the averages of the points on 22 imaginary circles centered on the thinnest point with increased diameters at 0.4 mm steps. Corneal-volume distribution is calculated by measuring the corneal volume is within diameters from 1.0 mm to 7.0 mm with 0.5 mm steps centered on the thinnest point.[3] In the CTSP graph following things can be seen:

- *Vertical axis*: The percentage of thickness increment
- *Horizontal axis*: It represents the location as circles centered on the thinnest location
- *Red color line*: Represents the curve of the examined cornea
- *Black dashed line*: It represents the result of the standard value study
- *The upper and lower line*: Both these lines represent the double standard deviation (SD) (95%) of the corneal thickness.

Interpretation

The red curve must fall within the normal range, and its course should be parallel to the normal range. If the red curve deviates as or after the 6 mm circle, it is normal. A quick downward deviation is a risk factor as it means that the corneal center is relatively thin in relation to the periphery.

Advantages

As the measurements are centered on the thinnest point rather than the anatomical corneal center, the thickness profile change is abrupt from center to the periphery. This is especially important for early detection of corneal ectasia.

D Value

Five new terms (Df, Db, Dp, Dt, Dy) have been added.

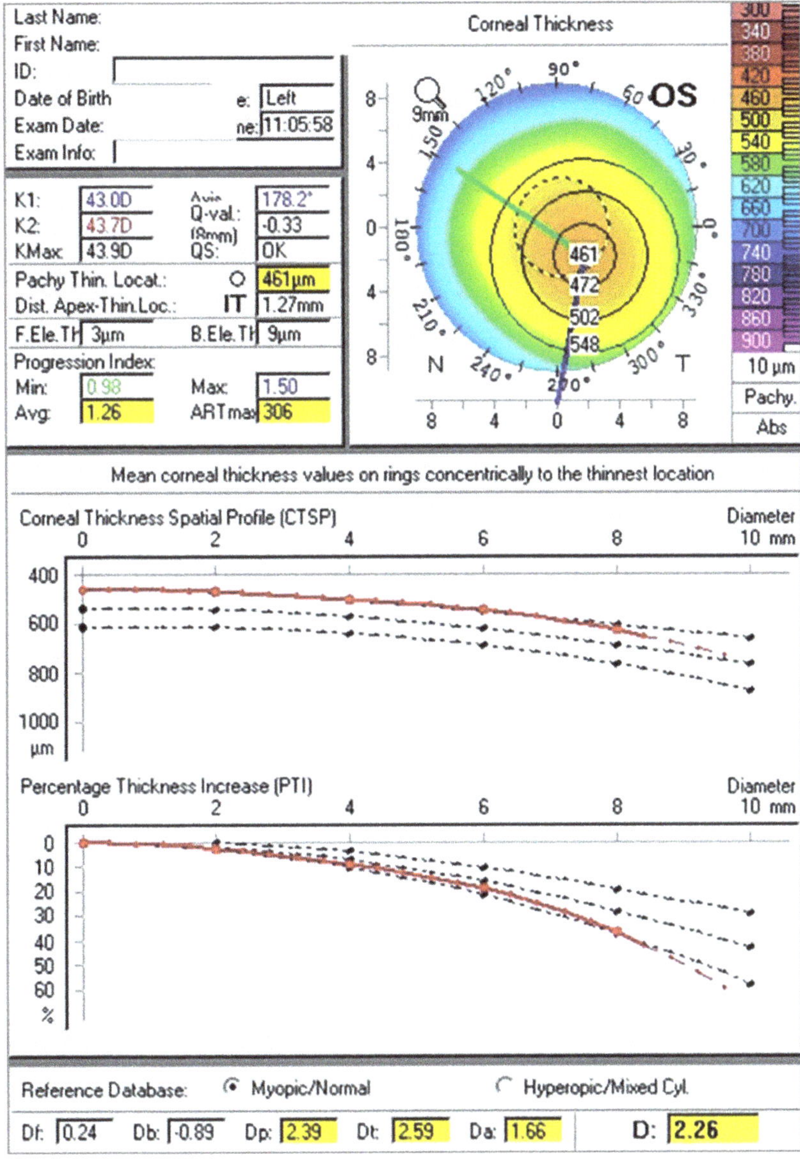

Fig. 2.3.9: Pentacam map with Belin Ambrosio enhanced ectasia display (BAD) display.

1. **Df** for the front surface
2. **Db** for the back surface
3. **Dp** for pachymetric progression
4. **Dt** for the thinnest point
5. **Dy** for thinnest point displacement.

Each of these and their final D number are depicted as the SD from the mean with the help of colors in the interpretation map.

The parameter is indicated in the following colors:

- *White color*: D less than 1.6 SD, suggests normal
- *Yellow color*: D more than 1.6 SD, suggests suspicious
- *Red color*: D more than 2.6 SD, suggests abnormal.

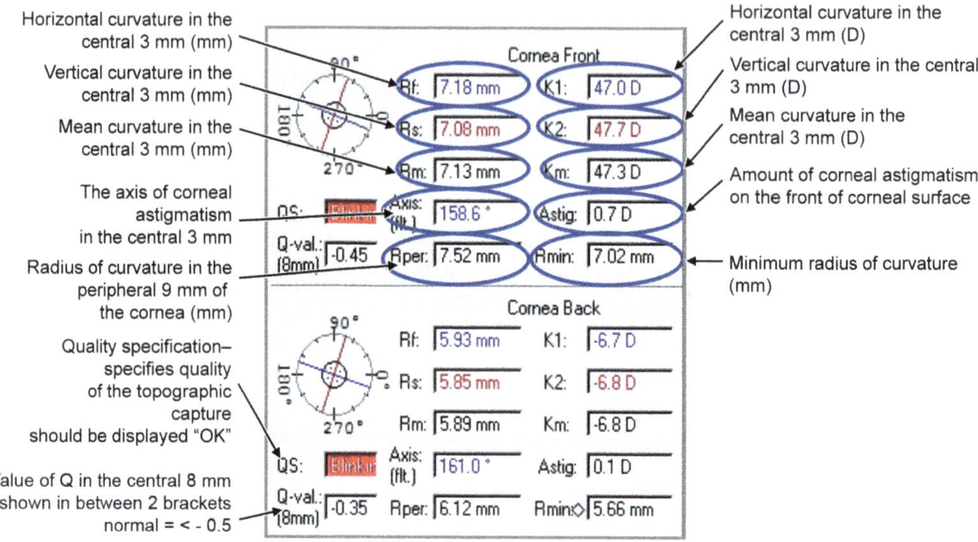

Fig. 2.3.10: Corneal parameters.

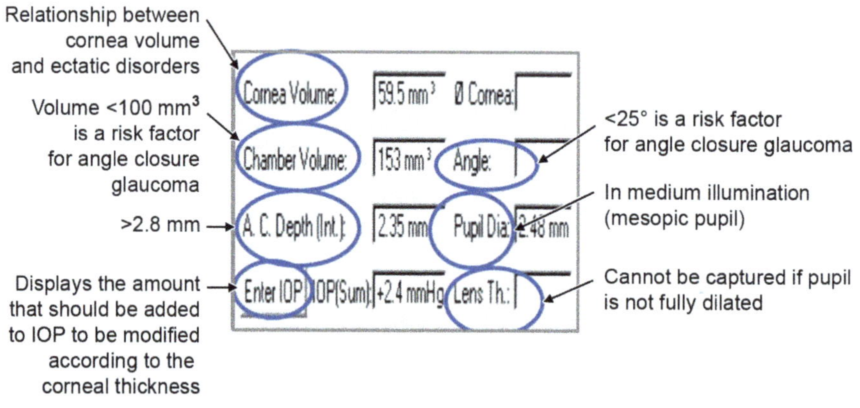

Fig. 2.3.11: Anterior chamber parameters. (IOP: intraocular pressure)

Figures 2.3.10 and 2.3.11 display various other parameters studied on the Pentacam.

CLINICAL APPLICATIONS AND EXAMPLES

Indications of Pentacam

When to get it done:

- Complain of frequent change of glasses
- Defective vision even with refraction
- Patients with a history of long-standing vernal keratoconjunctivitis (VKC) or allergic conjunctivitis
- Basic refractive surgery workup
- Abnormal keratometry
- Slit-lamp examination suggestive of thinning.

Why to get it done:

- Diagnosis and baseline topography
- Progression of the ectasia
- Classification of the disease.

Applications

Screening and Diagnosis of Ectatic Disorders

The Pentacam system helps in identifying forme fruste keratoconus (FFKC) and aids in diagnosis and grading progression of KC and other ectatic disorders like PMD and Terrien marginal degeneration (TMD). The global consensus on KC and ectatic diseases[4] identified the following findings as mandatory to diagnose KC.

- Abnormal posterior elevation
- The abnormal corneal thickness distribution
- Clinical noninflammatory corneal thinning.

Other findings suggestive of KC are increased area of corneal power surrounded by concentric areas of decreasing power, inferior-superior power asymmetry and skewing of the steepest radial axes (AB/SRAX). The AB/SRAX pattern only occurs in 0.05%[5] of the healthy patient population, but it is almost universal in patients with KC. Figures 2.3.12 and 2.3.13 show the Pentacam quad map and BAD display of a patient with KC. Table 2.3.2 summarizes the points that point towards a diagnosis of early KC.[6]

In cases of PMD, the classic topographic pattern is of IS which is most dramatic between the 4 and 8 o'clock positions, with superior flattening. Described as a "crab-claw" or "lobster-claw" pattern. The thinnest point does not coincide with the point of maximal steepening (Fig. 2.3.14). However, the claw-shaped topography is not diagnostic of PMD; it can also be seen in cases of KC.

Refractive Surgery

Corneal topography has become an indispensable tool for pre- and postrefractive surgery corneal evaluation. They help in identifying individuals with high risk of

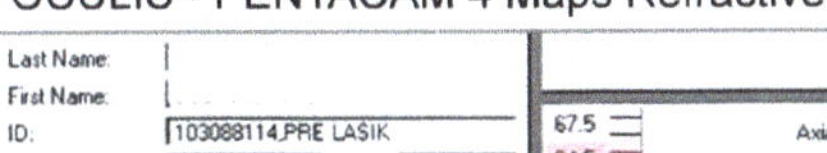

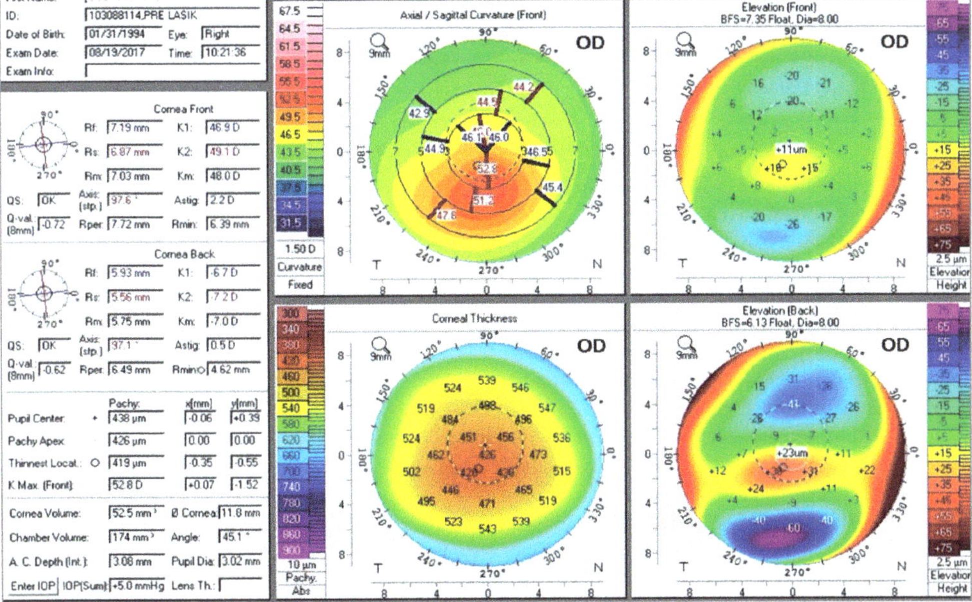

Fig. 2.3.12: The curvature map demonstrating corneal astigmatism with inferior steepening, elevation maps with abnormal anterior and posterior elevation and pachymetry map showing corneal thinning.

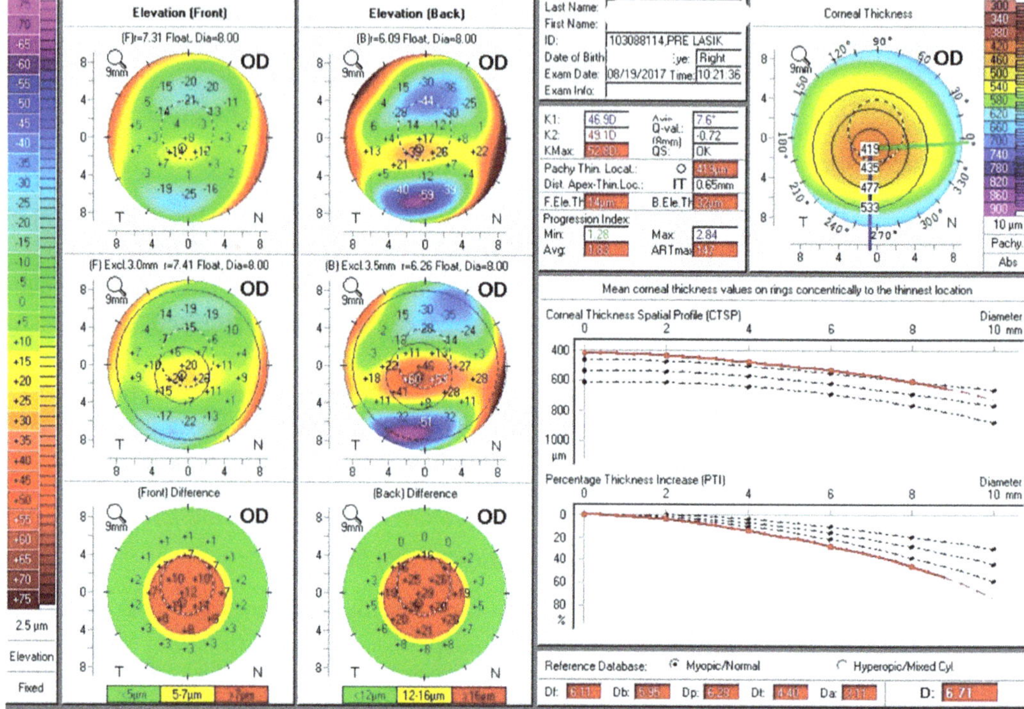

Fig. 2.3.13: The Pentacam Belin Ambrosio enhanced ectasia display (BAD) display showing corneal graph lying outside 2 standard deviation (SD) with abnormal D value.

Table 2.3.2: Pentacam parameters for diagnosis of early keratoconus (KC)/forme fruste KC (FFKC).
Findings on the sagittal map
Central K-readings ≥ 48 D SRAX ≥ 22° Superior-inferior difference (S-I) on the 5 mm circle ≥ 2.5 D Inferior-superior difference (I-S) ≥ 1.5 D Corneal astigmatism ≥ 6 D
Findings on the thickness map
Thinnest location < 470 µ Y coordinate value of the thinnest location ≥ –500 µ Pachymetry apex-thickness at thinnest location ≥ 10 µ Superior-inferior at 5 mm circle ≥ 30 µ Difference in thickness between both eyes at thinnest locations ≥ 30 µ
Findings on the elevation maps
Isolated focal island of ectasia (BFS mode) on either surface Values ≥ 12 µ within the central 5 mm on the anterior elevation map (BFTE mode) Values ≥ 15 µ within the central 5 mm on the posterior elevation map (BFTE mode)

(BFS: best-fit sphere; BFTE: best-fit toric ellipsoid; FFKC: forme fruste keratoconus; SRAX: skewed radial axis)

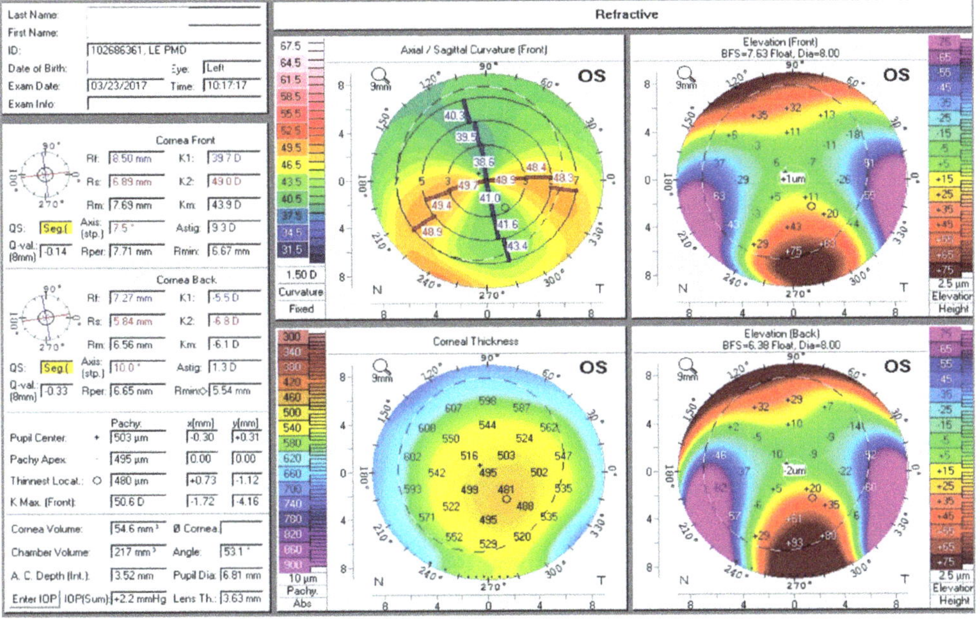

Fig. 2.3.14: Pentacam quad map of a patient of pellucid marginal degeneration (PMD) with crab claw appearance. Note that the thinnest point does not coincide with the point of maximal steepening.

developing post-LASIK ectasia, thus helping us to counsel them and provide other alternatives like phakic intraocular lenses (IOLs). Important risk factors include:[7]

- Abnormal topography
- Abnormal pachymetry: Residual corneal bed thickness
- Percentage tissue altered (PTA) more than 40%

[PTA = (FT + AD)/CCT], where FT: flap thickness; AD: ablation depth; and CCT: preoperative central corneal thickness.

- Young age
- The topographic asymmetry between two eyes.

Figure 2.3.15 illustrates a case of a myopic patient who developed ectasia after undergoing LASIK.

Glaucoma Evaluation

Various parameters like anterior chamber depth (ACD) (both central and peripheral), AC volume, CCT, and inbuilt intraocular pressure (IOP) correction formulae can be used for glaucoma screening (Fig. 2.3.11).

Contact Lens Fitting

The Pentacam helps in the improved fitting of contact lens is irregular corneas. Topography helps to identify the corneal apex, cone diameter, corneal astigmatism, thereby helping the diagnostic lens selection. Various preprogrammed contact lens fitting software is available.

Cataract Evaluation

Pentacam also has the Pentacam Nucleus Staging (PNS) Module which helps in objective quantification of lens opacities (densitometry) in 2D and 3D and graduation of lens opacities.[8] It also helps in visualization of lens opacities and posterior capsular opacities (PCOs). Cataract can be graded from grade 0 to 5.

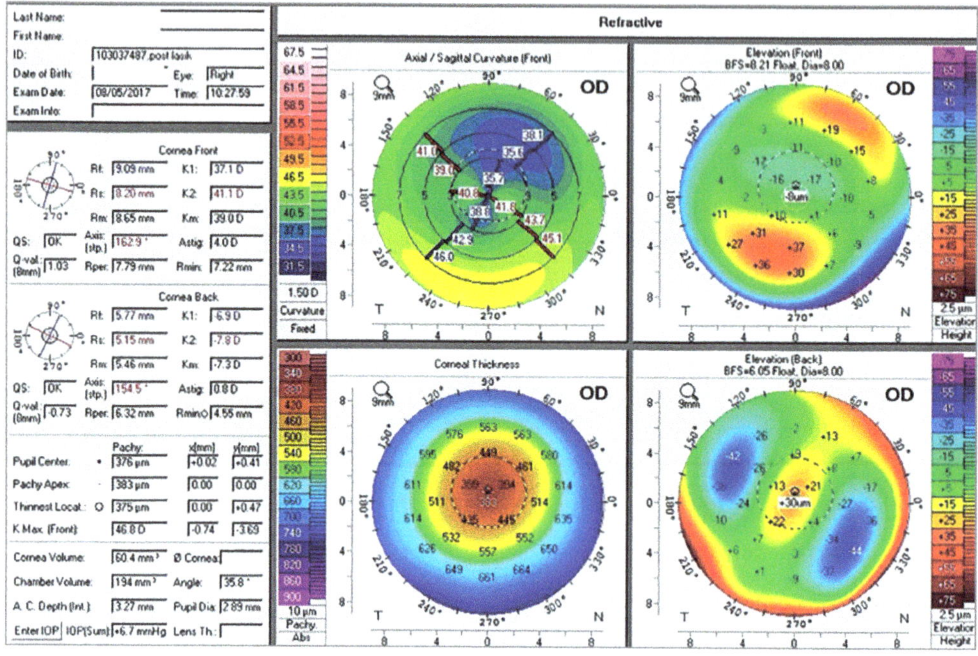

Fig. 2.3.15: Post-LASIK ectasia. Note the abnormal posterior elevation.

Intraocular Pressure Power Calculation

Previously, postmyopic LASIK, overestimation of keratometry led to an underestimation of IOL power resulting in hyperopic outcomes and vice versa. The Holladay report[9] incorporated in the Pentacam software helps in calculating optimal IOL refractive power for postrefractive surgery patients. It determines total corneal power, as equivalent keratometry readings (EKRs) for different zones of the cornea. These EKRs can be entered in the IOL calculation formulae to get a correct IOL power.

Corneal Optical Densitometry Display

Scheimpflug images alone can never give the exact location of corneal pathologies because the ocular structures often do not lie within a flat plane and structures at similar depths in the cornea appear at different depths in the tomography.[2] Corneal densitometry map (Fig. 2.3.16) is handy in such cases as it presents all structures located at the same relative distance from the corneal surfaces.[2] Thus, making it a useful tool for assessing the depth and position of scattering phenomena occurring within the cornea.[2]

Clinical utility of corneal densitometry includes:

- Reproducible measurements of corneal haze
- Following up corneal haze or opacity (objective assessment) in patients post-LASIK or post-photorefractive keratectomy (PRK), or with infectious keratitis, corneal dystrophy, and KC.

Limitations: It is difficult to perform in cases where the cornea is opaque or very hazy as the backscatter will be too high and the measurements unreliable. Scleral backscatter

OCULUS - PENTACAM Cornea Densito

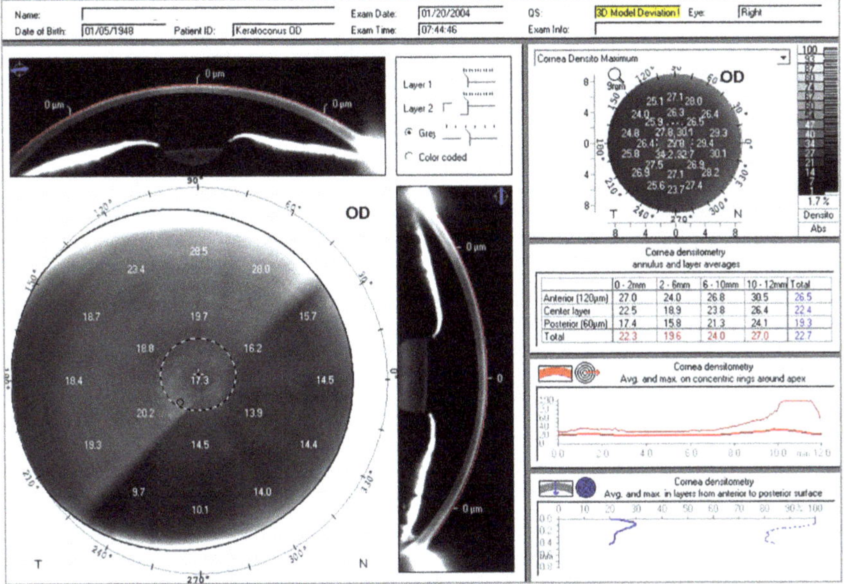

Fig. 2.3.16: Corneal optical densitometry display.

can artificially elevate the densitometry values near the limbus (10–12 mm from central fixation).

Intracorneal Ring Segments Implantation

Pentacam gives exact location of cone, higher-order aberrations (HOAs) (fitting of corneal rings in reference to the axis of the coma) as well as corneal thickness at 5–7 mm zone, hence useful for preoperative as well as postoperative follow-up of cases of corneal ectasia undergoing intracorneal ring segments (ICRS) (Intacs or Kerra) (Fig. 2.3.17).

Corneal Aberration

Pentacam provides Zernike analysis of the cornea based on the principle of ray tracing (Fig. 2.3.18). It provides the calculation of the corneal wavefront of the entire cornea (anterior and posterior surface) and is thus independent of the shape of the cornea [e.g. post-LASIK, PRK, lamellar keratoplasty (LKP), penetrating keratoplasty (PKP), etc.].[2] Besides, it can be shown for the anterior and posterior surface of the cornea.

Uses

- Selection of aspheric IOLs for correction of corneal spherical aberrations (Z4.0)
- Fitting of corneal rings in reference to the axis of the coma
- Determination of low- and high-order aberrations.[2]

CONCLUSION

The Pentacam topography system is a rapid scanning, reproducible and easy to use imaging system. It helps in a comprehensive evaluation of the anterior segment of the eye making it a useful tool for both diagnosis and surgical planning.

VIVA QUESTIONS

1. What are the Pentacam parameters for diagnosis of early KC/FFKC?

Ans. Refer to Table 2.3.2.

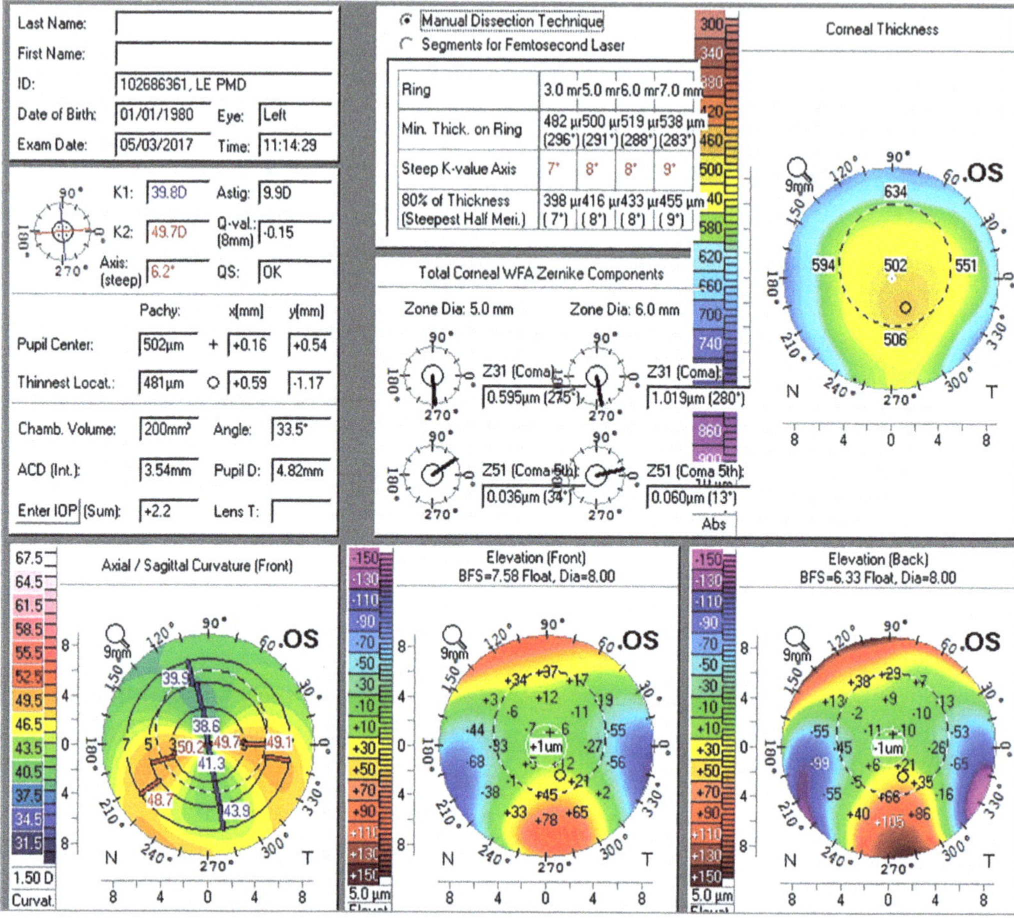

Fig. 2.3.17: Corneal rings in Pentacam.

2. What is the difference between Pentacam and Orbscan?

Ans. Refer to Table 2.3.3.

3. What is the clinical utility of corneal densitometry?

Ans. Refer to text.

4. Difference between Pentacam and Galilei.

Ans. The Pentacam Scheimpflug analyzer (Oculus Optikgeräte GmbH, Wetzlar, Germany) uses a single Scheimpflug camera to acquire multiple photographs of the anterior segment of the eye. The Galilei dual-Scheimpflug analyzer (V4.01 Ziemer, Port, Switzerland) uses dual Scheimpflug cameras and a Placido disc to improve the accuracy of corneal power and pachymetric measurements. Both the instruments show good correlation in all measured parameters except AC angle, AC volume, and average pupil diameter.[10] It is important to remember that these devices cannot be used interchangeably.

5. What is Pentacam AXL?

Ans. The Pentacam AXL determines the axial length of the eye as well as the data of

OCULUS - PENTACAM Zernike Analysis

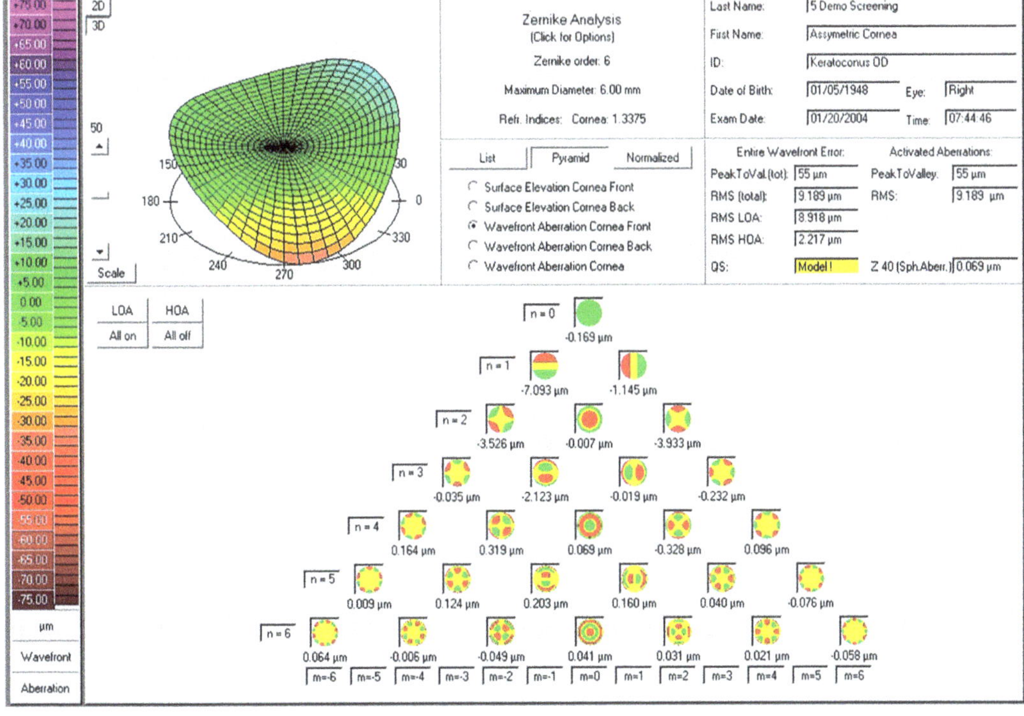

Fig. 2.3.18: Zernike analysis of the cornea in Pentacam.

Table 2.3.3: Pentacam versus Orbscan.

Pentacam	*Orbscan*
Based on Scheimpflug principle	Based on scanning slit and Placido disc system
Maintains the central point (the thinnest point) of each meridian. Thus, can reregister these central points and eliminate the effect of eye movements. Thus, it is 10 times more accurate than Orbscan	Takes multiple vertical images which have no common point. Thus, it cannot reregister for any eye movement
Posterior elevation data are more accurate	Less accurate

the anterior eye segment, from the anterior corneal surface to the posterior surface of the crystalline lens, all in a single measurement. In doing so it makes combined use of the Pentacam technology and an equally proven interferometry-based biometry technique. Various functions of Pentacam AXL are:

- Intraocular lens calculator for:
  - Both treated and untreated eyes
  - Spherical, aspherical multifocal, and toric IOL calculation
  - Toric IOL calculation based on the total corneal refractive power
- Fast screening report
- Belin/Ambrósio Enhanced Ectasia Display
- Topographical keratoconus classification (TKC)
- Qualitative assessment of the cornea:
  - Topography and elevation maps of the anterior and posterior corneal surface
  - Overall pachymetry
  - Corneal optical densitometry

- Glaucoma screening:
  - Pachymetry-based IOP correction
  - Chamber angle and chamber volume
- Elevation data
- Pentacam Nucleus Staging and 3D cataract analysis
- Premium IOL selection in four steps
- Comparative displays for follow-up
- Comparison and superimposition of Scheimpflug images
- Contact lens fitting.

REFERENCES

1. Scheimpflug T. Der photoperspektrograph und seine anwendung. Photogr Korr. 1906;43:516-31.
2. Pentacam. Interpretation guideline: 3rd edition. [online] Available from: https://www.pentacam.com/fileadmin/user_upload/pentacam.de/downloads/interpretations-leitfaden/interpretation_guideline_3rd_edition_0915.pdf [Accessed January, 2019].
3. Ambrósio R, Alonso RS, Luz A, et al. Corneal-thickness spatial profile and corneal-volume distribution: tomographic indices to detect keratoconus. J Cataract Refract Surg. 2006;32(11):1851-9.
4. Gomes JAP, Tan D, Rapuano CJ, et al. Global consensus on keratoconus and ectatic diseases. Cornea. 2015;34(4):359.
5. Matalia H, Swarup R. Imaging modalities in keratoconus. Indian J Ophthalmol. 2013;61(8):394-400.
6. Sinjab MM. Classifications and patterns of keratoconus and keratectasia. Berlin, Heidelberg: Springer; 2012. pp. 13-58.
7. Randleman JB, Woodward M, Lynn MJ, et al. Risk assessment for ectasia after corneal refractive surgery. Ophthalmology. 2008;115(1):37-50.
8. Nixon DR. Preoperative cataract grading by Scheimpflug imaging and effect on operative fluidics and phacoemulsification energy. J Cataract Refract Surg. 2010;36(2):242-6.
9. Holladay JT, Hill WE, Steinmueller A. Corneal power measurements using scheimpflug imaging in eyes with prior corneal refractive surgery. J Refract Surg. 2009;25(10):862-8.
10. Baradaran-Rafii A, Motevasseli T, Yazdizadeh F, et al. Comparison between two Scheimpflug anterior segment analyzers. J Ophthalmic Vis Res. 2017;12(1):23-9.

2.4 ABERROMETERS

Deepali Singhal, Siddhi Goel, Prafulla Kumar Maharana

INTRODUCTION

An aberrometer is a device that measures the ocular aberrations. Based on the principle used, they can be categorized into following types:[1]

- Hartmann-Shack aberrometry
- Tscherning's aberrometry
- Ray tracing aberrometry
- Automated retinoscope.

Based on the ray projection type aberrometers can be classified into:[2]

- *Backward or outgoing projection type:* Hartmann-Shack aberrometer
- *Forward or ingoing projection type:* Ray tracing aberrometer, Tscherning's aberrometer, and automated retinoscope.

iTRACE SYSTEM

The iTrace aberrometer (Tracey Technologies, Houston, Tx) is a combination of Placido disc corneal topography and ray tracing aberrometry (Fig. 2.4.1). It measures the total aberrations of the eye. It is a serial, double pass, and forward projection type retinal image aberrometer. A topographer is added in the same unit as the aberrometer to measure the corneal aberrations.

The Principle of iTrace[3]

Ray tracing aberrometry is a more physiological method of measuring the aberrations since it measures the forward aberrations of the light going through the eye that is analyzing along the natural trajectory of the light. Figure 2.4.2 shows a diagram of the ray tracing technique.

This method uses a laser beam parallel to the line of sight through the pupil. It measures the exact site where the laser beam reaches the retina utilizing the retroreflected light captured by reference lineal sensors. An unexpanded laser beam is scanned so that it enters the eye sequentially through different pupil locations. One marginal (dotted line) and the principal ray (solid line) are shown. Each retinal image (A, O) is projected onto a charge-coupled device (CCD) camera (A', O'). The displacement of the image with respect to a reference (A', O'), is proportional to the local derivative of the wave aberration. Local aberrations in the path of the laser beam through the cornea and the internal structures cause a shift in the location on the retina. Once the first position has been determined the laser beam is shifted to another position, which is then located in the retina. This process continues until several distinct points are projected into the entrance pupil and reconstruction of the real wavefront (WF) error is done.

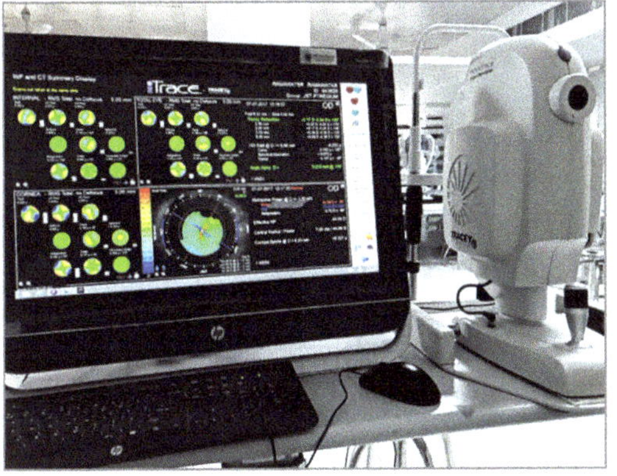

Fig. 2.4.1: The iTrace aberrometer.

The iTrace uses this principle of ray tracing where a series of infrared rays (on the order of 100 microns and a 785 nm wavelength each) are projected sequentially through pupil parallel to the eye's line of sight. 64 laser beams are projected through the pupil four times each (256 points) at

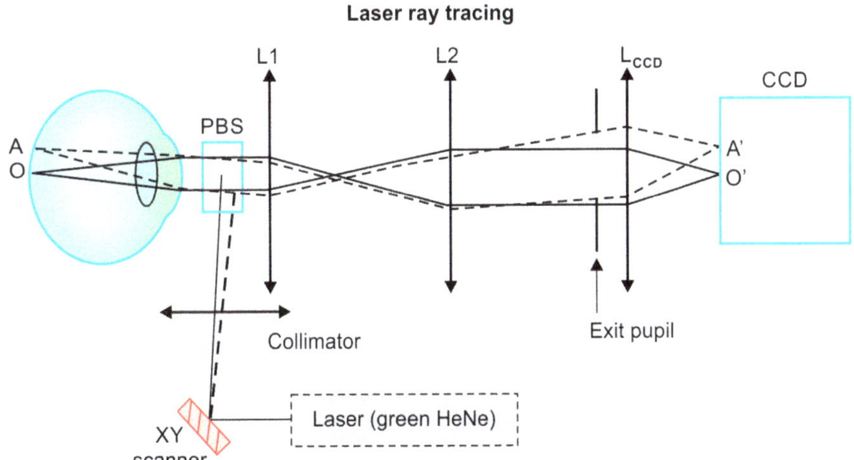

Fig. 2.4.2: Wavefront verification display showing the RSD (bottom left) with the horizontal point profile and the vertical point profile in the center. (RSD: retinal spot diagram)

a high speed (approximately 250 ms). All 256 points would be concentrated at a single point in the fovea in an emmetropic eye.

INTERPRETATION/DATA ANALYSIS[4]

- Wavefront analysis
- Topographic analysis.

Wavefront analysis: WF analysis is based on the concept of retinal spot diagram (RSD), which consists of a set of points projected through the pupil onto the retina. RSD provides all relevant information related to refraction, aberrations, and point spread function (PSF) of the patient. RSD is used to find the modulation transfer function (MTF) and PSF. The size of the RSD is inversely proportional to the concentration of photons that reaches the retina.

Point spread function shows the image of a point source of light formed in the retina. A sharper and smaller PSF is considered to be better. The MTF measures the transfer of contrast from the subject to the image by an optical system at different spatial frequencies. It measures how accurately the details from the object are transferred to the image produced by the lens. Thus, RSD simulates the vision of the patient.[5]

Interpretation/Basic Data Graphs

Reading an iTrace map should be done in the following manner:[5]

- *Wavefront verification display*: This display shows the data on limbus-to-limbus diameter, pupil size, and scan diameter. The pupil diameter can be selected manually to determine the aberrations. The left side of this display shows the RSD, which shows the retinal image of all the points projected. In an emmetropic eye, all 256 points should be concentrated on the fovea, which will be seen as a single point RSD. In the center of this display, the horizontal and the vertical point profile are seen. They show the position of each point reflected on the retina, taking the center of each profile in the X- and Y-axis. It represents the quality of the signal captured and the measurement is not accurate if it is irregular (Fig. 2.4.3). The top right of this display shows the multizone refraction analysis depending on the size of the pupil. This iTrace refraction has been reported to be highly correlated with the manifest refraction.[6]
- *Wavefront map total and higher-order aberrations (HOAs):* This is a color-coded map that shows the WF aberrations of the eye in microns. Warm colors on this map show that the WF is in front of the reference plane and cool colors show the retardation. This indicates what kind of aberrations are the main causes of low vision.
- *The root mean square (RMS)*: This map gives the magnitude of aberrations. Total aberrations of the eye are measured as the RMS value. It also displays the total lower and HOAs separately along with a specific value for each Zernike term or component of the eye aberrations (Fig. 2.4.4).
- *Total refractive and HOA refractive maps:* This map displays the refractive power of the eye in diopters referring to the whole eye and not just the corneal power. Emmetropia is represented in green, while myopia in red and hypermetropia in blue.
- *PSF total and HOA PSF*: This represents the quality of an image of a point source of light at the retina. Greater aberrations show a higher defocus effect on the image (Fig. 2.4.5).
- *Snellen letters total and HOA*: This represents the actual simulation of the

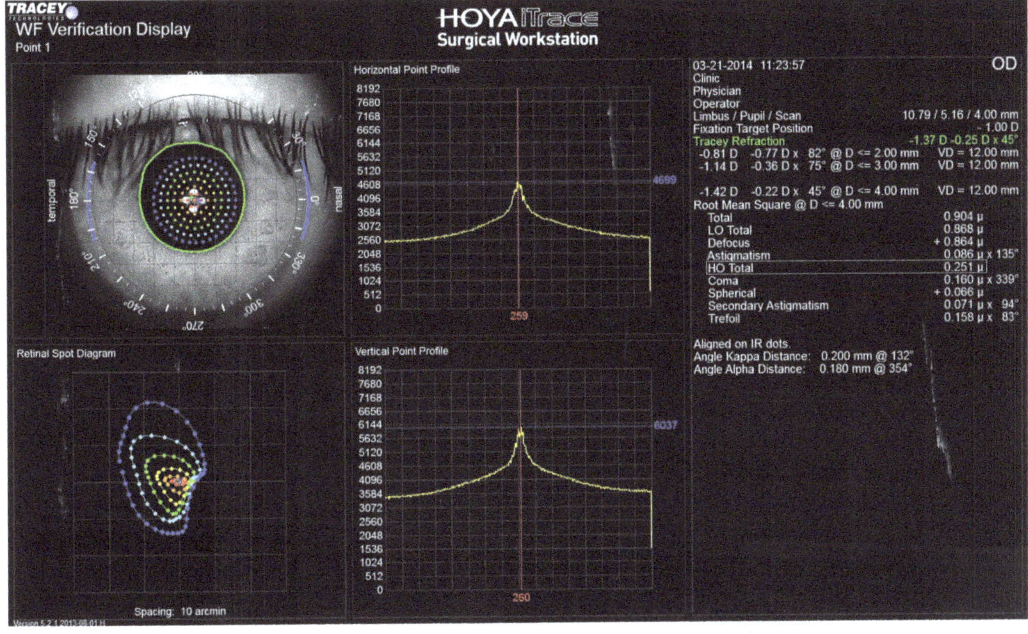

Fig. 2.4.3: Wave front verification display showing the RSD (bottom left) with the Horizontal Point Profile and the Vertical Point Profile in the center.

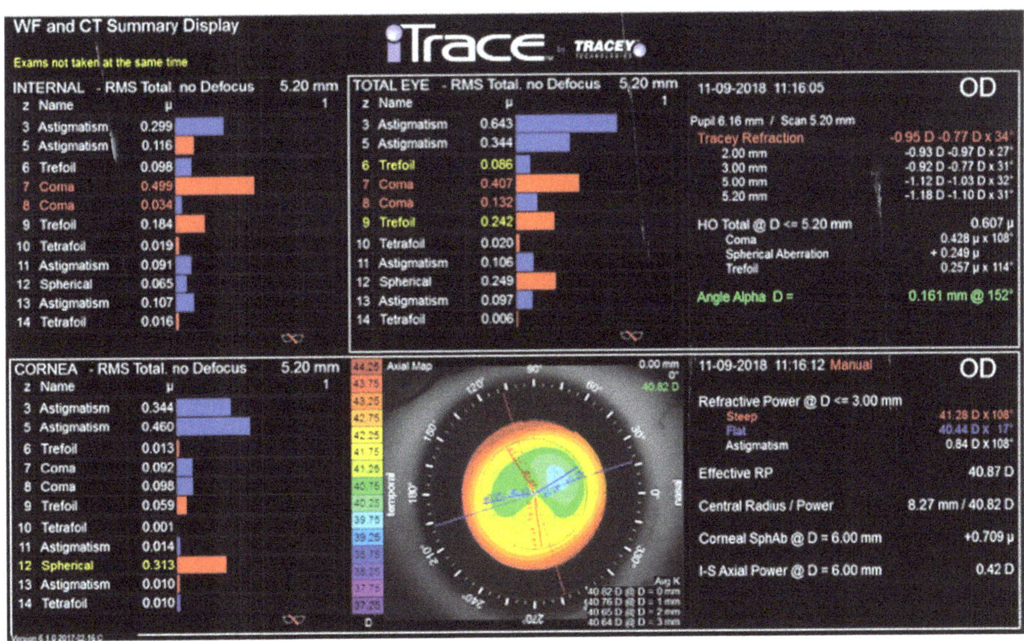

z	Name (INTERNAL)	µ
3	Astigmatism	0.299
5	Astigmatism	0.116
6	Trefoil	0.098
7	Coma	0.499
8	Coma	0.034
9	Trefoil	0.184
10	Tetrafoil	0.019
11	Astigmatism	0.091
12	Spherical	0.065
13	Astigmatism	0.107
14	Tetrafoil	0.016

z	Name (TOTAL EYE)	µ
3	Astigmatism	0.643
5	Astigmatism	0.344
6	Trefoil	0.086
7	Coma	0.407
8	Coma	0.132
9	Trefoil	0.242
10	Tetrafoil	0.020
11	Astigmatism	0.106
12	Spherical	0.249
13	Astigmatism	0.097
14	Tetrafoil	0.006

z	Name (CORNEA)	µ
3	Astigmatism	0.344
5	Astigmatism	0.460
6	Trefoil	0.013
7	Coma	0.092
8	Coma	0.098
9	Trefoil	0.059
10	Tetrafoil	0.001
11	Astigmatism	0.014
12	Spherical	0.313
13	Astigmatism	0.010
14	Tetrafoil	0.010

Fig. 2.4.4: Total RMS values, total LOA and total HOA (bottom right), and decomposition in each of the Zernike polynomials represented in red and blue bars depending on the value of the sign. (HOA: higher-order aberration; LOA: lower-order aberration; RMS: root mean square)

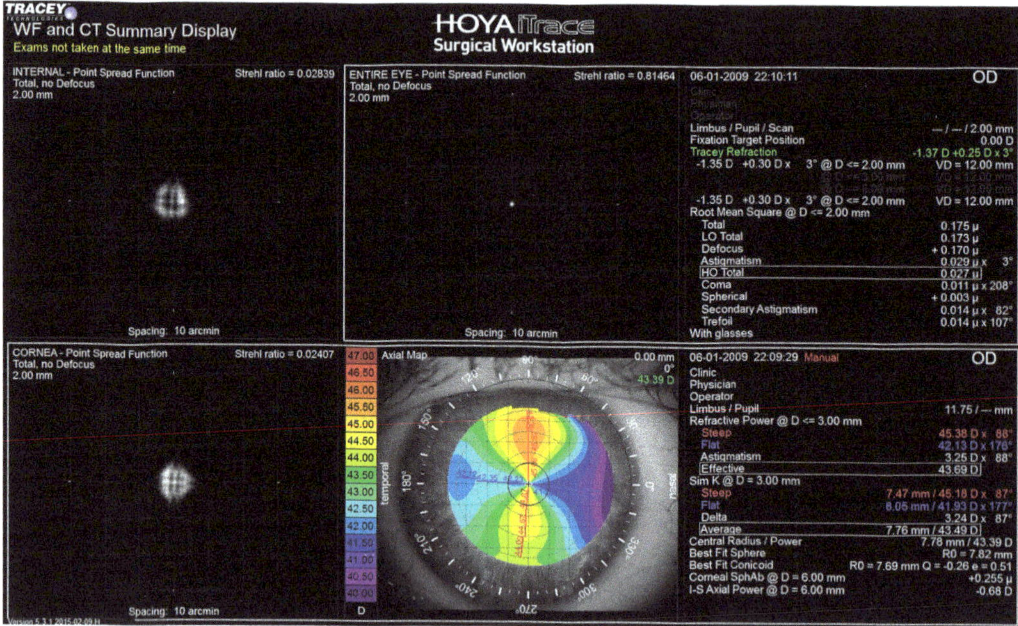

Fig. 2.4.5: Point spread function of a patient showing the compensation of corneal aberrations with internal optics.

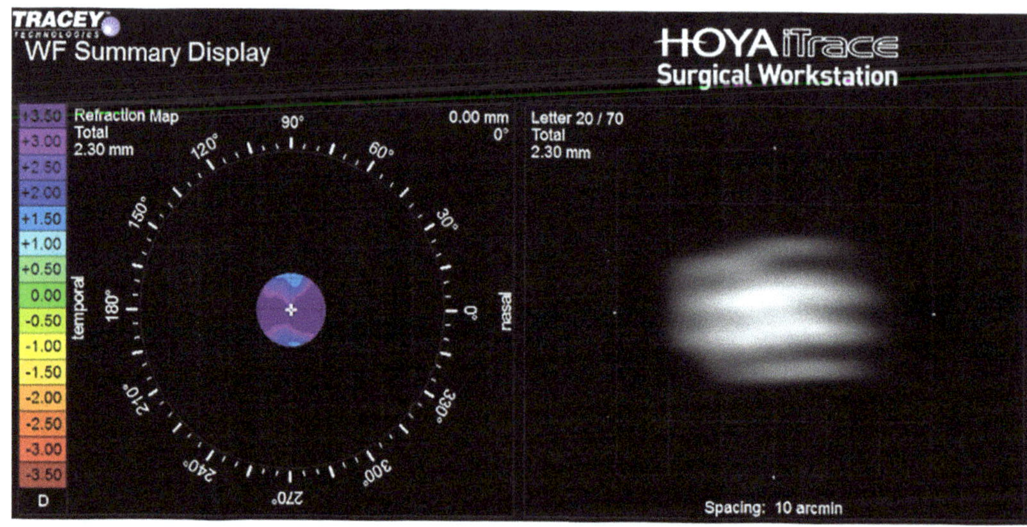

Fig. 2.4.6: Snellen letter equivalent of a patient with cataract reporting blurring of vision with glare.

patient's vision in the form of Snellen's E letter (Fig. 2.4.6).

- *Zernike polynomials bar graph*: This bar graph gives a detailed analysis of all total, corneal, and internal aberrations. iTrace shows the Zernike polynomials up to the 6th order (27 items).

Optical Alignment for Premium Intraocular Lenses

Angle alpha is the angle between the center of the limbus and the visual axis, whereas angle kappa is the angle between the center of the pupil and the visual axis (Fig. 2.4.7). Angle alpha is less commonly used since it is more difficult to measure. Premium intraocular lenses (IOLs) are being used increasingly to achieve an excellent refractive outcome after cataract surgery, which requires good centration relative to the visual axis.[7] Thus, angle alpha is an important determinant to decide whether these IOLs can be used or not. iTrace can be used to measure angle alpha and kappa with color coding. An angle ≤ 0.3 mm is green, 0.3–0.5 mm is yellow and > 0.5 mm is red. A green angle alpha has the maximum chances that the patient will be looking through the center of the central optic zone, as intended. It is not preferable to use these IOLs in cases with red angle alpha.

Cornea or Lens?

iTrace can separate the total aberrations between corneal and internal aberrations. Any significant internal aberrations indicate dysfunction of the lens. Thus it helps to identify dysfunctional lens syndrome that is characterized by difficulty in seeing at a distance or at near due to congenital ametropia or due to aging and progressive presbyopia, respectively. It also provides the dysfunctional lens index (DLI) that is calculated based on a number of factors like internal HOAs, pupil size, and contrast sensitivity. In patients with this syndrome and without any significant corneal aberrations, it would be advisable to perform a refractive lens exchange for a better outcome.

Wavefront Analysis Screens

- *Visual function analysis (VFA) summary display*: This includes the WF higher-order (HO) total or the refraction map HO total along with refraction in diopters, the

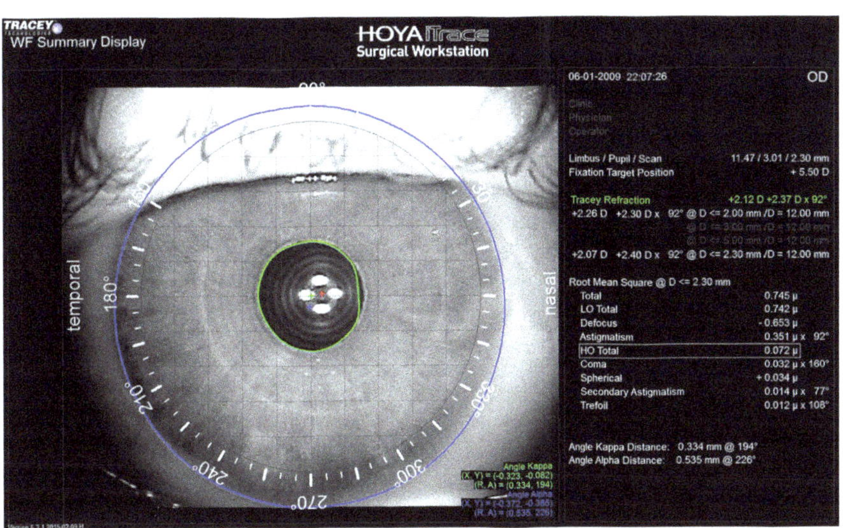

Fig. 2.4.7: Optical alignment using iTrace. The iTrace measures the distance between the visual axis, as estimated by the center of the first Purkinje reflex (red crosshair), and the center of the pupil (green crosshair), which is useful for laser-assisted in situ keratomileusis (LASIK). The angle alpha is the distance from the visual axis to the center of the limbus (blue crosshair), which is useful for intraocular lens (IOL) implantation.

RMS, Snellen letter, PSF, and potential visual complaints (nocturnal myopia, glare, halos, defocus, and double vision).

- *Wavefront comparison map*: This display is used to compare the two WF maps in a patient. It can be used to compare the status of the aberrations before and after refractive surgery and also to measure accommodation.

Uses of Aberration Analysis

- In case of high total aberrations, it helps to decide that refractive procedure would be better in cornea or lens.
- Pre- and post-cataract surgery analysis help to study the effect on the aberrations induced or compensated by the IOL.
- It also helps to identify which type of IOL will be suitable and to analyze different types of IOL.
- The contribution of an opacified lens in total ocular aberrations can be measured.
- Measurement of angle alpha and angle kappa to plan for premium IOLs.
- To evaluate the corneal and total astigmatism.
- Planning of toric IOL (Fig. 2.4.8).

CORNEAL TOPOGRAPHIC ANALYSIS (COMPUTED TOMOGRAPHY)

This is based on a Placido disc format named as Vista, which covers up to 10 mm of peripheral cornea.[5]

This provides:

- Standard keratometric readings at 3 mm zone
- Refractive power of cornea in central 3 mm zone
- Inferior-superior asymmetry corneal index (I-S)
- Topographic maps:
  - Standard axial map
  - Tangential curvature map
  - Refractive map
  - Elevation map
  - Corneal WF map.

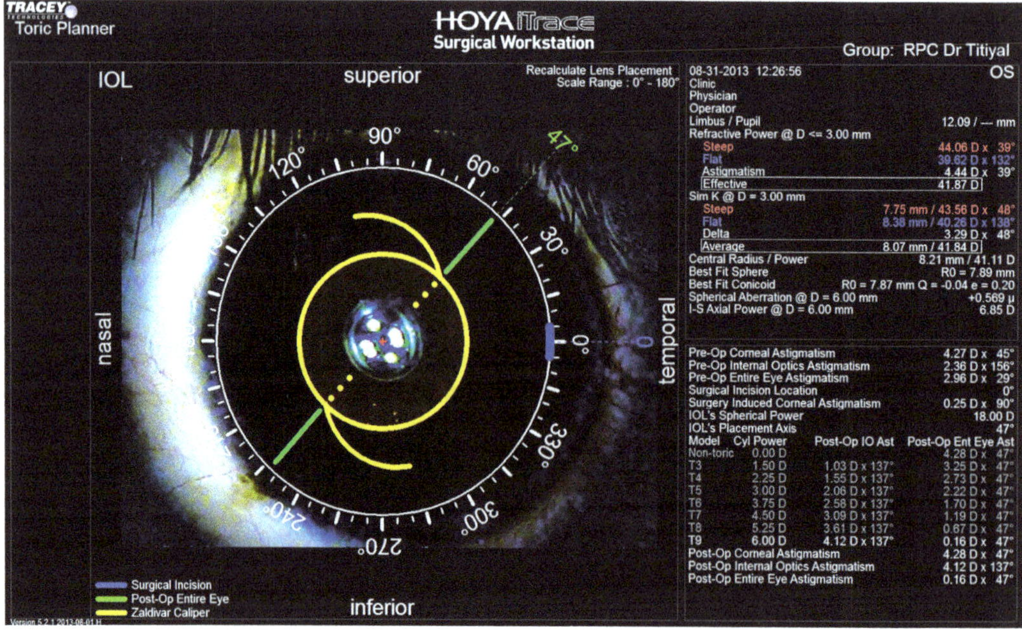

Fig. 2.4.8: Toric intraocular lens (IOL) planning with iTrace.

ADVANTAGES OF RAY TRACING ABERROMETRY

- It allows sequential capture of data with each point being processed separately and sequentially to avoid any confusion.
- The pattern of laser beams projected adjusts to the pupil size.
- Highly accurate and has a high resolution since each point is measured separately using linear detectors.
- iTrace is less susceptible to eye motion and tear film artifacts.

CLINICAL EXAMPLES

Case 1: Lenticonus

Here we analyze a case of Alport syndrome with anterior lenticonus showing a distorted RSD with the refraction of –4.37 D sphere with astigmatism of +2 D, and RMS HOA total of 1.5 microns (Fig. 2.4.9). On analyzing further to know from where the astigmatism is coming from the WF, and computed tomography (CT) summary display shows that the significant contribution of all lower-order aberration (LOA) and HOA is from the internal optics or the lens (Fig. 2.4.10). Similar results are seen with total Snellen eye (Fig. 2.4.11), thus this patient would benefit from a lens-based procedure.

Case 2: Corneal Astigmatism

Hereby we analyze a WF and CT summary display of a case with against the rule astigmatism. On separating the aberrations of cornea and lens, it is seen that the main contribution of astigmatism is from the cornea (Fig. 2.4.12).

Case 3: Balancing of Corneal and Internal Optics

This WF and CT summary display show that the internal aberrations compensate the corneal aberrations. Thus, the visual quality may get worsened if any procedure is done (Fig. 2.4.13).

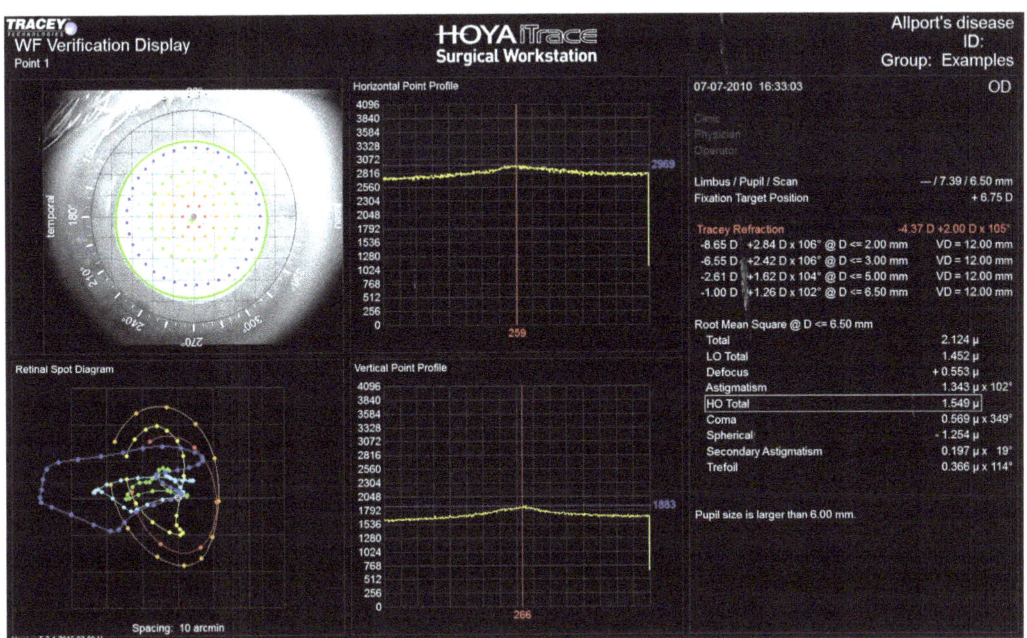

Fig. 2.4.9: Wavefront verification display of a case of Alport syndrome with anterior lenticonus showing the distorted RSD (bottom left) with the refraction of –4.37 D sphere and +2 D cyl, and RMS HOA total of 1.5 microns.

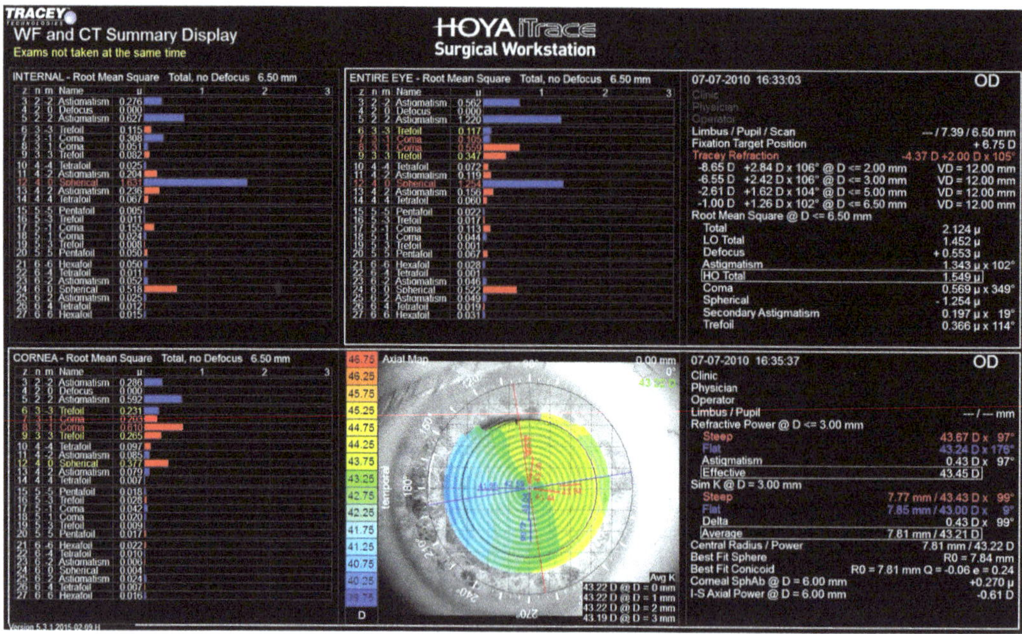

Fig. 2.4.10: Computed tomography display of a case of Alport syndrome with anterior lenticonus showing that there is a significant contribution of internal (lenticular) HOA to the total eye HOA mainly spherical aberration.

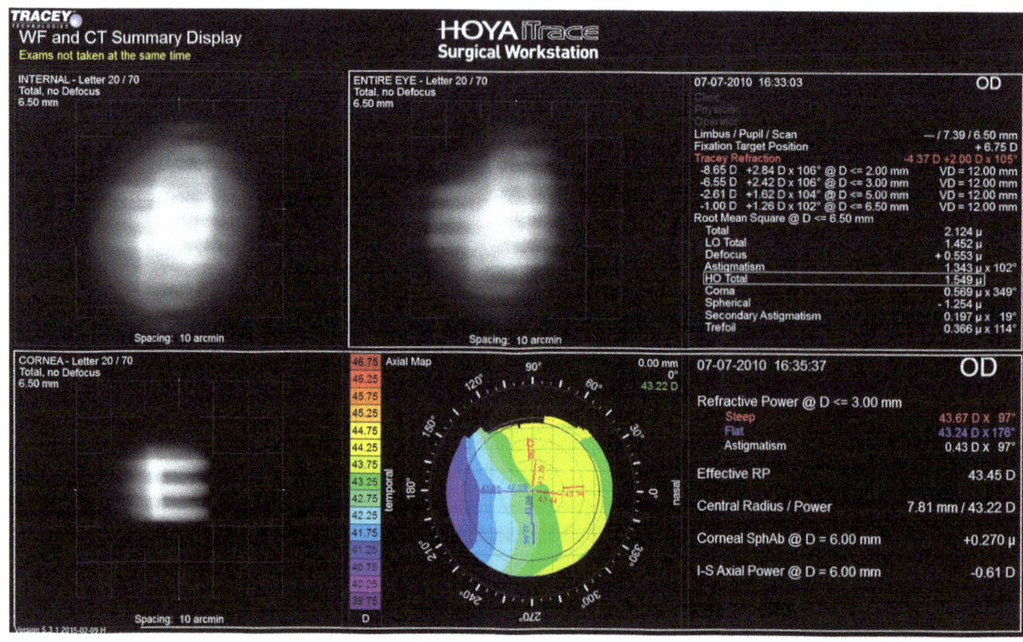

Fig. 2.4.11: Computed tomography display of a case of Alport syndrome with anterior lenticonus showing that major contribution of the distortion in Snellen E letter is due to internal aberrations and not due to corneal.

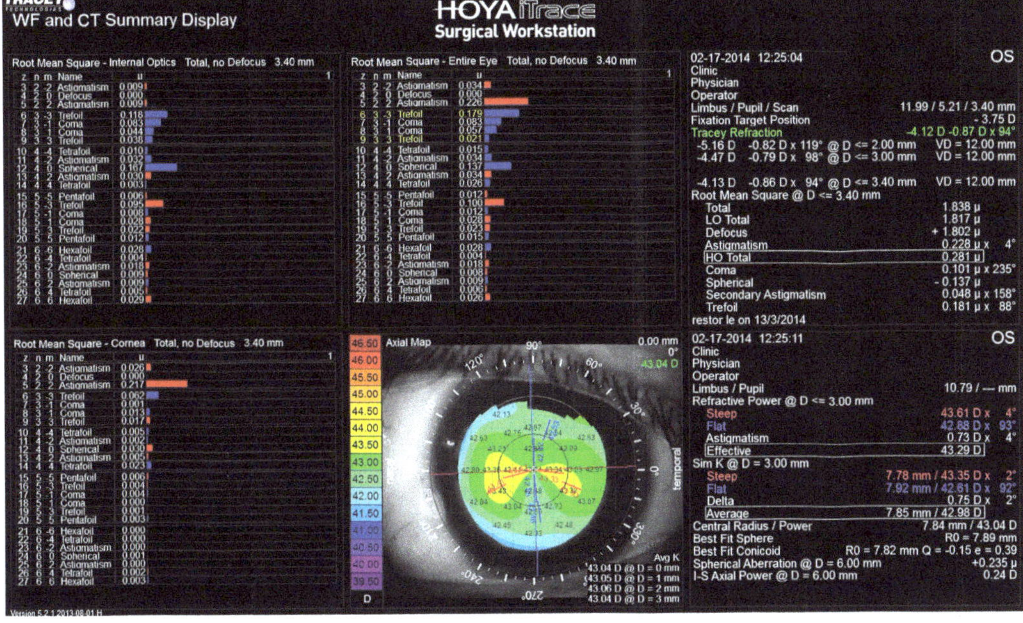

Fig. 2.4.12: A WF and CT display of a case of corneal astigmatism showing that the main contribution of total eye aberrations is from corneal aberrations especially astigmatism.

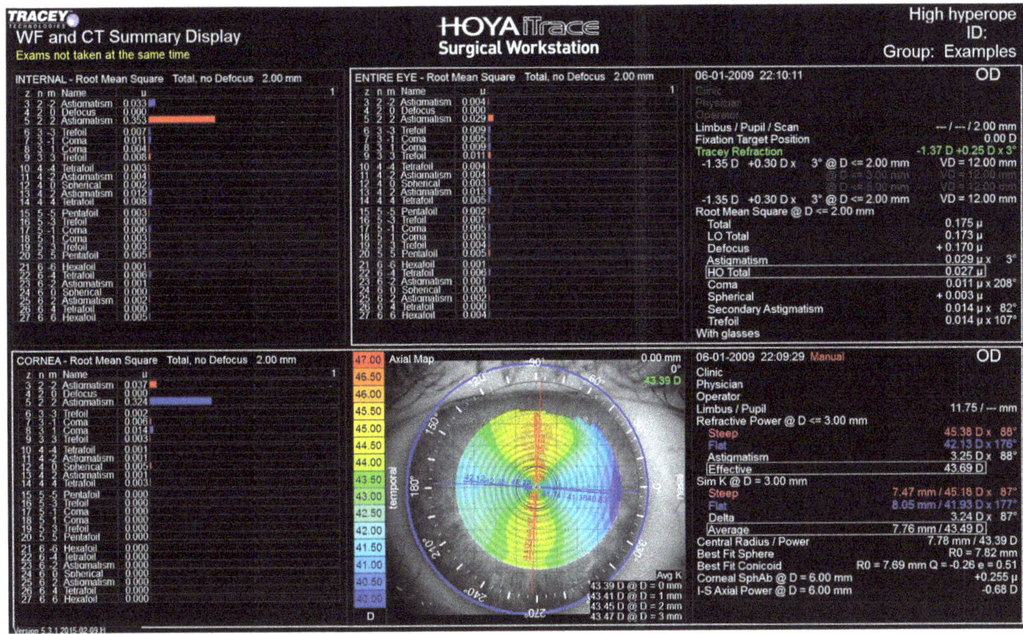

Fig. 2.4.13: A WF and CT summary display of a case showing that the internal eye aberrations are compensated with the corneal aberrations.

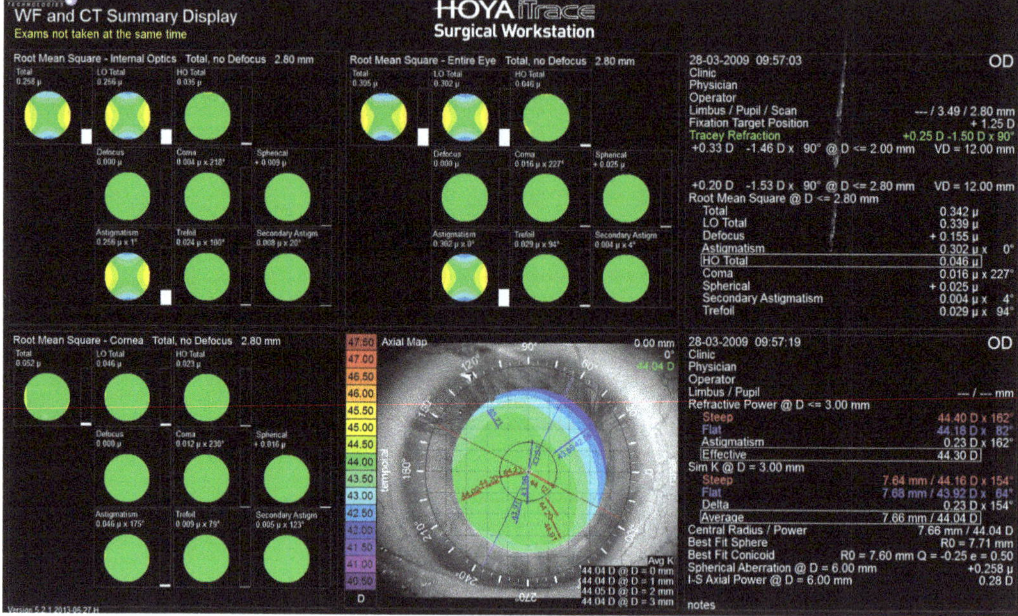

Fig. 2.4.14: The WF summary map of a case with astigmatism of 1.5 D on manifest refraction, showing that the axial map of corneal topography (bottom right) does not correspond to the map of the entire eye and the main contribution of astigmatism is from internal eye or the lens.

Case 4: Astigmatism

This case has an against the rule astigmatism of −1.5 D which is the leading cause of blurring of vision. On analyzing the WF summary map, we can see that the axial map of corneal topography (bottom right) does not correspond to the map of the entire eye. However, the internal optics maps correspond to that of the entire eye suggesting that the main contribution of astigmatism and HOAs is from the lens (Fig. 2.4.14). Thus, this patient would benefit from a lens-based procedure.

CONCLUSION

Thus, ray tracing aberrometry is an important tool that helps the surgeon at all stages of patient management. This includes preoperative planning and evaluation to achieve the best possible outcome along with evaluating the postoperative performance. At the same time, it can also help to find out the cause of low vision in a dissatisfied patient. Moreover, this technology being user friendly has made the understanding of a complex science easy and widely applicable.

VIVA QUESTIONS

1. What is aberration?

Ans. Aberration originates from the Latin "aberratio", which means going off track or deviating. Aberration is the difference between an ideal image and that achieved with the actual optical system. WF aberrations are most commonly specified by Zernike polynomials and these may be positive or negative in value leading to predictable alterations in the image quality. The magnitude of these aberrations is expressed as a RMS error that is the deviation of the WF averaged over the entire WF. The higher the RMS value is, the greater the overall aberration for a given eye. Majority of the population has a total RMS value of less than 0.3 μm.

2. Till what grade aberration can be corrected?

Ans. Aberrations can be corrected surgically till 4th order that is spherical aberrations (SAs).

3. What type of aberration is seen most commonly in keratoconus?

Ans. The most common aberration seen in keratoconus is vertical coma.

4. Mention the type of aberration in following:

a. **Cataract**

Ans. In the case of cortical cataract, the most common type of aberration reported is SA while in nuclear cataract it is coma.[8]

b. **Aging**

Ans. With aging, the major changes occur in HO and SAs only. This is mainly contributed by the changes in the lens with age, while there is a minimal contribution by the cornea. So, cornea does not affect significantly the changes in ocular aberrations seen with aging. In a young patient, the corneal aberrations are compensated by internal optics. Since the cornea has a positive SA, it is partially compensated by the negative SA of the clear lens. As the age increases, the SA of the lens becomes less negative leading to a net increase in the total ocular SA. Also, there is an increase in the horizontal coma and other third order aberrations as well. Thus, HOAs increase with age due in part to a decoupling of cornea and lens. In particular, lateral coma remains compensated in most of the older eyes due to angle kappa remaining stable with age and the lens shape factor only experiencing small changes.[9,10]

c. **Myopia**

Ans. In eyes with myopic astigmatism, primary horizontal trefoil, SA, and primary vertical coma are the predominant HOAs in descending order of frequency. A significant correlation has been seen between spherical equivalent refractive error and primary horizontal coma and the RMS of SA.[11]

REFERENCES

1. Maeda N. Clinical applications of wavefront aberrometry: a review. Clin Exp Ophthalmol. 2009;37:118-29.
2. Thibos LN. Principles of Hartmann-Shack aberrometry. J Refract Surg. 2000;16:S563-5.
3. Molebny VV, Panagopoulou SI, Molebny SV, et al. Principles of ray tracing aberrometry. J Refract Surg. 2000;16:S572-5.
4. Wakil JS, Padrick TD, Molebny S. The iTrace combination corneal topography and wavefront system by Tracey technologies. In: Wang M (Ed). Corneal Topography in the Wavefront Era. Thorofare, NJ: SLACK Inc.; 2006. pp. 177-88.
5. Gomez AC, Rey AVD, Bautista CP, et al. Principles and clinical applications of ray-tracing aberrometry (part I). J Emmetropia. 2012;3:96-110.
6. Wang Li, Wang Nan, Koch DD. Evaluation of refractive error measurements of the WaveScan Wavefront system and the Tracey wavefront aberrometer. J Cataract Refract Surg. 2003;29:970-9.
7. Park CY, Oh SY, Chuck RS. Measurement of angle kappa and centration in refractive surgery. Curr Opin Ophthalmol. 2012;23(4):269-75.
8. Rocha KM, Nosé W, Bottós K, et al. Higher-order aberrations of age-related cataract. J Cataract Refract Surg. 2007;33(8):1442-6.
9. Athaide HV, Campos M, Costa C. Study of ocular aberrations with age. Arq Bras Oftalmol. 2009;72(5):617-21.
10. Berrio E, Tabernero J, Artal P. Optical aberrations and alignment of the eye with age. J Vis. 2010;10(14):34.
11. Karimian F, Feizi S, Doozande A. Higher-order aberrations in myopic eyes. J Ophthalmic Vis Res. 2010;5(1):3-9.

2.5 ANTERIOR SEGMENT OPTICAL COHERENCE TOMOGRAPHY

Sourabh Verma, Talvir Sidhu, Deepali Singhal, Namrata Sharma

INTRODUCTION

Huang et al. first described optical coherence tomography (OCT) as high resolution imaging modality for cross-sectional analysis of retina.[1] Since its conception, OCT technology has dramatically improved resulting in more accurate and detailed reconstruction of images, which has revolutionized our understanding of retinal pathologies. More recently, a modification of OCT technology known as anterior segment optical coherence tomography (ASOCT) was described by Izzat et al. as a useful diagnostic tool for analyzing more anterior structures such as cornea, angle anatomy, association between iris and lens, intraocular masses and tumors, abnormalities of lens, etc.[2]

Anterior segment OCT is a noncontact and noninvasive optical imaging modality with a resolution much higher than ultrasound or ultrasound biomicroscopy (UBM). It is done in sitting position and requires no anesthesia. Currently most commonly available commercial models include Visante (by Carl Zeiss Meditec) and slit lamp OCT which are time domain (TD) OCT and CIRRUS HD-OCT 5000/500 (Carl Zeiss Meditec, Inc. Dublin, USA), CASIA SS-1000 OCT (by Tomey, Japan), which is a SS-OCT.

PRINCIPLES AND SPECIFICATIONS

Anterior segment OCT is based on principle of low coherence interferometry. A two-dimensional image of anterior structures of eye is produced by scattering of light by internal tissue microstructures. It makes use of longer wavelength (1,310 nm; Visante) or shorter wavelength (810 or 840 nm; Optovue). This results in less scattering through opaque media and deeper penetration through limbus and sclera.

Visante (Fig. 2.5.1) has a 16 mm scan width and 6 mm scan depth, which is more than spectral domain-OCT (SD-OCT) systems in which only a small component of anterior segment is captured. It has an axial resolution of 15–20 microns.

CASIA ASOCT (Fig. 2.5.2) uses a single detector and a rapidly tunable laser, taking about 30,000 A-scans per second. It can achieve an axial and transverse resolution of 10 and 30 microns, respectively. CASSIA is also capable of producing a 360-degree image of angle in 128 cross sections in about 2.4 seconds. SD-OCT devices have a horizontal scan width of 3–6 microns and lesser scan depth than TD-OCT devices.

Ultrahigh-resolution OCT (Fig. 2.5.3) has been recently introduced with axial resolution up to 1–3 microns, but they are used mostly for research purposes and are yet to find widespread clinical use. These devices have a scan depth of 5–12 microns.

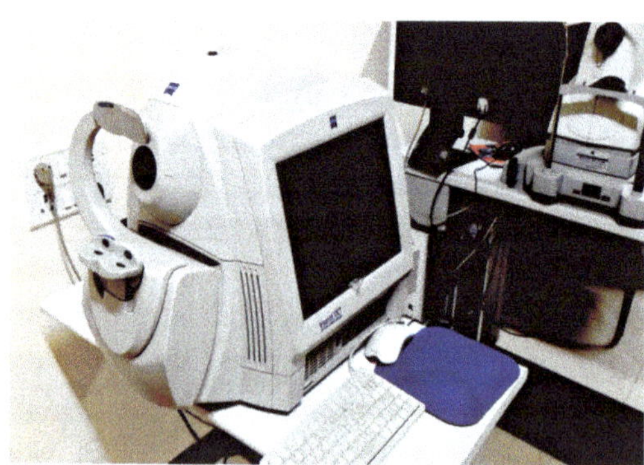

Fig. 2.5.1: Visante anterior segment optical coherence tomography (time domain).

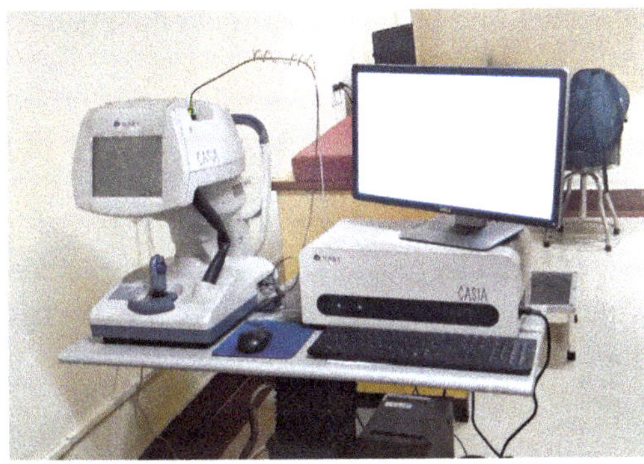

Fig. 2.5.2: CASIA anterior segment optical coherence tomography (Fourier domain).

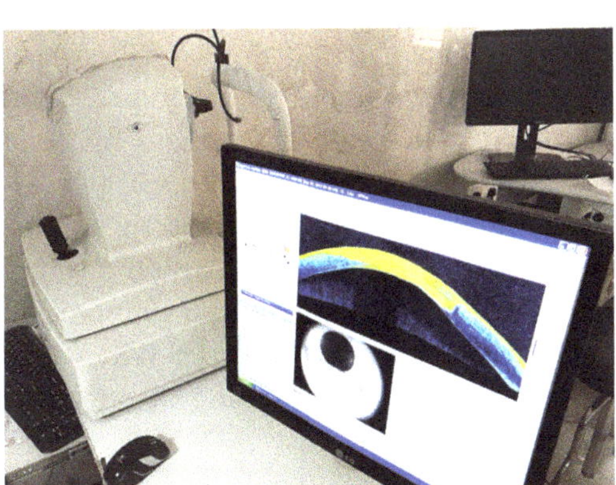

Fig. 2.5.3: Ultrahigh resolution anterior segment optical coherence tomography.

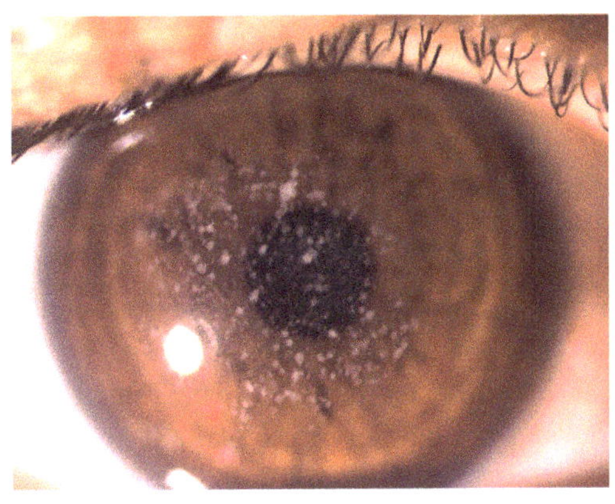

Fig. 2.5.4: Diffuse slit lamp corneal image of granular corneal dystrophy.

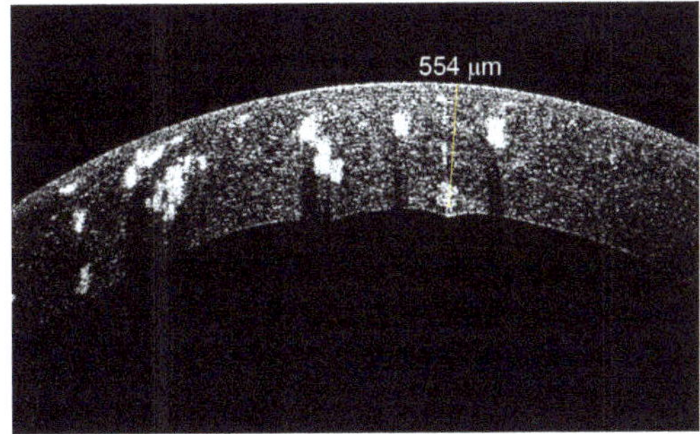

Fig. 2.5.5: Anterior segment optical coherence tomography showing multiple stromal cornea opacities in granular corneal dystrophy.

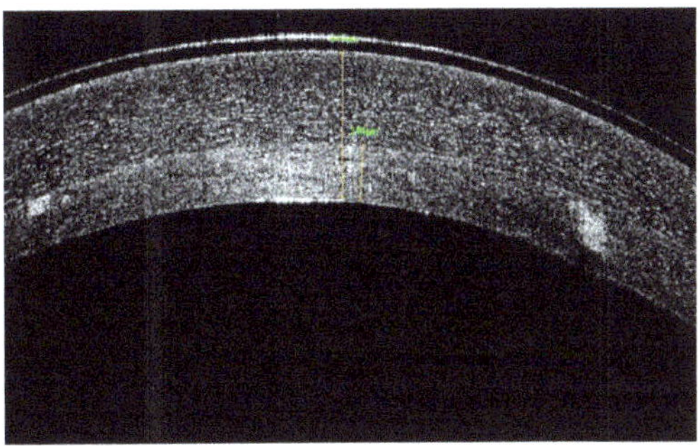

Fig. 2.5.6: Anterior segment optical coherence tomography (ASOCT) image post-anterior lamellar therapeutic keratoplasty clearly showing graft host junction and residual opacity in host cornea outside the visual axis.

INDICATIONS OF ANTERIOR SEGMENT OPTICAL COHERENCE TOMOGRAPHY

Anterior segment OCT is most useful for glaucoma and cornea specialists to diagnose, treat, and follow patients.

Applications in Corneal Conditions

Corneal Opacity

It can be used for determining depth and extent of corneal opacities. Such information is of great help when deciding for the level of lamellar keratoplasty procedure (Figs. 2.5.4 and 2.5.5). In addition, residual cornea opacities can be evaluated in postoperative period (Fig. 2.5.6).

Penetrating Keratoplasty

It has been used to study wound apposition and healing postpenetrating keratoplasty (PK). Any graft host junction malposition can be picked up. Studies have shown that such malposition can result in postoperative astigmatism, myopia, and faulty intraocular pressure (IOP) measurements. ASOCT has been used for studying wound healing pattern in various configurations of femto-assisted PKs and zigzag configuration has been found to be most stable with minimum astigmatism.

It has also been used for evaluating postoperative complications. ASOCT-based studies have proved that incomplete excision of Descemet membrane can result in postoperative glaucoma.

Anterior Lamellar Keratoplasty

Anterior lamellar keratoplasty offers several advantages over PK such as lesser chances of graft rejection and a closed globe procedure. Based on level of abnormality, different types of anterior lamellar procedures such as superficial anterior lamellar keratoplasty (SALK) and automated lamellar therapeutic keratoplasty (ALTK) can be done (Fig. 2.5.6). In deeper opacities and ectatic conditions, procedure such as deep anterior lamellar keratoplasty (DALK) can produce similar outcome as PK with minimal complications. Not only ASOCT helps in decision making, but it also helps in diagnosing possible complications like Descemet membrane detachment, double or triple anterior chamber (AC), and interface keratitis.[3]

Endothelial Keratoplasty

Optimal apposition between donor and host corneal components can be confirmed with ASOCT and resolution of corneal edema can be studied. Complications such as donor graft dislocation, epithelial ingrowth, interface opacities, and persistent lamellar fluid can be diagnosed.[3]

Eye Bank

It can also be used for screening eyes for evidence of any previous refractive procedure, which is a contraindication for being used as donor tissue.

Intraoperative Optical Coherence Tomography

It can be used to confirm apposition between lamellae in lamellar procedures and analyze the interface. Intraoperative Descemet membrane detachment can be visualized and effectively managed with intracameral air or gas injections. Intraoperative OCT (iOCT)-based studies have shown that an optimal donor–host apposition reached within minutes after Descemet stripping automated endothelial keratoplasty (DSAEK) thus reducing time for positioning in operation theater (OT).

Others

Keratoconus eyes have demonstrated donut-shaped configuration of epithelial thickness profile when examined through ultrahigh-resolution OCT. Epithelium over cornea is thinned, but epithelium in surrounding 3–4 mm zone is thickened. Other features, which are seen, include hyper-reflectivity and interruptions in Bowman's membrane, stromal thinning, and scarring in advanced cases. Descemet membrane tear and corneal hydration can be visualized in cases with corneal hydrops (Fig. 2.5.7).

Vanathi et al. used ASOCT to monitor acute hydrops in a patient with pellucid marginal degeneration.[4] Igbree et al. used it to measure AC cells.[5] Corneal re-epithelization can be monitored with the help of ASOCT with epithelium being hyper-

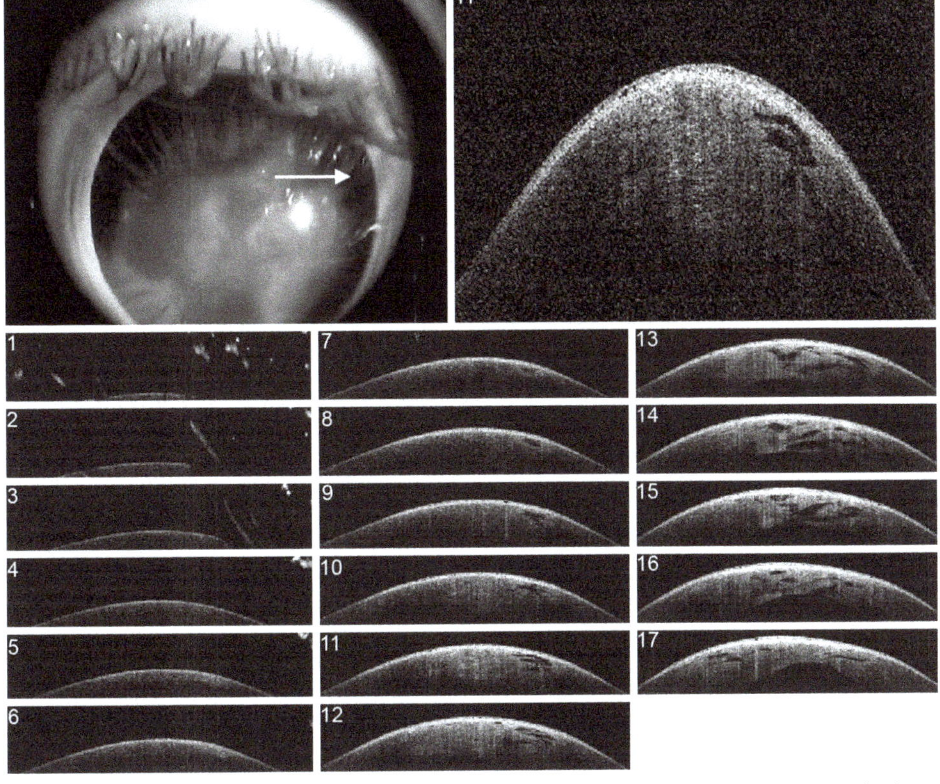

Fig. 2.5.7: Anterior segment optical coherence tomography image of corneal hydrops showing multiple stromal fluid clefts and markedly increased corneal thickness.

reflective (Fig. 2.5.8). Depth and extent of infiltrate in corneal ulcers can be visualized (Fig. 2.5.9).

Applications in Ocular Surface Diseases

Conjunctival Diseases

In conjunctivochalasis, it can be used to measure cross-sectional area of prolapsed tissue in tear meniscus. Pterygium and pinguecula appear as hyper-reflective wedge-shaped masses with thinned out epithelium. In lymphoma, hyper-reflective uninvolved epithelium and hyporeflective subepithelial lesion is seen. In conjunctival melanoma and nevi, hyper-reflectivity at basal epithelial layer and cysts can be seen.

Anterior Segment Tumors

Anterior segment OCT has been extensively used to evaluate ocular surface squamous neoplasia (OSSN). Extent of OSSN can be determined by hyper-reflective thickened epithelium of lesion and its abrupt transition to normal epithelium in uninvolved area. Depth of lesion can also be determined; however, UBM has proved to be superior in this regard. Deep intraocular penetration can warrant enucleation in place of medical management. Normalization of epithelial appearance has been seen with resolution of OSSN with medical management. Tumors of iris, angle, and ciliary body can be visualized but UBM has proved to be superior and a more reproducible modality to image and follow-up response to treatment.

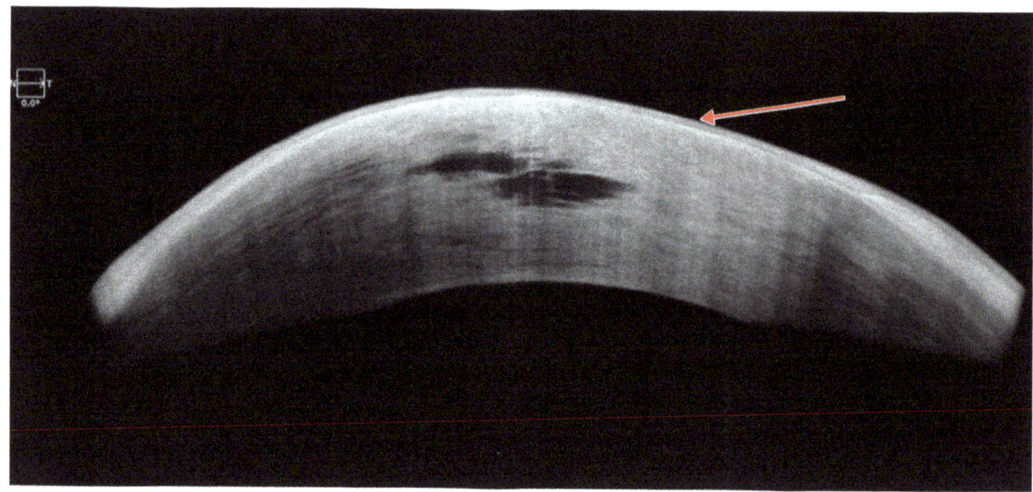

Fig. 2.5.8: Anterior segment optical coherence tomography (ASOCT) showing completely epithelialized surface as shown by red arrow.

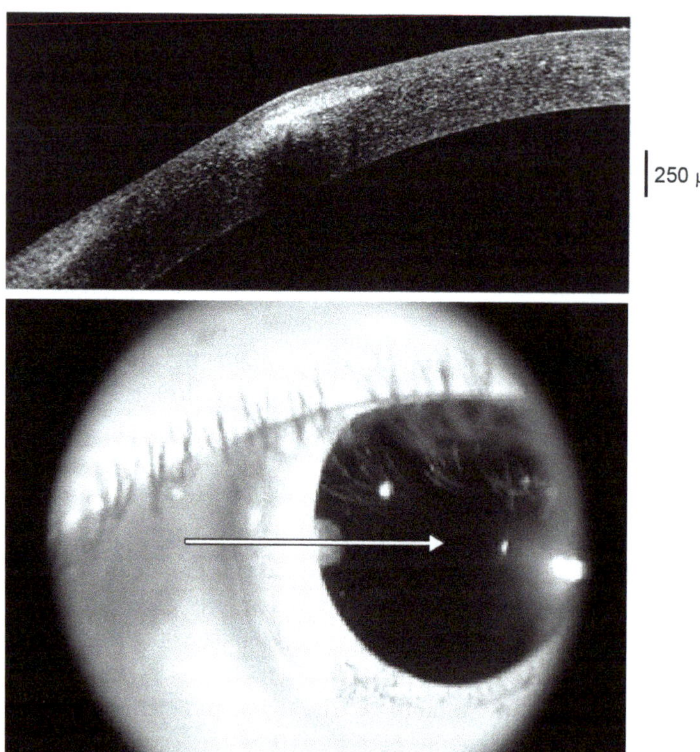

Fig. 2.5.9: Subepithelial corneal infiltrate as seen on anterior segment optical coherence tomography.

Dry Eye

Studies using ASOCT have shown that it is a useful tool for evaluation of tear film thickness, tear meniscus height, and can be used to follow-up response of management of dry eye (Fig. 2.5.10). Recently, it has been used to reconstruct three-dimensional images of meibomian glands thus proving its potential worth in managing meibomian gland disorders.

Anterior Segment Trauma

History of any ocular trauma or a suspected open globe injury is a contraindication for any contact procedure. ASOCT can be used to examine any corneal or scleral perforations and determining size, shape and position of any intraocular foreign body in anterior segment of eye. It is useful for determining the extent of injury in case of media opacity and monitoring response to medical management or amniotic membrane graft (AMG) in cases with thermal or chemical injuries.

Applications in Refractive Surgeries

Anterior segment OCT enables precise measurement of corneal thickness, flap thickness, and residual stromal bed thickness. This is especially useful in cases where a laser-assisted in situ keratomileusis (LASIK) enhancement is planned and can avoid any postoperative ectasia. It has been used to evaluate corneal wound healing responses, interface smoothness, and apposition after manual and laser-assisted LASIK. It can be used in diagnosis and management of postrefractive surgery complications. Interface fluid syndrome is a flap-related complication of LASIK which is characterized by fluid collection in interface, flap edema, and haze.[6]

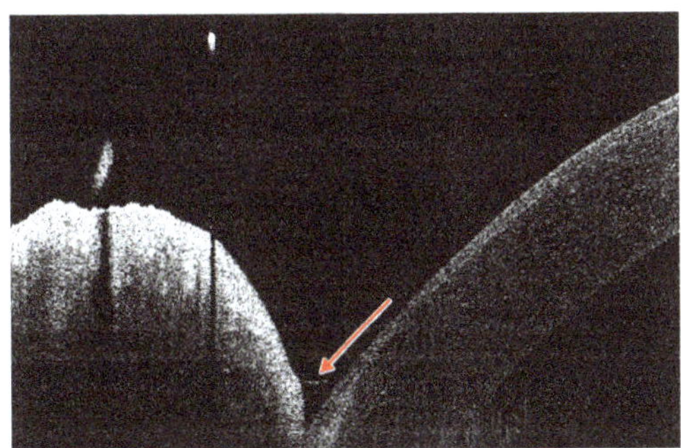

Fig. 2.5.10: Tear meniscus as visualized on anterior segment optical coherence tomography.

Anterior segment OCT has been used to determine implantable collamer lens (ICL) vault. Ideal lens vault varies between 250 microns and 750 microns and anything beyond this range may warrant a replacement procedure.

Applications in Cataract Surgeries

It can be used for evaluation of corneal biometry, lens, AC, and angle structures. Corneal power as measured with ASOCT can be used for calculating IOL power. Tang et al. showed that in patients with previous myopic laser correction, IOL power calculation with ASOCT-based biometry is equally or more accurate than current standard.[7]

Lens density measurement with ASOCT is highly reproducible and correlates well with lens opacity classification system III (LOCS III). It has been used to study corneal incisions and epithelial remodeling after cataract surgeries. Localized Descemet membrane detachments can be visualized at incision sites which are otherwise very difficult to observe clinically.[6]

Applications in Glaucoma

It is useful in quantifying angle closure glaucoma and important landmarks include scleral spur, Schlemm's canal, Schwalbe's line, and trabecular meshwork (Fig. 2.5.11). ASOCT can help in identifying occludable angles and quantifying extent of peripheral anterior

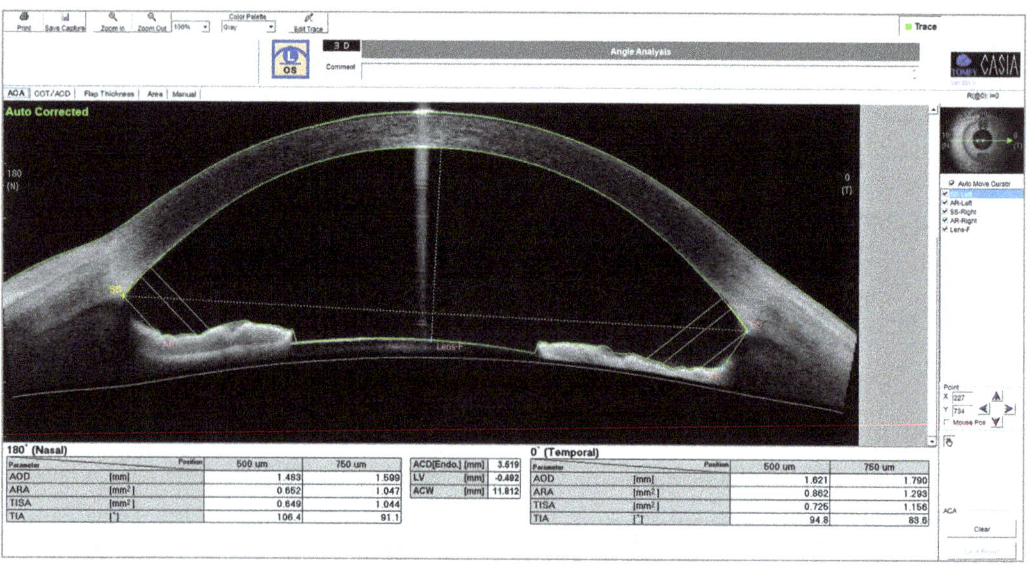

Fig. 2.5.11: Angle details on anterior segment optical coherence tomography.

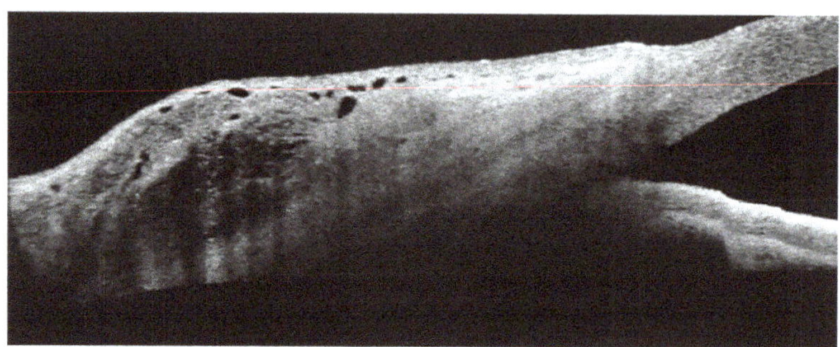

Fig. 2.5.12: Elevated bleb with microcysts.

synechiae. Pre- and post-laser peripheral iridotomy (LPI) ASOCT shows opening up of angles due to posterior falling of iris. It can also be used to confirm patency of peripheral iridotomies and study its healing response.

Pigment dispersion syndrome is characterized by open angle and posterior bowing of peripheral iris giving a typical "S-shaped configuration". "Sinusoidal configuration" of iris in plateau iris syndrome can be picked up. Opening up of AC angle after cataract surgery and IOL implantation can be seen on ASOCT.

It can also be used to study bleb morphology. It can visualize bleb dimensions, bleb wall thickness, flap, bleb cavity, patency of ostium, cysts within the bleb (Fig. 2.5.12), and Ologen implant (Fig. 2.5.13). It can help in identification of failing bleb and its cause so that a timely management is possible.

Failing bleb can show occlusion of ostium, apposition of conjunctiva and episclera to sclera, and absence of bleb wall thickening (bleb wall thickening is a sign of successful bleb). In cases where glaucoma drainage devices (GDDs) have been used, it can be

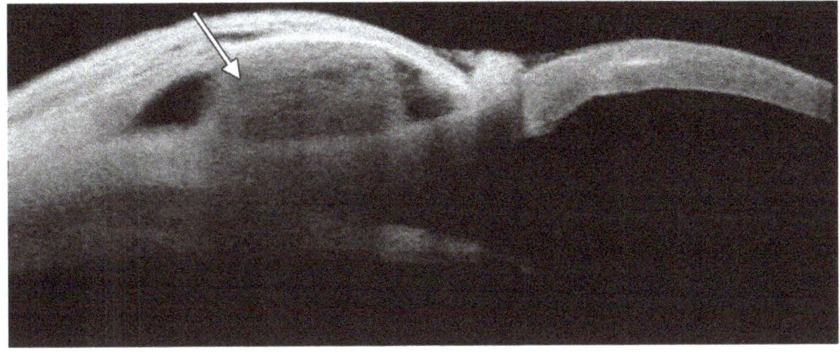

Fig. 2.5.13: Bleb with subconjunctival ologen (arrow).

used to know the position, patency, and state of drainage of GDD tube. Any excessive contact with iris or cornea can be picked up and appropriate management can be done.[8] Biodegradable collagen implants (Fig. 2.5.13) can be visualized in situ with ASOCT and has been used to study implant-tissue interaction.

Use in Squint Surgery

Ocular muscle insertions cannot be evaluated by ocular sonography or by computerized tomography. ASOCT can be used to look at the anterior part of the ocular muscles and muscle insertion. The distance of muscle insertion or absence may be accurately determined using ASOCT.[9-11]

LIMITATIONS

- Inability to visualize beyond iris. It is of no use in conditions where ciliary body imaging is required for diagnosis such as ciliary body tumors, misdirected ciliary processes, etc.
- It is unable to visualize beyond densely opaque media.
- Upper and lower eyelid interferes in imaging of superior and inferior angles thus reducing the amount of data obtained.
- Limited cost-effectiveness.

VIVA QUESTIONS

1. Role of ASOCT in early detection of keratoconus.

Ans. Refer to text.

2. ASOCT classification of keratoconus:

Ans. Keratoconus can be classified into five distinct stages based Fourier-domain OCT findings as proposed by Sandali et al.[12]

1. *Stage 1*: Thinning of apparently normal epithelial and stromal layers at the conus.
2. *Stage 2*: Hyper-reflective anomalies occurring at the Bowman's layer level with epithelial thickening at the conus.
3. *Stage 3*: Posterior displacement of the hyper-reflective structures occurring at the Bowman's layer level with increased epithelial thickening and stromal thinning.
4. *Stage 4*: Pan-stromal scar.
5. *Stage 5*: Corneal hydrops:
    - *Stage 5a, acute onset*: Descemet's membrane rupture with separation of collagen lamellae with large fluid-filled intrastromal and fluid-filled cysts.
    - *Stage 5b, healing stage*: Pan-stromal scarring with a remaining aspect of Descemet's membrane rupture.

3. Difference between TD and SD.

Ans. Refer to Table 2.5.1.

Table 2.5.1: Difference between time domain and spectral domain ASOCT.		
Characteristics	*Visante anterior segment OCT*	*Cirrus HD-OCT [RTVue-OCT (Optovue)]*
Wavelength	1,310 nm	840 nm
Scanning	• 6 mm depth by 16 mm width • 256 A-scan per B-scan • 3 mm depth by 10 mm width 512 A-scan per B-scan • 2,048 A-scans per second	• Cube: 4 × 4 mm, 512 A-scan • 5-line raster: 3 mm, 4,096 A-scans • 26,000 A-scans per second
Resolution	Transverse—60 μm Vertical—18 μm	Transverse—5 μm Vertical—8 μm
Advantage	Can penetrate deeper into the sclera, iris, and cornea than FD-OCT, owing to longer wavelength of its detector	High scan speed, improved resolution, significantly reduces motion artifacts, and increases signal-to-noise ratio
Principle	Time-domain OCT	Fourier-domain OCT

(ASOCT: anterior segment optical coherence tomography; FD-OCT: frequency domain optical coherence tomography; OCT: optical coherence tomography)

4. What is swept source OCT and its role in anterior segment imaging?

Ans. Refer to text.

5. Role of ASOCT in corneal dystrophy classification.

Ans. ASOCT imaging has been included in 2015 update of International Committee for Classification of Corneal Dystrophies (IC3D) classification of corneal dystrophies. It is useful in determining depth and extent of corneal opacities and depositions.

6. Role of ASOCT in Tear film assessment.

Ans. Refer to text.

7. What are DISCOVER and PIONEER study and their impact in anterior segment surgeries?

Ans. Determination of feasibility of Intraoperative Spectral domain microscope combined/integrated OCT Visualization during En face Retinal and ophthalmic surgery (DISCOVER) study examined microscope-integrated OCT systems in ophthalmic surgery.[13] It concluded that real-time iOCT can influence decision-making during Descemet membrane endothelial keratoplasty (DMEK) and is especially useful for novice surgeons. iOCT findings resulted in additional surgical maneuvers in 41% of patients and around 50% of cases, the iOCT provided information that was discordant to surgeon impression.

Prospective Intraoperative and Perioperative Ophthalmic ImagiNg with Optical CoherEncE TomogRaphy (PIONEER) established the feasibility of microscope-mounted portable OCT system.[14] PIONEER study evaluated use of iOCT in both anterior and posterior segment surgeries like lamellar corneal procedures and membrane peeling and concluded that it can influence decision making in both types of surgeries. This technology helps in confirming correct graft orientation, ruling out any interface separation and reduces need of resurgeries. iOCT identified residual persistent fluid in 48% of eyes that resulted in additional surgical maneuvers. In 18% of cases, the surgeon believed there were residual fluids but iOCT confirmed complete apposition, mitigating the need for additional maneuvers.

8. Role of ASOCT post-corneal cross-linking (CXL) of cornea.

Ans. ASOCT has been used to evaluate depth of demarcation line (DL) created after corneal collagen crosslinking procedures. Depth of DL does not depend upon osmolarity of riboflavin. Average depth of DL after epithelium off CXL using Dresden protocol or accelerated protocol is around 300 microns. In transepithelial procedures, it is much shallower and lies at around 100 microns depth.

9. Role of ASOCT in corneal hydrops.

Ans. In corneal hydrops, ASOCT can be used to assess corneal edema, rolled edges, and extent of Descemet detachment. It can be used to monitor resolution of corneal edema and attachment of Descemet membrane after intracameral gas or air injection.

10. ASOCT finding in pigment dispersion syndrome.

Ans. Wide open angle with posterior bowing of iris can be seen on ASOCT (Fig. 2.5.14).

11. Role of ASOCT in detecting lens-induced secondary angle closure glaucoma.

Ans. Thick lens can push iris anteriorly causing narrowing of angle predisposing to angle closure that can be visualized by ASOCT (Fig. 2.5.15).

12. Role of ASOCT in supraciliary effusion.

Ans. ASOCT can be used to detect supraciliary effusion as shown in Figure 2.5.16.

13. Role of ASOCT in keratitis.

Ans. ASOCT can be used to assess depth and extent of corneal infiltrates in keratitis. It can be used to determine location and extent of

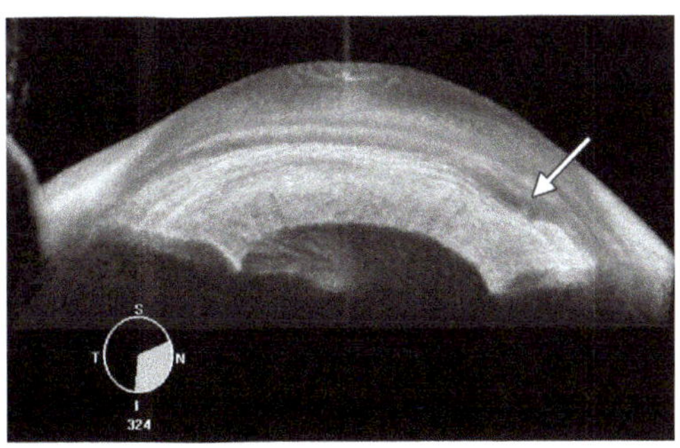

Fig. 2.5.14: Pigment dispersion syndrome showing wide-open angle with posterior bowing of iris.

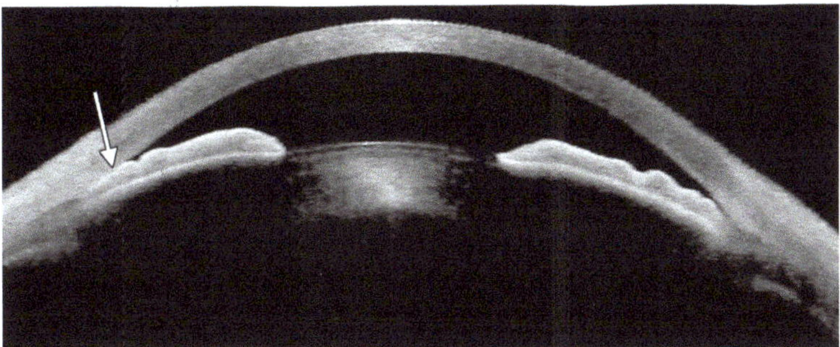

Fig. 2.5.15: Appositional angle closure in primary angle-closure glaucoma (PACG) (arrow).

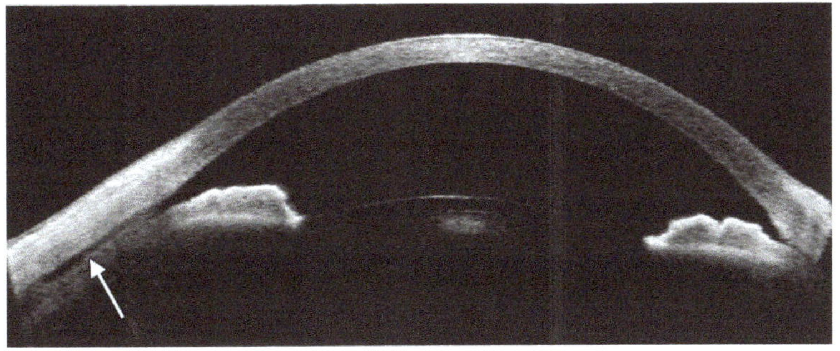

Fig. 2.5.16: Shallow choroidal detachment after trauma (arrow).

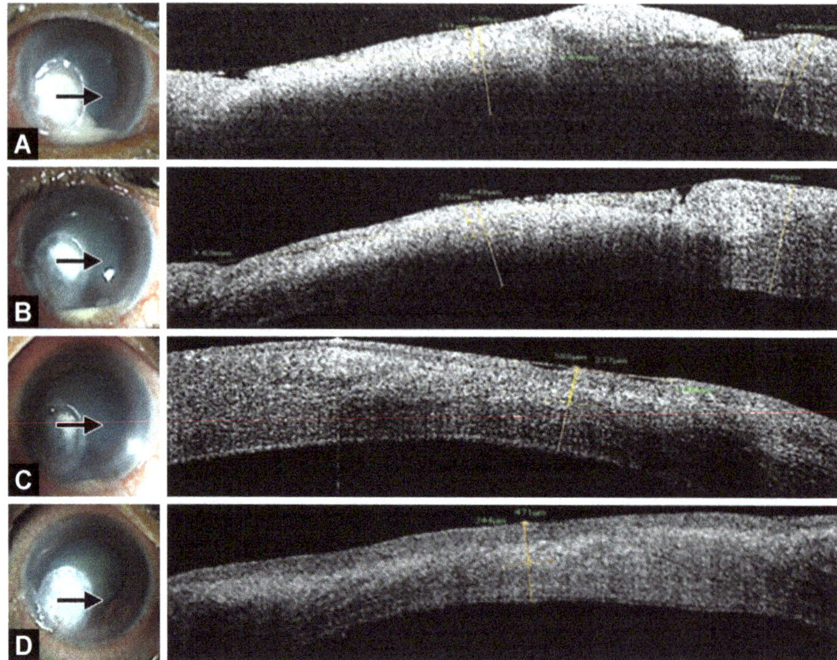

Figs. 2.5.17A to D: Location and extent of corneal infiltrate, thinning, and monitor of healing on anterior segment optical coherence tomography.

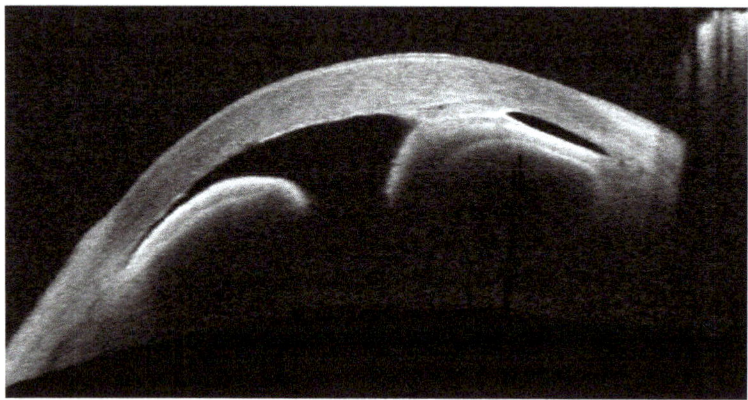

Fig. 2.5.18: Sequel of corneal ulcer such as adherent leukoma visualized on anterior segment optical coherence tomography.

corneal thinning and monitor healing (Figs. 2.5.17A to D). Sequelae of corneal ulcer such as adherent leukoma can be visualized on ASOCT (Fig. 2.5.18).

REFERENCES

1. Huang D, Swanson EA, Lin CP, et al. Optical coherence tomography. Science. 1991;254(5035):1178-81.
2. Izatt JA, Hee MR, Swanson EA, et al. Micrometer-scale resolution imaging of the anterior eye in vivo with optical coherence tomography. Arch Ophthalmol. 1994;112(12): 1584-9.
3. Nesi TT, Leite DA, Rocha FM, et al. Indications of Optical Coherence Tomography in Keratoplasties: Literature Review. J Ophthalmol. 2012;2012:1-6.
4. Vanathi M, Behera G, Vengayil S, et al. Intracameral SF6 injection and anterior

segment OCT-based documentation for acute hydrops management in pellucid marginal corneal degeneration. Contact Lens Anterior Eye. 2008;31(3):164-6.
5. Igbre AO, Rico MC, Garg SJ. High-speed optical coherence tomography as a reliable adjuvant tool to grade ocular anterior chamber inflammation. Retina. 2014;34(3):504-8.
6. Han SB, Liu YC, Noriega KM, et al. Applications of Anterior Segment Optical Coherence Tomography in Cornea and Ocular Surface Diseases. J Ophthalmol. 2016;2016:4971572.
7. Tang M, Wang L, Koch DD, et al. Intraocular lens power calculation after previous myopic laser vision correction based on corneal power measured by Fourier-domain optical coherence tomography. J Cataract Refract Surg. 2012;38(4):589-94.
8. Maslin J, Barkana Y, Dorairaj SK. Anterior segment imaging in glaucoma: An updated review. Indian J Ophthalmol. 2015;63(8):630-40.
9. Paciuc-Beja M, Salcedo-Villanueva G, Quiroz-Mercado H. The accuracy of anterior segment optical coherence tomography (AS-OCT) in localizing extraocular rectus muscles insertions. J AAPOS. 2015;19(5):489-90.
10. Park KA, Lee JY, Oh SY. Reproducibility of horizontal extraocular muscle insertion distance in anterior segment optical coherence tomography and the effect of head position. J AAPOS. 2014;18(1):15-20.
11. Pihlblad MS, Erenler F, Sharma A, et al. Anterior Segment Optical Coherence Tomography of the Horizontal and Vertical Extraocular Muscles With Measurement of the Insertion to Limbus Distance. J Pediatr Ophthalmol Strabismus. 2016;53(3):141-5.
12. Sandali O, El Sanharawi M, Temstet C, et al. Fourier-domain optical coherence tomography imaging in keratoconus: a corneal structural classification. Ophthalmology. 2013;120(12):2403-12.
13. Ehlers JP, Goshe J, Dupps WJ, et al. Determination of feasibility and utility of microscope- integrated optical coherence tomography during ophthalmic Surgery: The DISCOVER Study RESCAN Results. JAMA Ophthalmol. 2015;133(10):1124-32.
14. Ehlers JP, Dupps WJ, Kaiser PK, et al. The prospective intraoperative and Perioperative Ophthalmic ImagiNg with Optical CoherEncE TomogRaphy (PIONEER) study: 2-Year Results. Am J Ophthalmol 2014;158(5):999-1007.

2.6 SPECULAR MICROSCOPE

Pranita Sahay, Mohamed Ibrahime Asif, Divya Agarwal, Prafulla Kumar Maharana

INTRODUCTION

Specular microscope (Fig. 2.6.1) images light that is reflected in a mirror-like fashion off the tissue interface from the incident light.[1] When light strikes a surface it can undergo three types of changes namely reflection, transmission or absorption. In general, it undergoes a combination of all the three effects. Specular reflection occurs when the angle of reflection is equal to the angle of incidence. This reflected light is captured by the microscope. As the reflection can occur from any surface, there are multiple interfaces such as corneal epithelium, stroma, endothelium, and lens. The most important surface for evaluation is between endothelium and aqueous.

David Maurice in 1968[2] described the first specular microscope which was later modified by Laing et al.[3] Subsequently various designs have been introduced that varies in the light projected (stationary slit, moving slit, and moving spot) or optical design (confocal

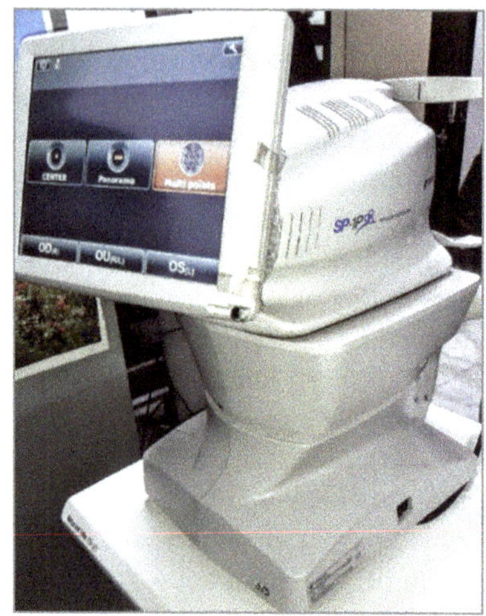

Fig. 2.6.1: Specular microscope.

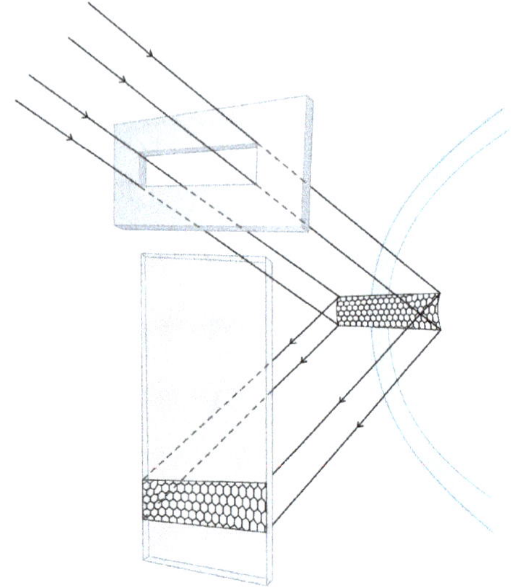
Fig. 2.6.2: Specular reflection.

or non-confocal) or the interface (contact or non-contact).

OPTICAL PRINCIPLE

As discussed specular reflection occurs when the angle of the incident light is equal to the angle of the reflected light at the interface (Fig. 2.6.2).[4] The reflected light is estimated to be about 0.02% of the incident light at the endothelium and aqueous interface. Reflected light from epithelium and stroma can obscure the reflected light from endothelial surface; hence, a narrow slit-beam of light is used for illumination. Laing described that specular microscopy yields image with three or four distinct zones depending on the width of the illuminating slit such as:[3,4]

- *Zone 1*: Epithelium/lens-coupling fluid
- *Zone 2*: Corneal stroma
- *Zone 3*: Corneal endothelium
- *Zone 4*: Aqueous humor.

The boundary between zones 2 and 3 is usually bright called "bright boundary", and the boundary between zones 3 and 4 is almost dark and is termed as "dark boundary".

TYPES OF SPECULAR MICROSCOPES

- *Contact specular microscope*: A contact lens with coupling fluid of refractive index similar to the cornea is needed to eliminate the corneal surface reflection. In such arrangements, corneal thickness also includes contact lens thickness.

  Advantages: Provides good resolution and magnification.

  Disadvantages: Patient discomfort, the risk of spread of infection, artifacts are produced during manipulation.

  Example: HAI Labs, Inc. Lexington (CL-1000xyz), Heidelberg Engineering Vista-confocal contact immersion (corneal module HRT), Nidek Fremont-confocal contact immersion (Confoscan 4).
- *Non-contact specular microscope*: In this, the reflection from the anterior corneal surface is eliminated by increasing the angle of incidence, so the reflection is moved to the side covering less of specular reflection from endothelium.

Advantages: Greater patient comfort, no risk of corneal trauma/infections, a broader field of view.

Disadvantages: Decreased resolution and magnification due to uncontrolled eye movements.

Example: CEM-530, confoscan 4.

- *Wide-field specular microscope*: Standard specular microscope is modified using a scanning mirror which increases the field to 800 microns diameter with no loss in contrast.

  Advantages: 10–15 times increased field of view, improved resolution of endothelium, endothelial topography is more easily evaluated with easier visualization of a specific region, improved optics so decreased annoying reflections.

PROCEDURE

The patient is explained about the procedure. Then, the patient is seated comfortably that is very important to obtain a good scan. In non-contact, the patient is asked to blink so that the corneal surface remains wet and smooth before capturing image. If using contact microscope, topical anesthesia is employed. Once contacted, punctate epithelial erosions can be seen; however, they disappear within a few hours. An internal fixation target is used to keep the patient's eye straight.

The image can be captured in three ways, such as:

1. *Automated*: This mode is quick and requires virtually no training as both alignment, and auto firing are automated. It is convenient for any user.
2. *Semi-automated*: In this mode, the user has better control over the area of examination while automatic mode simplifies the capture. It is useful in patients with fixation difficulty or irregular cornea.
3. *Manual*: Offers total control to the examiner as both alignment and firing are manual. This mode is useful in corneas with weak reflection or other anomalies.

Analytic Measurements

The qualitative examination involves analysis of the cell borders, configuration, cell intersections, guttae, intracellular bodies, vacuoles or bleb.[3,4]

Quantitative analysis includes calculation of cell area, density, polymegathism, and pleomorphism.[3,4]

Qualitative Analysis

Cell conformation: Normal endothelium is quasi-hexagonal/quasi-regular with side lengths equal and angle of intersection approximately 120°.

Cell boundaries: Often boundaries appear as dark, narrow lines.

Quantitative Analysis

- *Endothelial cell density (ECD)*: ECD is calculated as cells/mm^2. ECD can be determined by various methods like:
  - *Comparison method*: By comparing cells imaged with a standard set of hexagonal cell size design
  - *Frame method*: All cells within a frame are counted and are expressed as cells/mm^2. The problem is the need for adjustment of cells overlying the border by counting partial cells as full cells on two adjacent frames. It can be a fixed-frame or a variable-frame method (Figs. 2.6.3A and B).
  - *Corner method*: Cell border corners are taken into account to determine cell area from a polygon digitization.
  - *Center method*: The center of contiguous cells is marked to facilitate counting.

Endothelial cell density does not reflect the status of endothelial function accurately. This is evidenced by a clear cornea, even with

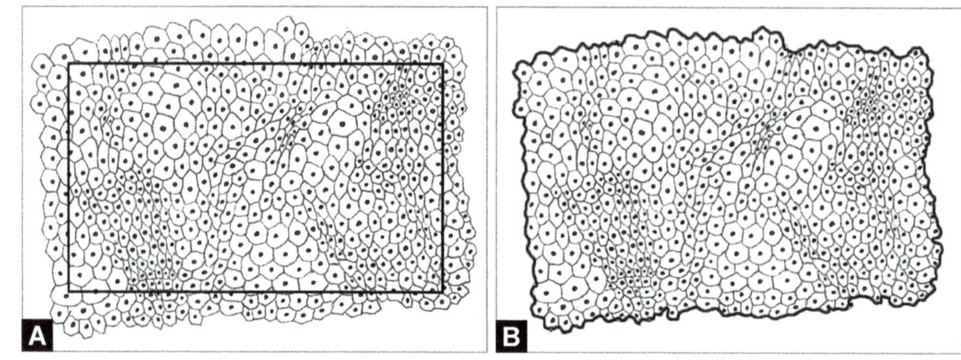

Figs. 2.6.3A and B: (A) Fixed frame analysis; (B) Variable frame analysis.

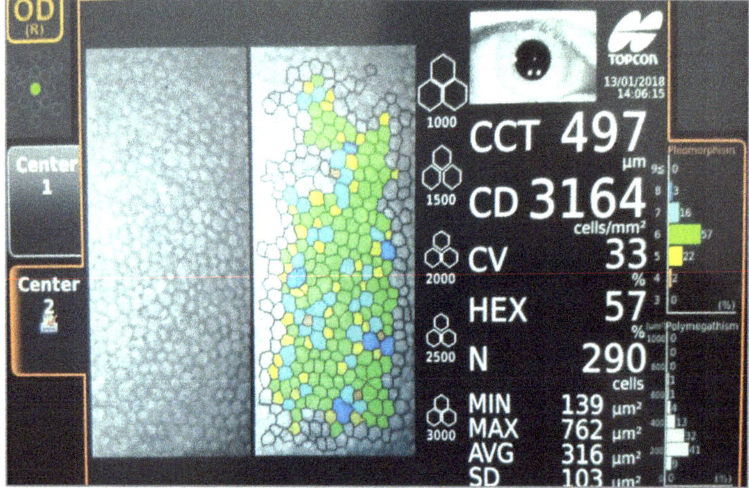

Fig. 2.6.4: Specular microscopy of a normal corneal endothelium.

ECD as low as 500 cells/mm². Theoretically, coefficient of variation (CV) and percentage of hexagonal cells are a better indicator for corneal endothelium dysfunction.

The coefficient of variation: Mean cell area is measured as µm²/cell. The CV is determined by measuring the areas of a population of cells and calculating the coefficient of variance which is the standard deviation of mean cell area divided by mean cell area. Normal coefficient of variation is 0.40. Anything above 0.4 is considered abnormal.

Pleomorphism: It is usually measured as a percentage of six, less than six or more than six-sided cells. Percentage of hexagonal cells endothelial mosaic in a healthy cornea is around 70–80% (Fig. 2.6.4).

CLINICAL APPLICATIONS

- *Specular microscopy is useful in the following*:
    - *Diagnosis of diseases*: For example, Fuchs endothelial dystrophy, posterior (Fig. 2.6.5) polymorphous dystrophy (PPMD) and bullous keratopathy.
- *Research and monitoring of endothelium*: For assessment of changes in the endothelium associated with:

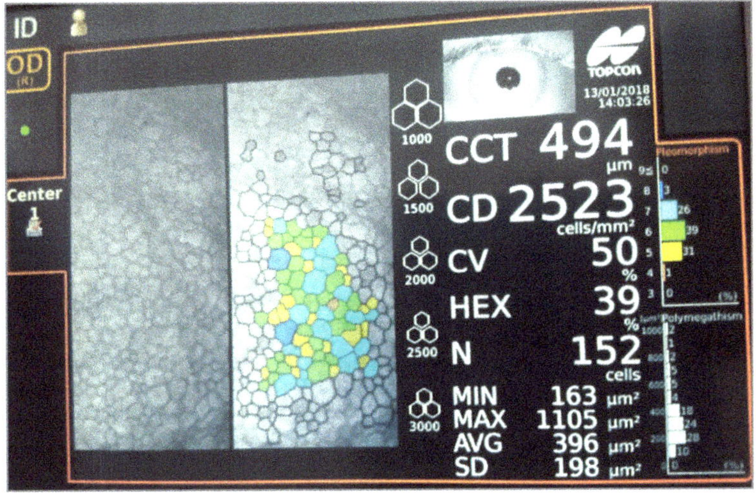

Fig. 2.6.5: Specular microscopy of a case with abnormal findings.

- Aging
- Surgical procedures like keratoplasty, cataract surgery, and LASIK (laser-assisted in situ keratomileusis)
- Pathological conditions like glaucoma, uveitis, and trauma
- Contact lens use
- Endothelial cell culture
- Comparison of different surgical procedures.

▪ *Eye banking*: For assessment of endothelium in donor corneas and the effect of preservation—Grading of donor cornea in eye bank is done on the basis of ECD of the donor cornea. A minimum of 2,000 cells/mm^2 is required to grade a donor cornea as an optical grade. A higher ECD is required for endothelial keratoplasty (2,300–2,500 cells/mm^2).

▪ *Surgery*: *Decision-making*—for example,
- ECD < 1,000 may be a relative contraindication (CI) for cataract surgery.
- Less than 1,500 is a CI for putting an ACIOL.
- Less than 2,500 is a CI for phakic IOL (ICL)
- Less than 800 is an indication to go for Descemet's stripping automated endothelial keratoplasty (DSAEK) triple in cases of Fuchs endothelial corneal dystrophy (FECD) with cataract.

▪ *For assessment of the long-term effect of surgeries*: efficacy of cataract surgery; comparison of different forms of endothelial keratoplasty [DSAEK vs Descemet's membrane endothelial keratoplasty (DMEK), penetrating keratoplasty (PKP) versus deep anterior lamellar keratoplasty (DALK)].

▪ *For measuring the corneal thickness (with contact type)*

▪ *For assessment of epithelium and lens.*

Common conditions and their specular findings: This has been summarized in Table 2.6.1.

VIVA QUESTIONS

1. What is the principle of a specular microscope?

Ans. Refer to text.

Table 2.6.1: Common conditions and their specular findings.

Conditions	*Specular findings*
Keratoconus	Stretched cells with long axis in the direction of the apex of the cone. Dark bodies inside normal appearing cell can also be seen
Lattice corneal dystrophy	Branching criss-cross lines in the stroma which are believed to be amyloid deposits. A crater form appearance has also been described
Posterior polymorphous corneal dystrophy	Vesicles with dark, thick border yielding doughnut appearance, appears to lie anterior to undistorted endothelial cells
Fuchs endothelial corneal dystrophy	Guttae (excrescences) with adjacent distorted endothelial cells. They appear as dark spots sometimes with central bright corneal reflections
Iridocorneal endothelial syndrome	ICE/ICE-berg cells look like PPMD vesicles within endothelium. There is loss of cellular definition and increased granularity and can eventually become completely blacked out areas. A reversal pattern may develop with black central and white borders
Glaucoma	Decreased endothelial count
Intraocular inflammation	Mononuclear inflammatory cells are seen between endothelial cells. Endothelial cells are generally unharmed
Contact lens wear	• Within minutes—small dark endothelial blebs occur but disappear quickly if lens is removed • Long-term-increased polymegathism that does not reverse, depends on duration and type of contact lens use
Diabetes	• Decreased cell density with age, increased polymegathism and pleomorphism and decreased hexagonality. • Topical aldose reductase inhibitor reverses this morphologic changes

(ICE: iridocorneal endothelial syndrome; PPMD: posterior polymorphous corneal dystrophy)

2. What is the normal endothelial cell count at birth and amount of loss with aging?

Ans. Normal endothelial cell density at birth is around 6,000 cells/mm^2. The count falls by 26% in the first year of life and a further decrease of 26% over the next 11 years. This rapid loss is partly due to the enlarging globe. It stabilizes from the age of 20 years through 50 years. After 60 years, on an average endothelial loss is approximately 0.5% per year.

3. What is bi-exponential decay model for endothelial cell loss?

Ans. The loss of endothelial cells follow a bi-exponential decay, i.e. a phase of rapid loss followed by a phase of the slow rate of endothelial loss.[5] Although this theory is not well established, it is supported by the results of most of the studies exploring endothelial cell loss. The proposed rates have been described in Table 2.6.2.

Table 2.6.2: Phases of endothelial loss.

Condition	*Rapid*	*Slow*
Age	14–15 years	Rest of the life
Cataract	6 months	21 years
Penetrating keratoplasty	4 years	26 years

4. What are the different rates of endothelial loss following ocular surgeries?

Ans. Refer to Table 2.6.3.[6-13]

5. What are the parameters measured using a specular microscope and its significance?

Ans. Refer to text.

Table 2.6.3: Different rates of endothelial loss following ocular surgeries.

Surgery	*EC loss*
Phacoemulsification	5–8% at 3 weeks and 6 months[10] 10.5% at 1 year[6]
ECCE	9.1% at 1 year[6]
SICS	4.21% at 6 weeks (4.72% for ECCE and 5.41% for phacoemulsification)[7]
ICCE	15–50%[8]
PKP	11% ± 20% at 6 months and 20% ± 23% at 12 months[9]
DALK	14.2% ± 11.7% at 1 month (the loss was 8.6% at 1 year and 13.9% at 5 years compared to the 1 month endothelial cell density)[10]
DSAEK	34% ± 22% at 6 months 38% ± 22% at 1 year[9]
DMEK	35% at 6 months, 38% at 1 year, 43% at 2 years, 55% at 5 years[11]
PPV	9.0% ± 14.6% at 3 months[12]
Trabeculectomy	7% after penetrating surgery and 2.6% after nonpenetrating surgery at 3 months (non-combined surgeries)[13]

(DALK: deep anterior lamellar keratoplasty; DMEK: Descemet membrane endothelial keratoplasty; DSAEK: Descemet stripping automated endothelial keratoplasty; ECCE: extracapsular cataract extraction; ICCE: intracapsular cataract extraction; PKP: penetrating keratoplasty; PPV: pars plana vitrectomy; SICS: small incision cataract surgery)

6. What are different methods of estimating endothelial cell count?

Ans. Refer to text.

7. What are the changes seen in specular microscopy in Fuchs corneal dystrophy?

Ans. Specular microscopy of FECD demonstrates the following changes.[14]

- *Stage 1*: Characterized by the presence of Guttae which are small to begin with, and more numerous centrally. The surrounding cells are normal. The sides of excrescences appear dark while their apex is bright.
- *Stage 2*: Size of the guttae becomes equal to that of endothelial cells.
- *Stage 3*: Guttae grow in size and become considerably larger than that of endothelial cells. The borders of the endothelial cell become blurred due to the presence of guttae.
- *Stage 4*: Guttae coalesce, blurring the adjacent boundaries. Multiple apical bright spots can be seen (coalesce of adjacent guttae). In advanced disease, complete disorganization of the adjacent endothelial mosaic is seen (few authors call it stage 5).

8. What are the changes seen in specular microscopy in iridocorneal endothelial (ICE) syndrome?

Ans. Specular microscopy of FECD demonstrates the following changes:

- Rounding off of cell angles
- Loss of shape, many pentagonal cells are evident
- Cells appear more granular
- The appearance of central dark areas in endothelial cells
- In advanced cases, loss of endothelial mosaic
- The typical appearance of central black with bright borders is reversed, i.e. there will be black central areas and white borders (also known as ICE cells).

9. What are the changes seen in specular microscopy in diabetes?

Ans. The following changes can occur in diabetes:
- A rapid decrease in ECD with age
- Normal corneal thickness
- Increased polymegathism
- Increased pleomorphism
- Decreased percentage of hexagonality.

10. How do guttae appear in specular microscopy?

Ans. Corneal guttae are focal excrescences of collagenous basement membrane material which have accumulated on Descemet's membrane, across the central cornea.[15]
- Corneal guttata are focal droplet-like accumulations of non-banded collagen on the posterior surface of Descemet's membrane that appear as dark areas in between the bright endothelial cells.[16]
- These are commonly found in elderly people (9.6% of people older than 40 years and 3.3% of those between 20 years and 40 years old had corneal guttata without edema).[16]
- Most common corneal disorder with gutta formation includes Fuchs' corneal endothelial dystrophy.

Other conditions where guttae are seen include: trauma, congenital glaucoma, macular dystrophy and corneal dystrophy resulting from βig-h3 R124H mutation (granular dystrophy, Reis-Bücklers dystrophy, lattice dystrophy and Avellino dystrophy).[16]

11. What is pseudogutta?

Ans. These are transient guttata-like features, usually found in cases of trauma, or intraocular inflammation. Pseudoguttaise considered to be formed due to endothelial edema or pigmentation.

12. How to void error in specular microscopy?

Ans. The following precautions may reduce the amount of error:
- By taking an average of multiple readings from the same reason using the same settings
- By keeping the image analysis method similar at every follow-up
- By measuring both density and morphology
- Regional variations must be kept in mind such as the ECD is higher in paracentral and peripheral areas compared to the central area.

REFERENCES

1. Hu V, Hughes EH, Patel N, et al. The effect of aqualase and phacoemulsification on the corneal endothelium. Cornea. 2010;29(3):247-50.
2. Maurice DM. Cellular membrane activity in the corneal endothelium of the intact eye. Experientia. 1968;24(11):1094-5.
3. Laing RA, Sandstrom MM, Leibowitz HM. Clinical specular microscopy. II. Qualitative evaluation of corneal endothelial photomicrographs. Arch Ophthalmol Chic Ill 1960. 1979;97(9):1720-5.
4. Laing RA, Sandstrom MM, Leibowitz HM. Clinical specular microscopy. I. Optical principles. Arch Ophthalmol Chic Ill 1960. 1979;97(9):1714-9.
5. Armitage WJ, Dick AD, Bourne WM. Predicting endothelial cell loss and long-term corneal graft survival. Invest Ophthalmol Vis Sci. 2003;44(8):3326-31.
6. Bourne RRA, Minassian DC, Dart JKG, et al. Effect of cataract surgery on the corneal endothelium: modern phacoemulsification compared with extracapsular cataract surgery. Ophthalmology. 2004;111(4):679-85.
7. George R, Rupauliha P, Sripriya AV, et al. Comparison of endothelial cell loss and surgically induced astigmatism following conventional extracapsular cataract surgery, manual small-incision surgery and phacoemulsification. Ophthalmic Epidemiol. 2005;12(5):293-7.
8. Neetens A, Dierens M, Delgadillo R. Endothelial Cell Damage after Intracapsular

Cataract Extraction and Primary Anterior Chamber Pseudophakos Implantation. Ophthalmologica. 1983;187(2):114-7.
9. Price MO, Gorovoy M, Benetz BA, et al. Descemet's Stripping Automated Endothelial Keratoplasty Outcomes Compared with Penetrating Keratoplasty from the Cornea Donor Study. Ophthalmology. 2010;117(3): 438-44.
10. Zhang Y, Wu S, Yao Y. Long-term comparison of full-bed deep anterior lamellar keratoplasty and penetrating keratoplasty in treating keratoconus. J Zhejiang Univ Sci B. 2013;14(5):438-50.
11. Baydoun L, Tong CM, Tse WW, et al. Endothelial cell density after descemet membrane endothelial keratoplasty: 1 to 5-year follow-up. Am J Ophthalmol. 2012;154(4): 762-3.
12. Koushan K, Mikhail M, Beattie A, et al. Corneal endothelial cell loss after pars plana vitrectomy and combined phacoemulsification-vitrectomy surgeries. Can J Ophthalmol J Can Ophtalmol. 2017;52(1):4-8.
13. Arnavielle S, Lafontaine PO, Bidot S, et al. Corneal endothelial cell changes after trabeculectomy and deep sclerectomy. J Glaucoma. 2007;16(3):324-8.
14. Jackson AJ, Robinson FO, Frazer DG, et al. Corneal guttata: a comparative clinical and specular micrographic study. Eye Lond Engl. 1999;13 (Pt 6):737-43.
15. Die Sichtbarkeit des lebenden Hornhautendothels | SpringerLink [Internet]. [cited 2018 Jan 7]. [online] Available from https://link.springer.com/article/10.1007/BF02004299 [Accessed Jan., 2019].
16. Akimune C, Watanabe H, Maeda N, et al. Corneal guttata associated with the corneal dystrophy resulting from a βig-h3 R124H mutation. Br J Ophthalmol. 2000;84(1):67-71.

2.7 ULTRASONIC PACHYMETER

Pranita Sahay, Mohamed Ibrahime Asif, Namrata Sharma

INTRODUCTION

Pachymetry is derived from the Greek word: *Pachos* meaning thick and *metry* meaning to measure. It refers to the measurement of corneal thickness. Central corneal thickness (CCT) is an indirect indicator of endothelial cell function. Pachymetry is used prior to refractive surgery, for screening ectatic corneal diseases and for glaucoma suspects.

Normal range: In healthy eyes, it ranges from 0.49 mm to 0.56 mm at the center, 0.52 mm to 0.57 mm in the paracentral region, and 0.7 mm to 0.9 mm at the limbus. Also, the thinnest quadrant is the temporal cornea followed by inferior. In general, a CCT of more than or equal to 0.7 mm suggests corneal endothelial cell dysfunction. Also, if the thickness of the center of the cornea is more than the midperipheral cornea, it points towards endothelial cell dysfunction.

PRINCIPLES

Broadly, pachymeters are based on either ultrasonic principles or optical principles. Most modern pachymeters are based on optical principle. The ultrasonic measurement is based on the reflection of ultrasonic waves from the anterior and posterior corneal surfaces. The time difference (transit time) between the echoes of the reflected ultrasonic signal from the anterior and posterior surface of the cornea to the transducer is used to measure the corneal thickness.

Corneal thickness is calculated by following the simple formula:

Corneal thickness = (Transit time × Propagation velocity) / 2

The speed of sound in the cornea is 1,640 m/s.

An ultrasonic pachymeter has the following important components (Figs. 2.7.1 and 2.7.2):

- *Probe handle*: Which constitutes piezo-electric crystal that emits an ultrasonic beam of 20 MHz.
- *Transducer*: Which sends ultrasonic waves and receives echoes from the corneal surface.
- *Tip*: Having a diameter not more than 2 mm.

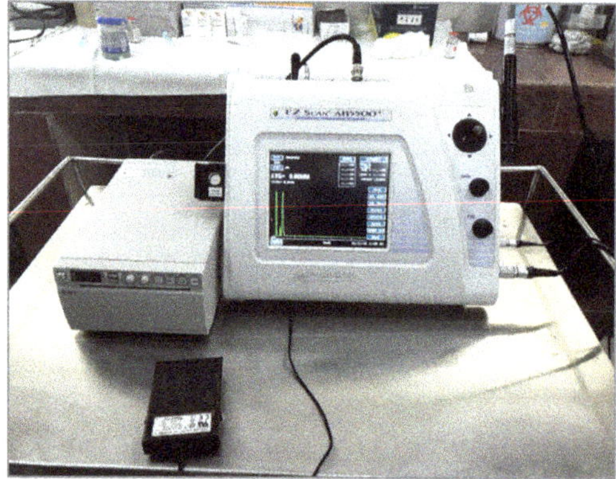

Fig. 2.7.1: A-scan pachymeter.

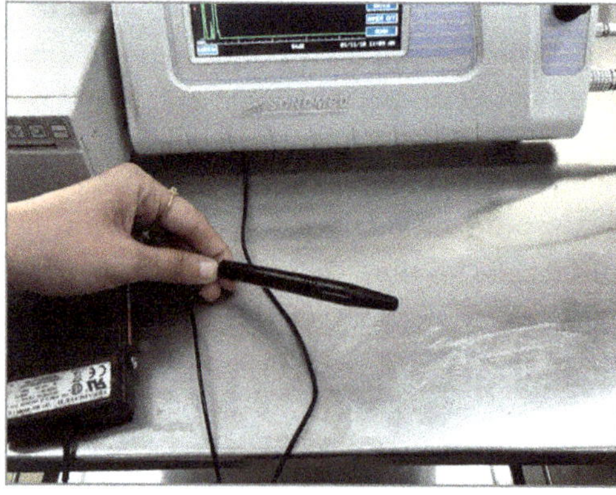

Fig. 2.7.2: Pachymeter probe.

TECHNIQUES OF PACHYMETRIC MEASUREMENTS

There are two types of pachymetric techniques:

1. *Spot measurements*: This technology is used in traditional optical pachymetry, specular microscopy, confocal microscopy, ultrasound pachymetry, and optical low-coherence reflectometry.
2. *Wide area mapping:* This technique provides the ability to map a wide area of the cornea and includes slit scanning optical pachymetry and very high-frequency ultrasound imaging. Pachymetric mapping provides several advantages over spot measurements:
   - Mapping technique might helps to reveal corneal abnormalities such as keratoconus and pellucid marginal degeneration.
   - It also allows preoperative planning for corneal surgeries that primarily do not concern just the center of the cornea, such as astigmatic keratotomy, intracorneal ring segment (ICRS) implantation, deep anterior lamellar keratoplasty (DALK), and phototherapeutic keratectomy.

Despite these advantages, conventional ultrasound spot pachymetry is still the gold standard because of its reliability, ease of use, and relatively low cost.

OTHER TECHNIQUES OF PACHYMETRY

Methods of pachymetry (Flowchart 2.7.1) include the following:

- Ultrasonic techniques:
  - Conventional ultrasonic pachymetry
  - Ultrasound biomicroscopy (UBM)
- Optical techniques:
  - Manual optical pachymetry
  - Specular microscopy

Flowchart 2.7.1: Pachymetry techniques.

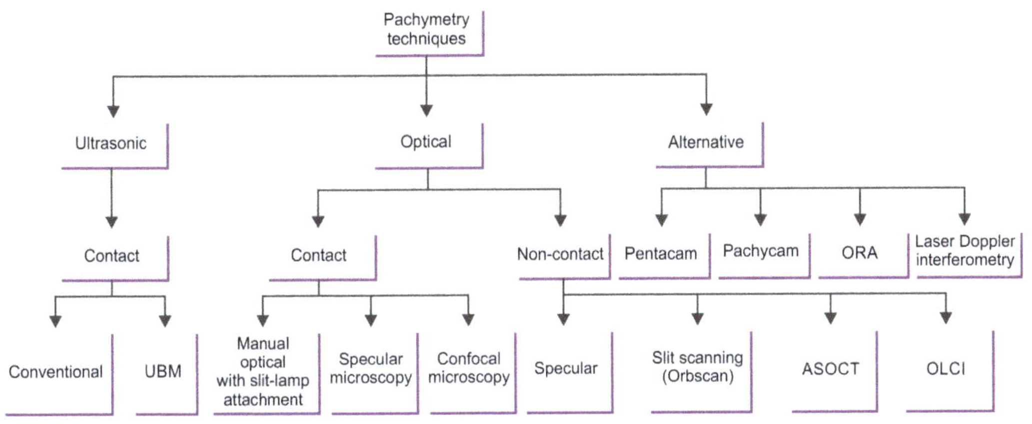

(ASOCT: anterior segment optical coherence tomography; OLCI: optical low coherence interferometry; ORA: ocular response analyzer; UBM: ultrasound biomicroscopy)

- Scanning slit technology
- Optical coherence tomography (OCT) [anterior segment OCT (ASOCT), IOLMaster 700]
- Optical low coherence interferometry (OLCI) [Lenstar)
- Confocal microscopy
- Laser Doppler interferometry
- Partial coherence interferometry (PCI)

- Alternative measurements:
  - Pentacam
  - Pachycam
  - Ocular response analyzer (ORA).

Ultrasonic method is regarded as the gold standard by Henderson and Kremer introduced it in 1980. Older units were more expensive and subject to alignment errors. With the improvement in ultrasound technology, these instruments give less intersession and intraobserver variation with consistent and repeatable readings when compared to optical pachymetry.[1] They can be used intraoperatively and require no coupling medium. However, ultrasound pachymetry comes with a few disadvantages. Being a contact procedure; topical anesthesia is required so, is most undesirable in the early postoperative period. They have poor resolution and have limited accuracy, as the probe is handheld. Indentation on the cornea can lead to underestimation of CCT. Modern ultrasound pachymeters are lightweight with good portability, have memory storage capability, intraocular pressure (IOP) correction factor, high accuracy of ±5 microns, and resolution of 1 micron.

Maurice and Giardini first described optical methods of pachymetry as early as in 1951. These methods used various equations depending upon variables, such as corneal refractive index and anterior radius of curvature, to calculate corneal thickness and often had variable accuracy. The major advantages include relatively low cost and a noncontact technique. Specular microscopes were later designed to measure corneal thickness using electromechanical devices. Other optical methods utilize rotating three-dimensional (3D) Scheimpflug camera (available in Pentacam and Galilei devices) to obtain corneal tomography images noninvasively and provide a highly reproducible measure of CCT along with helping in the evaluation of regional changes in corneal thickness.

Anterior segment OCT (ASOCT) is an easy and comfortable method for patients since it is a noncontact procedure and allows rapid image acquisition. It allows quantification of structures including corneal epithelium and images through corneal opacity. However, it may not always be used interchangeably with ultrasound pachymetry for CCT measurement.

The Orbscan device uses slit-scanning technology and measures the corneal thickness along with anterior and posterior corneal elevations. It, however, overestimates corneal thickness by almost 5%.

Optical low coherence interferometry methods use a diode laser beam and are attached to slit lamps. They measure only the CCT and have a precision of up to 1 micron.

Confocal microscopy is unique as it uses a computerized scanning system to provide total corneal thickness while evaluating cornea at high magnification (20X–500X). It has moderate to good repeatability and has slower data acquisition as compared to other methods.

USES

- *Refractive surgeries*: CCT is used while planning refractive surgeries[2] as adequate preoperative thickness is critical in reducing the risk of developing postrefractive surgery ectasia. Residual stromal bed thickness of 250–300 µm is recommended before going for laser-assisted in situ keratomileusis (LASIK) surgery. Patients with thinner corneas should be considered for surface ablation procedures.
- *Glaucoma suspects*: Corneal thickness influences IOP. Tonometry often overestimates or underestimates IOP in eyes with thicker and thinner corneas, respectively. Thin CCT is an independent risk factor for the development of glaucomatous optic neuropathy.[3] A correction factor of 0.7 must be used and deducted or added for every 10 µm above or below, respectively, from the average corneal thickness (530 µm for Indian population).
- *Congenital glaucoma*: CCT has been reported to be higher in cases of primary congenital glaucoma.[4] Pachymetry is essential for management of pediatric glaucoma.
- *Post-keratoplasty patients*: Pachymetry measurement tells about the health of a transplanted cornea. Serial measurement of CCT can be used for follow-up of post-keratoplasty patients to record the progress of corneal deturgescence. Besides, increase in CCT is an early indication of endothelial dysfunction or graft failure. Serial CCT measurement following an acute episode of graft rejection helps in detecting the response to pulse steroid therapy.
- *Contact lens*: Prolonged contact lens wear can cause corneal edema and hypoxia. This is seen most commonly with daily wear, extended wear, and therapeutic lenses.
- *Corneal ectasia*: Pachymetry helps to determine and to monitor abnormalities of corneal structure or function. Corneal thinning is noted in disorders like keratoconus and pellucid marginal degeneration while corneal thickening is seen in cases of endothelial dystrophy and other causes of endothelial dysfunction.
- *Corneal decompensation*: Corneal thickening is seen in endothelial dysfunction due to Fuchs endothelial corneal dystrophy (FECD) and herpetic endotheliitis. In cases of FECD with corneal stromal swelling of 20% or CCT more than 640 µm, the risk of corneal decompensation after cataract surgery is significant.[5]

- *Decision making*: Computed tomography (CT) is an essential determinant for deciding upon the type of surgery, e.g. in cases of keratoconus [to decide for corneal collagen cross-linking, automated lamellar therapeutic keratoplasty (ALTK), deep anterior lamellar keratoplasty (DALK) or intrastromal corneal ring segment (ICRS)]. Similarly, CCT is essential to decide whether to go for a triple procedure or only Descemet stripping automated endothelial keratoplasty (DSAEK) in cases of FECD with cataract.

VIVA QUESTIONS

1. What is Artemis digital ultrasound?

Ans. Artemis is a very high frequency (VHF) digital ultrasound that uses a 50 MHz VHF ultrasound transducer with immersion scanning technology. These waves are swept in an arc by a high precision mechanism to acquire B-scans, which follow the surface contour of anterior or posterior segment structures. Artemis possesses an adjustment mechanism for the radius of curvature to enable maximum perpendicularity and enhanced signal to noise ratio. Digital signal processing significantly enhances the signal to noise ratio compared to analog processing by a factor of 3 thereby, reducing the noise. Its axial resolution is 21 micron, and 3D-layered pachymetry (using multiple meridional scans) has precision less than 1.0 micron.

2. What is layered corneal pachymetry?

Ans. Layered corneal pachymetry is measuring the individual thickness of different components of the cornea like the epithelium, stroma, cornea, flap, and residual stromal bed. This can be done using Artemis VHF ultrasound, which has high repeatability.

3. What is normal corneal thickness?

Ans. Mean CCT is 515 microns (410-625 microns). In the paracentral region, the corneal thickness varies from 522 microns inferiorly to 574 microns superiorly while in the peripheral zone, thickness varies from 633 microns inferiorly to 673 microns superiorly.

4. Impact of CCT on IOP measurement.

Ans. Deviations from average CCT are a source of error in the measurement of IOP. In cases with corneal edema, IOP is often underestimated. Similarly, in patients with normal corneas, IOP is often overestimated in thicker corneas whereas, underestimated in thinner corneas. Ehler and colleagues have reported that the average error is 0.7 mm Hg per 10 microns of deviation from the mean 520 microns.

REFERENCES

1. Salz JJ, Azen SP, Berstein J, et al. Evaluation and comparison of sources of variability in the measurement of corneal thickness with ultrasonic and optical pachymeters. Ophthalmic Surg. 1983;14(9):750-4.
2. Marsich MW, Bullimore MA. The repeatability of corneal thickness measures. Cornea. 2000;19(6):792-5.
3. Kass MA, Heuer DK, Higginbotham EJ, et al. The Ocular Hypertension Treatment Study: a randomized trial determines that topical ocular hypotensive medication delays or prevents the onset of primary open-angle glaucoma. Arch Ophthalmol. 2002;120(6):701-13.
4. Lopes JE, Wilson RR, Alvim HS, et al. Central corneal thickness in pediatric glaucoma. J Pediatr Ophthalmol Strabismus. 2007;44(2):112-7.
5. Seitzman GD, Gottsch JD, Stark WJ. Cataract surgery in patients with Fuchs' corneal dystrophy: expanding recommendations for cataract surgery without simultaneous keratoplasty. Ophthalmology. 2005;112(3):441-6.

2.8 ORBSCAN

Alisha Kishore, Pranita Sahay, Ritu Nagpal

INTRODUCTION

A wide range of devices are available for performing corneal topography. Adequate knowledge is needed about the advanced computerized systems along with the normal ranges of various parameters for evaluation. "Orbscan" (Bausch and Lomb Inc, Rochester, NY, USA) and "Pentacam" (Oculus GmBH, Wetzlar, Germany) are the most common systems in use. Orbscan is scanning slit, noncontact tomography system.[1]

PRINCIPLE

Scanning Slit System

A series of slit-lamp beams are compiled across the cornea to create a profile of the cornea. The curvature of the anterior surface of the cornea along with posterior surface and anterior surface of the lens and iris can be assessed. The concept of "*slit scanning*" and "*triangulation*" is used to extrapolate the actual spatial location of multiple points on the surface.

The entire cornea is covered with 40 vertical slits, 20 from the right and 20 from the left (Figs. 2.8.1A and B), normal to the surface at each point of acquisition capturing the backscattered light. Each of the slits has 240 points, so a total of 9,600 points and data for points in between is interpolated. The acquisition time is 1.5 seconds.

Orbscan II combines both a scanning slit and Placido disc system. Orbscan IIz is integrated with a Shack-Hartmann aberrometer in the Zyoptix workstation.

INTERPRETATION OF DIFFERENT MAPS

There are four different maps known as quad map. It includes the anterior elevation map, posterior elevation map, curvature map, and the pachymetry map.[2] The map should be read in the following order.

Details of the Patient

Check the *details* of the patient which includes name, date, and eye. Check the scale range and step interval which can be absolute or normalized.

Absolute scale (standardized): There is same dioptric power step on every map. The advantage is that it allows a direct comparison of two different maps and rapid pattern recognition of topographic maps is possible.

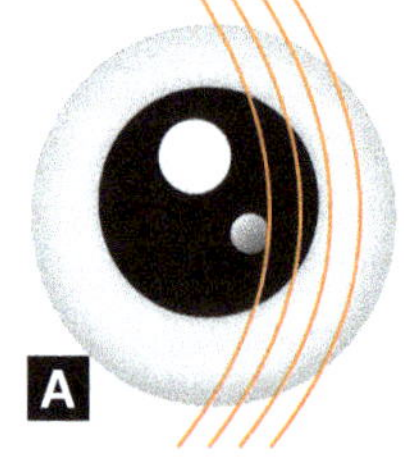

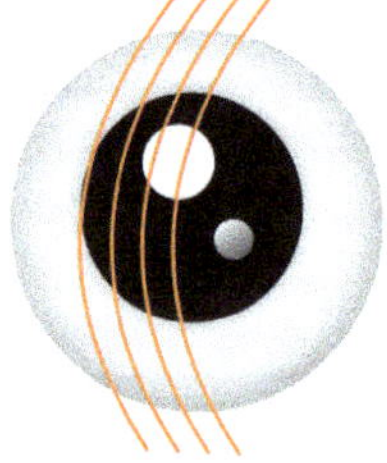

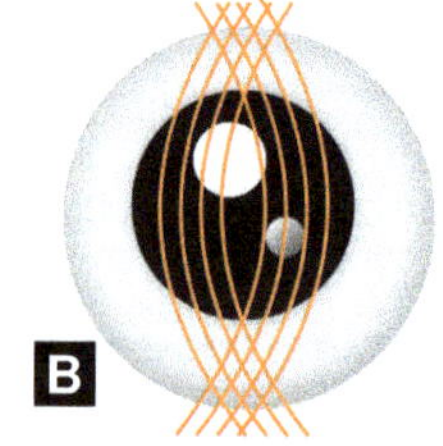

20 slits to the right and 20 slits to the left

Overlapping images (40 total)

Figs. 2.8.1A and B: Scanning slit imaging in Orbscan.

The disadvantage is that because of large steps it does not show subtle changes. It should be used for routine clinical analysis.

Normalized scale (relative): In this, the dioptric power step is based on the patient's cornea. The advantage is that since the dioptric power is smaller, therefore, it will show more detailed changes. However, the disadvantage is that the two maps cannot be compared directly. It is more sensitive and useful for research.[3]

Color scale: In all the four maps (i.e. power, curvature, elevation, and pachymetry) color scale is used using the concept of the best-fit sphere (BFS) as explained below, where:

- Red—is towards the higher side
- Blue—is towards the lower side for power, curvature, elevation, and pachymetry
- Green—denotes the reference surface.

Data Overview

This includes (Fig. 2.8.2):[4]

- *Simulated keratometry (Sim K):* Maximum power of the surface along any axis and the power orthogonal to that axis (Sim K1 and Sim K2) in the central 3 mm area. The difference between Sim K1 and Sim K2 gives the value for astigmatism.
- *Irregularity index at 3 mm and 5 mm zone*: Keratoconus screening and higher order aberrations.
- *White-to-white diameter*: Measures the horizontal corneal diameter from limbus to limbus. The normal value is between 11 mm and 13 mm. It provides essential clinical information for diagnostic purposes (for example, microcornea and relative anterior microphthalmos) as well as for surgical procedures:
  - Haptic size calculation in anterior chamber intraocular lens and phakic intraocular lens
  - Size of capsular tension ring (CTR)
  - Intraocular lens power calculation in cataract surgery using third-generation formulas
  - Endothelial keratoplasty: Corneal endothelial graft size should be 3 mm less than the smallest diameter of the recipient cornea as larger graft are more challenging to unfold
  - Corneal refractive surgeries: Mesopic pupil diameter is closely related to horizontal white-to-white so more stringent approach in preoperative evaluation for ablation zone planning.
- *Pupil diameter*: Photopic pupil size
- *Thinnest point of the cornea*
- *Anterior chamber depth*: From corneal endothelium to the lens. The normal value is between 2.5 mm and 3.5 mm.
- *Angle kappa*: It is the angle formed between the visual axis (line connecting fixation point with the fovea) and pupillary axis (the line that passes perpendicularly through the center of cornea and center of the pupil). It is crucial in refractive surgery as proper centration is required for optimal

Case, 10
N2 Y249984 M32
20.04.01 11:26:15
Screen

Sim K's: Astig:	-1.6 D	@ 36 deg
Max:	44.9 D	@ 126 deg
Min:	43.3 D	@ 36 deg
3.0 MM Zone:	Irreg:	± 1.9 D
Mean Pwr	44.0	± 1.2 D
Astig Pwr	1.7	± 1.4 D
Steep Axis	119	± 38 deg
Flat Axis	16	± 38 deg
5.0 MM Zone:	Irreg:	± 2.5 D
Mean Pwr	43.0	± 1.8 D
Astig Pwr	0.7	± 1.7 D
Steep Axis	90	± 44 deg
Flat Axis	21	± 44 deg

White-to-White [mm] : 11.3
Pupil Diameter [mm] : 4.5
Thinnest : 510 um @ (-0.7, -0.7)
ACD (Endo): 2.87 mm
Kappa : 6.75° @ 199.55°
Kappa Intercept : -0.72, -0.04

Fig. 2.8.2: Data overview.

results as a large angle kappa may lead to alignment errors during photoablation in laser refractive surgery as well lens decentration in intraocular refractive surgery. The decentration of ablation zones can lead to undercorrection and irregular astigmatism. Decentration of intraocular lenses may cause photic phenomenon and decreased lens effectiveness. A positive angle kappa causes pseudoexotropia, and a negative angle kappa causes pseudoesotropia. The normal value is 5°.

Elevation Map

This uses the concept of the BFS (Fig. 2.8.3).[5] In this a hypothetical sphere is calculated that resembles the shape of the cornea to be measured as close as possible and then compares the real surface to the hypothetical sphere. Areas above the surface of the sphere appear in warm colors (red) and areas below in cool colors (blue) in the color scale (Fig. 2.8.4). Both anterior (top left of the quad map) and posterior elevation maps (top right of the quad map) are there, also known as the anterior and posterior float.

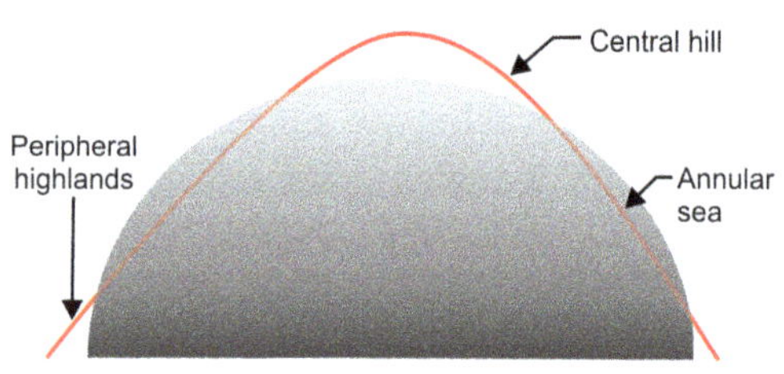

Fig. 2.8.3: The concept of best-fit sphere.

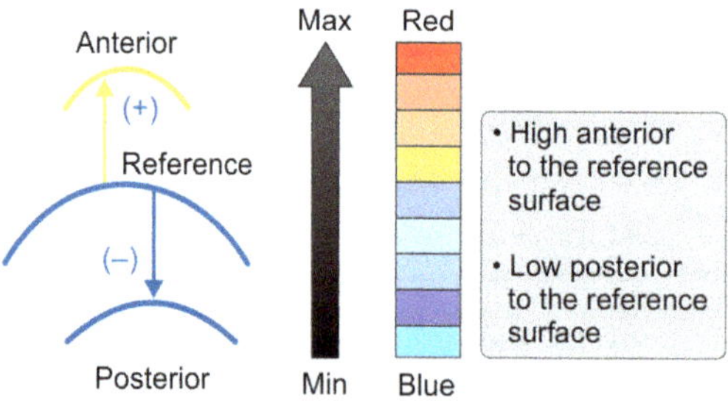

Fig. 2.8.4: The concept of color scale.

Anterior elevation map provides an overall diagnostic view of the cornea. Besides, it is important for contact lens trial.

Orbscan does not measure the posterior surface, but calculates it from the anterior surface and then produces a posterior elevation map. Relative elevation measures height difference in microns from a best fitting reference sphere. Posterior elevation map is vital for early diagnosis of cases of corneal ectasia. It is used for screening of cases of suspected or forme fruste keratoconus (FFKC) cases before any refractive surgery. A posterior float elevation of more than 40 μm is suggestive of posterior ectasia.

The normal cornea is *prolate* which means that the meridional curvature decreases from the center to the periphery. It causes the normal cornea to rise centrally above the reference surface resulting in a central hill. Immediately surrounding the hill is an annular sea where cornea dips below the reference surface. In the far periphery, the prolate cornea again rises above the reference surface producing peripheral islands (Fig. 2.8.5).

The regular astigmatic cornea is toric which means that the meridional curvature has maximum and minimum directions which are 90° apart. The steep part falls below the reference surface. The flat part rises above the reference surface resulting in central saddle topography (Fig. 2.8.6).

The anterior elevation and posterior elevation map should be studied carefully and together to understand the shape of the cornea and look for any abnormal shape. Elevation patterns can be either "regular ridge, irregular ridge, incomplete ridge, island or unclassified". Amongst these patterns, the

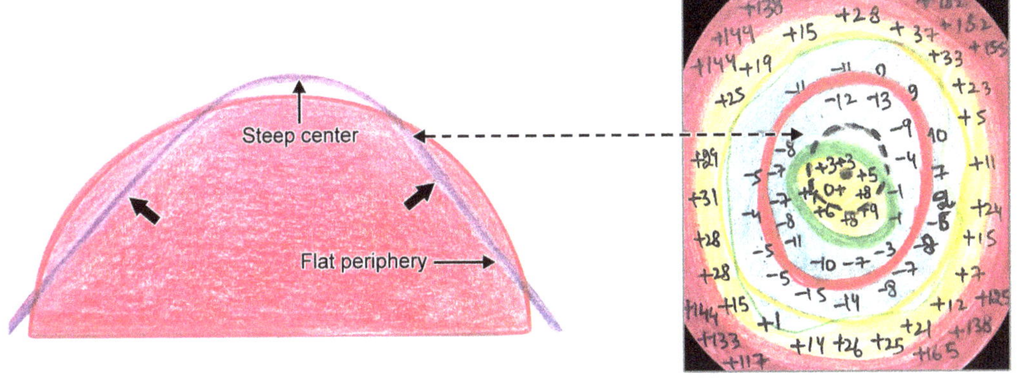

Fig. 2.8.5: Normal anterior elevation map of the cornea (prolate shape).

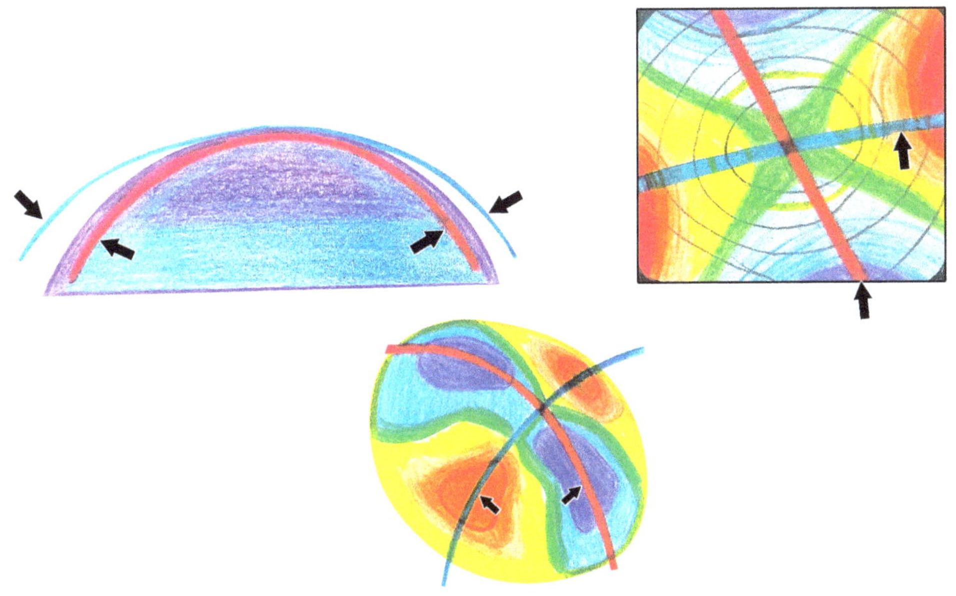

Fig. 2.8.6: Astigmatic elevation map.

most commonly seen on anterior elevation map is incomplete ridge and island and on posterior elevation is island. On the elevation maps, abnormally elevated areas can be seen and further accuracy depends upon the color scale and step size. Tanabe et al. suggested 10 and 20 µm scale range on the anterior and posterior elevation maps, respectively. According to them, maps with three or more colors in the central zone (3 mm) were considered to be abnormal. Fam et al. reported that posterior elevation of 40 µm or more has a sensitivity of 57.7% and specificity of 89.9%. They have suggested anterior elevation ratio which is anterior elevation/anterior BFS. If this is 0.5122 or less, it is more significant compared to posterior elevation alone.

Curvature Map

Axial keratometry map or sagittal curvature map which is the bottom left map on the quad map (Fig. 2.8.7). A fixed center of curvature is used for calculating the power at all points. The values are directly comparable to keratometry. The color scale as for the elevation map is also used for the keratometry map. This map is important for diagnosis and grading of ectatic corneal disorders such as keratoconus and contact lens fitting.

Pachymetry Map

It is calculated by the distance between the anterior and posterior surface. It is the bottom right map on the quad map (Fig. 2.8.7). The color scale is used to denote the pachymetry values.

It is important to note that the hot color represents increased thickness (or otherwise near normal thickness) while cool colors denote decreased corneal thickness (or otherwise ectatic cornea). These findings are just opposite to curvature map where hot colors denote ectatic cornea.

Pachymetry map is significant for treatment planning of cases of keratoconus. Some of the crucial points to remember are as follows:

- Automated lamellar therapeutic keratoplasty (ALTK)—minimum thickness 400 microns
- Deep anterior lamellar keratoplasty (DALK)—increased risk of perforation if thinnest pachymetry is less than 250 microns
- Intacs—contraindicated if the thickness is less than 350 microns in mid-periphery
- Laser-assisted *in situ* keratomileusis (LASIK)—minimum thickness if more than 499 microns (for microkeratome,

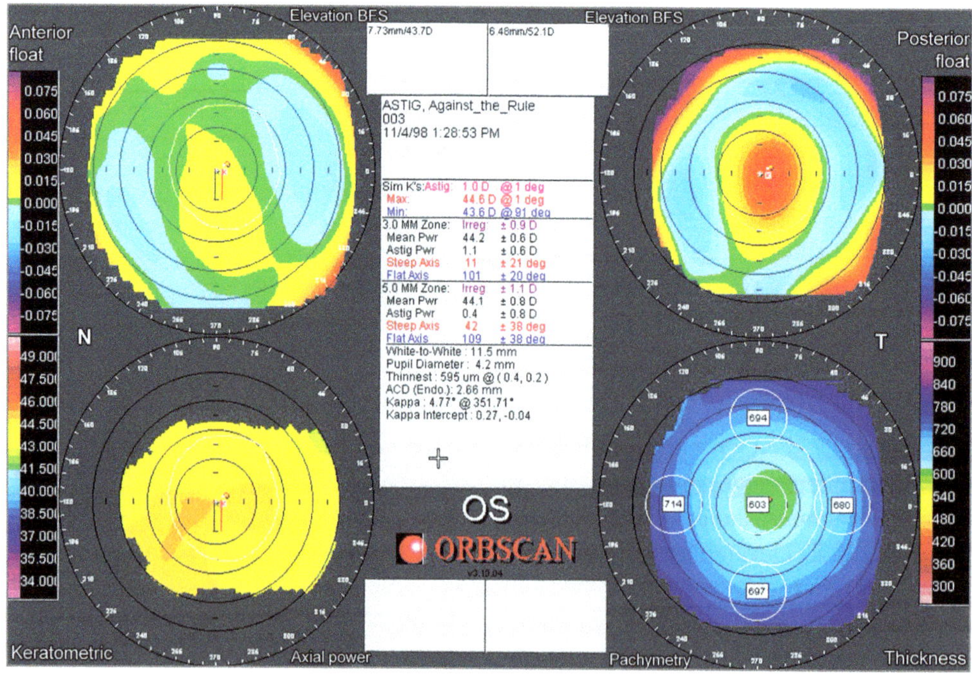

Fig. 2.8.7: Orbscan quad map (top left is the anterior elevation map, top right is the posterior elevation map, bottom left is the curvature map, and bottom right is the pachymetry map).

although it varies from surgeon to surgeon)
- Corneal collagen cross-linking—5% decrease in corneal thickness in 6 months suggests progression.

Compare

Always *compare* previous maps of the same eye and also compare with the other eye.

CLINICAL APPLICATIONS

Orbscan is used in the following conditions:
- Detection of irregular corneal astigmatism in:
  - Keratoconus
  - Contact lens-induced corneal warpage
  - Pellucid marginal degeneration
- Preoperative evaluation:
  - Laser-assisted in situ keratomileusis
  - Astigmatic keratotomy (AK)
  - Intrastromal corneal ring segments (Intacs)
  - Penetrating keratoplasty
- Applications to contact lens fitting:
  - Routine rigid gas permeable (RGP) fitting: Preprogrammed protocol and simulated fitting.

HOW TO READ AN ORBSCAN MAP OF KERATOCONUS

This is an Orbscan quad map (Fig. 2.8.8) of a patient X of the left eye showing anterior elevation map at the top left and posterior elevation map at the top right side with color scale steps of 0.005 mm. The bottom left map is the axial curvature map with color steps of 1 D and the bottom right map is the pachymetry map with color steps of 20 μm. The simulated keratometry maximum is 59.9 D at 149, and simulated keratometry minimum is 54.7 D at 59° with astigmatism of 2.2 D at 149°. The irregularity index along the 3 and 5 mm zones are given. The white-to-white is 11.9 mm with a pupil diameter of 3.9 mm. The thinnest pachymetry is 437 μm which is located inferotemporally as shown by the plus mark position. The anterior chamber

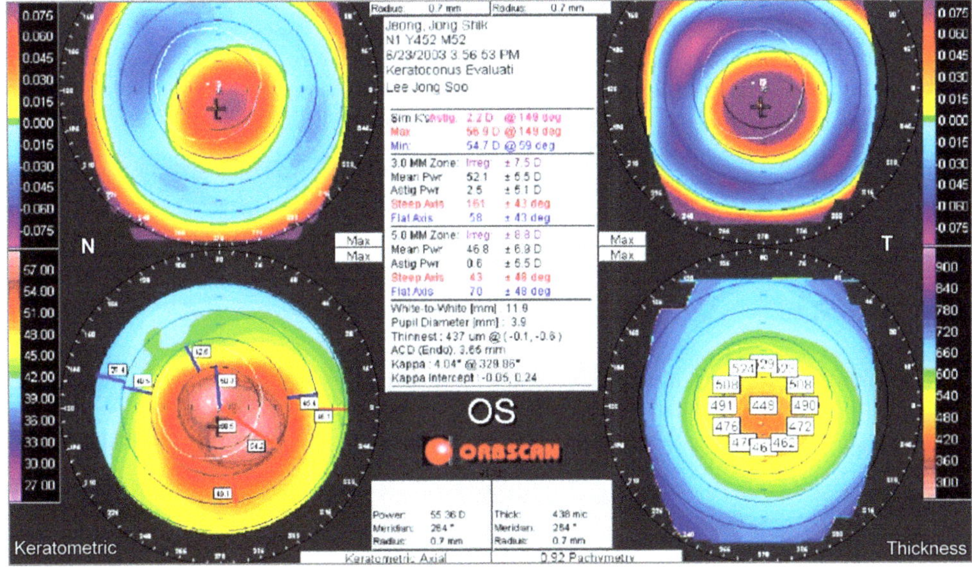

Fig. 2.8.8: Orbscan of a case of keratoconus.

depth is 3.65 mm, and the angle kappa is 4.04° which is normal.

The anterior elevation map shows inferotemporal steeping as shown by the red color with corresponding steepening on the posterior elevation map. The axial curvature map shows asymmetric bow tie pattern with skewing of radial axis. The pachymetry map shows thinning along the corresponding area. On correlating it with the clinical picture this is most likely a case of keratoconus. Also, it is important to compare with the fellow eye and any previous records if available for progression.

LIMITATIONS

- It lags in accuracy and reproducibility to the Scheimpflug devices and the readings were not interchangeable.
- Inaccurately identifies the postoperative posterior corneal surface and routinely locates the surface anteriorly.

VIVA QUESTIONS

1. Compare the different topography systems.

Ans. Different topography systems include:

- Placido disc (reflection) based
- Elevation based:
  - Slit scanning (Orbscan)
  - Scheimpflug imaging (Pentacam and Galilei)

  Refer to Tables 2.8.1 and 2.8.2 for details.

2. Importance of white-to-white diameter in corneal surgery.

Ans. Refer to text.

Table 2.8.1: Difference between Placido and slit scanning technologies.

	Placido based	*Slit scanning based*
Number of images scanned	One image, one surface	Multiple images, multiple surfaces
Mechanism	Angle dependent specular reflection	Omni direction diffuse backscatter
Measures	Measures slope (as a function of distance between mires)	Measures triangular elevation
Data on the central cornea	Missed	Present
Accuracy	Able to acquire limited data points so less accurate	More number of data points and hence more accurate

Table 2.8.2: Difference between Pentacam and Orbscan.

	Pentacam	*Orbscan*
Principle	Scheimpflug	Scanning slit and Placido disc system
Number of measured data points per scan	>25,000	9,600
Effect of eye movement	Maintains the central point (thinnest point) of each meridian. Thus can reregister these central points and eliminate eye movement	Takes a vertical image separate slice which has no common point. Thus cannot reregister for any eye movement
Accuracy	10 times more accurate	Less accurate
Lens details	Measures anterior and posterior lens shape, lens thickness and lens densitometry	Measures only anterior lens shape

Table 2.8.3: Signs suggestive of early keratoconus on Orbscan.	
Parameter	*Criteria*
Pachymetry	Thinnest point <470 µm
	A difference of >100 µm from the thinnest point to the values of the 7 mm optic zone implies a steep gradient of thinning from mid periphery to the thinnest point
	Thinnest point on cornea should correspond with the highest point of elevation on the posterior corneal surface
Posterior elevation map	Posterior high point >50 µm above the best fit sphere
	Best fit sphere with a power >55 D on the posterior profile
	Roush criteria: relative difference > 100 µm between the highest and lowest point on the posterior elevation map
Power map	Keratometric mean power map >46 D
	Bow tie pattern or lazy C on the axial power map is suspect when astigmatism shifts > 20° from a straight line
	Change within the central 3 mm optic zone of the cornea >3 D from superior to inferior can be correlated to the presence of vertical coma (commonest aberration in keratoconus)
Composite integrated information	Highest point on the posterior elevation coincides with the highest point on the anterior elevation, the thinnest point on pachymetry and point of steepest curvature on the power map
	Efkarpides criteria: ratio of the radii of anterior and posterior best-fit sphere of the cornea should be more than 1.21. Between 1.23 and 1.27 would be suspect and >1.27 is diagnostic
	Astigmatic discrepancy of >1.5 D in 3 mm zone and discrepancy >2 D in the 5 mm zone

3. Importance of angle Kappa.

Ans. Refer to text.

4. Various cutoffs for diagnosis of keratoconus in Orbscan.

Ans. Refer to Table 2.8.3.

5. What is the irregularity index and mention its clinical importance?

Ans. Irregularity index is proportional to the standard deviation of the curvature of the surface. Orbscan calculates this index in the 3 mm and the 5 mm zone. Any further improvement of vision which cannot be corrected with refraction can be correlated with this index. Higher the value more is irregular astigmatism or higher order aberration. The index is considered to be significant and suggestive of keratoconus if it is more than 1.5 D in the central 3 mm zone or more than 2–3 D in the 5 mm zone. However, this should always be correlated clinically.

6. Advantages of Orbscan pachymetry over ultrasonic pachymeter.

Ans. Advantages of Orbscan include:

- Noncontact method
    - Less chance of infection
    - Error due to the eccentricity of the probe is minimized
- Measurement of several parts of the cornea
- Simultaneous analysis of anterior and posterior corneal surfaces and pachymetry
- Less technician dependent
- Repeatability.

7. Importance of BFS.

Ans. The posterior surface of the cornea is first to be involved in corneal ectasia. A value of 51 D or more is suggestive of primary posterior corneal elevation and 55 D or more for FFKC. The ratio of anterior to posterior BFS is also important. If it is more than 1.27, it is a contraindication for refractive surgery. Below 1.21 is acceptable and between 1.21 and 1.27 is considered as keratoconus suspect.

REFERENCES

1. Marinez CE, Klyce SD. Keratometry and Topography. In: Krachmer (Ed). Cornea: Fundamentals, Diagnosis and Management, 3rd edition. Amsterdam: Mosby Elsevier; 2011. pp. 161-75.
2. DOS Times. (2014). Topography for the Refractive Surgeon. [online] Available from http://dos-times.org/pulsar9088/20140424040901240.pdf [Accessed January, 2019].
3. Roberts C. Corneal topography: A review of terms and concepts. J Cataract Refract Surg. 1996;22(5):624-9.
4. DOS Times. (2013). Corneal Topography. [online] Available from http://dos-times.org/pulsar9088/20131113064559307.pdf [Accessed January, 2019].
5. Dharwadkar S, Nayak BK. Corneal topography and tomography. J Clin Ophthalmol Res. 2015;3:45-62.

2.9 APPLIANCES AND INSTRUMENTS IN CORNEA

Pranita Sahay, Mohamed Ibrahime Asif, Devesh Kumawat, Namrata Sharma

KERATOPLASTY

Globe Fixation Rings

Flieringa Ring (Fig. 2.9.1)

It is made of stainless steel and is useful for maintaining the architecture of the globe once the host corneal button has been removed. They are available in 11 sizes from 12 mm to 22 mm.

Uses:
- Vitrectomized eyes
- Pediatric cases, as the eyeball has a tendency to collapse in these cases after trephination due to low sclera rigidity
- Aphakic eyes
- Ocular hypotony
- Penetrating keratoplasty (PK) combined with cataract surgery (optical triple procedure).

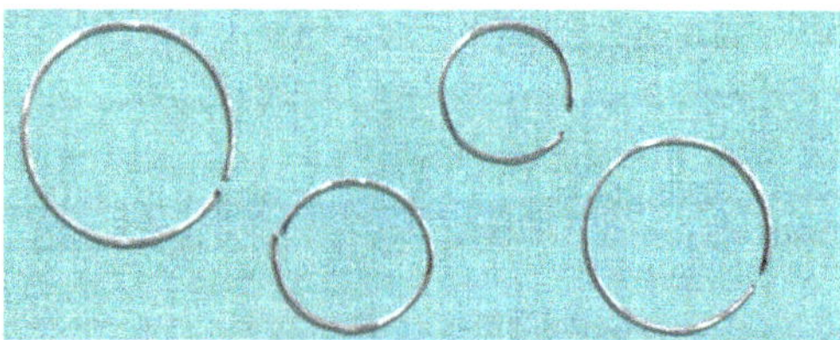

Fig. 2.9.1: Flieringa ring.

Disadvantage:
- It can distort the shape of the eyeball and causes an oval cut during trephination and subsequent high astigmatism.
- Very rarely, it can result in sclera perforation while passing sutures to fixate the ring.
- Subconjunctival hematoma.

McNeill-Goldman Ring (Fig. 2.9.2)

It provides support at four strategically placed sutures. The ring features medial and temporal openings for greater access to the surgical field and two lid retractors to prevent

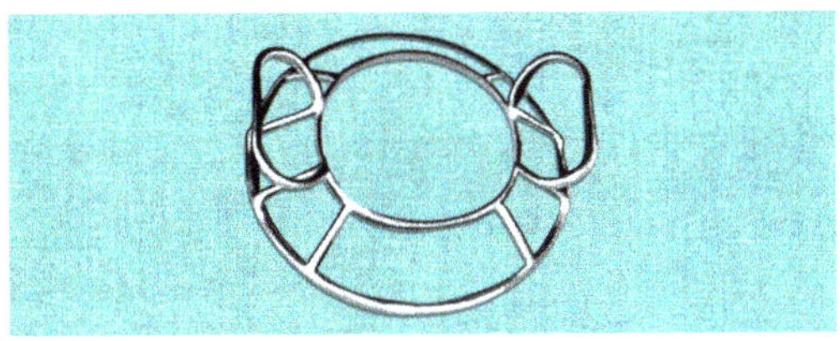

Fig. 2.9.2: McNeill-Goldman ring.

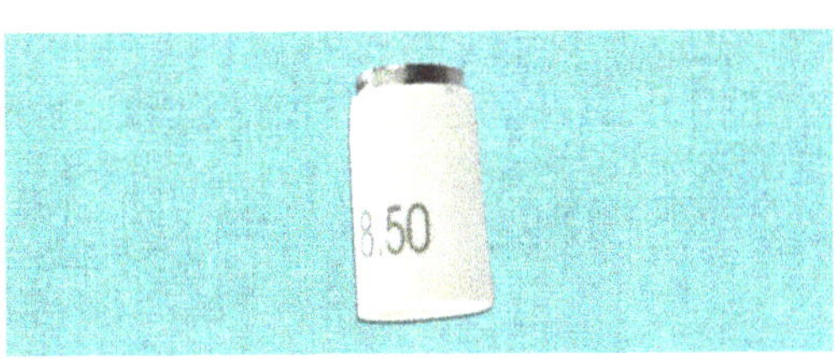

Fig. 2.9.4: Handheld.

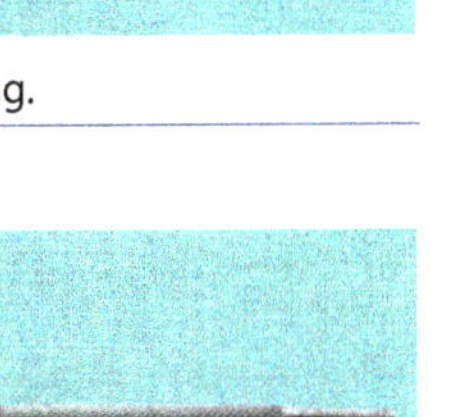

Fig. 2.9.3: RK marker.

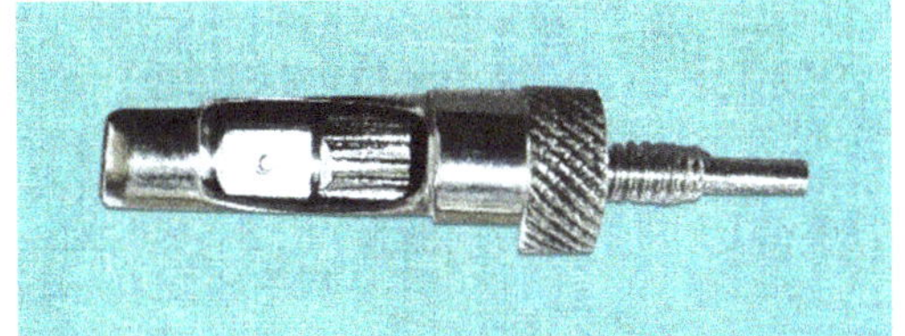

Fig. 2.9.5: Castroviejo trephine.

eyelid closure by the patient. It is available in three sizes—small, medium, and large. The adult size has an inner diameter of 17 mm and outer diameter of 24 mm. It is made of stainless steel.

Corneal Marking Instruments

Radial keratotomy (RK) marker (Fig. 2.9.3), Vajpayee corneal marker (20 radial arms), and Anis corneal marker (8 radial arms) are the various instruments that guide the optimal placement of sutures in keratoplasty.

Corneal Trephines

Different types of trephines are discussed below:

Conventional Circular Cutting Trephines

- Handheld (Fig. 2.9.4):
  - Ranging from 3 mm to 17 mm diameter
  - In some trephines, there is a central obturator, which can be adjusted to select the depth of the corneal cut and hence an inadvertent entry into the anterior chamber. However, the obturator obscures the view of central cornea which may result in inaccurate centration during the trephination of the recipient's cornea.
  - Examples of handheld trephines with obturator are the Castroviejo trephine (Fig. 2.9.5) and the Grieshaber-Franceschetti trephine.
- *Mechanized*: The disadvantages associated with motor driven trephines include corkscrew edge effect in the corneal stroma.
- *Suction-fixation type*: It is devised to obtain a perpendicular cut in the recipient cornea. These trephine systems essentially consist of an outer corneal suction ring for fixation and an inner circular cutting blade.
  - Hessburg-Barron trephine (Fig. 2.9.6) has a cross hair device for improved centration and an outer ring of corneal marks at equal intervals to assist in suture placement. It is available in diameters 6.0–9.0 in 0.5 mm increments as well as diameter of 7.75 mm. For each spoke (90°) turned, the blade is lowered or raised approximately 0.06 mm.

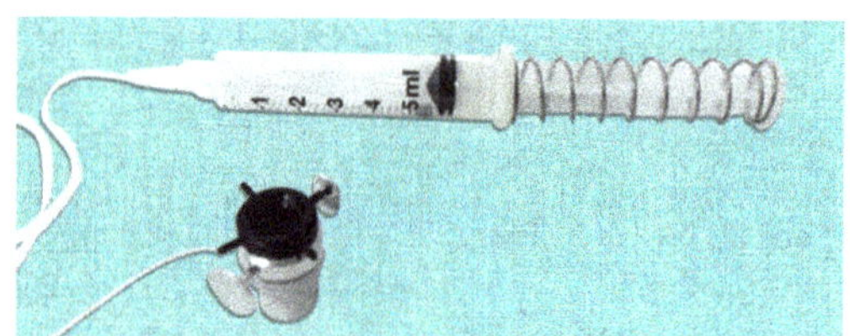

Fig. 2.9.6: Hessburg-Barron trephine.

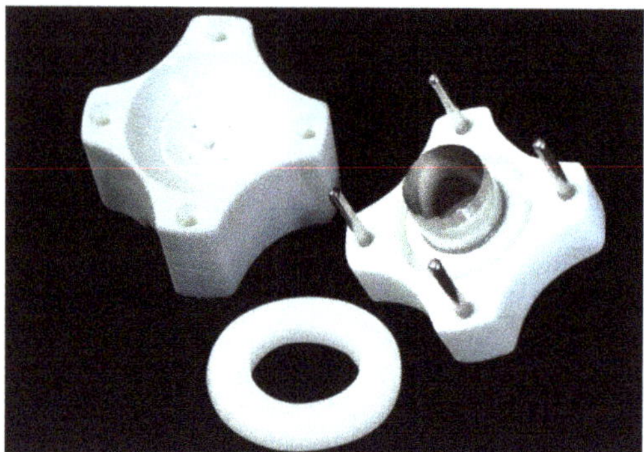
Fig. 2.9.7: Barron vacuum punch.

- Barron vacuum punch (Fig. 2.9.7) features a solid stainless steel blade which is permanently mounted in nylon housing. Four steel guide posts align with four corresponding holes in the cutting block base, automatically centering the blade over the donor cornea.

- *Special-purpose type*: *The Olson calibrated cornea trephine system* used to trephinate both the donor and recipient corneas. The system consists of an anterior chamber maintainer, reusable blade holder (with micrometer setting), and suction ring. One revolution of the micrometer is equivalent to 500 microns.
  - *Skin biopsy punches*: The skin biopsy punches, which have been used in dermatological practice, are especially useful in harvesting of small patch grafts used for tectonic purposes in cases of impending/frank perforation.

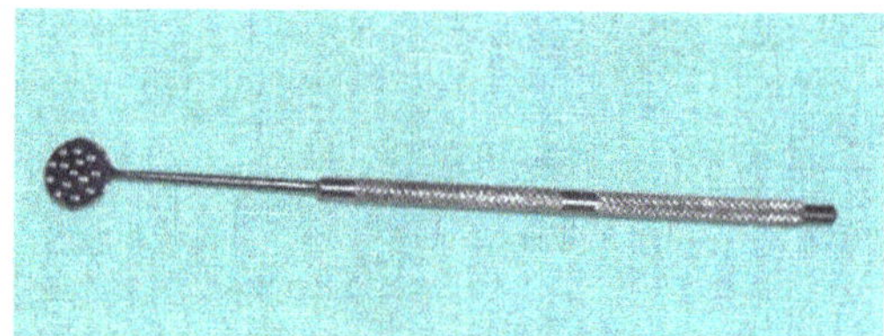
Fig. 2.9.8: Graft holder (Paton Spatula).

Single Point Cutting Trephines

The single point cutter trephines were designed to decrease corneal torsion, e.g. *Leiberman single point cutter.*

Combination Trephines

Hanna trephine system has got a circular razor-cutting blade and incorporates many of the salient features of single point cutting trephines.

Noncontact Trephines (Lasers)

Laser noncontact trephination eliminates corneal topography distortion provides the visualization of the entire cornea and enhances centration.

Graft Holder (Paton Spatula) (Fig. 2.9.8)

The graft is placed over viscoelastic and is kept covered till the recipient dissection is complete.

Cutting Blocks

The various cutting blocks available for corneal grafting are Paraffin block, Teflon block (Fig. 2.9.9), and Polycarbonate and nylon blocks.

- *The Kaufmann corneal cutting block*: This is the simplest design which consists of a Teflon block with metal cover.
- *The Brightbill polytef cutting block*: This modern, compound curved block

Fig. 2.9.9: Teflon block.

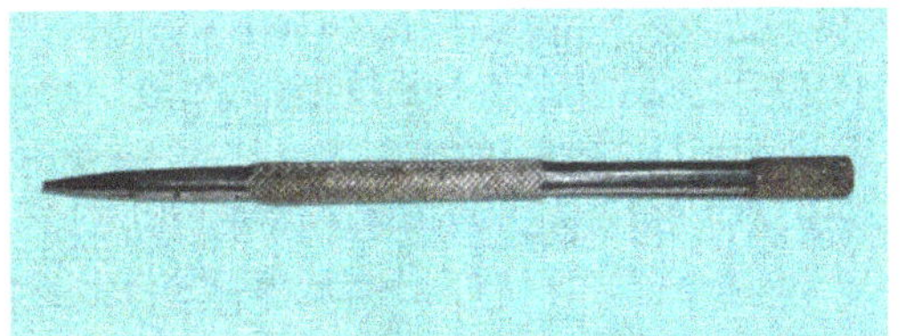

Fig. 2.9.10: Blade breaker.

approximates the central, midperipheral, and peripheral curvature of donor. The Brightbill polytef cutting block uses three wells, each with a different radius of curvature and diameter. Two concentric inlays of colored polytef are present. The outer black polytef zone has a chord length of 12.5 mm and corresponds to the limbus and a second white polytef inlay with an 8 mm chord length corresponds to the central zone of the donor cornea. Slippage of the moist donor cornea at the time of cutting can cause oval graft. This can be prevented by repeated drying of the well in which the donor is placed or by using a thin, slightly moistened layer of cotton in the well.

Corneal Endothelial Punches

To cut a donor button from endothelial side corneal punches are also available which use disposable trephine blades. The advantage of corneal punch is that they yield sharp vertical cuts without beveling.

- *Cottingham corneal punch*: It is a metal punch with a universal style handle. Additionally, it also has two replaceable base plugs.
- *Troutman corneal punch*: It incorporates a centered block and a piston carrier with a central piston. The piston accommodates blades of 7-9 mm. This relies on the surgeon's thumb to incise the cornea.
- *Iowa PK press corneal punch*: It incorporates a spring-loaded piston with an expandable edge to accommodate 6-9.5 mm trephines to harvest various sizes the donor graft from the endothelial side. It has a unique two color cutting block, which aids in centration of the donor tissue. The recessed base assumes that the block is held centrally under the trephine block.
- *Lieberman gravity-action punch*: It is a guillotine-style punch with a heavy head, which uses the force of gravity rather than the surgeon's hand to punch the cornea.
- *Rothman-Gilbard corneal punch*: It uses a piston which is not spring loaded. The suction block has eight evenly spaced suction holes which anchor the corneal button firmly so that there is minimal movement during trephination. The button has eight precisely placed marks and can be sutured into the host bed by suturing every mark on the button with the marks placed on the host bed.

There are four trephine assemblies, which use artificial anterior chamber (AAC). These include *Krumeich, Hanna, Olson*, and *Lieberman* systems. This involves cutting the donor corneas from the epithelial side rather than the endothelial side. Pressure in the AAC is adjusted to the intraocular pressure with the help of attachments of the infusion tubing.

Cutting Instruments

Blade Breaker (Fig. 2.9.10)

A disposable razor blade is broken and mounted on the tip of a metallic pencil handle. This is one of the best instruments available for cutting tissues in straight or curved lines. Blade breaker is used to enter the anterior chamber in a controlled manner after a deep cut has been created in the recipient's cornea by a trephine. Blunt side of the blade can sometimes be used for blunt dissection of adherent iris.

Diamond Knife (Fig. 2.9.11)

This is the sharpest cutting instrument and available in various sizes and shapes. It is the most durable instrument and useful for stab incisions as well as to complete the trephine cuts.

Corneal Scissors (Fig. 2.9.12)

Ideally, all corneal scissors should have an immobile lower blade. Troutman microscissor is the prototype, which has blades 5 mm in length and is curved on a radius of 5 mm. The lower handle, which controls the upper blade, has a flexible spring. This is a very light and fine scissors and mainly used to complete the cutting of the trephine incision. The blades should be kept vertical and must be curved to follow the curvature of the trephine, while cutting the host cornea. It is often used to remove the irregular tags from the wound margin. Corneal scissors are used to complete the trephination of the host cornea after creation of the circular cut following anterior chamber entry. Curved Vannas scissors can also be used for the same.

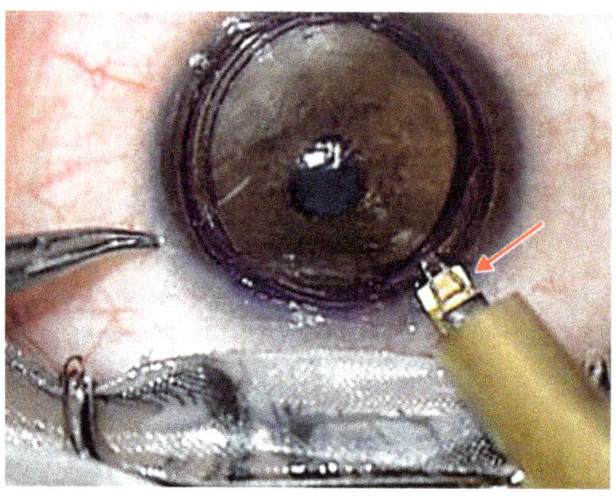

Fig. 2.9.11: Diamond knife.

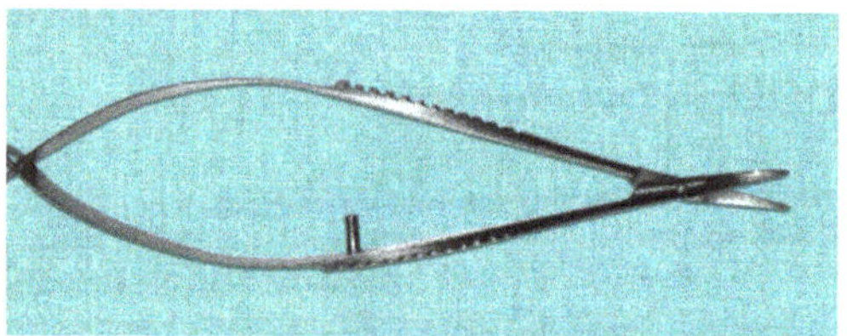

Fig. 2.9.12: Corneal scissors.

Holding Instruments

Needle holders used in ophthalmic microsurgery consists of two handles, which are supported between index finger and thumb. Needle holder, which is lightweight, with nonslip curved handle and curved jaws is preferred for PK. The curvature of the jaw varies from a uniform smooth to a hockey stick shape. The jaws should be atraumatic to the steel needles, but the grip should be firm. Barraquer's curved needle holder (Fig. 2.9.13) is an example.

Grasping Instruments

Varieties of forceps are used for PK. However, they can be broadly classified into toothed, nontoothed or forceps used for special purposes.

Toothed Forceps

- *Pierse-Hoskins forceps (Fig. 2.9.14)*: It is a fine toothed tissue holding forcep used

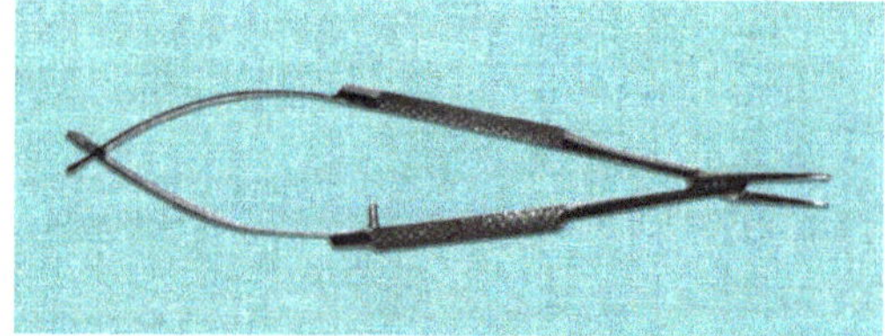

Fig. 2.9.13: Barraquer's curved needle holder.

to hold the corneal tissue firmly. Pierse-Hoskin's forceps is the most frequently used tissue holding forceps in corneal grafting surgery. It is a 2 × 1 fine toothed lightweight instrument and extensively used for suture tying.

- *Colibri forceps (Fig. 2.9.15)*: This is another example of tissue holding forceps. The advantage of this instrument is that it is less likely to damage surrounding tissues due to its curved shape.

Nontoothed Forceps

The nontoothed forceps have flat edges that help in holding or picking up structures like 10-0 nylon suture. McPherson forceps (Fig. 2.9.16) is the prototype of this variety. It can be used for suture tying and for burying the suture knots.

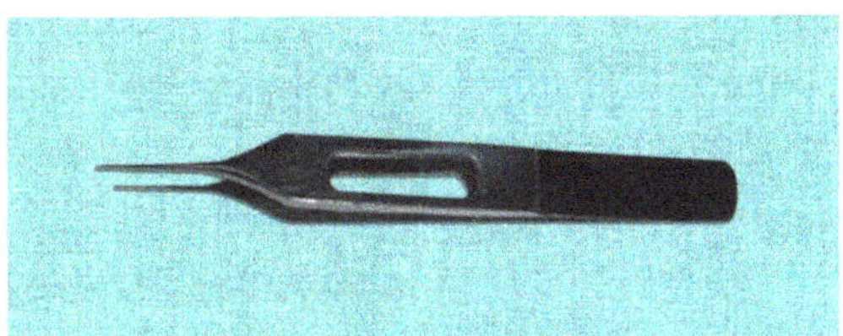

Fig. 2.9.14: Pierse-Hoskins forceps.

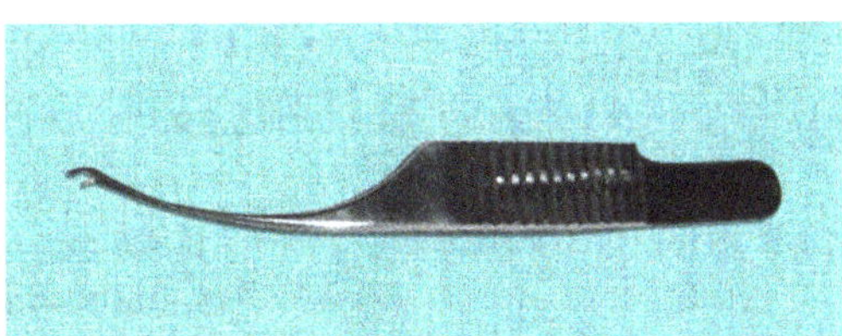

Fig. 2.9.15: Colibri forceps.

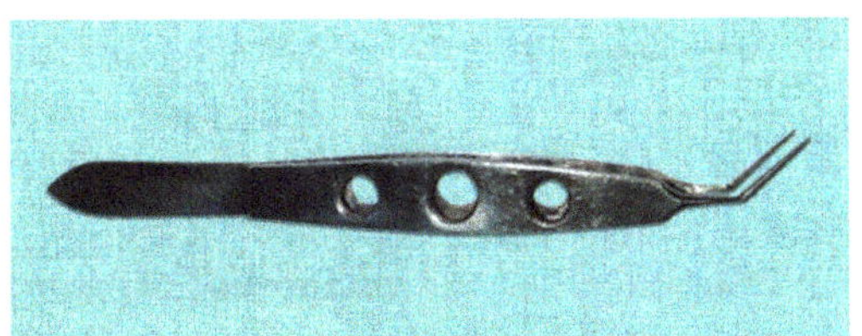

Fig. 2.9.16: McPherson forceps.

Forceps with Special Functions

- *Double corneal forceps, Colibri style*: It has two 2.75 mm long tips separated 1 mm with 0.4 mm Pierse tips. It is 72 mm long and has a serrated handle.
- *Colibri style Polack double corneal forceps (Fig. 2.9.17)*: It is used for the first corneal suture. The cut edge of the graft is gently grasped at the junction of the epithelium and stroma with fine toothed forceps.

Spatulas and Hooks

These are mainly used in the reconstruction of the anterior chamber, the manipulation of the iris, and assistance in intraocular lens (IOL) placement. A double-ended iris repositor (Fig. 2.9.18) is useful for lysis of synechiae between the iris and lens capsule, dissection of iris from retrocorneal membranes and iris supported implants, lysis of broad based anterior synechiae, and sweeping the donor tissue to undermine its edges below the host tissue. IOL manipulators such as Sinskey (Fig. 2.9.19) and Lester hooks are very useful for placing and stabilizing an anterior chamber lens.

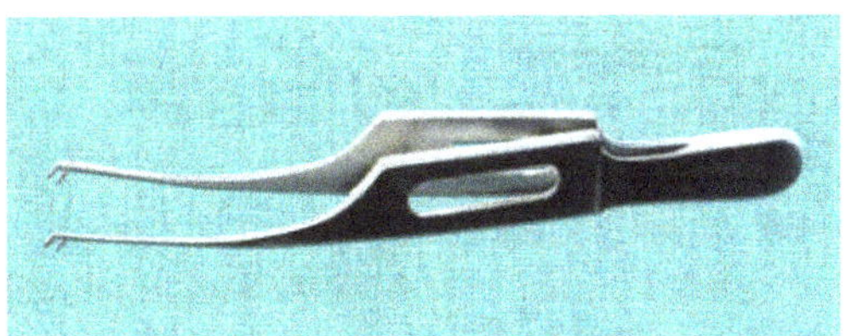

Fig. 2.9.17: Polack double corneal forceps.

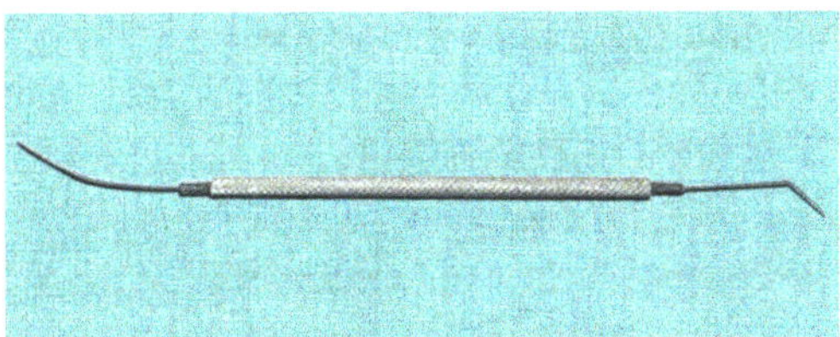

Fig. 2.9.18: Double-ended iris repositer.

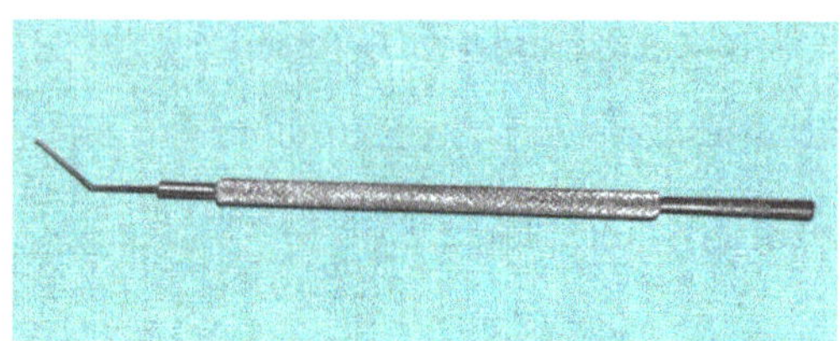

Fig. 2.9.19: Sinskey.

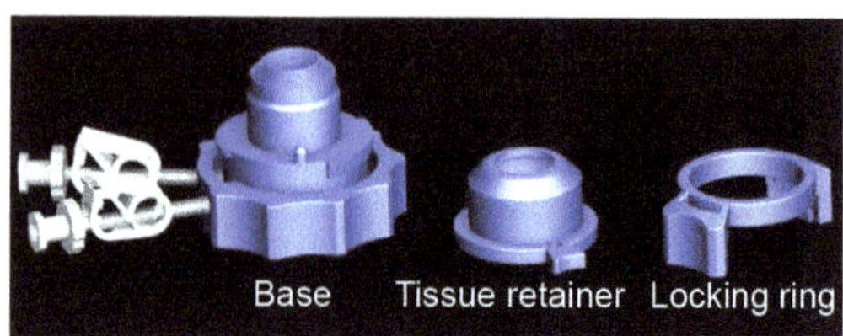

Fig. 2.9.20: Barron's.

Qualitative Keratometers

The keratometers are very helpful to assess the degree of corneal toricity at the end of the surgery. These can be of two types depending on whether they are attached to the microscope or they are hand-held.

Keratometers with Microscopic Attachment

There are a number of surgical keratometers like *Smirmaul, Troutman,* and *Terry* that are physically attached to the microscope and work by reflecting projected light off the surface of the cornea. However, these are not portable and require a regular smooth refracting surface to reflect the image and are quite expensive.

Handheld Keratometers

Simpler, cost-effective, and portable methods as Mandel intraoperative keratometer and *Maloney* keratometer are available which work by reflecting a circle from the corneal surface. Maloney keratometer is a titanium cone-shaped instrument, which is designed to reflect the microscope light in rings on the cornea to detect astigmatism. In the absence of the expensive intraoperative surgical keratometers, a safety pin can also be used to monitor the intraoperative astigmatism. The circle of the safety pin is reflected off the corneal surface and any observed ovality implies excessive curvature in the axis of the shortest diameter of the oval. This is used for readjusting and replacement of the sutures and helps to reduce astigmatism intraoperatively and postoperatively.

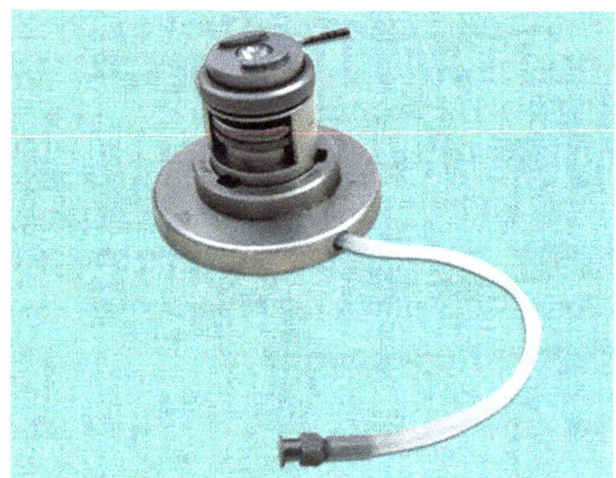

Fig. 2.9.21: Moria's.

Instruments for Donor Cornea Dissection in Lamellar Keratoplasty

- *Artificial Anterior Chamber and Clamp [Barron's (Fig. 2.9.20), Moria's (Fig. 2.9.21), etc.]:* The chamber is used to mount the donor tissue and maintain adequate pressure while lamellar dissection or full thickness trephination is being performed. It is designed in a bright blue color to provide a high contrast background for visualizing the cornea and aiding in the lamellar dissection of the cornea.

  The chamber is composed of three pieces: (1) base with tissue pedestal, (2) tissue retainer, and (3) locking ring. The base has two ports with silicone tubing: (1) in-line pinch clamps and (2) Luer Lock connectors. Either port may be used to inject or aspirate viscoelastic material, balanced salt solution, preservation media, or air.

- King's clamp (Fig. 2.9.22).

Lamellar Dissectors

- *Tooke's knife (Fig. 2.9.23)*: The pocket for the initiation of the lamellar dissection may be performed with a Tooke's knife. It has a smooth blade at one end, which can be inserted intralamellarly to create a pocket.
- *Paufique's knife (Fig. 2.9.24)*: It has a double-edged sharp angled blade that helps in outlining the graft, making the pocket, and dissecting the lamellar plane.
- *Desmarre's lamellar dissector*: It is used in the open type of dissection, which has a curve in its vertical meridian and it is used to sweep across the fibers in a cutting and teasing motion. A duckbill shape lamellar dissector is used for closed type of dissection, which is curved in the horizontal dimension.
- *Gill's lamellar dissector*: It has a 3 mm wide blade which can be either straight or curved.
- *Guarded diamond knife*: It is a micrometer adjusted guarded diamond knife, useful for obtaining irregular shaped lamellar grafts.
- *Crescent knife (Fig. 2.9.25)*: This is another useful instrument for the lamellar dissection. It has a 2.0 mm blade. It is also used in pterygium surgery and small incision cataract surgery (SICS).

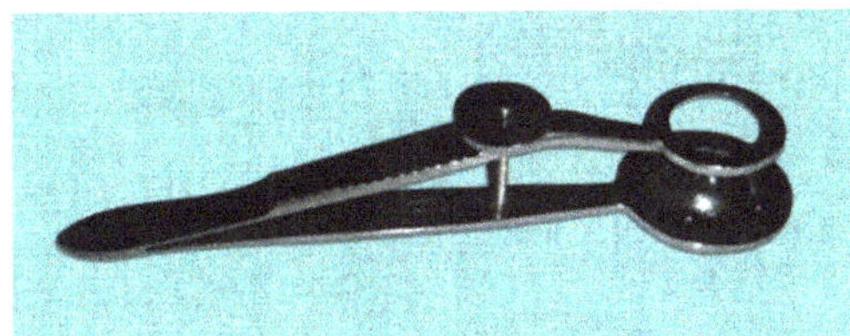

Fig. 2.9.22: King's clamp.

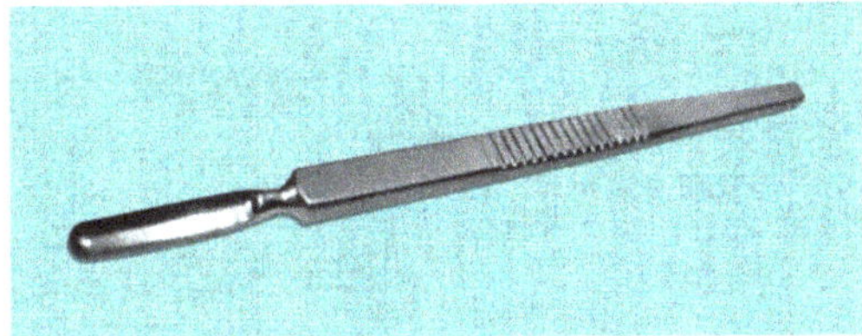

Fig. 2.9.23: Tooke's knife.

Automated Lamellar Therapeutic Keratoplasty Machine

The Moria automated lamellar therapeutic keratectomy microkeratome system utilizes the Moria Carriazo-Barraquer (CBm) microkeratome (Fig. 2.9.26) and an artificial chamber which is manually driven by the surgeon. Multiple microkeratome heads may be used to achieve dissection of various thicknesses ranging from 130 μm to 350 μm (130, 150, 250, 300, and 350 μm). The Moria automated lamellar therapeutic keratoplasty (ALTK) AAC requires a donor scleral rim that is symmetrically greater than 16 mm (max 19 mm) in diameter to provide proper

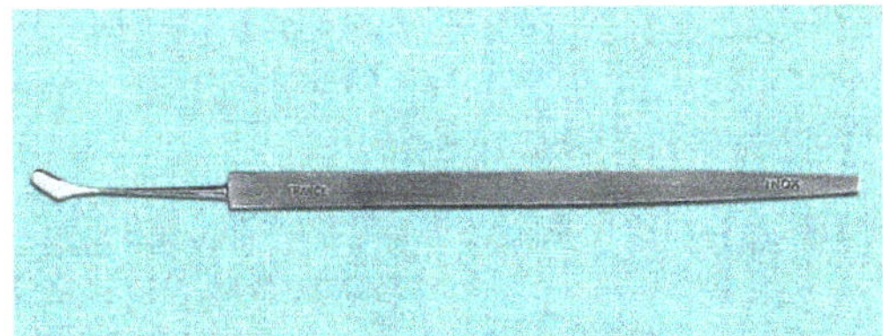

Fig. 2.9.24: Paufique's knife.

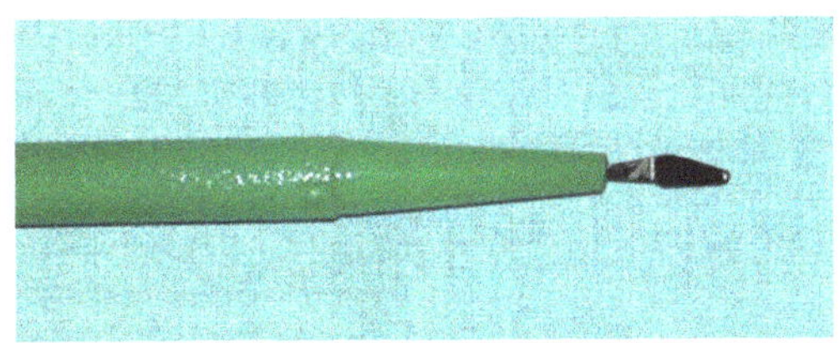

Fig. 2.9.25: Crescent knife.

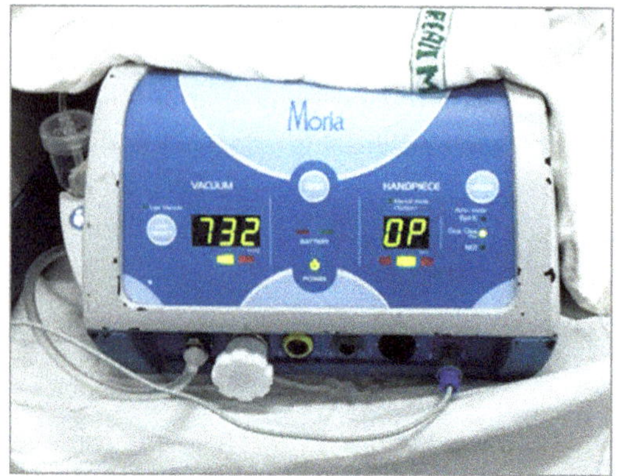

Fig. 2.9.26: Microkeratome.

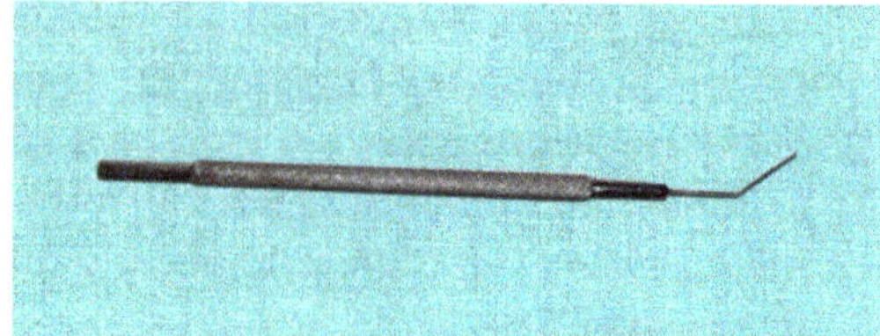
Fig. 2.9.27: Reverse Sinskey hook.

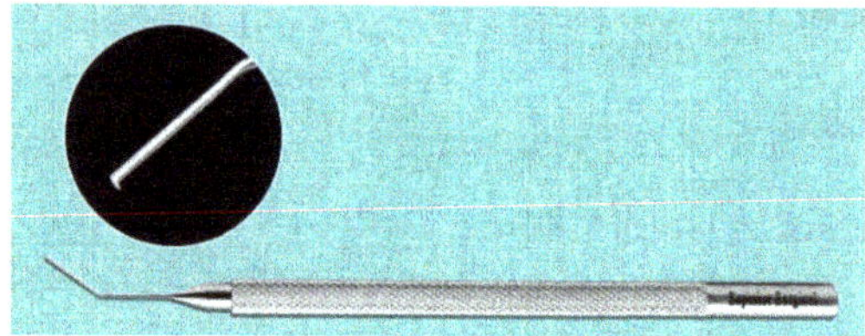
Fig. 2.9.28: DSAEK scraper.

vacuum during the microkeratome pass. The surgical time is greatly reduced as compared to manual dissection technique.

Another machine available is the Amadeus II microkeratome with an AAC (Ziemer Group). The assembly unit comes equipped with four interchangeable suction units (with diameters of 8.5, 9.0, 9.5, and 10.0 mm) and a choice of five blade holders (for a flap thickness of 200, 250, 350, 400 or 450 µm).

Descemet Stripping Automated Endothelial Keratoplasty Instruments

For Donor Dissection

Donor tissue can be prepared manually as in Descemet stripping endothelial keratoplasty (DSEK), using an automated microkeratome as in Descemet stripping automated endothelial keratoplasty (DSAEK) or with the aid of femtosecond laser. Irrespective of the mode of tissue dissection, an AAC is required to aid dissection. Donor tissue can be prepared at the time of surgery or preprepared by surgeon or eye bank staff (precut tissue).

For Recipient Preparation

- *Instruments for making incision*: Blades such as 15, 30, and 45° for inserting anterior chamber maintainer. Alternatively one can use microvitreoretinal (MVR) blade for this purpose. A crescent blade with straight sides and rounded tip is used for making scleral tunnel.
- *Instruments for Descemet scoring and scraping*:
  - Reverse Sinskey hook (Fig. 2.9.27).
  - Descemet's stripper such as Melles stripper, Steinert Descemet stripper, and Gorovoy irrigating stripper can be used instead of Sinskey hook.
  - DSAEK scraper (Fig. 2.9.28) such as Terry scraper, Rosenwasser scraper, Melles PLK scraper or Daya Descemet scraper have angled broad smooth tip with sharp edge and can be used to score as well as take out the host Descemet membrane.
  - Stripping forceps such as Snyder stripping forceps, tips of which are angled upwards, often serrated to grasp the edge of Descemet membrane to complete stripping technique.

For Graft Insertion

- Forceps techniques
  - Taco folding technique (60:40 overfold/40:60 underfold/50:50) using

compression forceps or nonappositional DSEK forceps
    - Trifold or burrito fold technique with forceps
- Needle assisted technique
- Rosenwasser shovel
- Suture pull—through insertion technique
- Donor glides—Busin glide (Fig. 2.9.29), TAN EndoGlide, and Sheets glide
- Donor inserters—EndoSerter, Neusidl corneal inserter, and EndoInjector (EndoShield)
- Others—Macaluso DSAEK endothelial lenticule inserter, Daya Endostar, IDEEL injector, Rieck Glide, and Al-Ghoul vacuum-assisted injector

DSAEK Spatula (Stripper)

It is designed to strip the recipient's Descemet's membrane during the DSAEK procedure. The DSAEK strippers are available in 45° and 90° angled models, in both irrigating and nonirrigating versions. The angled tips facilitate the efficient dissection and removal of Descemet's membrane without inadvertent damage to the stroma. The strippers are made of surgical steel.

Busin Glide (Fig. 2.9.29)

It allows insertion of the taco by pull through technique through 3.2 mm incision. It facilitates the unfolding of the graft and simplifies centration of the donor button in the anterior chamber. It helps to minimize intraoperative manipulation of the graft and the possibility of endothelial loss.

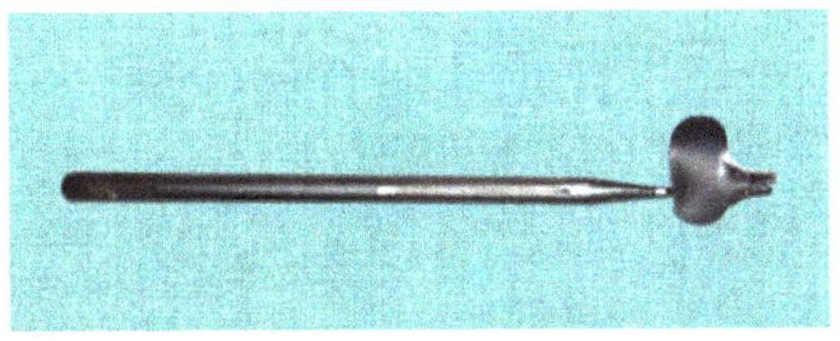

Fig. 2.9.29: Busin glide.

DSAEK Busin Forceps

It is a microincision forceps with 20 G diameter and distal action. It is designed to position the graft in the glide and to pull it from the glide into the anterior chamber. Its tips have been designed specifically to contact the periphery of the graft such that the endothelial and the stromal surfaces remain untouched in the optical zone.

Descemet Membrane Endothelial Keratoplasty Instruments

For Graft Insertion

- Modified IOL injection cartridges (Alcon B cartridge)
- Staar microinjector
- Viscoject IOL injector
- Modified AMO Emerald IOL injector and tip
- Glass injectors—Descemet membrane endothelial keratoplasty (DMEK) Jones tube and Geuder glass injector (Figs. 2.9.30A and B)

To Check Orientation of the Graft before Injection

- Staining the graft with 0.06% trypan blue
- Veldman Venn technique
- S-stamp on the stromal side (Fig. 2.9.31).

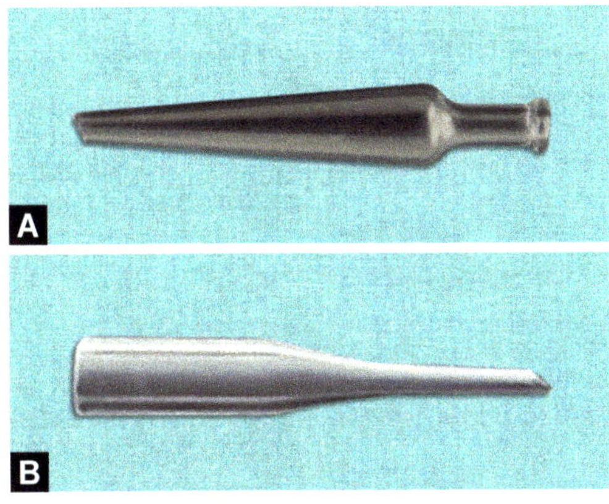

Figs. 2.9.30A and B: Glass injectors—DMEK Jones tube and Geuder glass injector.

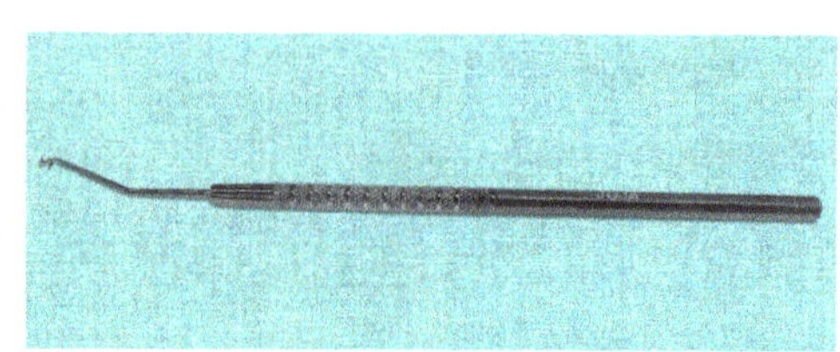

Fig. 2.9.31: S-stamp.

To Check Orientation after Insertion

- Moutsouris sign
- Handheld slit lamp—described by Bukhart et al.
- Endoilluminator or light probe—described by Agarwal et al.
- Intraoperative optical coherence tomography (iOCT).

VIVA QUESTIONS

1. What are the indications for use of Flieringa ring?

Ans. Refer to text.

2. Classify corneal trephines.

Ans. Refer to text.

3. What are the advantages of using suction trephine?

Ans. The following are the advantages of using suction trephine:

- Precise depth of trephination (250 microns for full rotation in Hessburg-Barron vacuum trephine)
- Better stabilization and less chance of slippage due to suction that is maintained during trephination
- Less endothelial cell loss compared with the posterior punch in donor tissue preparation.

4. What are the types of lamellar dissector?

Ans. Refer to text.

5. What are open and closed type of lamellar dissection?

Ans. In *closed method* of lamellar dissection the plane of dissection is not under direct visualization because the anterior lamellar flap is maintained in its original position close to the stromal bed and the dissector is advanced between the two layers. The advantage of this technique is, it results in an even dissection plane with an increased likelihood that the dissection stays in the same plane throughout. However, the chances of corneal perforation are high when compared to open method. In *open method* of lamellar dissection the plane of dissection is visualized by lifting the overlying corneal flap vertically. Slight traction of this flap caused tractional splitting of the stromal fibers at the leading edge of this dissection and the lamellar dissector is then applied in a pressing or sweeping motion at the base of the stromal fibers under traction.

6. What are different techniques of DALK?

Ans. Refer ophthalmology clinics (Part 1).

7. What are the different techniques of donor tissue insertion in DSAEK?

Ans. Refer to text.

8. Conditions where host Descemet membrane scoring is not required.

Ans. There are two school of thoughts in this regard. However, most of the cornea surgeons believe that host Descemet membrane peeling is not routinely indicated except in cases of scarred or wrinkled Descemet membrane, Descemet folds, and prominent guttae that can impair the postoperative visual function. It should be absolutely avoided in cases of regraft following PK. In few cases the Descemet membrane may be either absent or adherent to the underlying stroma making it extremely difficult to score under the hazy overlying corneal stroma.

9. What are the different techniques of donor tissue insertion in DMEK?

Ans. Refer to text.

3

CHAPTER

Cataract

3.1 INTRAOCULAR LENS MASTER

Deepali Singhal, Alisha Kishore, Arpit Sharma, Prafulla Kumar Maharana

INTRODUCTION

Method of optical biometry was introduced by Carl Zeiss Meditec in 1998. It is the gold standard in optical biometry and measures the distance from the corneal apex to the retinal pigment epithelium.

PRINCIPLE

IOLMaster 500 (Fig. 3.1.1) is based on the concept of partial coherence interferometry. It measures the time required for the infrared light to travel to the retina. The recently introduced IOLMaster 700 uses first swept source optical coherence tomography (OCT)-based biometry.

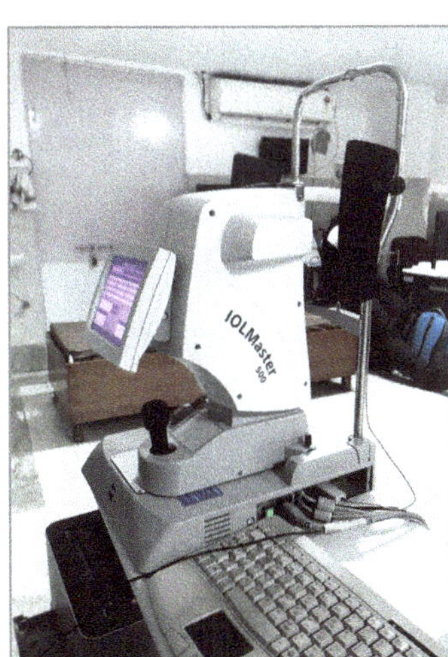

Fig. 3.1.1: IOLMaster 500.

USES

The following parameters can be measured:[1]

- *Axial length*—in the range from 14 mm to 38 mm with the interval scale of 0.01 mm.
- *Radius of curvature of cornea*—in the range from 5 mm to 10 mm with the interval scale of 0.01 mm. It determines the value by measuring the relative position of six spots on the cornea. These are projected in hexagonal pattern with a diameter of 2.5 mm.
- *Anterior chamber depth*—in the range from 1.5 mm to 6.5 mm with the interval scale of 0.01 mm.
- *White-to-white diameter*—in the range from 8 mm to 16 mm with the interval scale of 0.1 mm.
- *Intraocular lens (IOL) power calculation formulas*—SRK II, SRK/T, Holladay 1 and 2, Hoffer Q, and Haigis formula are integrated (Fig. 3.1.2). For calculating IOL power after laser *in situ* keratomileusis (LASIK)/photorefractive keratectomy (PRK)/laser epithelial keratomileusis (LASEK), Haigis-L formula is used. Phakic

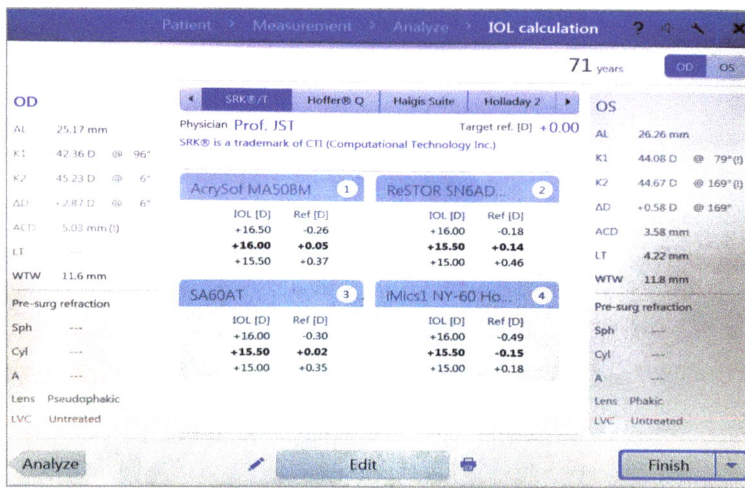

Fig. 3.1.2: IOLMaster 700 with different IOL power calculation formula.

lens power calculation is also integrated. Constants of various IOL are optimized. Also with the Holladay 2, only the postoperative refraction of the patient is needed. All the other information is filled automatically. There is no need for the data to be exported.

ADVANTAGES

- Integrated device which measures axial length, keratometry, and IOL power calculation with wide range of options for calculating power.
- All measurements are done along visual axis for accurate axial length measurement. It is useful even in cases of staphyloma, pseudophakics, eyes filled with silicone oil, and patients with phakic lens.
- Faster acquisition time. Both keratometry and axial length can be measured simultaneously in the dual mode. Different modes can be changed automatically and is user independent.
- Patient comfort since the measurements are distance independent. It is, therefore, useful in patients with poor fixation.
- Higher success rate compared to other devices as there is better cataract penetration. The signals to noise values are also increased, thereby increasing the reliability. It should be more than 2.0.
- The IOLMaster can be integrated with CALLISTO eye for better management in the operating room. It helps in toric IOL alignment without marking the cornea. It can also be connected with A-scan ultrasound device for quick axial length measurement.

INTERPRETATION OF INTRAOCULAR LENS MASTER (FIG. 3.1.3)

This is an IOLMaster of a patient named X with ID 163638 and date of birth 24/05/1968. The examination was done on 28/11/2017 under the surgeon Y. The formula used for IOL power calculation is SRK/T with the target refraction as plano which means emmetropic. The axial length of the right eye is 22.66 mm and the left eye is 22.44 mm which is within normal limit and the difference between the two eyes is less than 0.3 mm. The keratometry value of the right eye is 42.88/43.38 D @ 166°/76° with an astigmatism of 0.50 D at 76°. The right eye is pseudophakic. The keratometry value of the left eye is 42.67/43.10 D @ 147°/57°

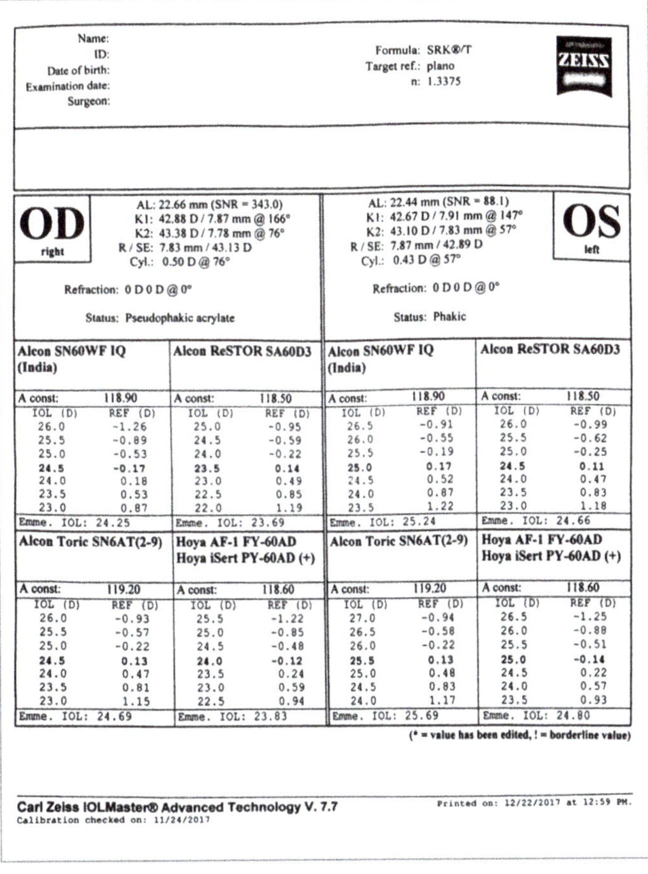

Name:
ID:
Date of birth:
Examination date:
Surgeon:

Formula: SRK®/T
Target ref.: plano
n: 1.3375

ZEISS

OD right

AL: 22.66 mm (SNR = 343.0)
K1: 42.88 D / 7.87 mm @ 166°
K2: 43.38 D / 7.78 mm @ 76°
R / SE: 7.83 mm / 43.13 D
Cyl.: 0.50 D @ 76°

Refraction: 0 D 0 D @ 0°

Status: Pseudophakic acrylate

OS left

AL: 22.44 mm (SNR = 88.1)
K1: 42.67 D / 7.91 mm @ 147°
K2: 43.10 D / 7.83 mm @ 57°
R / SE: 7.87 mm / 42.89 D
Cyl.: 0.43 D @ 57°

Refraction: 0 D 0 D @ 0°

Status: Phakic

OD: Alcon SN60WF IQ (India)		OD: Alcon ReSTOR SA60D3		OS: Alcon SN60WF IQ (India)		OS: Alcon ReSTOR SA60D3	
A const:	118.90	A const:	118.50	A const:	118.90	A const:	118.50
IOL (D)	REF (D)	IOL (D)	REF (D)	IOL (D)	REF (D)	IOL (D)	REF (D)
26.0	-1.26	25.0	-0.95	26.5	-0.91	26.0	-0.99
25.5	-0.89	24.5	-0.59	26.0	-0.55	25.5	-0.62
25.0	-0.53	24.0	-0.22	25.5	-0.19	25.0	-0.25
24.5	**-0.17**	**23.5**	**0.14**	**25.0**	**0.17**	**24.5**	**0.11**
24.0	0.18	23.0	0.49	24.5	0.52	24.0	0.47
23.5	0.53	22.5	0.85	24.0	0.87	23.5	0.83
23.0	0.87	22.0	1.19	23.5	1.22	23.0	1.18
Emme. IOL: 24.25		Emme. IOL: 23.69		Emme. IOL: 25.24		Emme. IOL: 24.66	

OD: Alcon Toric SN6AT(2-9)		OD: Hoya AF-1 FY-60AD Hoya iSert PY-60AD (+)		OS: Alcon Toric SN6AT(2-9)		OS: Hoya AF-1 FY-60AD Hoya iSert PY-60AD (+)	
A const:	119.20	A const:	118.60	A const:	119.20	A const:	118.60
IOL (D)	REF (D)	IOL (D)	REF (D)	IOL (D)	REF (D)	IOL (D)	REF (D)
26.0	-0.93	25.5	-1.22	27.0	-0.94	26.5	-1.25
25.5	-0.57	25.0	-0.85	26.5	-0.58	26.0	-0.88
25.0	-0.22	24.5	-0.48	26.0	-0.22	25.5	-0.51
24.5	**0.13**	**24.0**	**-0.12**	**25.5**	**0.13**	**25.0**	**-0.14**
24.0	0.47	23.5	0.24	25.0	0.48	24.5	0.22
23.5	0.81	23.0	0.59	24.5	0.83	24.0	0.57
23.0	1.15	22.5	0.94	24.0	1.17	23.5	0.93
Emme. IOL: 24.69		Emme. IOL: 23.83		Emme. IOL: 25.69		Emme. IOL: 24.80	

(* = value has been edited, ! = borderline value)

Carl Zeiss IOLMaster® Advanced Technology V. 7.7
Calibration checked on: 11/24/2017
Printed on: 12/22/2017 at 12:59 PM.

Fig. 3.1.3: IOLMaster of a right eye pseudophakic patient for left eye cataract surgery.

with an astigmatism of 0.43 D at 57°. The left eye is phakic. So, the patient is for left eye cataract surgery. IOL calculations for Alcon IQ, ReSTOR, Toric, and Hoya have been calculated. The IOL, which has been used in the right eye, should be used in the left eye. For example, if Alcon IQ of 24.5 D was used in the right eye then in the left eye, Alcon IQ of power 25.5 D should be used which will give a refraction of -0.19 which will comparable to the right eye of -0.17 at 24.5 D. It is important to correlate the findings clinically.

VIVA QUESTIONS

1. What is the difference between LenStar and IOLMaster?

Ans. Refer to Table 3.1.1.

2. Advantages of IOLMaster 700.

Ans. IOLMaster 700 (Fig. 3.1.4) has integrated swept source OCT and Barrett suite.[2] Its various advantages include:

- Refractive surprises are less
- Repeatability
- Integration of swept source OCT provides measurement based on image. It provides longitudinal section of the eye. It helps in identifying conditions such as lens tilt
- Accurate measurement since image of the fovea (Fig. 3.1.5) tells about the fixation
- Central corneal thickness and lens thickness can be measured additionally
- More effective in cases of posterior sub-capsular cataract (PSC) and dense nuclear cataract as compared to IOLMaster 500.

Table 3.1.1: Difference between LenStar and IOLMaster.

	LenStar	*IOLMaster*
Manufacturer	Haag-Streit	Zeiss
Principle	Optical low-coherence reflectometry	Partial coherence interferometry
FDA approved	October 2009	March 2000
Laser used	Superluminescent diode (820 nm)	Infrared diode laser (780 nm)
Measurement	Dual zone keratometer with a total of 32 marker points on two concentric rings of 1.65 mm and 2.3 mm in diameter	It measures the relative position of six spots on the cornea. These are projected in hexagonal pattern with a diameter of 2.5 mm
Pupillometry	Can be measured	Cannot be measured
Lens thickness	Can be measured	Cannot be measured
Central corneal thickness	Can be measured	Cannot be measured

(FDA: Food and Drug Administration; IOL: intraocular lens)

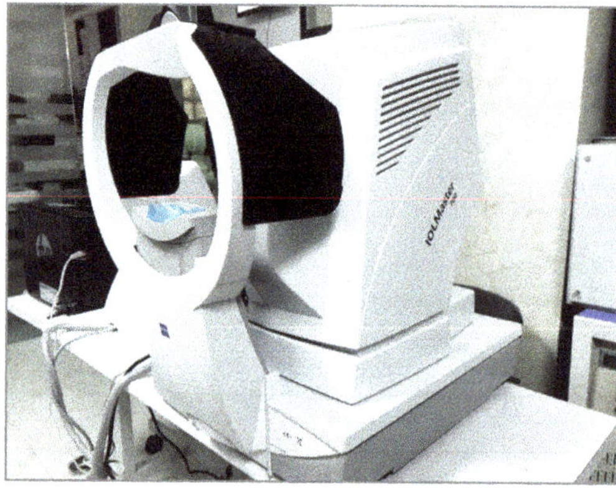

Fig. 3.1.4: IOLMaster 700.

3. Difference between IOLMaster 500 and IOLMaster 700.

Ans. Refer to Table 3.1.2.[3]

4. Difference between A-scan and IOLMaster for axial length (AL) measurement.

Ans. Refer to Table 3.1.3.[4]

5. What is partial coherence interferometry?

Ans. Partial coherence interferometry uses a low coherene length infrared light of 780 nm and is split into two parts by an external Michelson interoferometer. A coaxial dual beam is produced out of which one goes to a reference mirror and the other component is reflected at several intraocular interfaces that separate media of different refractive indices. For the measurement of axial length, reflection sites are the anterior surface of the cornea and the retinal pigment epithelium. If the delay of these two components produced by the interferometer equals an intraocular distance within the coherence length of the light source, an interference signal (called partial coherence interferometry signal) is detected, similar to that of ultrasound A-scan, but with a very high resolution and precision.

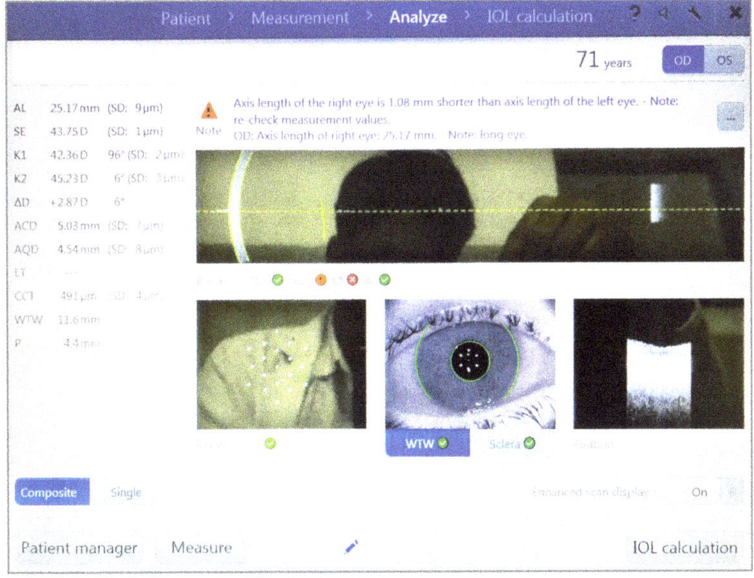

Fig. 3.1.5: IOLMaster 700 showing foveal image.

Table 3.1.2: IOLMaster 700 versus 500.

Parameters	*500*	*700*
AL measurements	PCI	Swept source OCT
LT and central corneal thickness (CCT)	Not available	Possible
ACD measurements	Optical section through the anterior chamber by means of a slit-illumination system	Swept source OCT images
	Not possible in pseudophakic eyes	Possible
	Prone to error	More accurate
Identify irregular eye geometries	Not possible	Possible
Dense PSC/dense cataracts	Inaccurate measurement	Accurate
Patients with poor fixation, irregular eye geometries	Inaccurate	Useful

(AL: axial length; IOL: intraocular lens; OCT: optical coherence tomography; PCI: partial coherence interferometry; PSC: posterior subcapsular cataract; ACD: anterior chamber depth; LT: lens thickness)

Table 3.1.3: Difference between AL measurement using A-scan and IOLMaster.

	A-scan	*IOLMaster*
Signal transmission	Ultrasound waves	Laser
Measurement	• From corneal apex to the internal limiting membrane • Measures along the anatomical axis	• From corneal apex to retinal pigment epithelium • Measures along the visual axis
Contact procedure	Contact	Noncontact
Accuracy	• Less resolution • Approximately 0.10–0.12 mm	• Better resolution and more accurate • Approximately 0.012 mm

(AL: axial length; IOL: intraocular lens)

6. What is swept source OCT?

Ans. Swept source OCT utilizes longer wavelength of 1,040 nm compared to 840 nm in spectral domain OCT. This overcomes the scattering of light by the retinal pigment epithelium. Also, there is deeper penetration into the choroid allowing more accurate imaging of vitreous, retina, and the choroid. The axial resolution is increased and there is faster acquisition time.

REFERENCES

1. Meditec CZ. (2016). IOLMaster 500 from ZEISS: Defining Biometry. [online] Available from https://applications.zeiss.com/C1257A290053AE30/0/6D036B2F9E9161C8C1257BF30033EF8F/$FILE/IOLMaster_500_Brochure_EN_32_010_0022II.pdf. [Accessed January, 2019].
2. Meditec CZ. (2017). ZEISS IOLMaster 700: Getting Fewer Refractive Surprises. [online] Available from https://zeiss.taimaz.com/wp-content/uploads/2018/06/TAIMAZ_iolmaster_700_brochure_en_32_010_0009v-.pdf. [Accessed January, 2019].
3. Akman A, Asena L, Güngör SG. Evaluation and comparison of the new swept source OCT-based IOLMaster 700 with the IOLMaster 500. Br J Ophthalmol. 2016;100:1201-5.
4. Holladay JT. Ultrasound and optical biometry. Cataract Refract Surg Today Eur. 2009;26:18-9.

3.2 LENSTAR

Yogita Gupta, Deepali Singhal, Prafulla Kumar Maharana

INTRODUCTION

LenStar LS900 (Fig. 3.2.1) is a high-resolution, noncontact, and noninvasive optical biometry device. When it was first introduced in 2009[1] by Haag-Streit manufacturer, it became popular as the first optical biometry device which could measure crystalline lens thickness.

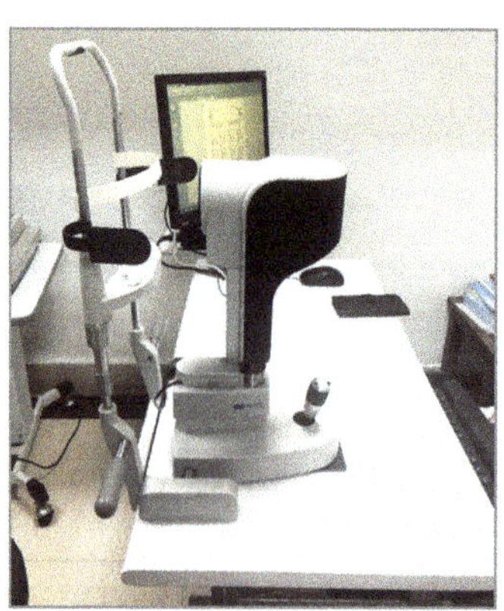

Fig. 3.2.1: LenStar LS900 device for optical biometry.

PRINCIPLE

The LenStar is based on optical low-coherence reflectometry (OLCR).[2] Like the IOLMaster, it uses the effect of time domain interferometric or coherent superposition of light waves to measure ocular lengths of the eye in a similar technique to one-dimensional optical coherence tomography. The IOLMaster uses a diode laser, whereas the LenStar uses 820 μm superluminescent diode[2] with a Gaussian-shaped spectrum which allows a higher axial resolution; hence, the terminology OLCR, rather than partial coherence interferometry, has been coined.[1]

EQUIPMENT

LenStar obtains measurements after user focuses or aligns the image of the eye on the computer monitor while patient fixates on a flashing red light (Fig. 3.2.2).

Central corneal topography is obtained using two rings of diameters 1.65 mm and 2.3 mm of 16 light spots each, reflected off the air/tear interface. These 32 closely spaced measurement points give a dual-zone keratometry system.

The retinal thickness can also be determined from the scans by subjective alignment of the cursor. The horizontal iris width [white-to-white (WTW)] is measured as the horizontal diameter of a best fit circle to the iris boarder and the pupil diameter is measured as the diameter of a best fit circle to the pupil boarder.

USES

LS900 measures nine parameters: (1) axial length (AL), (2) keratometry, (3) lens thickness, (4) corneal thickness, (5) retinal thickness, (6) anterior chamber depth (ACD), (7) WTW diameter, (8) pupil diameter, and (9) eccentricity of the visual axis with respect to the center of cornea (Fig. 3.2.3). Besides it also gives: aqueous depth, radii for flat and steep meridian, and axis of flat meridian.

ADVANTAGES

- The Dense Cataract Measurement (DCM) Mode allows penetration through dense cataract and allows biometry in aphakic, pseudophakic, or silicone oil-filled eyes.
- LenStar Pro version has Automated Positioning System (APS) that tracks

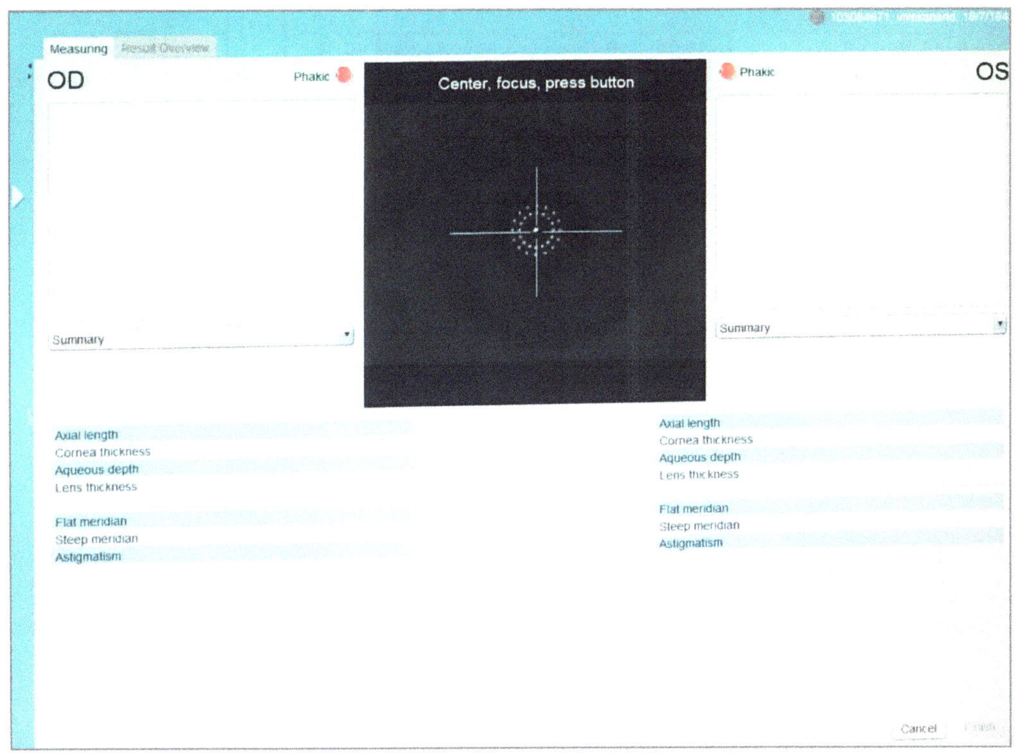

Fig. 3.2.2: Patient fixation in LS900.

Page 1 of 1

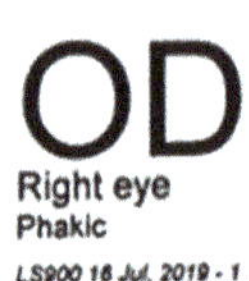

OD

Right eye
Phakic

LS900 16 Jul, 2019 - 1

AL [mm] 25.42[1]
CCT [µm] 516
AD [mm] 2.99
ACD [mm] 3.51
LT [mm] 4.09

R1[mm/D/°] 8.08 / 41.75 @ 93
R2[mm/D/°] 7.56 / 44.66 @ 3
R [mm/D] 7.82 / 43.15
+AST [D/°] 2.91 @ 3
n 1.3375
WTW [mm] 12.18

Warnings:
1: Significant difference between OD and OS

Target Refraction: 0.00 *Template: Room No. 279*

SN60WF
Alcon

IOL [D]	Eye [D]
14.50	0.73
15.00	0.41
15.50	**0.08**
16.00	-0.25
16.50	-0.58

SRK/T
A=119.00

AcrySof MA60AC
Alcon

IOL [D]	Eye [D]
15.00	0.51
15.50	0.19
16.00	**-0.13**
16.50	-0.46
17.00	-0.79

SRK/T
A=119.20

Tecnis 1 ZCB00
AMO

IOL [D]	Eye [D]
15.00	0.57
15.50	0.25
16.00	**-0.07**
16.50	-0.40
17.00	-0.73

SRK/T
A=119.30

CT LUCIA 601P/PY
Zeiss

IOL [D]	Eye [D]
15.00	0.51
15.50	0.19
16.00	**-0.13**
16.50	-0.46
17.00	-0.79

SRK/T
A=119.20

ReSTOR SN6AD1/3
Alcon

IOL [D]	Eye [D]
14.50	0.73
15.00	0.41
15.50	**0.08**
16.00	-0.25
16.50	-0.58

SRK/T
A=119.00

Symfony ZXR00
AMO

IOL [D]	Eye [D]
15.00	0.57
15.50	0.25
16.00	**-0.07**
16.50	-0.40
17.00	-0.73

SRK/T
A=119.30

OS

Left eye
Phakic

LS900 16 Jul, 2019 - 1

AL [mm] 26.03[1]
CCT [µm] 519
AD [mm] 3.03
ACD [mm] 3.55
LT [mm] 3.71

R1[mm/D/°] 8.17 / 41.31 @ 88
R2[mm/D/°] 7.54 / 44.75 @ 178
R [mm/D] 7.86 / 42.96
+AST [D/°] 3.43 @ 178
n 1.3375
WTW [mm] 11.92

Warnings:
1: Significant difference between OD and OS

Target Refraction: 0.00 *Template: Room No. 279*

SN60WF
Alcon

IOL [D]	Eye [D]
13.00	0.66
13.50	0.34
14.00	**0.02**
14.50	-0.31
15.00	-0.64

SRK/T
A=119.00

AcrySof MA60AC
Alcon

IOL [D]	Eye [D]
13.00	0.75
13.50	0.44
14.00	**0.12**
14.50	-0.21
15.00	-0.53

SRK/T
A=119.20

Tecnis 1 ZCB00
AMO

IOL [D]	Eye [D]
13.50	0.49
14.00	0.17
14.50	**-0.15**
15.00	-0.48
15.50	-0.81

SRK/T
A=119.30

CT LUCIA 601P/PY
Zeiss

IOL [D]	Eye [D]
13.00	0.75
13.50	0.44
14.00	**0.12**
14.50	-0.21
15.00	-0.53

SRK/T
A=119.20

ReSTOR SN6AD1/3
Alcon

IOL [D]	Eye [D]
13.00	0.66
13.50	0.34
14.00	**0.02**
14.50	-0.31
15.00	-0.64

SRK/T
A=119.00

Symfony ZXR00
AMO

IOL [D]	Eye [D]
13.50	0.49
14.00	0.17
14.50	**-0.15**
15.00	-0.48
15.50	-0.81

SRK/T
A=119.30

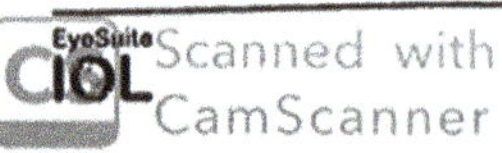

EyeSuite™ IOL, V4.3.2
SID: 1800

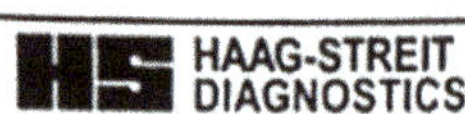

Fig. 3.2.3: A report of LS900.

eye movement to capture reliable measurements in one click.

- When planning for toric or premium IOLs, the Pro version of the LS900 can be used to measure 6-mm optical zone with the option of adding T-cone Toric Platform, a double-ring placido disc topographer, which improves refractive outcomes.
- It helps in determination of the appropriate IOL power by including the modern IOL formulae like: Barrett Universal II, Barrett True-K, Haigis, Hoffer Q, Holladay 1, SRK/T, SRK II, Masket, Modified Masket and Shammas No-history, and Hill RBF methods. The option of EyeSuite IOL toric planner software also includes the Barrett Toric Calculator.
- It is patient-friendly and high-speed device with each scan capturing all measurements in 30 seconds.[3]
- It uses a separate external PC, which allows good memory for storage and enables regular software updates.
- It has excellent intra- and intersession repeatability and good accuracy, comparable with the IOLMaster and ultrasonic biometry.

VIVA QUESTIONS

1. What is the principle of LenStar?

Ans. Refer to text.

2. What are the advantages over IOLMaster?

Ans. Refer to text and also chapter on IOLMaster.

REFERENCES

1. Buckhurst PJ, Wolffsohn JS, Shah S, et al. A new optical low coherence reflectometry device for ocular biometry in cataract patients. Br J Ophthalmol. 2009;93:949-53.
2. Haag-Streit Diagnostics. (2017). LENSTAR LS 900: Improving Outcomes. [online] Available from https://www.haag-streit.com/fileadmin/Haag-Streit_USA/Lenstar/Landing/papers/Brochure_Lenstar_eng.pdf. [Accessed January, 2019].
3. Haag Streit LENSTAR®. (2017). LENSTAR LS 900® The First Optical Biometer Of The Entire Eye. [online] Available from https://www.doctor-hill.com/lenstar_haag_streit/lenstar_main.htm. [Accessed January, 2019].

3.3 A-SCAN

Srujana D, Mohamed Ibrahime Asif, Pranita Sahay, Ritu Nagpal

INTRODUCTION

A-scan ultrasound (Fig. 3.3.1) is a one-dimensional amplitude modulation scan, used commonly to determine the axial length (AL) of the eye. Measurement of AL is an important component of any intraocular lens (IOL) calculation formula prior to cataract surgery. Besides, A-scan is also used in conjunction with B-scan imaging to measure the size and characterize the ultrasonic properties of any mass lesion located in the posterior segment or in orbit.

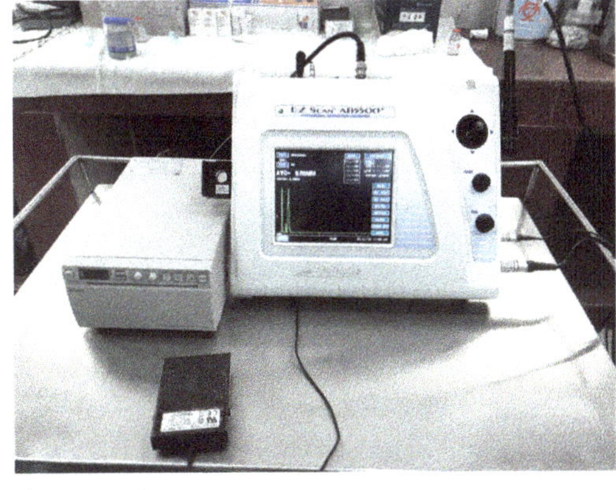

Fig. 3.3.1: A-scan.

PRINCIPLE

A-scan ultrasonography is based on the principle of calculating the time required for the sound waves to go across the eye using a 10-MHz ultrasound transducer (Fig. 3.3.2) and conversion of it to a quantitative (linear) value through a velocity formula.

Using an estimated average velocity through the various ocular media: cornea (1,620 m/s), aqueous (1,532 m/s), lens (1,641 m/s), and vitreous (1,532 m/s), the biometric software calculates the AL. This value should be altered when velocities differ as in performing AL measurements in aphakia, pseudophakia, and silicon-filled eye. Special precaution must be taken in silicone oil-filled eyes. The refractive index of silicone oil is considerably less than vitreous humor; hence this must be taken into consideration along with the type of IOL while calculating the IOL power in silicone oil-filled eyes.

While performing A-scan, multiple spikes are seen in the display, each representing reflection of the waves from different parts such as the cornea, anterior surface of the lens, posterior surface of the lens, and the retina. The gap between the spikes from the corneal and retinal surface provides the AL of the eye (Fig. 3.3.3).

METHOD

After instilling topical anesthetic, the ultrasound probe (6 mm in diameter) of A-scan is placed gently over the apex of the cornea. The patient is asked to fix a target light on the probe or is asked to fixate his thumb raised by the technician to keep the eye aligned along the pupil-macular axis. High spikes are obtained when the sound beam is perpendicular to the ocular interfaces. If the beam strikes the optic nerve instead of the macula, scleral and orbital fat spikes are absent. Hence, alignment of the probe is critical as incorrect alignment can give erroneous readings. Patients with poor vision, such as dense cataracts or due to other pathology, are less likely to fixate accurately, causing errors. To avoid any error, the average of 10, most reliable readings with 100% spike must be calculated.

In the manual mode when an acceptable scan is obtained, the operator has to freeze the scan with a foot pedal. The gates (corneal and retinal) should then be moved to the correct place and the reading taken. While doing this, it is advisable to keep the gain at the lowest level at which a high-quality reading is obtained.

In automatic mode, the machine freezes the image when the spikes fall in a certain range. However, prior to measurement, the

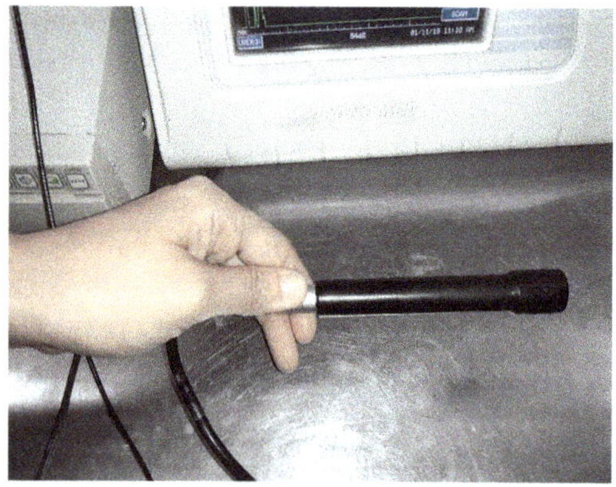

Fig. 3.3.2: Ultrasonic probe.

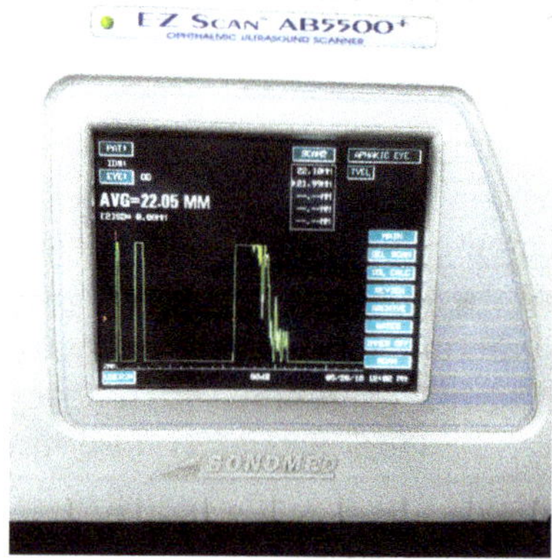

Fig. 3.3.3: Display of contact A-scan showing spikes at various ocular interfaces.

machine must be calibrated, and the velocity settings must be appropriately chosen depending upon the condition of the eye. It is important not to apply too much pressure over the cornea, or else compression of the cornea could lead to an underestimation of the measured AL. For example, in the case of Sanders-Retzlaff-Kraff (SRK) formula, an error of 1.0 mm will result in approximately 2.50 D postoperative refractive surprise. This may further increase while measuring AL in short or long eyes. Thus, in case of an underestimation of AL, there will be a myopic surprise while in case of an overestimation, there will be a hyperopic surprise in the postoperative period. It is important to note that a greasy corneal surface due to prior application of ointment or lubricants can also lead to an error in IOL power calculation.

Another source of error is not choosing the right IOL mode. The velocity of the sound wave is more in cases of polymethylmethacrylate (PMMA)/acrylic/silicon IOL than through the crystalline lens. Hence, in these eyes, pseudophakic mode has to be used.

Repeat scan: Repeat scan is indicated in the following situations:

- Axial length less than 22 mm or more than 25 mm. In short or long eyes, the indentation effect can lead to significant error; hence, it is better to repeat the measurement several times till reliable results are obtained.
- Eyes with posterior staphyloma.
- If the difference is measured, AL between the two eyes is more than 0.3 mm.
- *If repeated measurements vary by more than 0.2 mm, discrepancy between patients refractive status and the measured AL*: It is always a good practice to compare the refractive error of the patient with the AL. For example, an AL of 30 mm having an error of +2.00 D, one should repeat measurements of A-scan.

A-SCAN IN SPECIAL SITUATIONS

- *Silicon oil-filled eye*: The speed of ultrasound wave in silicon oil is around 987 m/s (with a viscosity of 1,000 centistokes and 1,040 m/s for 5,000 centistokes) while in vitreous humor, it is 1,532 m/s; hence, the AL measured is usually falsely high in oil-filled eye. Theoretically, the correction factor comes out to be 0.64 mm. Murray et al. derived the conversion factor of 0.71 for silicon oil of viscosity 1,300 centistokes.[1]

The second major challenge in oil-filled eyes is the difficulty in identifying the ocular interfaces accurately. The identification of the retinal interface is challenging in oil-filled eyes due to sound attenuation. Besides, the majority of oil-filled eyes are myopic and may be having posterior staphyloma, which further can amplify the error.

The situation becomes worse when the eye is partially silicone oil-filled. The oil bubble moves with movement of the eye producing shifting retinal echoes. In the supine position, often the routinely followed technique, the oil bubble would rest on the retina while the liquefied vitreous will stay on top of it. If the measurements are taken in this position, the ultrasound wave will cross the layer of liquefied vitreous first, prior to crossing the silicone oil-filled portion. Thus, separate measurements must be taken for these two parts to calculate the vitreous cavity depth accurately. The best approach to deal with such cases is to perform the measurement with the patient in a seated position. The liquefied vitreous will shift superiorly leaving only the silicone oil in the optical axis through which the ultrasound beam would pass. Also, with contact A-mode, the echoes from the tip of the probe merge with the echoes from the cornea to become a single broad echo, leading to difficult identification of the anterior corneal spike. Further, lens opacities also generate additional echoes that interfere with the instrument's ability to detect the posterior capsule spike and to measure the proper lens thickness.

- *Posterior staphyloma*: In the presence of staphyloma, the anatomic AL (corneal apex to the most posterior portion of the globe) may not correspond to the refractive AL (corneal apex to the center of the macula). This could lead an erroneous AL measurement.
- *Others*: Several other factors can also produce errors in AL measurement on A-scan. The difficulty in delineating the anterior and posterior corneal surfaces can lead to an error in exact positioning of the anterior spike for AL measurement. Similarly for lenticular opacities, the presence of IOL can produce multiple echoes that can lead to errors in AL measurement.

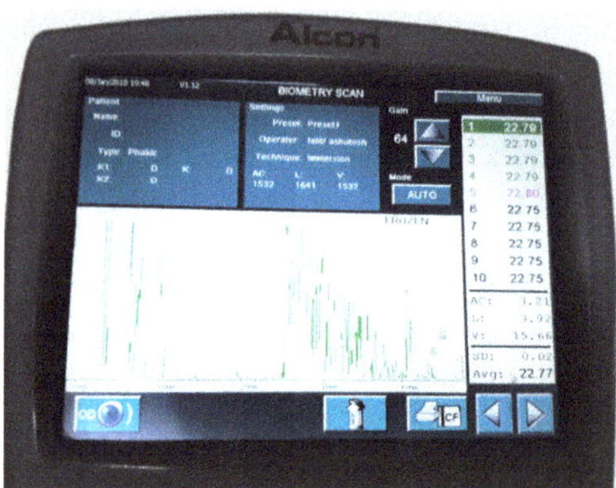

Fig. 3.3.4: Display of immersion A-scan showing spikes at various ocular interfaces.

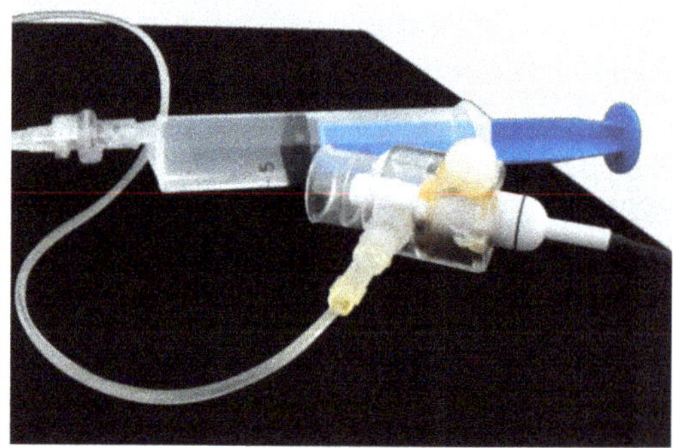

Fig. 3.3.5: Prager Scleral Shell.

IMMERSION SCAN

In this, the coupling fluid rather than the ultrasound probe comes into contact with the corneal apex. This excludes any compression of the cornea and hence avoids any errors in AL measurement (Fig. 3.3.4). The coupling fluid requires a Prager Scleral Shell (Fig. 3.3.5), or a set of Ossoinig or Hansen Scleral Shells to be placed within the palpebral aperture. A shell of size 20 mm usually fits most eyes, a larger cup may be required for the bigger eye with large palpebral fissure, and a smaller cup for eyes with a narrow palpebral fissure.

For performing the scan, the patient is asked to lie down supine, looking up at the ceiling. The Prager Shell is placed between the eyelids. Normal saline or lubricant eye drop is used to fill the shell that acts as the coupling media. The ultrasound beam is then aligned with the macula by asking the patient to look at the fixation light, and the measurements are taken. Although both saline and a higher concentration of methylcellulose 1% can be used as coupling fluid, 1% methylcellulose is the best as saline is too thin and a higher concentration of methylcellulose is too thick.

Accuracy

The accuracy of immersion scan is within 0.12 mm. Thus, the use of this technique could lead to a refractive surprise of approximately 0.28 D. This error may be more in short or long eyes.

Advantages

Immersion scan has following advantages:

- Better reproducibility and accuracy.
- Avoids corneal compression thereby displaying true anterior chamber depth and exact AL.
- Possible to identify anterior corneal spike clearly (c.f. applanation A-scan).
- In posterior staphylomatous eyes, it is (immersion B-scan) extremely useful in identification of the macula in relation to staphyloma.
- Allows measurement of correct AL in oil-filled eyes by identifying retro silicon space accurately.
- Posterior staphyloma, recurrent retinal detachment (RD), epiretinal membranes, and retained perfluorocarbon (PFC) bubbles can be detected, and gates can be adjusted to give the exact AL.

VIVA QUESTIONS

1. What is Artemis very high-frequency (VHF) digital ultrasound?

Ans. Artemis uses a 50-MHz VHF ultrasound transducer with immersion scanning technology. It acquires high precision B-scans that approximately represent the surface contour of anterior or posterior segment structures. The radius of the curvature adjustment mechanism to enable maximum perpendicularity and enhanced signal-to-noise ratio allows for excellent precision. Its axial resolution is 21 μ, and three-dimensional (3D) layered pachymetry (using multiple meridional scans) has precision less than 1.0 μ.

2. What is the axial length (AL) at birth?

Ans. Axial length at birth is 14.5–15.5 mm.

3. Changes in AL with age.

Ans. The change in the AL of the eye occurs in three phases:

- *Phase 1 (birth to age 2 years)*: This is a period of rapid growth. In the first 6 months, the AL increases by 4 mm while in the subsequent 6 months, it increases by 2 mm.
- *Phase 2 (age 2–5 years)*: The growth slows down and the AL increases by 1 mm.
- *Phase 3 (age 5–13 years)*: The growth further slows down and the AL increases by another 1 mm.

4. Impact of cataract surgery on axial length in congenital cataract.

Ans. The impact of cataract surgery on AL change is controversial with few reports suggesting a reduction while few reporting increased axial elongation of the eye following cataract surgery. Unilateral cataract surgery, especially during infancy, has been reported to be associated with more axial elongation in the operated eye than bilateral cataract surgery.

5. The advantage of A-scan over IOLMaster.

Ans. Though IOLMaster is more precise than A-scan, it is disadvantageous in patients with dense cataract (media opacities), corneal opacity, dense vitreous hemorrhage, and if patients are not able to fix.

REFERENCE

1. Murray DC, Durrani OM, Good P, et al. Biometry of the silicone oil-filled eye: II. Eye Lond Engl. 2002;16:727-30.

3.4 APPLIANCES AND INSTRUMENTS IN CATARACT SURGERY

Pranita Sahay, Prafulla Kumar Maharana

VON GRAEFE'S KNIFE (FIG. 3.4.1)

It is a long, narrow, and thin blade with a sharp tip with cutting edge on one side. It was used for making the corneoscleral entry in cataract surgery.

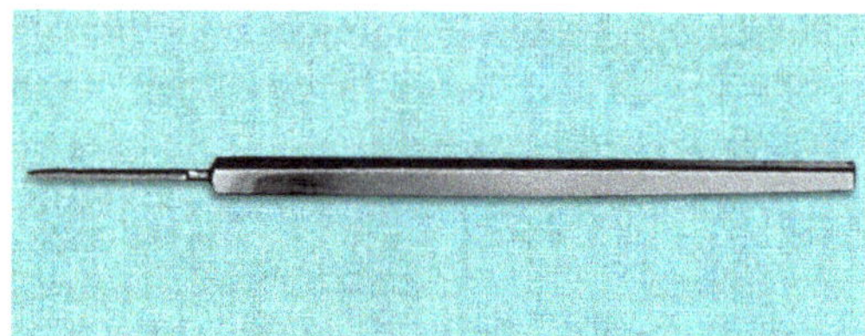

Fig. 3.4.1: Von Graefe's knife.

KERATOMES (FIG. 3.4.2)

It is a thin blade with a diamond-shaped apex and cutting edge on both sides. It is available in both straight and curved design as well as in various sizes (2.2 mm, 2.8 mm, 3 mm, 3.5 mm, and 5.5 mm). It is used for making self-sealing corneal incisions in cataract surgery.

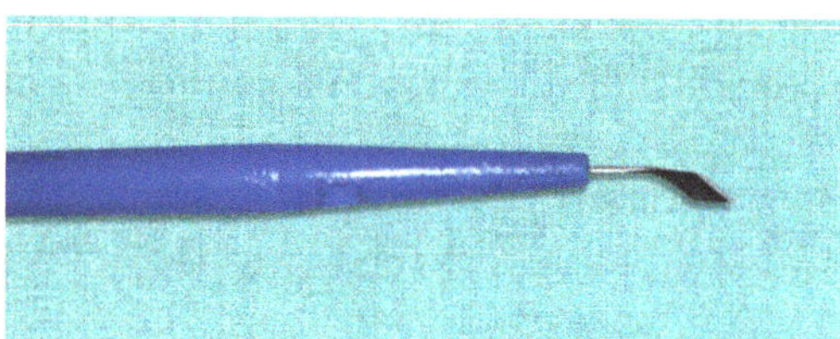

Fig. 3.4.2: Keratomes.

MICROVITREORETINAL OR V-LANCE BLADE (FIG. 3.4.3)

It is a fine straight instrument with triangular knife at its distal end having cutting edge on both the sides. It is used for making the side port entry at the limbus as well as sclerotomy for vitreoretinal surgery. The incision width with this blade is approximately 1.1 mm.

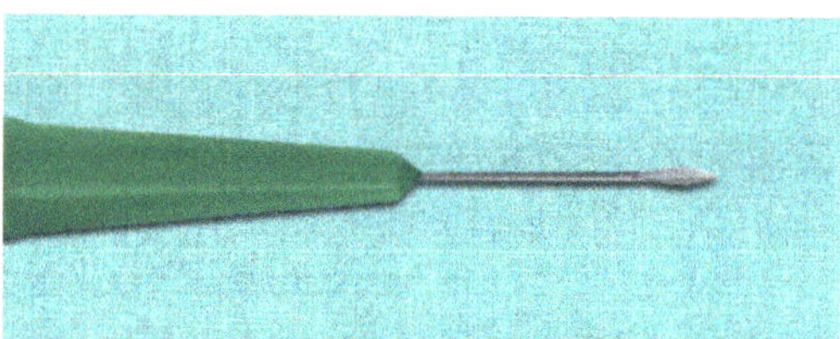

Fig. 3.4.3: Microvitreoretinal (MVR).

One special use of microvitreoretinal (MVR) is posterior-assisted levitation (PAL) technique, described by Charles Kelman to salvage a dropping nucleus during cataract surgery. In this technique, a pars plana sclerotomy is done at the 11 o'clock meridian, 3.5 mm behind the limbus using a MVR blade. A spatula is passed through the sclerotomy and placed behind the nucleus which is then elevated forward into the anterior chamber (AC) and subsequently managed by phacoemulsification or manual removal. The other special uses of MVR include transcorneal venting incisions in Descemet stripping automated endothelial keratoplasty (DSAEK) to drain residual interface fluid and stab incisions to drain intrastromal fluid pockets in cases of corneal hydrops.

The limitation of MVR is similar to other sharp instruments, i.e. chances of inadvertent prick injuries to the operating surgeon. During cataract surgery, it can lead to Descemet's membrane detachment and inadvertent damage to iris or lens capsule especially if the tip is bent or blunt.

CORNEAL SCISSORS (FIG. 3.4.4)

It is a fine curved scissor that works on spring action. The main differentiating feature of conjunctival scissor is that it is short and stout.

Uses

- To enlarge the corneal or corneoscleral incision for intracapsular cataract extraction (ICCE)/extracapsular cataract extraction (ECCE)
- To enlarge corneal incision in keratoplasty
- To cut the scleral tissue flap.

The main advantage of enlarging the corneal incision with corneal scissor is that it enlarges the wound exactly along the limbus. The limitation is that it may lead to ragged margins of the cut edges especially if the scissors are not sharp.

VANNAS SCISSORS (FIG. 3.4.5)

They are fine scissors that work on spring action. It has two wings to operate—(1) one sharp and (2) one blunt. These can be curved, straight, or angulated.

Uses

- For cutting sutures
- For performing anterior capsulotomy in ECCE
- For cutting the vitreous strand while performing anterior vitrectomy
- For excising the host corneal ledge during keratoplasty.

LENS SPATULA (FIG. 3.4.6)

It has a metallic handle with spoon-shaped end which is used to apply pressure at 12 o'clock position in Smith's technique and expression of nucleus in ECCE.

WIRE VECTIS (FIG. 3.4.7)

It is a wire loop attached to metallic handle.

Uses

It is used to remove subluxated lens in ICCE and nucleus in ECCE.

While it is extremely useful in retrieving the nucleus pieces in the event of posterior capsular rent (PCR) during cataract surgery, it can lead to complications like iridodialysis and giant retinal tear if performed blindly or when a desperate attempt is made to retrieve an already sinking nucleus from anterior vitreous cavity.

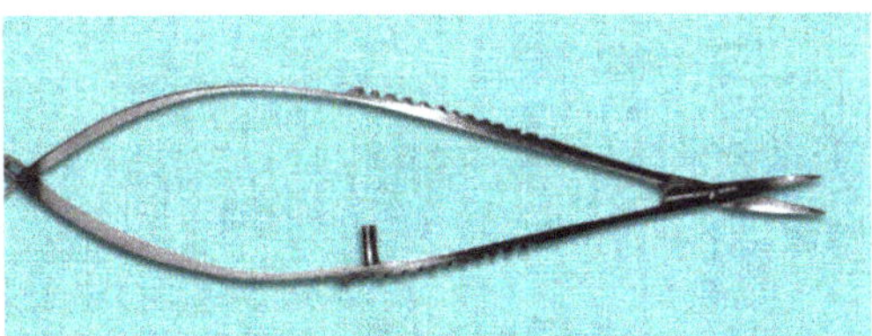

Fig. 3.4.4: Corneal scissors.

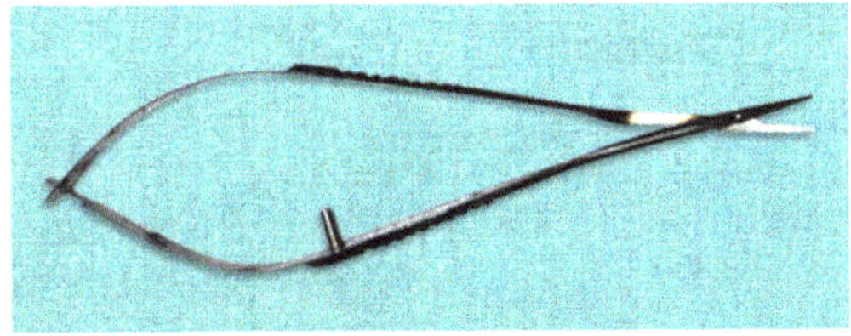

Fig. 3.4.5: Vannas scissors.

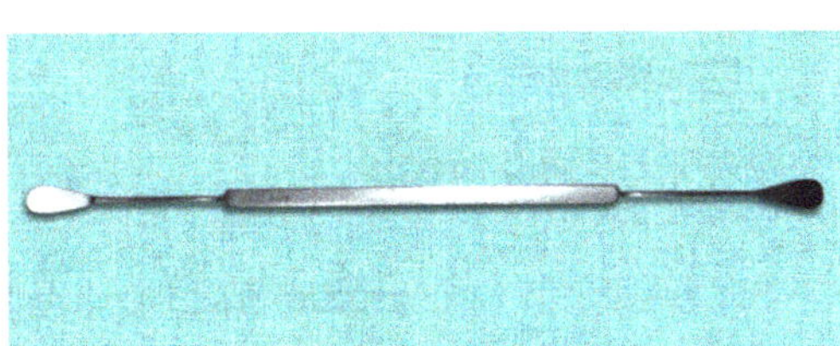

Fig. 3.4.6: Lens spatula.

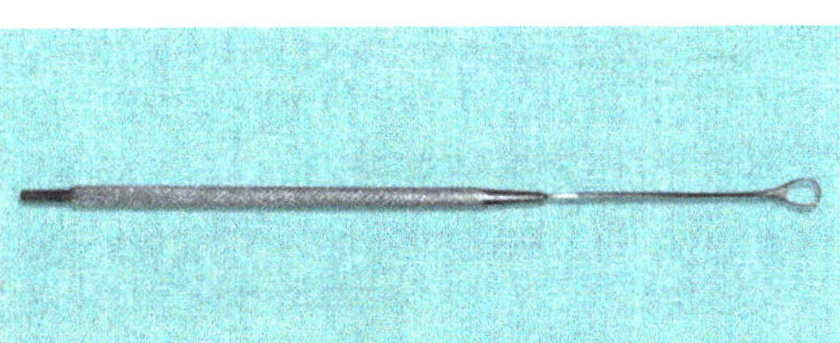

Fig. 3.4.7: Wire vectis.

IRRIGATING WIRE VECTIS (FIG. 3.4.8)

It is a modification of the wire vectis and has a hollow rim with a 0.3-mm opening at the anterior end and a hollow handle at the posterior end which is attached to a hub similar to that of a hypodermic needle through which fluid can be injected. The advantage of using irrigation is that there is a less chance of pulling unaimed structures like iris during nucleus delivery.

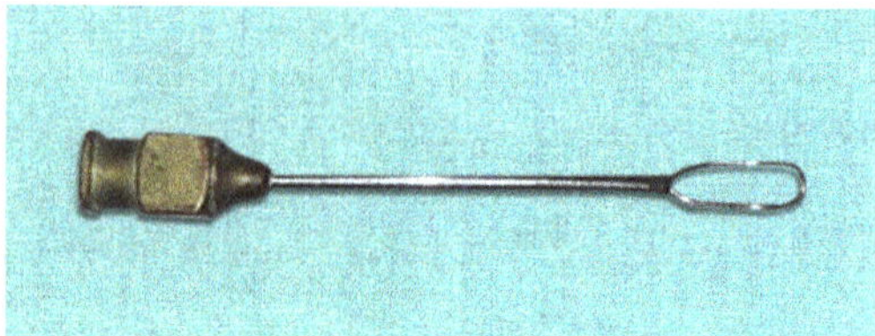

Fig. 3.4.8: Irrigating wire vectis.

Use

It is used for hydro-/viscoexpression of the nucleus in ECCE and small-incision cataract surgery (SICS).

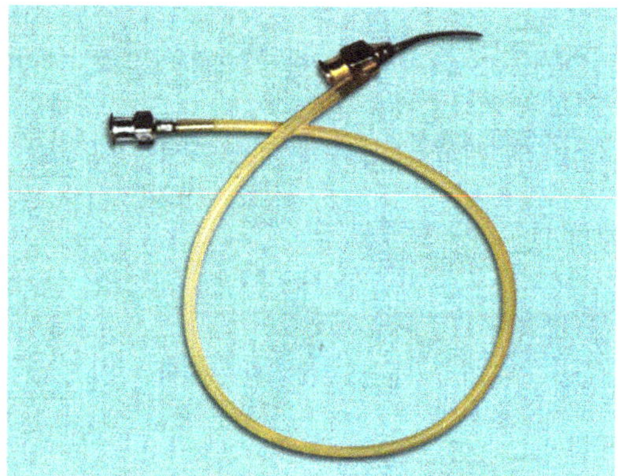

Fig. 3.4.9: Simcoe's irrigation and aspiration cannula.

SIMCOE'S IRRIGATION AND ASPIRATION CANNULA (FIG. 3.4.9)

It is available in the classical and reverse design with both right-handed and left-handed models available in each design. It has an irrigation system through the main port and aspiration system through the port on the side which is attached to a syringe through a silicon tube.

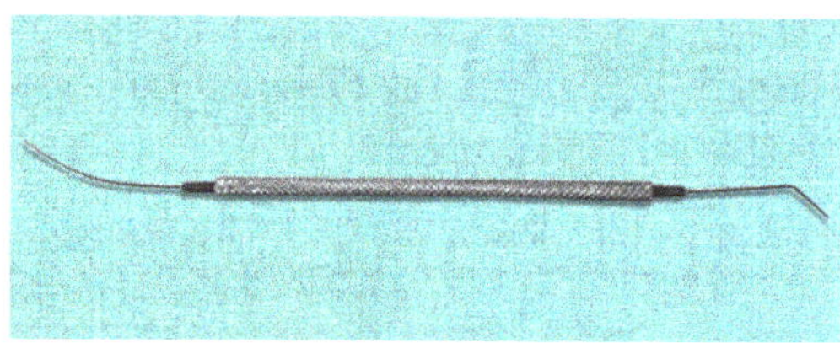

Fig. 3.4.10: Dastoor's iris repositor.

Uses

- For irrigation and aspiration of cortical matter in ECCE and open sky cataract surgery in keratoplasty
- For aspiration of hyphema.

Simcoe cannula is extremely useful in the setting of PCR with retained cortical matter. One modification to minimize vitreous loss is to remove the irrigation cannula and aspirating the retained lens matters after filling the AC with viscoelastics (dry IA). By removing the irrigating fluid, hydration of vitreous is prevented, thereby reducing further vitreous loss.

DASTOOR'S IRIS REPOSITOR (FIG. 3.4.10)

It is a flat and straight/bent blade with blunt edges.

Uses

- To reposit the iris in the AC
- To tuck the donor cornea underneath the host cornea in keratoplasty surgery.

CYSTOTOME NEEDLE (FIG. 3.4.11)

It is prepared with a 26-gauge needle by bending the needle tip down while holding

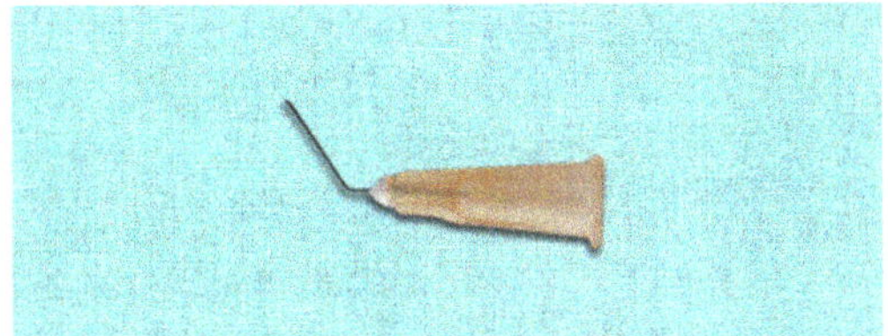

Fig. 3.4.11: Cystotome needle.

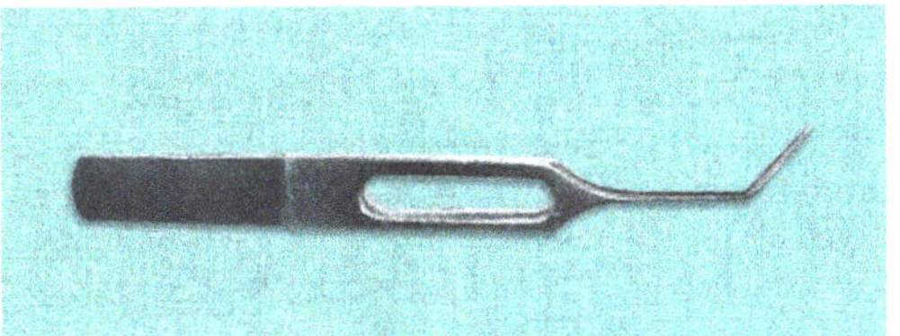

Fig. 3.4.12: Utrata capsulorhexis forceps.

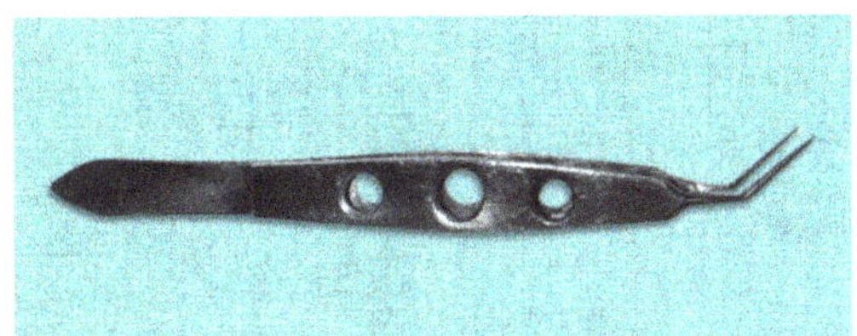

Fig. 3.4.13: McPherson's forceps.

the bevel up. Then, while maintaining this needle orientation, bend the needle up near the hub. Experience will aid in determining the optimal preferred angles. Most commonly, bends near 90° are common at the tip and slightly less than this angle at the hub. However, authors recommend a bend that is more than 90° so that the tip of the needle and its contact point with the anterior capsule are clearly visible. This would prevent capsulotomy-related complications like rhexis extension. Some surgeons introduce a third bend downward in the middle of the needle to get more vertical displacement of the tip to aid in reaching down into deep ACs.

The advantage of 26-gauge needle is that it is disposable (useful in camp/mass surgery setup), more controlled, and can be used through the sideport incision compared to utrata forceps. The limitation is that the torque generated is less compared to the utrata forceps hence, it is not preferred in cases like pediatric cataract where the capsule is extremely elastic and the chances of extension is high.

Uses

- It is used to make the anterior capsulotomy in ECCE as well as capsulorhexis in phacoemulsification
- To initiate posterior capsulorhexis in pediatric cataract surgery.

UTRATA CAPSULORHEXIS FORCEPS (FIG. 3.4.12)

The forceps have a fine precise tip with a sharp point that enables to initiate the capsular tear and then securely grasp the capsule to perform the capsulorhexis. It also has an "iris stop platform" to stop the shafts of the forceps from completely closing when tips are closed. This avoids inadvertent trauma to iris tissue. A 2.2-mm incision is required to insert this instrument into the AC. The force generated is much better compared to cystotome, hence preferred in pediatric cataract, intumescent lens, fibrosed capsule, lax capsule (subluxated lens), posterior capsulorhexis, and hypermature cataract. The limitation is that it needs a larger incision and chamber stability is often difficult in inexperienced hand.

MCPHERSON'S FORCEPS (FIG. 3.4.13)

It is a fine sharp tipped nontoothed forceps with angulation.

Uses

- Holding the intraocular lens (IOL) while implanting it
- Holding the suture while tying the knot
- Suture removal

- Removal of capsular tags/retained lens matters/foreign body (FB) from AC.

ARRUGA'S INTRACAPSULAR (CAPSULE HOLDING) FORCEPS (FIG. 3.4.14)

This forceps has a cup at inner side of the tip of each limb to create enough vacuum force for a tight grip. The edges of the cup are smooth and atraumatic to the lens capsule.

Uses

- It is used to remove the lens during forceps method of ICCE
- It is also used to remove the lens capsule remnant after accidental ECCE.

INTRAOCULAR LENS HOLDING FORCEPS (FIG. 3.4.15)

They are spring action forceps with short, blunt, and curved blades having smooth edges and tips.

Use

To hold the optic of non-foldable polymethylmethacrylate (PMMA) IOL during implantation.

SINSKEY HOOK OR INTRAOCULAR LENS DIALER (FIG. 3.4.16)

It is a fine instrument with a bent blunt tip. The tip can engage the dialing holes of the IOL.

Uses

- Dialing of the non-foldable PMMA IOL for proper positioning in the capsular bag or sulcus
- Also used in nucleus manipulation in phacoemulsification
- Useful to check for any vitreous strand by sweeping across the suspected area.

CHOPPER (FIG. 3.4.17)

It is similar in appearance to the Sinskey hook but the difference lies in the tip which is sharp with cutting edges in a chopper. A sharp chopper is useful in cases of hard cataract.

Use

To split or chop the nucleus into smaller pieces during phacoemulsification.

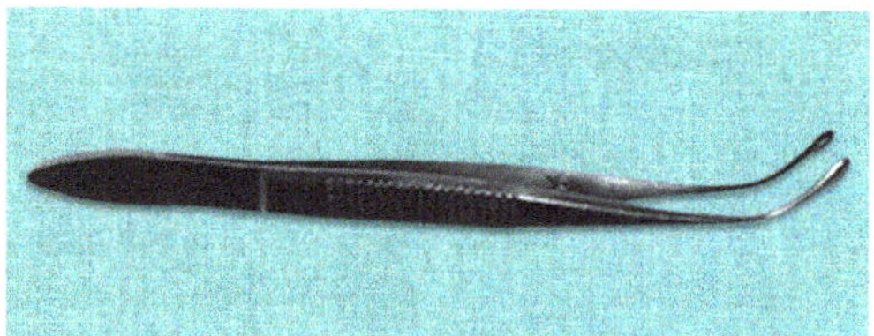

Fig. 3.4.14: Arruga's intracapsular (capsule holding) forceps.

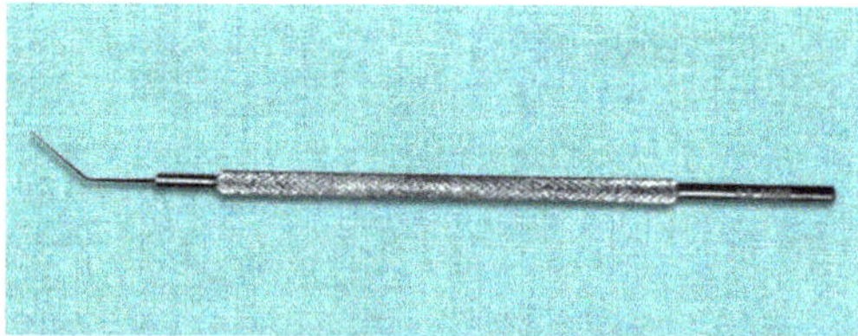

Fig. 3.4.16: Sinskey hook or intraocular lens (IOL) dialer.

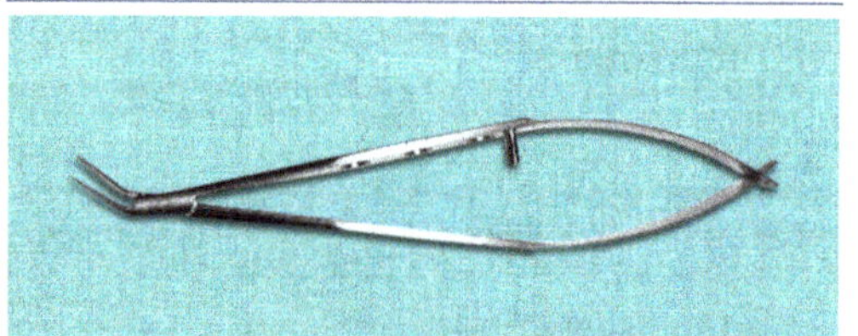

Fig. 3.4.15: Intraocular lens (IOL) holding forceps.

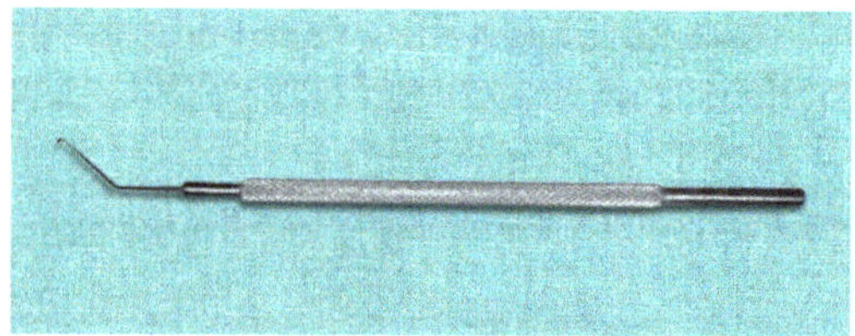

Fig. 3.4.17: Chopper.

PHACO NEEDLE TIP (FIG. 3.4.18)

It is made of titanium with a distal opening of 0.9 mm in diameter with a silicon sleeve which has two openings on the side 180° apart, through which the irrigation fluid flows. The phaco needle threads directly onto the phaco handpiece.

The tip can have bevel with 0°, 15°, 30°, 45°, or 60°. The greater is the angulation of the bevel tip, better is the sculpting effect and visibility of the tip but leads to poor occlusion. The 30° bevel offers the best compromise and leads to better sculpting, visibility as well as occlusion. The silicon sleeve acts as an insulator and the fluid flowing through the sleeve keep the tip cool and prevents wound burn.

The Kelman tip has a 22° angulation of the shaft of 3.5 mm from the tip. This enhances the emulsification as well as allows the surgeon to use the phaco tip in manipulating the nucleus during surgery. Kelman tip makes phacoemulsification faster; however, the chances of PCR are higher.

The Flared tip has an outer diameter of the tip greater at the tip than 1–2 mm behind it. This helps to enhance the emulsification effect and reduce the postocclusion surge.

The Cobra tip is bell-shaped tip, which increases the surface producing the ultrasound to reduce the level of energy required.

Balanced Tip

It is a phaco tip that has specially been designed for torsional ultrasound. Its design though similar to Kelman tip but has two curves near the tip. There is increased lateral movement at its tip but decreased lateral movement at the incision site compared to conventional phaco tips. Therefore, it is especially useful in cases with hard cataract as it reduces the cumulative dissipated energy, total ultrasound time, torsion amplitude, aspiration time, fluid used, and wound burn.

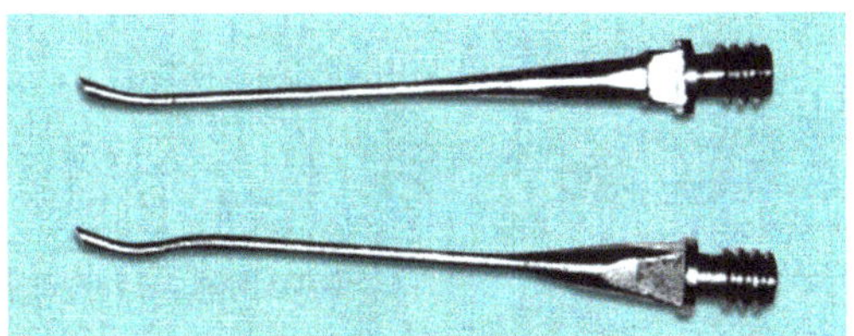

Fig. 3.4.18: Phaco needle tip. The 45° conventional tip with a 22° bend (top) and the new 45° balanced tip (bottom). Note the single bend in the conventional tip and two bends in the new balanced tip.

VIVA QUESTIONS

1. What are the different types of surgical incisions in cataract surgery?

Ans. The different surgical incisions for cataract surgery are:

- *Scleral*—It induces less astigmatism and is self-sealing but has increased risk of conjunctival ballooning and subconjunctival hemorrhage. Peritomy, cauterizing of blood vessels that are inherent to this incision, can increase the surgical time although marginally. In addition, it is difficult to perform under topical anesthesia. Best suitable for cases where a PMMA IOL is planned or when corneal diameter is less (e.g. IFC) or when endothelium status is compromised.
- *Limbal*—It has advantages of both corneal and sclera incisions. It induces less astigmatism, has good wound apposition, and less patient discomfort. The risk of iatrogenic limbal stem cell deficiency is very rare but is a possibility with large limbal incisions. Similar to scleral incision, it is difficult to perform under topical anesthesia.
- *Corneal*—It is easy to construct with minimal manipulation of conjunctiva but the disadvantages are that it induces astigmatism and has poor wound apposition. These kind of incisions are free of any bleeding (preferred for patients on anticoagulants) and most suited for surgery under topical anesthesia. Corneal

incisions are the most preferred incision for phacoemulsification.

2. What are the types of clear corneal incision?

Ans. The types of clear corneal incision are:
- *Uniplanar*—Easy to construct but poor self-sealing
- *Biplanar*—Relatively easy to construct with better self-sealing
- *Triplanar*—Relatively difficult to construct with better self-sealing but risk of Descemet's membrane detachment (DMD) is more
- *Hinged*—Very difficult to construct but best self-sealing.

3. What is hydrodissection and hydrodelineation?

Ans. Hydrodissection is separation of the cortex from lens capsule by injecting fluid while hydrodelineation is the separation of the epinucleus from the inner compact nucleus by injection of fluid.

4. What are soft-shell, ultimate soft-shell, and tri-soft shell techniques?

Ans.
- *Soft-shell technique*: A low viscosity dispersive ophthalmic viscosurgical device (OVD) (Viscoat) is injected first onto the surface of the lens, followed by a viscous cohesive, which pushes the dispersive up into a smooth layer against the endothelium, providing a protective layer.
- *Ultimate soft-shell technique*: Uses viscoadaptive (Healon 5) and balanced salt solution (BSS) instead of dispersive OVD. The BSS layer allows ease in turning the capsulorhexis, provides an area to place capsular dye, and provides area for circulation of BSS, thus avoiding phaco handpiece overheating and possible corneal burns.
- *Tri-soft shell technique*: Uses layers of dispersive against the cornea, viscous cohesive centrally to establish stability, and BSS on the lenticular surface for a low-viscosity surgical space.

5. What is the ideal size of capsulorhexis?

Ans. Ideally the rhexis should cover 0.5 mm of the IOL all around. Therefore, the ideal size is around 5–5.5 mm. 0.5 mm overlap prevents the posterior migration of "A" cells, thereby reducing the chances of posterior capsular opacification (PCO).

6. Concept of continuous curvilinear capsulorhexis was given by?

Ans. Howard Gimbel and Thomas Neuhann.

7. Name the various capsulotomy techniques that have been described in literature.

Ans. The different capsulotomy techniques are:
- *Vogt's technique*—Toothed forceps is used for grasping and ripping out a part of anterior capsule
- *Kelman's "Christmas tree" approach*—Cystitome is used to peel anterior capsule in a triangular or Christmas tree morphology
- *"Can-opener" technique*—Cystitome is used for interconnecting perforations of anterior capsule to create a circular window. This technique provides precise control of size and shape of the capsular opening
- *Galand "letterbox" technique*—Two steps procedure in which the anterior capsular opening is completed after implantation of the IOL.

8. Causes of capsulorhexis run out.

Ans.
- Shallow AC
- Inadequate viscoelastic injection
- Weak zonules [as in pseudoexfoliation (PXF) syndrome]
- High positive vitreous pressure (e.g. either due to excessive injection of anesthesia or inadequate anesthesia)

- Large continuous curvilinear capsulorhexis (CCC) that may disrupt the anterior zonules
- Intumescent cataract
- Hypermature cataracts
- *Pediatric cataracts*—with elastic anterior capsules.

9. What is capsulorhexis rescue technique?

Ans. In this technique, described by "Little et al.", a cohesive OVD is injected at the site of extending capsulorhexis to flatten the anterior capsule followed by grasping and pulling the extending edge of rhexis toward the center. After this maneuver, the rhexis can be continued regularly.

10. What are the various chopping techniques?

Ans. The classic "Nagahara technique" of *horizontal chopping* involves movement of both the phaco tip and chopper toward each other in the horizontal plane during the chop. The phaco tip is deeply buried in the center of the nucleus using high vacuum and insertion of chopper under the anterior capsule engaging the endonucleus near the equator followed by inward movement of the chopper toward the phaco tip to crack the nucleus into two pieces.

Vertical chopping involves burying the phaco tip in the center of the nucleus using high vacuum. After ensuring that the center of the nucleus is adequately impaled with the phaco tip, a chopper with a sharp tip is buried within the nucleus adjacent to the phaco tip. The phaco tip is then lifted up while the chopper is depressed down which results in cracking of the nucleus along the natural fault lines in the nucleus.

Stop and chop phaco involves creation of a central groove in the nucleus followed by division of the nucleus into two pieces through sculpting and cracking. This is followed by subsequent chopping of the two nucleus pieces.

11. Advantage of balanced phaco tip.

Ans. Refer to text.

12. What are the different techniques of performing intracapsular cataract extraction (ICCE)?

Ans.

- Verhoeff and Kirby described the use of forceps to hold the upper anterior surface of the capsule to deliver the upper pole first.
- *Arruga's capsule forceps method/tumbling technique*: Arruga's capsule holding forceps is used to hold the anterior surface of the lens capsule at 6 o'clock position. The lens is then lifted slightly with gentle sideways movements to break the zonules. The lens is then delivered by gentle sliding movements by the forceps along with pressure at 6 o'clock position near the limbus by a lens expressor.
- Barraquer described the use of *suction cup* for holding the lens capsule and subsequent delivering of the lens.
- *Indian Smith method*: The lens is delivered with tumbling technique by applying pressure on limbus at 6 o'clock position with lens expressor and counterpressure at 12 o'clock with the lens spatula. In this technique, the lower pole of lens is delivered first.
- *Cryoextraction*: In this technique, the tip of cryoprobe is placed on the anterior surface of the lens in the upper quadrant. With a temperature of -40°C, an adhesion is created between the lens capsule and the cryoprobe. With gentle rotator movements, the zonules are broken and the lens is extracted out by sliding movements. The upper pole of the lens is delivered first.
- *Irisophake* method.
- *Wire vectis method*: It is used in cases with subluxated or dislocated lens. In this technique, the loop of wire vectis is slid

below the subluxated lens, which is then lifted and delivered.

Alpha-chymotrypsin is used in cases where the zonules are found to be very resistant.

13. What are the different techniques for delivering the nucleus in small-incision cataract surgery (SICS)?

Ans.

- *Blumenthal's anterior chamber maintainer technique*: The nucleus is engaged into the corneoscleral tunnel followed by injection of OVD both above and below the nucleus. A lens glide is then passed behind the nucleus and with the help of intermittent hydropressure generated by the AC maintainer, the nucleus is delivered out of the tunnel's mouth.
- *Wire vectis technique*: Wire vectis is used to deliver the nucleus.
- *Irrigating vectis technique/Microvectis technique*: Irrigating wire vectis is used to deliver the nucleus by either hydroexpression or viscoexpression. The irrigating wire vectis is 4 mm in width and 9 mm in length. The anterior surface is concave with three 0.3 mm openings at one end. The other end is continuous with the main body and can be attached to a syringe or infusion set.
- *Phacofracture technique*: After the nucleus is prolapsed at the iris pupillary plane, a wire vectis is insinuated under the nucleus followed by positioning of a nucleotome on the anterior surface of nucleus. The *two* instruments are then maneuvered toward each other leading to cleavage of the nuclear substance. Nuclear forceps, which have a 9.0-mm long jaw (each having a double row of teeth), are used to deliver the nucleus fragments.
- *Fish hook technique*: In this technique, initially only the superior pole of nucleus is brought into the AC. OVD is injected both in front and behind the nucleus. The tip of 30 G needle is bent in the form of hook and is then maneuvered behind the nucleus to hook the undersurface of the nucleus. Once the nucleus is hooked, it is delivered by applying gentle pressure over the posterior lip of the tunnel.
- *Ruit's technique*: OVD is injected around the nucleus to prolapse it into AC. An irrigating Simcoe cannula is then inserted below it which aids in delivering the nucleus with hydropressure.
- *Phacosandwich technique*: In this technique, the nucleus is prolapsed into AC and delivered by sandwiching the nucleus between a dialer and vectis.
- *Viscoexpression*: Viscoelastic is continuously injected into AC to deliver the nucleus.

4 CHAPTER

Retina and Uvea

4.1 OPHTHALMOSCOPE

Alisha Kishore, Hannah Shiny R, Suman Meena, Pranita Sahay

BINOCULAR INDIRECT OPHTHALMOSCOPE

Introduction

Ophthalmoscopy, also called funduscopy, is a test that allows viewing inside the fundus of the eye and other structures using an ophthalmoscope. Broadly it can be categorized as direct and indirect. Marc Antonie Giracid Tenlon of France invented the first binocular indirect ophthalmoscope in 1861. Charles Schepens described the first binocular indirect ophthalmoscope in 1945 (Fig. 4.1.1).

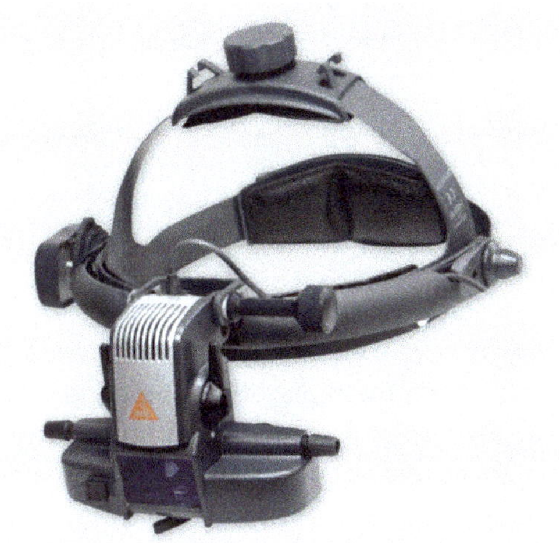

Fig. 4.1.1: Indirect ophthalmoscope.

Principle

The parts of an indirect ophthalmoscope are a headset with binocular viewing box and a light source which can be adjusted. The view box has prisms acting to optically reduce the interpupillary distance of the observer forming a binocular stereoscopic image. The light is brought to focus on an angled mirror, which is then reflected into the patient's eye. Light passes through the pupil and is reflected from the retinal surface. The reflected light is then brought to focus with a handheld convex lens (Fig. 4.1.2). Indirect ophthalmoscope works on the principle that by placing a convex lens in front, the eye is made highly myopic. The image is formed between the lens and the observer and is inverted and real.

In the emmetropic eyes, reflected light from the retina are parallel and is hence brought to focus by the condensing lens. An inverted image is therefore formed at the principal focus of the lens, which lies between the lens and the observer.[1]

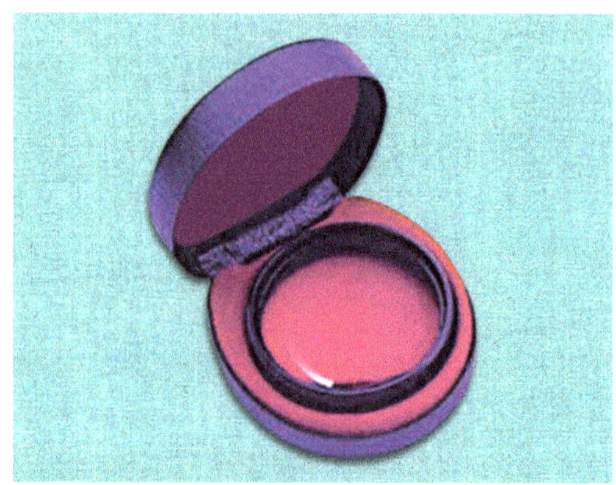

Fig. 4.1.2: 20 D lens.

Table 4.1.1: Field of view, magnification, and working distance of various lenses.

Lens	*Field of view*	*Magnification*	*Working distance*
14 D	36°/43°	4.30 x	75 mm
20 D	46°/60°	3.13 x	50 mm
28 D	53°/69°	2.27 x	33 mm
2.2 Pan retinal lens	56°/73°	2.68 x	40 mm

In hypermetropia, the emerging rays will diverge and appear to come from an imaginary enlarged upright image situated behind the eye. The condensing lens, therefore, uses this as an object and forms an inverted image of it. Since the rays are divergent, the final image will be situated in front of its principal focus.[1]

In the myopic eye the rays coming from the fundus are convergent and therefore an inverted image is formed in front of the eye. A second smaller image is then formed by the condensing lens at a point within its focal length.[1]

The most commonly used handheld lens is a 20 D aspheric lens. It has a field of view of 46°/60° and provides an image magnification of 3.13 x. The working distance is 50 mm.[2] The magnification of various lenses is described in Table 4.1.1.

Technique

The prerequisites for an indirect ophthalmoscopic examination are a dark room and fully dilated pupil of the patient. The procedure is explained to the patient and he is made to lie in the supine position or sit comfortably. Adjust the headset of the ophthalmoscope to a comfortable position. Move the eyepiece to set the interpupillary distance. The examination is carried out at an outstretched arms distance. The light of the ophthalmoscope, the condensing lens, the patient's pupil and the retina must fall on one line. A bright red reflex appears when the examiner aligns his viewing access with the patient's pupil. The handheld lens is then placed over the patient's eye and adjusted until an image is identified. The most convex surface of the lens must face the examiner. The opposite surface is marked on most lenses buy an unpainted edge and this must face the patient. The periphery of the retina is examined first because it is the least light-sensitive part. The examiner has to stand opposite to the clock hour position to be examined, for example, to examine the inferior quadrant the examiner stands toward the patients head.[2]

Scleral Indentation

The peripheral retina can be examined in detail, by performing scleral indentation. Schepens scleral indentor (Fig. 4.1.3), sockets indentor (Fig. 4.1.4) or a cotton tip applicator can be used.[2]

Instillation of topical anesthesia reduces the pain during the procedure. In order to visualize the superior peripheral retina, the scleral depressor is positioned vertically at 12 o'clock while the patient looks down. The patient is then asked to look superiorly, allowing the visualization of the indent of the depressor with indirect ophthalmoscopy. If the indent is not visible, it indicates that the depressor is placed too anteriorly or the indent is too less.

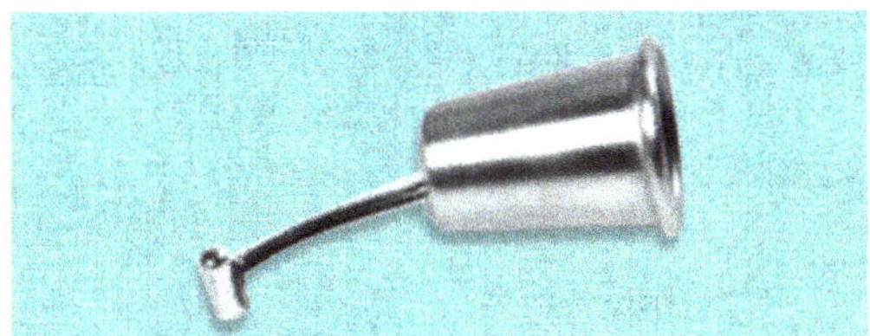

Fig. 4.1.3: Schepens scleral depressor.

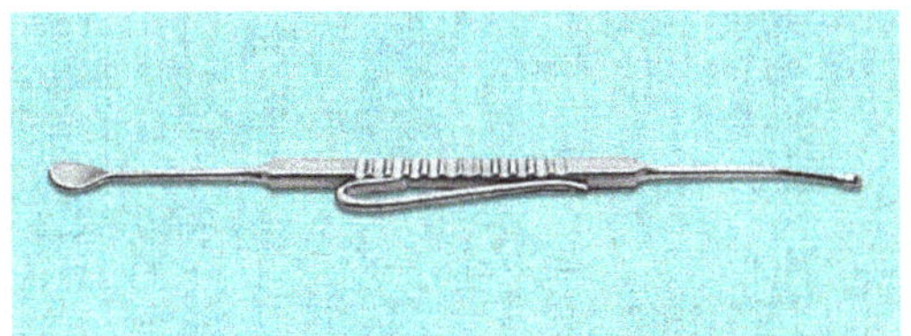

Fig. 4.1.4: Josephberg-Besser scleral depressor, double-ended.

The nasal and temporal periphery of the retina is the most difficult to indent because of lesser fornix space and presence of canthal ligaments.[2]

Indentation must be done very gently in patients who have undergone filtering surgeries as it can cause bleb leakage. Scleral depression is deferred in patients with globe rupture and hyphema following trauma.

DIRECT OPHTHALMOSCOPE

Introduction

Scientists discovered that using a coaxial illumination observation system, with the light source kept close to the eye, visualization of the retina is possible. Charles Babbage made the first practical ophthalmoscope. Following which Von Helmholtz in 1851 described the direct ophthalmoscope.[3,4] As the name indicates, a direct image is formed on the retina in a direct ophthalmoscope, and there is no intermediate image formation, unlike in an indirect ophthalmoscope.[3]

Parts

It consists of a metallic optical tube containing a lamp, aperture dial assembly, mirror/prism, objective and condensing lens (Figs. 4.1.5 and 4.1.6).[4]

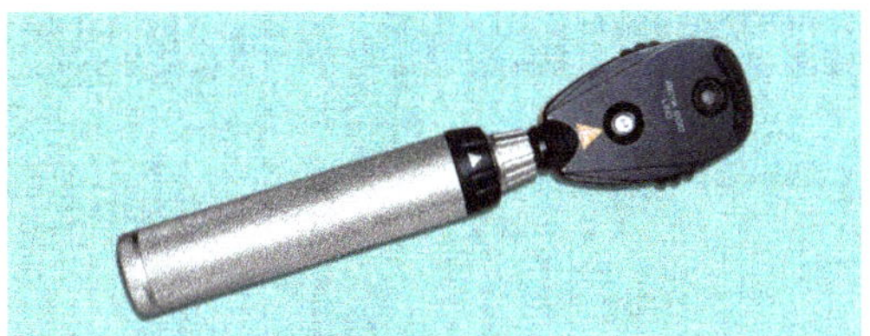

Fig. 4.1.5: Direct ophthalmoscope.

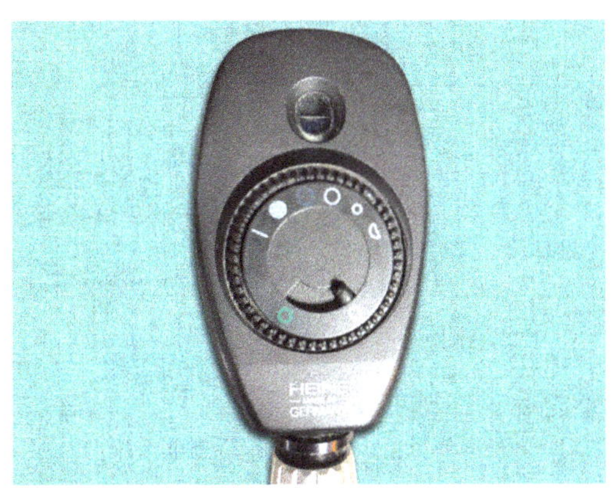

Fig. 4.1.6: Head of direct ophthalmoscope.

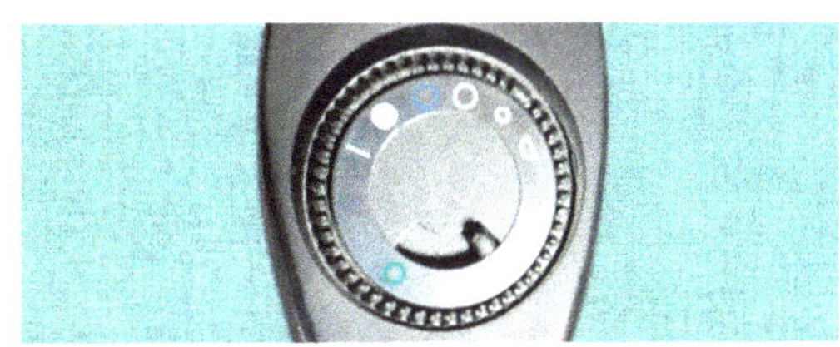

Fig. 4.1.7: Apertures of direct ophthalmoscope.

Illumination System

It consists of a halogen lamp powered by rechargeable battery, an aperture dial with different apertures including Linkz star, cobalt blue filter, medium and large spot, hemispot, slit and pinhole (Fig. 4.1.7). It has two condensing lenses, one on each side of the aperture dial. Also has angled mirrors at 45°, which are nowadays replaced in modern ophthalmoscope by prisms (Table 4.1.2).[4]

Table 4.1.2: Uses of various apertures in a direct ophthalmoscope.

Aperture type		*Use*
Small spot		For seeing through small pupil. Provides approximately a 5° cone
Large spot		For viewing in dilated pupil
Macular spot/pin hole		To observe only fovea, enables view through even 2 mm pupil
Hemispot or half-circle diaphragm		Reduces corneal reflex and improved depth of perception Avoid fundus reflection while examining the fundus It is also helpful in the observation of certain fine retinal details that are seen best in the transitional zone between illuminated and nonilluminated retina
Slit		Accurate evaluation of retinal elevation and depression (diagnosis of retinal detachment, tumors, disc edema), anterior chamber depth
Cobalt blue		For corneal abrasions To enhance the visibility of fluorescein, for use in fluorescein angioscopy and as a handheld light source for fluorescein staining of the cornea
Linkz star/fixation star with polar coordinates		Graduated cross-hairs for measuring eccentric fixation or locating lesions
Red free filter		Better visualization of blood vessel, hemorrhage, and retinal nerve fiber layer Differentiate between retinal and choroidal lesion It also makes small macroaneurysms and small hemorrhage standout more clearly Retinal nerve fiber layer (RNFL) defect Helpful in estimating C/D ratio

Note: Not all filters are present in every ophthalmoscope.

Observation System

It has condensing lens of power +1 to +10, +15, +20, +40, and −1 to −10, −15, −20, −25, −35, a viewing window with antireflective coating to avoid glare and a red-free filter to detect nerve fiber layer defects.[4]

Optical Principle

The image formed depends on the distance at which the ophthalmoscope is used. When used for distant direct ophthalmoscopy at a distance of 25 cm a real, inverted, unmagnified image is formed. When fundoscopy is done at a very near distance to the subject's eye, a virtual, erect image is formed.

The emergent rays of light from an emmetropic patient are parallel and are brought to focus on the observer's retina. If the patient is hypermetropia, the emergent rays are divergent and will be brought to focus on the observer's retina only if the latter accommodates or if a convex lens is used. On the other hand, if the subject is myopic, the emergent rays are convergent and should be interposed by a concave lens to bring them to focus on the observer's retina.

When the accommodation of the subject and the observer are at rest, and the refractive error of the observer is corrected fully, and mirror of the ophthalmoscope is held at the anterior focal point of the eye; 15.7 mm in front of the cornea, if the disc is seen then the eye is emmetropic. If the image formed is not clear, the convex lenses of increasing power are turned in front of the observer's eye and the highest power which produces a clear image give the measure of hypermetropia. If the image becomes progressively blurred with the convex lens, then the concave lens is turned on, and the highest power which forms a clear image gives the myopic power of the patient. If astigmatism is present, then the blood vessels are blurred unequally in different directions, and when spherical lenses are presented in the ophthalmoscope, only the vessels that are perpendicular to that meridian will become clear.

The direct ophthalmoscope magnifies images to 15 times. The field of view is 5° and is directly proportional to the size of the subject's pupil, the axial length of the patient and inversely proportional to the distance between subject and observer.[3]

Technique

First examine the patient from a distance of 1 m to look for abnormality of the lid, orbit, and ocular deviation. Then, the examination is carried out at 25 cm from the subject. A red reflex or any media opacity can be seen. To identify the position of the opacity, the patient is asked to look in all four gazes, and movement of the opacity is noted. Opacity lying behind the lens moves against the ocular movements, whereas any opacity lying in the cornea or anterior chamber moves along with ocular gaze. Any squint can be seen as an unequal reflex (Brückners test). One should also look for relative afferent pupillary defect (RAPD). The retina should be brought to focus by moving closer to the patient. As the retina gets focused, look for the blood vessels and trace them backward to reach the optic disc. The macula is focused by asking the patient to focus into the light. The right eye should be examined using the right eye of the observer and vice versa.

Modifications of ophthalmoscope include a panoptic ophthalmoscope which works on the principle of axial point source optics. This enables a large field of view and reduces corneal reflexes.[4,5]

VIVA QUESTIONS

1. At what distance is the distant direct ophthalmoscopy performed?

Ans. At 25 cm.

2. How will you quantify disc edema using direct ophthalmoscope?

Ans. The direct ophthalmoscope is first focused on the surface of the disc. The dioptric power at which the disc is focused clearly is noted and then the ophthalmoscope is used to focus on the adjacent retina for which the dioptric power is noted again. The difference between the two dioptric powers gives the amount of elevation. Every addition of +3 D equals to 1 mm elevation in phakics and 2 mm in aphakics.

3. Mention the differences between direct and indirect ophthalmoscope.

Ans. Refer to Table 4.1.3 .

4. Is there any light exposure hazard with the use of direct ophthalmoscope?

Ans. Prolonged exposure to intense light damages the retina. Hence, the minimum intensity of light which allows clear visualization of structures should be used.

Table 4.1.3: Difference between direct and indirect ophthalmoscope.

	Direct ophthalmoscope	*Indirect ophthalmoscope*
Stereopsis	Absent	Present
Magnification	15 times	5 times
Static field of view	2 disc diameter	8 disc diameter
Dynamic field of view	Up to equator	Up to ora serrata
Retinal image	Virtual, erect	Real, inverted
Technique	Easy	Difficult
Illumination	Good	Excellent
Uses	Diagnostic mainly	Diagnostic and therapeutic (laser)

Table 4.1.4: Recommended exposure to light with direct ophthalmoscope when operated at maximum intensity.

Distance from instrument to patient (mm)	*Duration (min)*
10	≤8–10*
50	≤3–8*
100	≤1–3*

*The higher duration is for LED bulbs.

Persons at risk are:
- Infants
- Aphakes
- Persons with retinal disease
- Eye exposed to retinal photography, the same procedure repeated within of 24 hours.

During operating conditions at a maximum light intensity, the duration of exposure should not exceed the durations as described in Table 4.1.4 (for HEINE direct ophthalmoscopes).

5. How will you optimize lamp life?

Ans. Keep on time less than 2 minutes with off-time not less than 15 minutes.

REFERENCES

1. Abrams D. Duke-Elder's Practice of Refraction, 10th edition. London: J & A Churchill Ltd; 1954.
2. Wirthlin RS, Young TA. Pearls on indirect ophthalmoscopy. Tech Ophthalmoscopy. 2005;3(3):138-40.
3. Yanoff M, Duker JS. Ophthalmology, 3rd edition. St Louis, United States: Elsevier Health Sciences; 2009.
4. Keeler CR. Babbage the unfortunate. Br J Ophthalmol. 2004;88:730-2.
5. Mark HH. On the evolution of binocular ophthalmoscopy. Arch Ophthalmology. 2007;125(6):830-3.

4.2 FUNDUS FLUORESCEIN ANGIOGRAPHY

Nasiq Hasan, Priyanka, Brijesh Takkar, Rohan Chawla, Atul Kumar

INTRODUCTION

Fundus fluorescein angiography (FFA) was devised by two medical students (Novotny and Alvis) in 1959.[1] Blood flow through vessels of retina can be visualized using this technique which allows sequential imaging with passage of time. It is a useful diagnostic modality that allows monitoring of posterior segment diseases and assesses the efficacy of retinal therapeutics.

The basic principle of FFA revolves around three phenomena:

1. *Luminescence* is the emission of light from any source not resulting due to high temperature.
2. *Fluorescence* is *luminescence* that is maintained by continuous excitation of electrons.
3. *Phosphorescence* continues to emit light even after the excitation is stopped.

There are earlier reports of performing FFA using oral fluorescein. However, in today's era, sodium fluorescein is injected intravenously. It is 80% protein bound and the molecules fluoresce on excitation at a particular wavelength. In a fundus camera, a blue excitation filter permits only the blue light from a white source to enter the retina and absorbs all other light. This blue light excites the fluorescein in the bloodstream, which starts emitting green-yellow light at 520–530 nm. A barrier filter keeps out the blue excitation light (all wavelengths < 520 nm) and allows only green-yellow light (all wavelengths > 520 nm) to be captured electronically as a digital image.

Pseudofluorescence is a phenomenon that occurs when nonfluorescent light cannot be filtered by the entire filter system as seen in the case of old worn-out filters.

SODIUM FLUORESCEIN

Properties

It has the following properties:

- It is a water-soluble orange-red crystalline hydrocarbon, also known as *resorcinol phthalein sodium* ($C_{20}H_{10}Na_2O_5$) or uranine ($C_{20}H_{12}O_5Na$).
- It has a molecular weight of 376.27 Da.
- It is excited by blue light (465–490 nm) and emits green light (520–530 nm).
- *80% of the dye is protein-bound*, and this fraction does not fluoresce, only the unbound 20% fluoresces.
- The commercial concentration of solutions available is 10 mL of 5% fluorescein, 5 mL of 10% fluorescein, and 3 mL of 25% fluorescein.
- The fluorescein diffuses through the choriocapillaris, but cannot diffuse through the inner or outer blood-retinal barriers.
- It is usually eliminated by the kidney within 24 hours, although can be found in the body for a few weeks.

Side Effects

Side effects include the following:[2]

- Transient nausea and vomiting
- Vasovagal attacks
- Pain due to extravasation of dye
- Inadvertent arterial injection
- Thrombophlebitis
- Anaphylaxis
- Seizures
- Cardiorespiratory arrest.

Contraindications

Contraindications include the following:

- Absolute contraindications:
  - Known history of allergy to the dye
  - Previous anaphylaxis to fluorescein angiography (FA)
- Relative contraindications:
  - The first trimester of pregnancy (although there are no reported complications)
  - Severe renal impairment
  - Recent cerebrovascular accident (CVA), myocardial infarction (MI), and unstable angina
  - History of heart disease, arrhythmia, and pacemakers are no contraindications.

FUNDUS CAMERA

The following systems have been used to acquire fluorescein images:

- Film-based fundus camera
- Digital fundus camera (Fig. 4.2.1)
- Confocal scanning laser ophthalmoscope (cSLO).

Confocal scanning laser ophthalmoscope uses a near-infrared laser beam instead of the flash bulb used in digital and film-based systems.[3] This helps in the quick scanning of the retina and producing *high-resolution and high-contrast images* in a very short span of time. They use *longer wavelength lasers* and hence can be used to obtain fundus autofluorescence (FAF) and indocyanine green (ICG) images too.

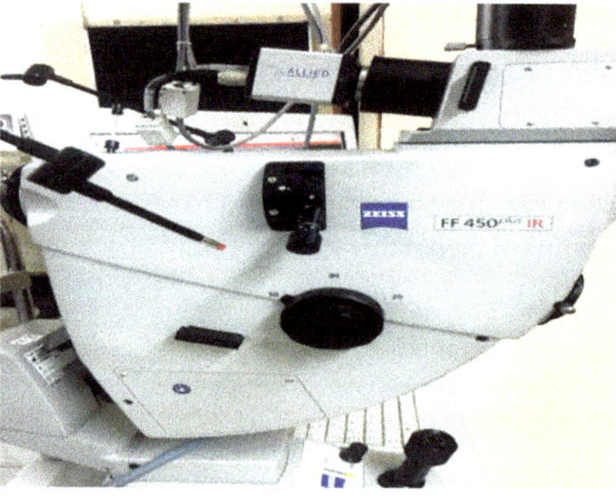

Fig. 4.2.1: Digital fundus camera.

Fundus cameras range from *30° to 50° field of view*; however, there are machines which can provide widefield and ultra-widefield images *up to 200°*. Montage system is used to capture peripheral angiograms with the conventional cameras; however simultaneous imaging of each fundus field is not possible.

The exciter filter transmits blue light at 465–490 nm which is the absorption peak of fluorescein excitation and the barrier filter transmits light at 525–530 nm which is the fluorescent or emitted peak of fluorescein.

TECHNIQUE

Following are the steps of FFA:

- Explain about the procedure to the patient and take informed consent.
- The patient should ideally be *fasting* while performing FFA given the high likelihood of nausea and vomiting during the procedure.
- The patient sits comfortably with a loose neck collar in front of the camera.
- The patient should be positioned for proper alignment, focus, and comfort.
- Color and monochromatic red-free filter images are obtained.
- Before injecting the dye, the illuminating beam of the fundus camera is centered within the dilated pupil.
- A bolus injection of the dye is administered in a peripheral vein (Fig. 4.2.2).
- Images are usually rapidly taken very second up till maximal fluorescence.
- After early phase, images of the fellow eye and retinal periphery may be clicked.
- When photography is done, the patient should be reassured about the discoloration of urine.

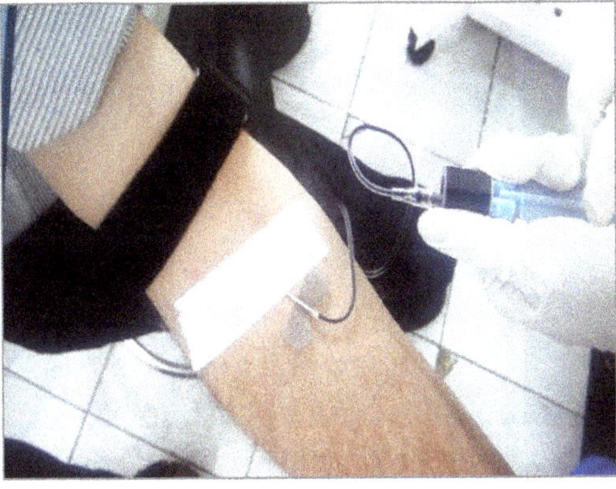

Fig. 4.2.2: Intravenous injection of fluorescein dye via the antecubital vein using a 24 G scalp vein attached to the 10 cc syringe.

PHASES OF FUNDUS FLUORESCEIN ANGIOGRAPHY

- Arm-to-retina circulation time: 10–12 seconds
- Posterior ciliary arteries: 9.5 seconds
- Choroidal flush (or prearterial phase): 10 seconds
- Retinal arterial phase: 0–12 seconds
- Arteriovenous phase (laminar stage or early venous stage): 14–15 seconds
- Venous phase: 16–17 seconds
- Late phase: 5 minutes.

The foveal avascular zone (FAZ) is relatively hypofluorescent due to the presence of dense xanthophyll pigments, taller and more retinal pigment epithelium (RPE) cells and absence of retinal capillaries in the center of fovea.

Choroidal Phase

It is due to the permeability of choriocapillaris to the dye, causing a widespread area of hyperfluorescence. A cilioretinal artery, if present, will fill during this phase as it is derived from posterior ciliary circulation.

Arterial Phase

It is seen 2 seconds later when dye enters into retinal arterioles.

Arteriovenous Phase

Next the retinal capillaries fill followed by the laminar flow in veins seen as thin columns of dye along their walls.

Venous Phase

The arteriovenous phase is followed by a venous phase where the venous columns become broader as the dye fills up the venous lumen.

Mid Phase

About 2-4 minutes after injection, the veins and arteries remain roughly equal in brightness.

Late Phase

Gradual removal of dye can be seen at ~10 minutes postinjection. Disc margin remains hyperfluorescent due to staining (Figs. 4.2.3A to C).

ABNORMAL FLUORESCEIN PATTERNS

Hypofluorescence: Reduced or absent normal fluorescence. It can be categorized to:

- Blocked fluorescence—masking of fluorescence (Fig. 4.2.4A):

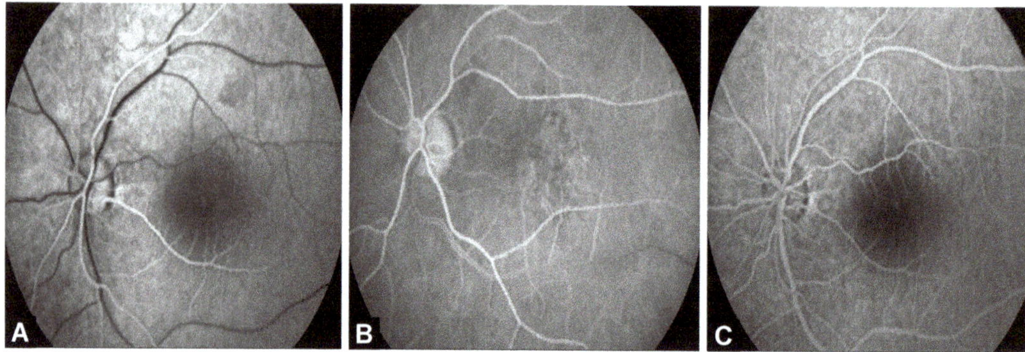

Figs. 4.2.3A to C: Normal fluorescein angiogram. (A) Arterial phase in which only the artery is filled with the dye; (B) Arteriovenous phase showing laminar flow along the walls of the veins; (C) Venous phase showing filling of veins also.

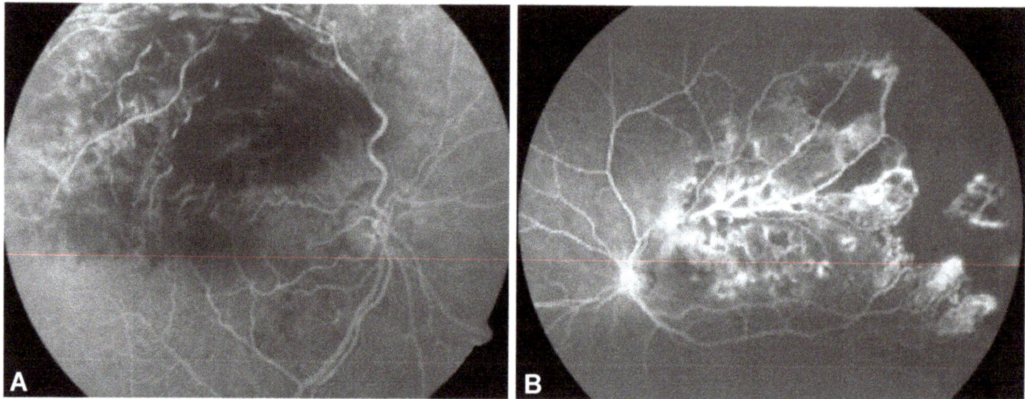

Figs. 4.2.4A and B: Hypofluorescence. (A) Blocked fluorescence where the underlying retinal vessels are obscured; (B) Vascular filling defects showing peripheral capillary nonperfusion areas in the temporal retina.

  - Any opacity anterior to the fluorescence like blood or media opacification.
  - Additionally, choroidal fluorescence can be blocked by occurrence of abnormal pigment in RPE cells.
- Vascular filling defects—absence of vascular circulation (Fig. 4.2.4B).

Hyperfluorescence: Increased fluorescence.

- *Leakage*: The area of fluorescence increases in both size and intensity with time (Fig. 4.2.5A), e.g. neovascularization and macular edema.
- *Pooling*: The area of fluorescence is the same, but the intensity increases with time in a confined anatomical space (Fig. 4.2.5B), e.g. focal serous retinal detachment and pigment epithelial detachment (PED).
- *Staining*: Increase in intensity over time in the late frame, but margins are irregular (Fig. 4.2.5C), e.g. macular scars, drusen, and laser mark.
- *Transmitted fluorescence (window defect)*: Increased fluorescence from the underlying choroidal vasculature due to the absence of overlying pigment (Fig. 4.2.6), e.g. geographical atrophy.
- *Autofluorescence*: Continuous emission of fluorescent light from ocular structures in the absence of fluorescein dye, e.g. optic nerve head drusen, astrocytic hamartoma, and lipofuscin.

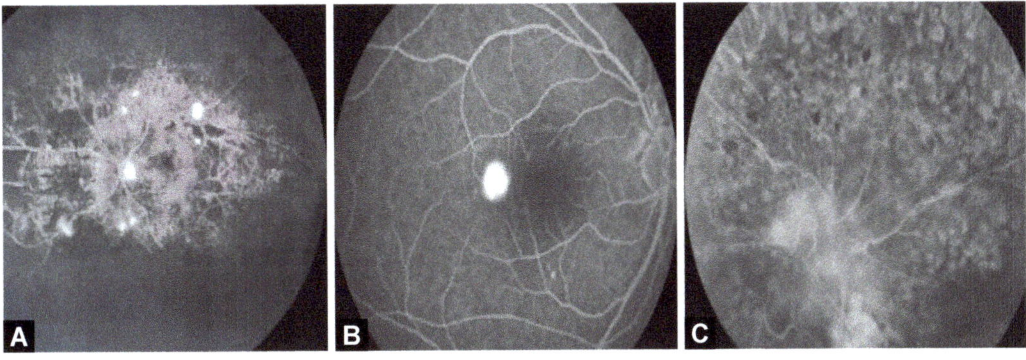

Figs. 4.2.5A to C: Hyperfluorescence. (A) Leak; (B) Pooling; (C) Stain.

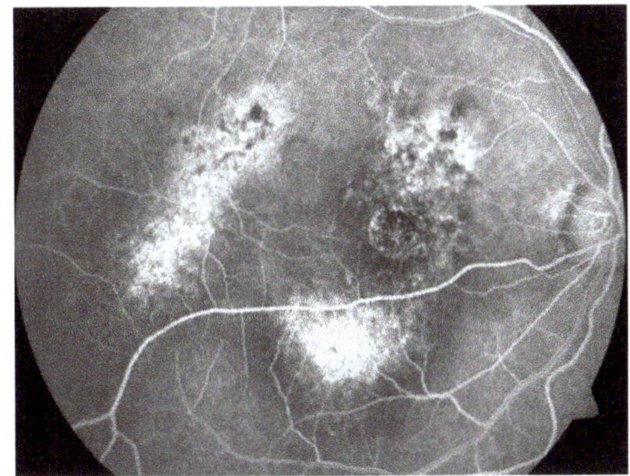

Fig. 4.2.6: Window defect is seen as hyperfluorescence as the overlying retinal pigment epithelium (RPE) shows atrophy.

CHARACTERISTIC FFA FEATURES OF CERTAIN CONDITIONS

1. *Central serous choroidopathy*: Two types of leakage patterns are seen on FFA:
   i. Smock stack pattern (Fig. 4.2.7)
   ii. Inkblot pattern (Fig. 4.2.8).
2. *Diabetic retinopathy*: Different stages of diabetic retinopathy (DR) can have the following presentation:
   - Nonproliferative diabetic retinopathy (NPDR):
     - Mild NPDR:
       - *Microaneurysms*: Appear as hyperfluorescent dots, which may leak in later phases (Fig. 4.2.9A).
     - Moderate NPDR:
       - *Microaneurysms*: Appear as hyperfluorescent dots, which may leak in later phases.
       - Superficial and deep retinal hemorrhages cause blocked choroidal fluorescence.
       - Hard exudates (Fig. 4.2.9B).
     - Severe NPDR:
       - All features as in mild NPDR.
       - *Capillary nonperfusion (CNP) areas*: Appear as areas of hypofluorescence and usually outlined by dilated capillaries (Fig. 4.2.9C).
       - Intraretinal microvascular abnormalities (IRMAs) are segmental

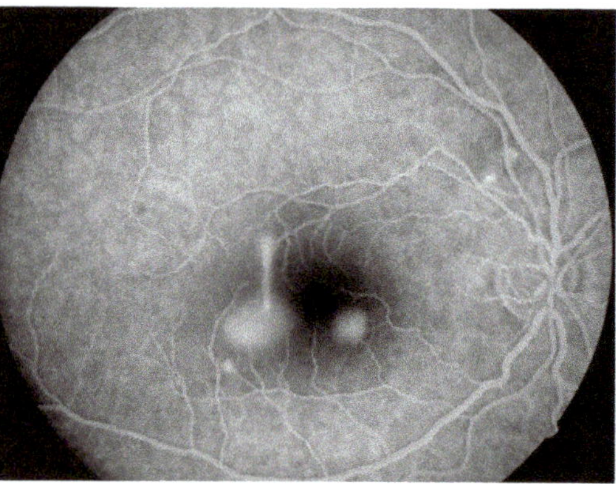
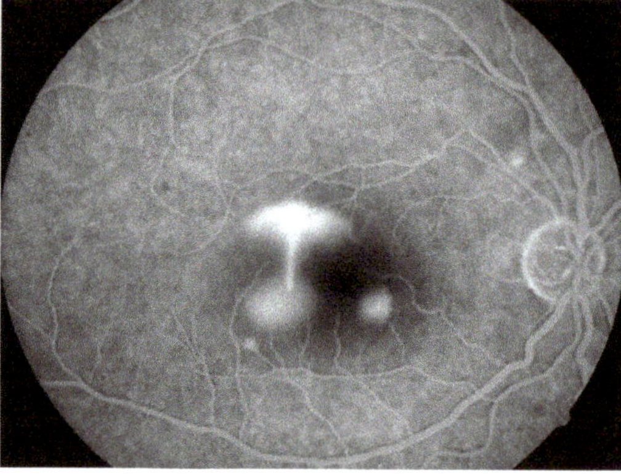

Fig. 4.2.7: Smock stack pattern of central serous chorioretinopathy (CSC) leak showing increasing hyperfluorescence in terms of area and intensity with time.

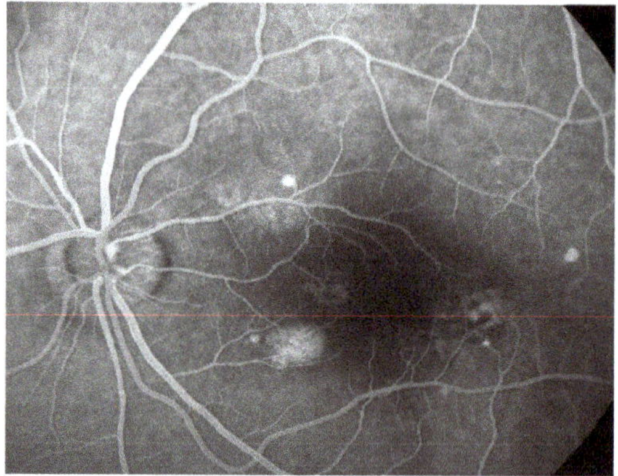

Fig. 4.2.8: A well-defined inkblot leak is seen superonasal to the fovea. A pigment epithelial detachment is seen temporal to the fovea. Additional areas of stippled hyperfluorescence are also visible.

and irregular dilatation of capillary bed lying within CNP areas. They may slightly leak in later phases at their growing tips.
- Soft exudates cause blockage of choroidal fluorescence.

- Proliferative diabetic retinopathy (PDR):
  - Neovascularization of the disc (NVD) or neovascularization elsewhere (NVE) (Fig. 4.2.9D) on the retinal surface. These cause leakage of dye profusely which increases in the late phase.
  - Preretinal (subhyaloid) hemorrhages block both retinal and choroidal fluorescence.
- Diabetic macular edema (DME) (Figs. 4.2.10A and B):
  - Focal diabetic maculopathy:
    - Focal leaks from microaneurysms in the macular area.
    - Hard exudates cause blocked choroidal fluorescence, may also show staining.
  - Diffuse diabetic maculopathy (cystoid):
    - Dilated retinal capillaries leak diffusely into the macular area.
    - Typical petaloid or honeycomb pattern of cystoid macular edema (CME) may also be seen (Fig. 4.2.10A).

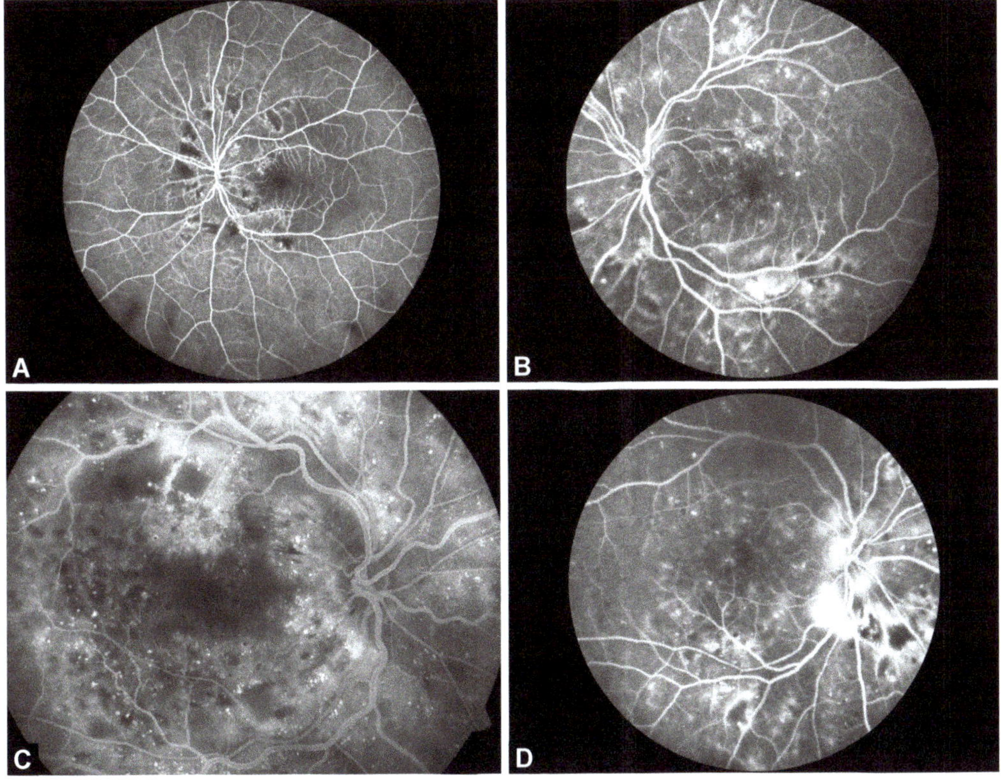

Figs. 4.2.9A to D: (A) Fluorescein angiogram of a diabetic patient showing focal hyperfluorescent microaneurysms; (B) Fluorescein angiogram of a diabetic patient showing multiple hard exudates, focal hyperfluorescent microaneurysms, and few areas of flame-shaped hemorrhages; (C) This is a late phase fluorescein angiogram of a diabetic patient showing diffuse leak at the macula. Hypofluorescent capillary nonperfusion areas are also visible. Focal hyperfluorescent microaneurysms are also seen. Neovascularization of the disc (NVD) or neovascularization elsewhere (NVE) is not seen; (D) Fluorescein angiogram of a diabetic patient showing multiple areas of leaking NVE and NVD along with other features of severe nonproliferative diabetic retinopathy (NPDR).

- *Ischemic diabetic maculopathy*: FAZ appears broken, i.e. CNP areas merge into FAZ.

3. *Age-related macular degeneration (AMD)*:
   - Dry AMD:
     - Geographical atrophy is usually seen as window defects with transmitted fluorescence from underlying choroid.
     - Drusen can be hyper (staining in late phase) or hypofluorescent depending on the concentration of lipid material.
   - Wet AMD:
     - Choroidal neovascular membrane (CNVM) can be seen as areas of the leak, serous PED as pooling and subretinal fibrosis/disciform scar as staining. Further submacular and intraretinal hemorrhage are seen as blocked hypofluorescence.
     - "Classic" choroidal neovascularization (CNV) is typically seen as a leak, in the early phase, which intensifies throughout the transit phase. It is uniform, with "lacy" margins (Fig. 4.2.11).

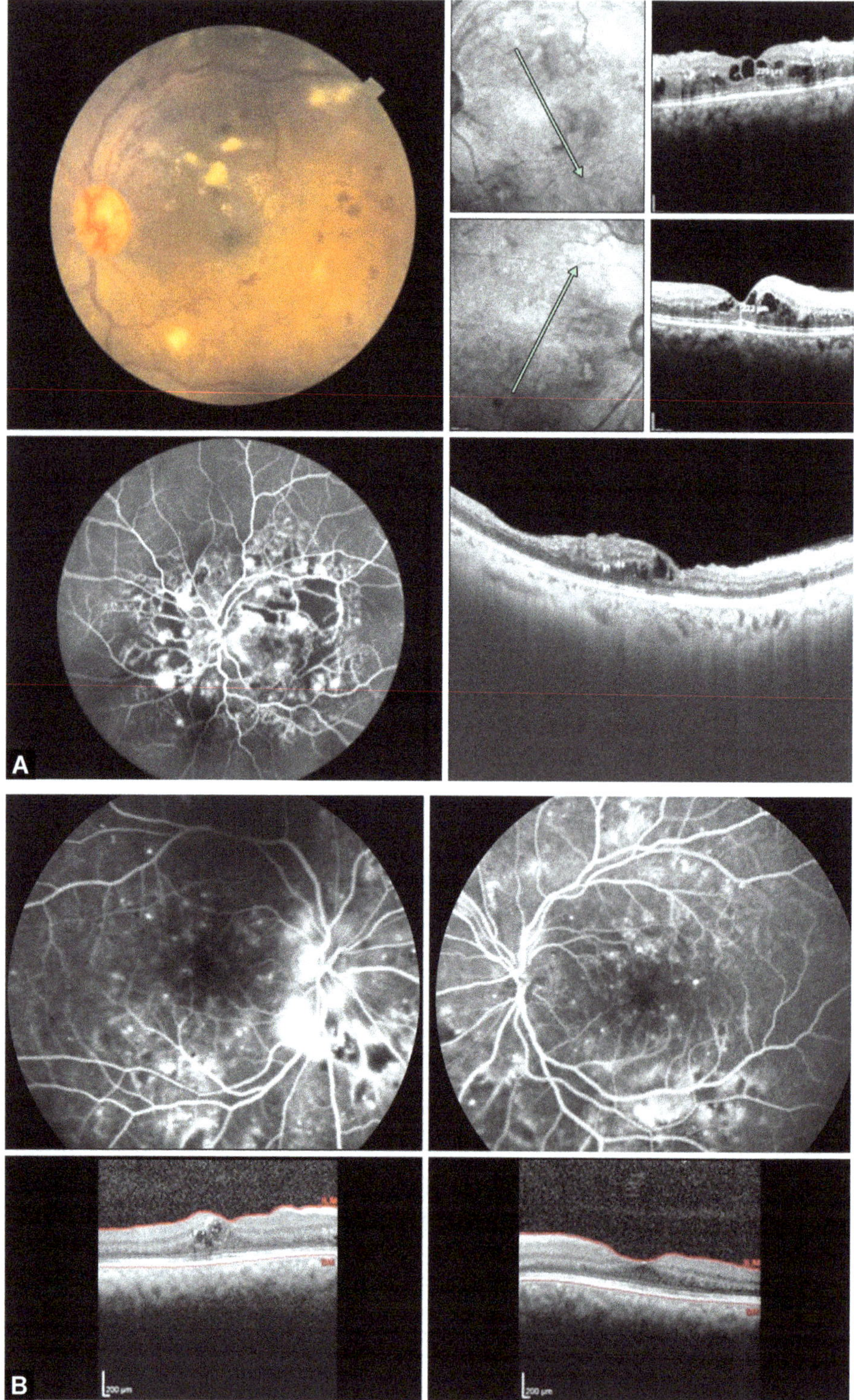

Figs. 4.2.10A and B: Diabetic macular edema corroborated with optical coherence tomography (OCT) findings.

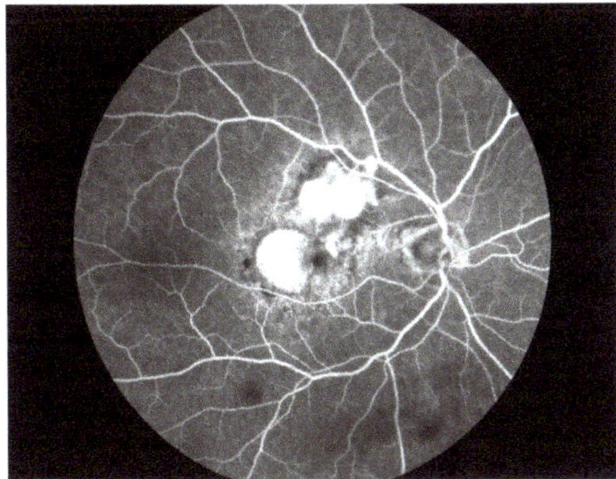

Fig. 4.2.11: Venous phase angiogram showing areas of well-defined hyperfluorescence, extrafoveal, and increasing with time. At the fovea, there is an area of pooling of fluorescein with an adjacent diamond-shaped area of leak. Associated stippled hyperfluorescence is also seen. Findings are suggestive of a combined type 1 and 2 choroidal neovascular membrane.

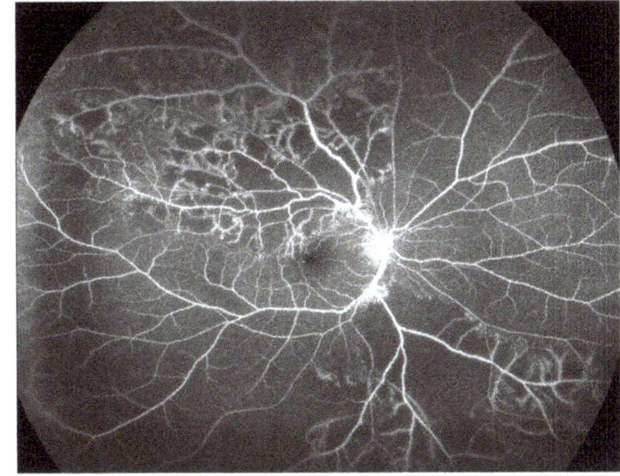

Fig. 4.2.12: This is a wide field (Optos) fluorescein angiogram showing two areas of vascular block (venous) one in the superotemporal quadrant and the other in the inferonasal quadrant. Both these areas show areas of capillary nonperfusion and few microaneurysms. Few focal leaking microaneurysms are also visible superior to the fovea. Neovascularization is not evident.

- "Occult" lesions are typically seen in the late phase of FA. It consists of two described forms on FA: (1) fibrovascular PED (FVPED) and (2) late leakage of undetermined source (LLUS).
- Fibrovascular PED is seen as an irregular elevation of the RPE with stippled or granular irregular fluorescence. Late leakage of the undetermined source is seen as areas of hyperfluorescence at the level of RPE seen in late phases.

4. *Vascular occlusion*: The characteristic findings are:
   - Delayed filling of the occluded retinal veins with areas of capillary nonperfusion (Figs. 4.2.12 and 4.2.13).
   - Blocked fluorescence from intraretinal or preretinal hemorrhages.
   - Leak from neovascularization or macular edema (Fig. 4.2.14).
   - Macular ischemia, which is seen as an increase in FAZ area (Fig. 4.2.15).

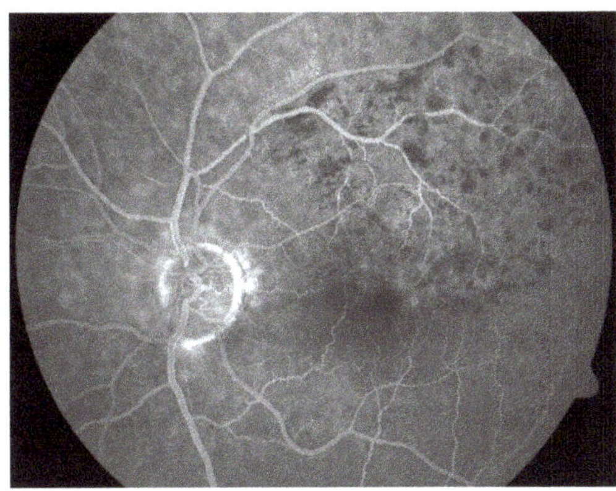

Fig. 4.2.13: Fresh superior-temporal branch retinal vein occlusion (BRVO) depicting scattered hemorrhages in the area of drainage of the major vein and maculae hemorrhages. Late fundus fluorescein angiography (FFA) picture showing blocked fluorescence in the area of the hemorrhages along with minimal leakage of the capillary bed.

Note: Fluorescein angiography is recommended *only* after the intraretinal hemorrhages have adequately cleared out from the retina. It is not advised in acute cases as dense intraretinal hemorrhages may make interpretation difficult due to blockage of fluorescence.

Ultra-widefield FA (UWFA)[4] has been recommended in vascular occlusion to look

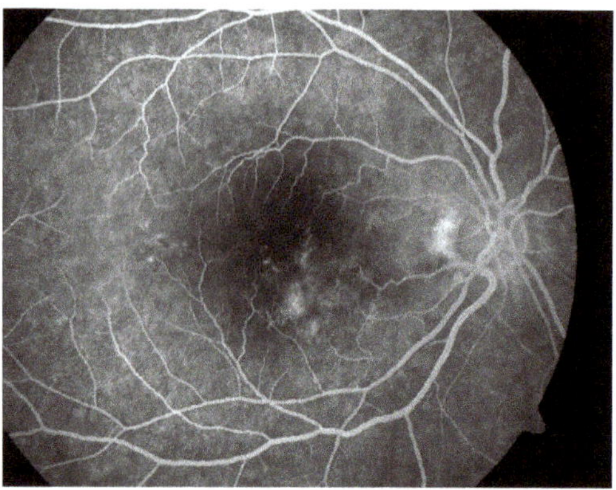

Fig. 4.2.14: Fundus image showing macular branch retinal vein occlusion, corresponding venous phase angiogram showing focal leakage at macula, and collateral formation.

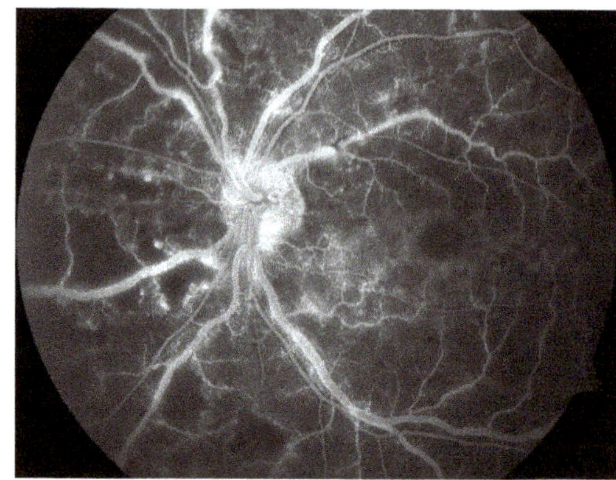

Fig. 4.2.15: Central retinal vein occlusion (CRVO) showing dilated veins with capillary nonperfusion areas involving the entire retina.

at the peripheral vascular status and presence of CNP areas and to mark the areas for targeted retinal photocoagulation or sectoral laser photocoagulation.

5. *Neuro-ophthalmology*: FFA has been used to study diseases like nonarteritic anterior ischemic optic neuropathy (NAION) extensively, and also helps in determining telangiectasia over the optic disc that is considered typical of diseases like Leber hereditary optic neuropathy (LHON).
6. *Cystoid macular edema*: CME shows petaloid appearance of fluorescence.

ADVANCES IN FUNDUS FLUORESCEIN ANGIOGRAPHY

Advances in FFA include following:

- *Confocal scanning laser ophthalmoscope:* Uses low-power laser beam to sweep through the retina and the reflected beam is recorded by a detector. The standard size is a field of 30° × 30°, but may be increased using attachments. Advantages include better resolution, reduction of noise, patient comfort through less bright light, and imaging in small pupil sizes.
- Ultra-widefield FFA is done using a camera which gives a *200° field* of view, which equates to 82.5% of the total retinal surface area. It uses a wide ellipsoid mirror to image retina through an undilated pupil. It can even be used in nondilating pupils that is typically difficult with older cameras. Pediatric sedation less imaging for diseases like retinopathy of prematurity (ROP), familial exudative vitreoretinopathy (FEVR), and Coats disease may also be done.[5] More importantly, it allows simultaneous imaging of near-total retina that was not possible with conventional FFA. Newer studies document its role in targeted laser photocoagulation of CNP areas in diseases like retinal vein occlusion (RVO), PDR, etc. Evaluations for retinal vasculitis have found it advantageous in determining the true extent and laterality of the disease. It also allows autofluorescence analysis and magnified central imaging.
- Retcam with FFA to look for vascular loops and adequacy of the laser in ROP babies. Wide field system is considered gold standard for pediatric imaging.

REFERENCES

1. Novotny HR, Alvis DL. A method of photographing fluorescence in circulating blood in the human retina. Circulation. 1961;24:82-6.
2. Lipson BK, Yannuzzi LA. Complications of intravenous fluorescein injections. Int Ophthalmol Clin. 1989;29(3):200-5.
3. Webb RH, Hughes GW, Delori FC. Confocal scanning laser ophthalmoscope. Appl Opt. 1987;26(8):1492-9.
4. Atkinson A, Mazo C. Imaged area of the retina. Dunfermline, UK: Optos PLC; 2015.
5. Friberg TR, Gupta A, Yu J, et al. Ultrawide angle fluorescein angiographic imaging: a comparison to conventional digital acquisition systems. Ophthalmic Surg Lasers Imaging. 2008;39:304-11.

4.3 OPTICAL COHERENCE TOMOGRAPHY

Priyanka Ramesh, Nawazish Shaikh, Nasiq Hasan, Atul Kumar

INTRODUCTION

Optical coherence tomography (OCT) is a noninvasive technique of imaging the retina and optic nerve. It gives high resolution images of the retina and optic nerve head. It is being used extensively in the diagnosis and management of many retinal and choroidal pathologies. It is also used in the diagnosis as well as follow-up of glaucoma.

The principle of "Michelson interferometry" or low-coherence interferometry is used in OCT. A ray of light is divided into a reference and a sample beam. The sample beam falls on the retina and is backscattered and interferes with the reference beam to form interference patterns. These interference patterns are used to reconstruct axial A-scans. Multiple A-scans are constructed at each point of the retina, and these are together reconstructed to give a two-dimensional cross-sectional image.

TYPES OF OPTICAL COHERENCE TOMOGRAPHY

- *Time-domain OCT*: It used a single-photon detector and moving mirror. This caused limitation in the speed of imaging. It had an axial resolution of 10 μm and a transverse resolution of 20 μm. The OCT could take 400 A-scans per second and used 820 nm wavelength light. For example, Stratus OCT (Carl Zeiss Meditec, Inc, Dublin, California).
- *Spectral-domain OCT*: It uses 840 nm wavelength of light. Also called Fourier-domain OCT or high-definition OCT (HD-OCT). It uses an array of detectors to acquire all the A-scans and hence it is faster than the time-domain OCT. A-scan rate is 27,000 Hz and has an axial resolution of 5–7 μm. For example, Cirrus HD-OCT (Carl Zeiss Meditec, Inc, Dublin, California).
- *Spectralis OCT (Heidelberg Engineering, Heidelberg, Germany)*: This is a machine that combines spectral-domain OCT and confocal scanning laser ophthalmoscopy. It has the eye-tracking technology and also the facility for fundus fluorescein angiography, autofluorescence, and indocyanine green angiography. It can take 40,000 A-scans per second and has an axial resolution of 8 μm.

- *Swept-source OCT*: This is a newer type of OCT which uses a broadband superluminescent diode light source of 1,050 nm wavelength. The longer wavelength has better penetration and therefore has better visualization of structures deep to the retinal pigment epithelium. The A-scan rate is 100,000 Hz. The axial resolution is 3–5 μm.

NEWER TECHNOLOGIES IN OPTICAL COHERENCE TOMOGRAPHY

- *Enhanced depth imaging*: This involves setting the choroid next to the zero-delay line to enhance imaging of the choroid and the choroid-scleral junction.
- *Optical coherence tomography angiography*: It is a noninvasive method of visualizing the retinal microvasculature. It does not require dye injection. It is based on the principle of "split-spectrum amplitude-decorrelation angiography". Here there is contrast created between the retina and the blood vessels by assessing the signal changes in the moving red blood cells (RBCs) in the blood vessels.

INTERPRETATION OF OPTICAL COHERENCE TOMOGRAPHY

First identify the name, age, type of OCT scan, and the date of acquisition. The OCT is read from inner layers to the outer layers.

- The vitreous has to be commented and the vitreoretinal interface.
- The different layers of the retina have to be seen.
- The retinal pigmented epithelium (RPE)-Bruch's membrane complex integrity has to be commented on.
- The choroid has to be seen for the thickness and normal pattern.
- The sclera-choroidal junction has to be seen.

The layers of retina seen in an OCT image are as follows (Fig. 4.3.1):

- Precortical vitreous
- Internal limiting membrane
- Nerve fiber layer
- Ganglion cell layer
- Inner plexiform layer
- Inner nuclear layer
- Outer plexiform layer
- Outer nuclear layer (Henle's layer in the macula)
- External limiting membrane
- Myoid zone
- Ellipsoid zone
- The outer segment of photoreceptors
- Interdigitation zone
- RPE-Bruch's complex
- Sattler's layer
- Haller's layer
- Choroid-sclera junction.

CLINICAL CASES/EXAMPLES

1. *Central serous chorioretinopathy (CSC)/ central serous retinopathy (Figs. 4.3.2A and B)*:
    - An elevation of the inner layers of the retina, which is suggestive of a neurosensory detachment.
    - There is also an elevation of the RPE and Bruch's complex, which is suggestive of a pigment epithelium detachment which is suggestive of CSC.
    - Acute CSC in which there is neurosensory detachment whereas the other retinal layers are not distorted.
    - Chronic CSC in which there are large cystic spaces in the retinal layers with RPE disruption.
2. *Cystoid macular edema (Figs. 4.3.3A to C)*: There is the presence of cystic spaces

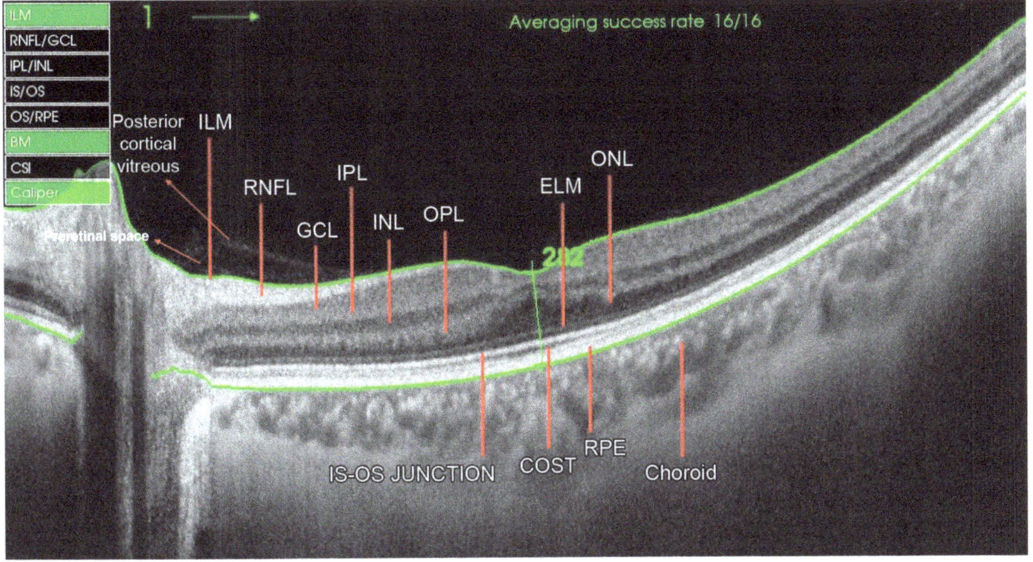

Fig. 4.3.1: Normal layers in OCT. (OCT: optical coherence tomography; RPE: retinal pigmented epithelium; ILM: internal limiting membrane; RNFL: retinal nerve fiber layer; GCL: ganglion cell layer; IPL: inner plexiform layer; INL: inner nuclear layer; ELM: external limiting membrane; ONL: outer nuclear layer; COST: cone outer segment tips also known as interdigitation zone; IS-OS junction: inner segment-outer segment junction).

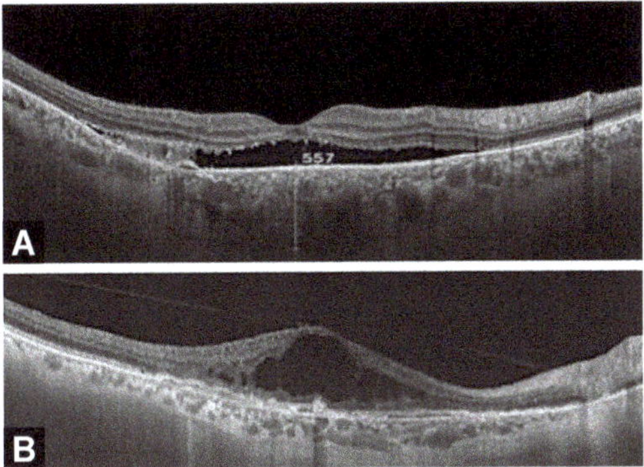

Figs. 4.3.2A and B: Central serous chorioretinopathy (CSC).

in the retina corresponding to the outer plexiform layer.

3. *Diabetic macular edema (Figs. 4.3.4A to C)*: There is the presence of cystic spaces in the inner retina. There is the presence of hyper-reflective dot-like lesions which correspond to hard exudates. There may be associated thickening of the posterior hyaloid which is seen as a hyper-reflective band called "thick taut posterior hyaloid".
4. *Macular hole (Figs. 4.3.5A and B)*:
   - Optical coherence tomography is showing a macular hole extending full thickness in the retina with cystic spaces in between the retinal layers.
   - There is a presence of a defect in all the layers of the retina except for the RPE-Bruch's membrane complex.
   - The different dimensions of the hole can be calculated like minimum diameter, height, basal diameter, and also the

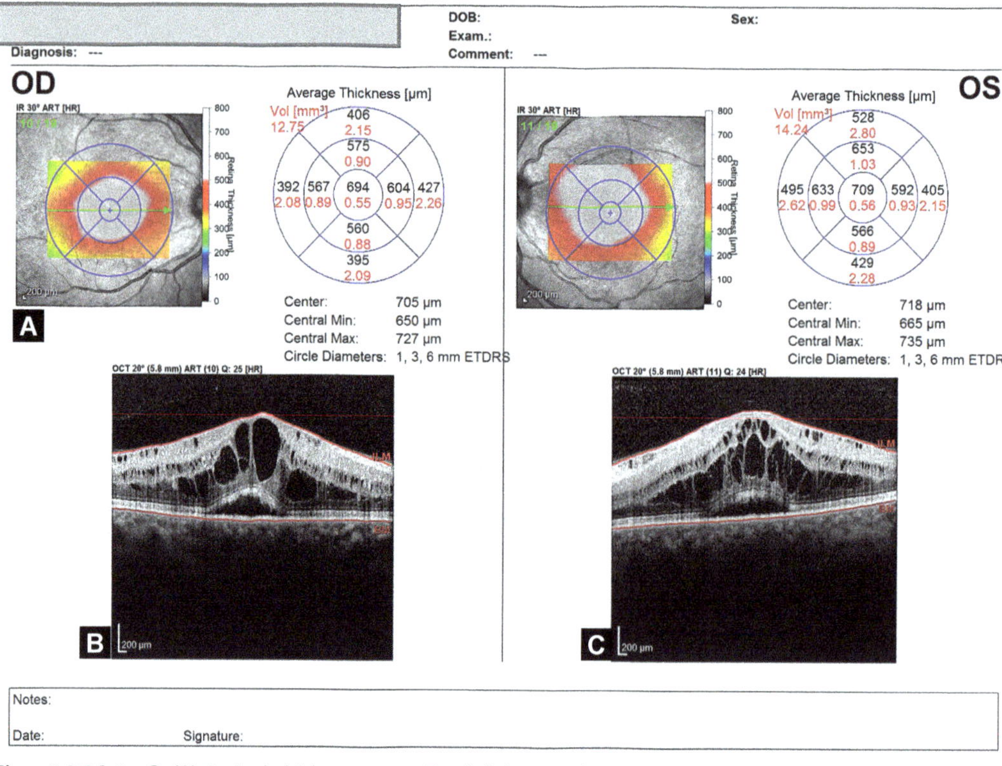

Figs. 4.3.3A to C: (A) Retinal thickness map: Top left image shows the color-coded macular thickness map showing thickening at the macular region and macular thickness values are seen in 1 mm, 3 mm and 6 mm circles in the top right image; (B and C) The corresponding spectral domain optical coherence tomography image of right eye and left eye respectively depicting cystoid macular edema.

different indices like diameter hole index, hole forming factor, tractional hole index, and macular hole index.

5. *Epiretinal membrane (Fig. 4.3.6)*: There is the presence of a hyper-reflective membrane on the surface of inner retina with associated distortion of the retinal architecture.
6. *Vitreomacular traction (Figs. 4.3.7A and B)*:
   - Optical coherence tomography showing focal attachment of the posterior hyaloid in the perifoveal area with separation in the macular area.
   - Vitreomacular adhesion (focal) in which the posterior vitreous cortex is attached only at the fovea and the foveal counter is normal.
   - Vitreoretinal traction in which the posterior vitreous cortex pulls the macula at the point of traction distorting the foveal contour.
7. *Choroidal neovascular membrane (Fig. 4.3.8)*: There is the presence of a discontinuity in the RPE-Bruch's membrane complex and hyper-reflective structure extending beneath the RPE-Bruch's complex. Also small area of neurosensory detachment.
8. *Polypoidal choroidal neovascularization (Fig. 4.3.9)*:
   - Polypoidal choroidal vasculopathy (PCV) is characterized by the presence of pigment epithelial detachments

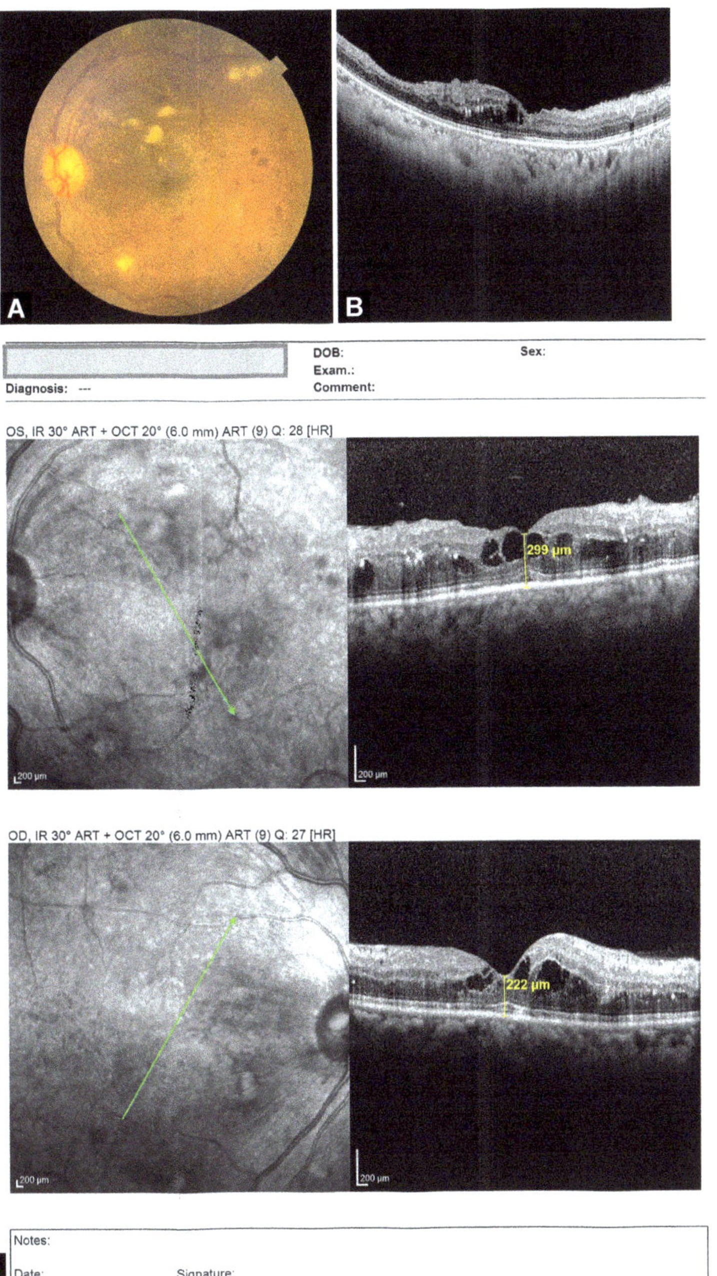

Figs. 4.3.4A to C: Diabetic macular edema.

which are steep and called "thumb-like polyps" (star).

- There is the presence of characteristic "double-layer sign" (arrow), which is because of the split of the RPE and Bruch's membrane due to the branching vascular network.

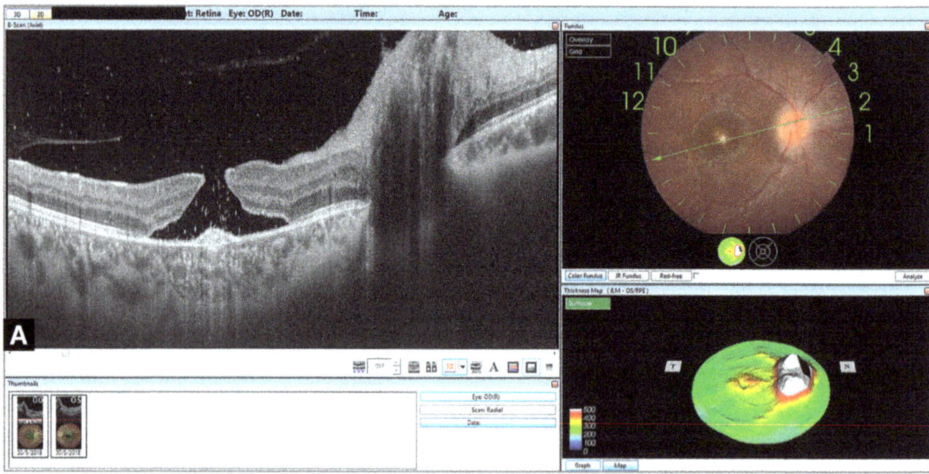

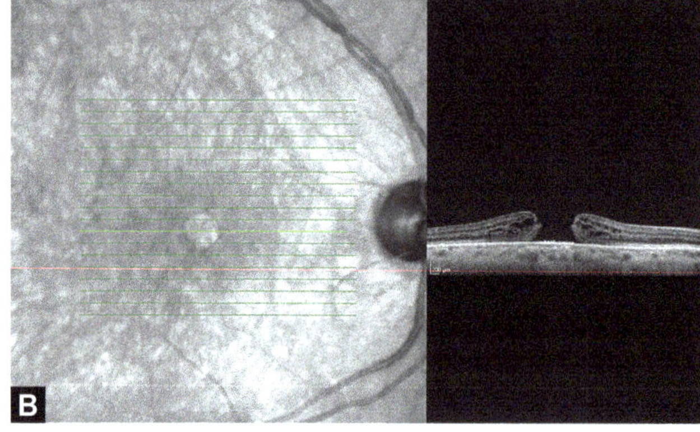

Figs. 4.3.5A and B: (A) Macular hole with choroidal neovascular membrane (CNVM); (B) Macular hole with cystoid changes.

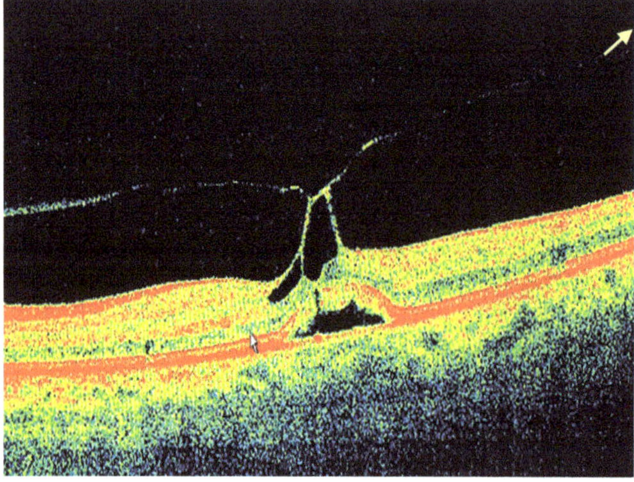

Fig. 4.3.6: Epiretinal membrane with vitreomacular traction (VMT).

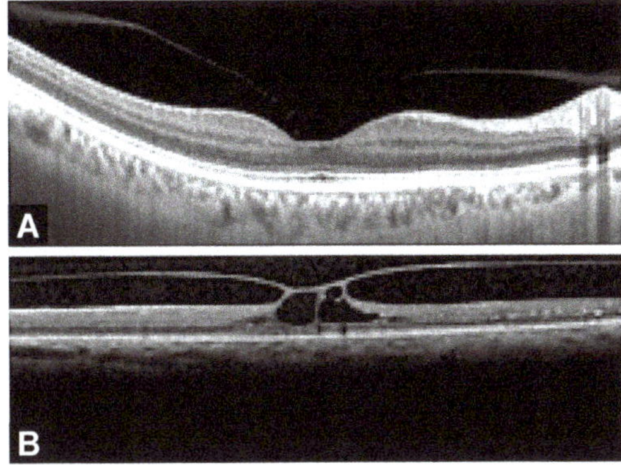

Figs. 4.3.7A and B: Vitreomacular traction.

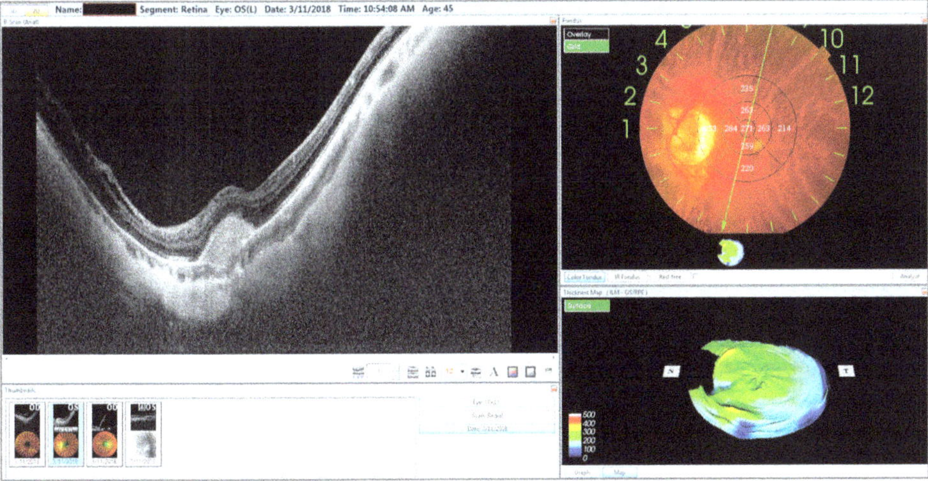

Fig. 4.3.8: Choroidal neovascular membrane.

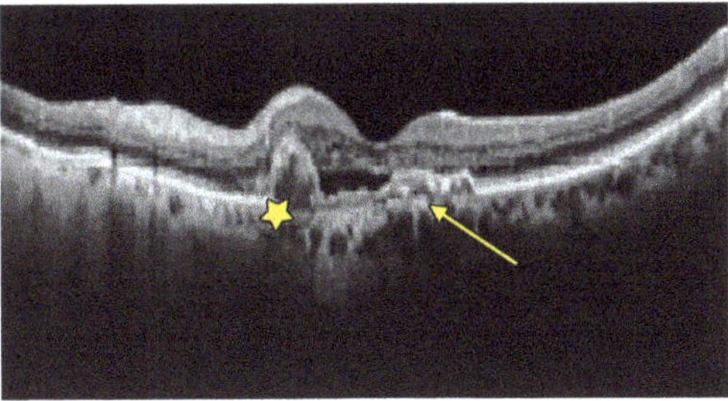

Fig. 4.3.9: Polypoidal choroidal neovascularization.

BIBLIOGRAPHY

1. Gao SS, Jia Y, Zhang M, et al. Optical coherence tomography angiography. Invest Ophthalmol Vis Sci. 2016;57(9):OCT27-36.
2. Ryan SJ. Retinal reattachment: general surgical principles and techniques. In: Ryan SJ (Ed). Retina, 5th edition. Philadelphia, PA: Elsevier Saunders; 2013. p. 1713.

4.4 INDOCYANINE GREEN ANGIOGRAPHY

Anusha Sachan, Nasiq Hasan, Atul Kumar

INTRODUCTION

Indocyanine green (ICG) is water soluble, tricarbocyanine anionic dye. Its first application was used in measuring cardiac output. Flower and Hochheimer performed the first intravenous ICG angiography to image the human choroid in 1972. Hayashi and coworkers worked on improved filter combinations in 1980. The dye has a molecular weight of 774.96 Da and has maximum absorption at 790 nm and emission at 835 nm in the near infrared wavelength. This allows penetration through macular pigment, blood, melanin, and pigments, thereby better angiography under challenging situations.[1-3]

Indocyanine green is 98% protein bound compared to 80% of that of sodium fluorescein. This allows the dye to stay within the larger choroidal circulation resulting in its enhanced definition. The dye is eliminated through the bile without metabolism. ICG is known to have more side effects than sodium fluorescein. Nausea, vomiting, and pruritis are the most common side effects. Urticaria and difficulty breathing can occur, hypotensive shock and anaphylactic shock can also occur rarely. It is usually contraindicated in patients with iodine and seafood allergy, liver disease, end-stage renal failure, and uremia. It is a category-C drug in pregnancy. Differences between fundus fluorescein angiography (FFA) and ICG have been summarized in Table 4.4.1.

Table 4.4.1: Differences between fundus fluorescein angiography (FFA) and indocyanine green (ICG) dye.

Features	*Fluorescein dye*	*ICG dye*
Molecular weight (kD, kilodalton)	375	775
Absorption wavelength (nm)	494	800
Emission wavelength (nm)	521	830
$t_{1/2}$ (minutes)	23	2.5
Excretion	Renal	Biliary
Waiting time after injection (minutes)	15	2
Side effects	++	+

ADMINISTRATION OF INDOCYANINE GREEN

Indocyanine green is used in the standard concentration of 25 mg/mL. Rapid IV injection is done with 5 mL saline flush and images are captured serially.

PHASES OF INDOCYANINE GREEN

1. Early phase—first 1-minute postinjection—shows choroidal arteries
2. Early mid-phase—(1-3 minutes)—choroidal veins and retinal vessels
3. Late mid-phase—(3-15 minutes)—choroidal vessels fading but retinal vessels are still visible.
4. Late phase—15-45 minutes—hypofluorescent choroidal vessels and gradual fading of retinal vessels.

The "hyper" lesions are described as hot spots.

The two technologies used for imaging ICG are the standard digital camera-based systems and SLO-based systems. The newer techniques of indocyanine green angiography (ICGA) are real-time ICGA (30 frames/sec), wide angle ICGA (160° field), digital subtraction ICGA. It has also been incorporated in ultra-widefield imaging (Optos) in the latest Optos California machines. Simultaneous FFA with ICG can also be done.[1-3]

ADVANTAGES OVER FUNDUS FLUORESCEIN ANGIOGRAPHY

- More useful in the presence of optical media opacification.
- More useful for the understanding of choroidal pathologies due to its ability to penetrate melanin. Example: CSCR, PCV, etc.
- Very useful in identifying feeder vessels of tumors and CNVMs.
- It was an excellent guide for the treatment of age-related macular degeneration (ARMD) when anti-VEGF therapy was unavailable.
- In cases, where background fluorescence is high or in cases with PEDs, differentiating pathologies may be difficult. In such cases, ICG was considered advantageous. However, with the advent of OCT-angiography, this advantage is now lost.

DISADVANTAGES OF INDOCYANINE GREEN

Side effects are much more common than FFA, and severe too. It cannot be used in patients with specific allergies and those with hepatic dysfunction.

CLINICAL APPLICATIONS

ARMD: Choroidal neovascularization has been classified depending on size and delineation into "focal hotspots" and "plaques". Plaques are further classified into well defined, poorly defined and a combination of both. The most common type was plaques (61% of the cases) and had a poor visual prognosis, compared to focal spots or "hot spots" (29%) which had a better prognosis, and they were considered to be potentially treatable by ICG-guided laser photocoagulation. ICGA also shows feeder vessels in its early phase.

Polypoidal choroidal vasculopathy: Indocyanine green angiography is very useful in detecting and characterizing polyps, which are seen as small hypercyanescent spots in early and late phase. ICGA helps in measuring the total size of the lesion, which includes polyps and branching vascular network (BVN) (Fig. 4.4.1) and allows us to select the spot size when considering photodynamic therapy (PDT).

Central serous chorioretinopathy: Indocyanine green angiography helps to assess the location of areas of hyperpermeability, which can be useful when considering treatment with verteporfin PDT.

Choroidal inflammatory disease: Indocyanine green angiography helps in staging and determining the activity of the disease. Active lesion show areas of hypocyanescence or cold spots with poorly defined margins whereas healed lesions show well-defined margins. Aggressive lesions show areas of late hypercyanescence or hot spots.

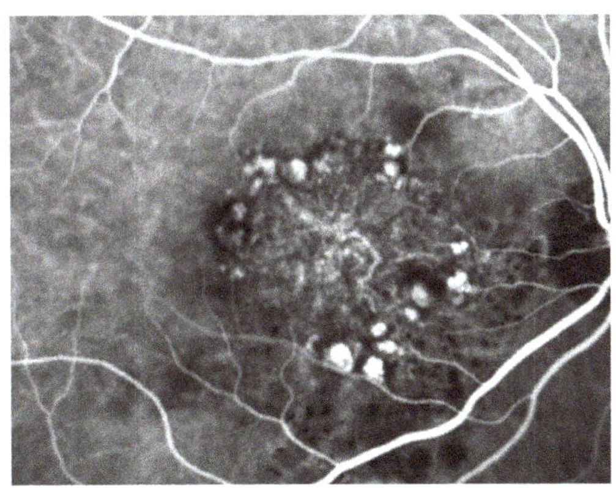

Fig. 4.4.1: Indocyanine green (ICG) frame reveals multiple polyps with branching vascular network (BVN) in an eye with polypoidal choroidal vasculopathy.

Choroidal tumors: Indocyanine green angiography is useful to diagnose choroidal tumors that cannot be diagnosed with FA. It shows the intrinsic vascular pattern of the tumors.

REFERENCES

1. Agrawal RV, Biswas J, Gunasekaran D. Indocyanine green angiography in posterior uveitis. Indian J Ophthalmol. 2013;61(4):148-59. [online]. Available from https://www.ncbi.nlm.nih.gov/pmc/articles/PMC3714951/ [Accessed January, 2019].
2. Ryan SJ. Retina, Fourth edition. Philadelphia: Elsevier; 2006. [online]. Available from https://books.google.co.in/books?id=au15FQb4P-sC&printsec=frontcover&dq=indocyanine+green+angiography+RYAN&hl=en&sa=X&ved=0ahUKEwjovvyblM_dAhVJpo8KHV3TBfQQ6AEIPjAE#v=onepage&q=indocyanine%20green%20angiography%20RYAN&f=false [Accessed January, 2019].
3. Regillo CD. The present role of indocyanine green angiography in ophthalmology. Curr Opin Ophthalmol. 1999;10:189-96.

4.5 ELECTRORETINOGRAM

Sourabh Verma, Lohith Rambarki, Divya Agarwal

INTRODUCTION

Electroretinogram (ERG) (Fig. 4.5.1) is a record of change in electric potential of the eye in response to light stimuli. Holmgren first described it in 1865, and first recording in humans was done by Dewar.[1] Riggs and Karpe made corneal electrodes mounted on contact lens with which clinical recording of ERG became possible.[1] Pattern ERG (PERG) and standard full-field ERG (referred to as ERG) have found widespread use in diagnosis and prognostication of retinal and macular diseases. They provide objective data, which can be interpreted according to set norms. However, as its findings may be similar for many conditions, a precise correlation with clinical context and history is necessary. International Society of Clinical Electrophysiology of Vision (ISCEV) has established guidelines to record and interpret its results.[2]

PHYSIOLOGY OF ELECTRORETINOGRAM

A potential difference of 1 mV exists between cornea and retina, cornea having a relative positive charge, called corneoretinal potential. Stimulation of retina by light leads to a generation of a cascade of electrical changes in the retina, which is recorded with the help of electrodes. ERG is a record of electrical activity from radially arranged retinal components, i.e. photoreceptors, bipolar cells, Müller cells, and retinal pigmented epithelium (RPE). Horizontally arranged cells such as amacrine cell and ganglion cell have minimal effect on it.

ERG waveform (Fig. 4.5.2) is composed of following parts:

- A-wave—it is the initial negative wave, which arises from *photoreceptors*. When recorded in isolation it is called Granit's P-III or late receptor potential.[3] Both

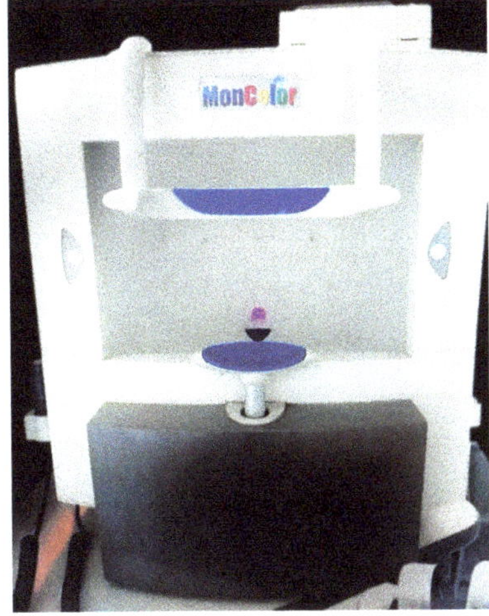

Fig. 4.5.1: Electroretinogram (ERG) machine.

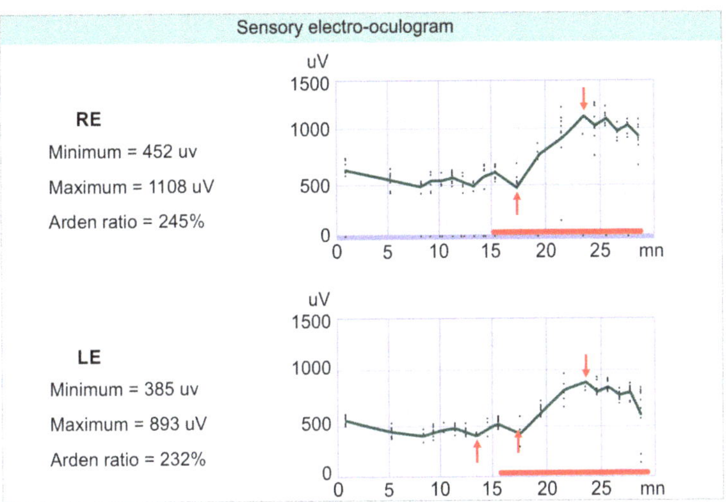

Fig. 4.5.2: Normal electroretinogram (ERG) wave. (RE: right eye; LE: left eye).

rods and cones contribute to it after light-induced hyperpolarization and using specific stimuli can separate their individual responses.

- B-wave (P-II component of Granit). It is a positive wave after a wave. It arises due to *Müller cell membrane* potential change in response to potassium released from photoreceptors during hyperpolarization. It represents the activity of *the bipolar cell layer.*

Small wavelets are found on the ascending limb of the b-wave, which represents a negative feedback circuit in the inner retina between amacrine cells, ganglion cells, and bipolar cells. They are recorded in the light-adapted retina using a bright flash of light and using filters to filter out low-frequency b-wave responses. Their frequency varies from 100 Hz to 150 Hz.

- C-wave (AKA P-I) component of Granit. It is a small positive wave after b-wave arising from RPE. Since predominantly rods are in contact with RPE cells in interdigitation zone, cones are believed to have no contribution to it.

There is no contribution of retinal components proximal to ganglion cells and optic nerve.

DEFINITION OF PARAMETERS

- *Amplitude*:
  - A-wave amplitude—measured from baseline to tip of a-wave.
  - B-wave amplitude—measured from trough of a wave to peak of b-wave.
- *Latency*: The time between stimulus and initiation of the wave. It is approximately 2 ms for a-wave.
- *Implicit time*: The time period between stimulus and peak of a- or b-wave.

TYPES OF ELECTRORETINOGRAM

- *On the basis of stimulus zone*:
  - Full field ERG
  - Multifocal ERG (mfERG)
- On the basis of stimulus type:
  - Single flash ERG
  - Red flash ERG
  - Flicker ERG
  - Blue filter ERG
  - Pattern ERG (PERG)
- On the basis of the state of retinal adaptation:
  - Photopic ERG (Fig. 4.5.3)
  - Scotopic ERG (Fig. 4.5.4)
  - Mesopic ERG.

Full-field Electroretinogram

International Society of Clinical Electrophysiology of Vision has given revised guidelines for recording ERG which are based on strength of stimuli (flash strength in cd s m^{-2}) and state of adaptation.[2]

Six protocols for recording ERG are as follows:

1. Dark-adapted 0.01 ERG—gives the rod driven response of bipolar cells.

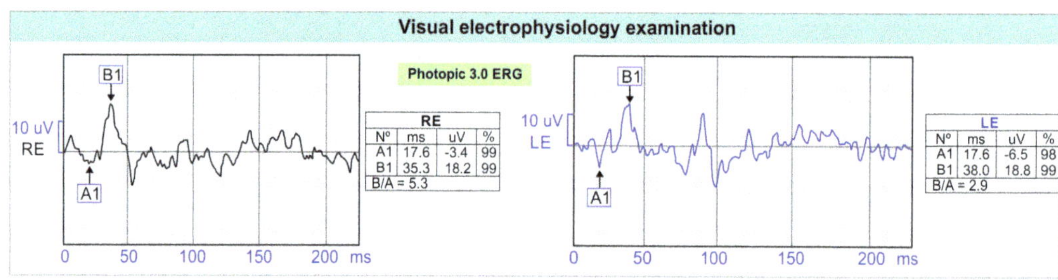

Fig. 4.5.3: Photopic electroretinogram (ERG).

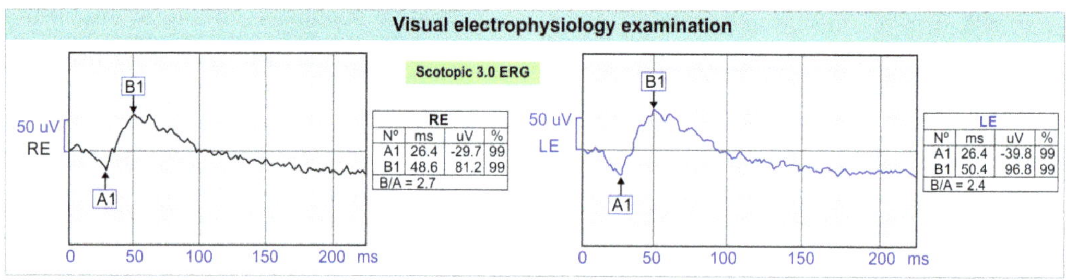

Fig. 4.5.4: Scotopic electroretinogram (ERG).

2. Dark-adapted 3 ERG—represents the combined response from both rod and cone-driven bipolar cells. The rod response is more predominant.
3. Dark-adapted 10 ERG—represents combined response from rods and cones. Prominent a wave is seen.
4. Dark-adapted oscillator potentials—it represents amacrine cell activity.
5. Light-adapted 3 ERG—represents cone response; a-wave from cones and cone off bipolar cells; b-wave from on and off cone bipolar cells.
6. Light-adapted flicker ERG (30 Hz)—it is cone driven response.

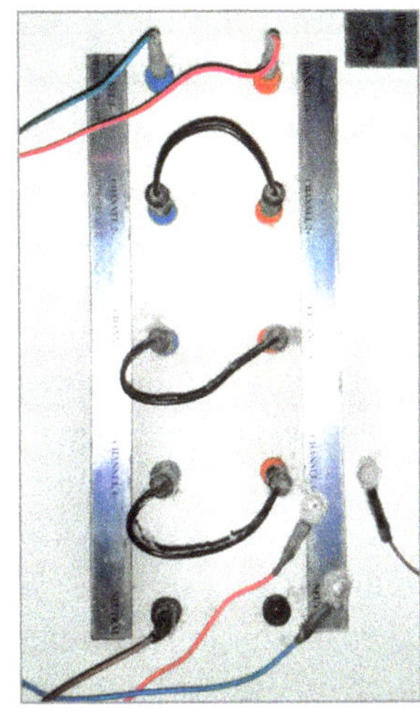

Fig. 4.5.5: Electroretinogram (ERG) leads.

Patient Preparation

The pupil should be dilated. Before recording, a period of 20 minutes dark adaptation for scotopic ERG and 10 minutes light adaptation for photopic ERG is required. Any investigation using bright light should be avoided before it; if done a 30-minute recovery period is required before recording. The patient is instructed to look at a fixation point. Scotopic ERG should be recorded before photopic ERG.

Electrodes

Active electrode: Different types are available which can be placed on the cornea, conjunctiva or skin of lower lid (Fig. 4.5.5). Most commonly used ones are embedded in the contact lens and placed on the cornea as they provide the most stable and reproducible recordings.

Reference electrodes: They serve as the negative pole. They can be placed on cornea conjunctiva or skin. Mostly they are placed on the lateral orbital rim. They should not be placed over muscle masses.

Ground electrode/common electrode: Placed on forehead, mastoid or earlobe.

Stimulus

A Ganzfeld field in the shape of a dome or integrating sphere to stimulate entire retina provides background illumination of about 17-34 candelas/m^2. A fixation spot is provided. Duration of flash stimulus should be less than 5 ms, which is shorter than the integration time of photoreceptors. Different wavelengths can be used to stimulate rods and cones separately or in a combined fashion. Standard strength of stimulus is 3 cd s m^{-2}.

Factors Affecting Electroretinogram

- Area of retina illuminated
- Duration of stimulus
- Strength of stimulus
- Interval between stimulus
- Size of pupil.

Abnormal Electroretinogram Responses and Associated Conditions

- Accentuated/supernormal response—characterized by the amplitude of a- and b-waves being greater than two standard deviations from the mean. It is seen in conditions such as early stages of siderosis bulbi, subtotal circulatory disturbance of retina and albinism.[4,5]

- Subnormal response—characterized by a- and b-wave amplitude less than two standard deviations of the mean. As ERG gives an estimate of total retinal function, a subnormal response is seen only when a large area of the retina is not functioning. It is seen in retinal detachment, chloroquine and quinine toxicity and early cases of retinitis pigmentosa. It can also found in systemic conditions such as vitamin A deficiency, anemia, and mucopolysaccharidosis.
- Extinguished response—a-and b-waves are not seen, and a flat ERG waveform is recorded (Fig. 4.5.6). It is seen in advanced cases of siderosis bulbi, old retinal detachment and retinitis pigmentosa. An extinguished response at birth characterizes Leber's congenital amaurosis. It can also be found in progressive conditions such as choroideremia, cancer-associated retinopathy, and chorioretinitis in later stages. Presence of an extinguished response signifies a poor visual outcome.
- Negative response—it is characterized by a large a-wave and absent b-wave (b/a<1) and signifies gross retinal dysfunction. It is seen in central retinal artery occlusion, X-linked retinoschisis, melanocyte-associated retinopathy, Goldmann-Favre syndrome, etc.[1]
- Absent oscillatory potentials—they are absent in patients of diabetic retinopathy and may point toward the conversion of NPDR to PDR. They are also abolished in other ischemic conditions of the retina such as CRAO.

Pattern Electroretinogram

It is a retinal response evoked by a contrast-reversing pattern, predominantly generated from ganglion cells driven by photoreceptors. Most commonly a black and white checkerboard pattern is used. The width of individual checks is 0.8° (±0.2°) their shape should be square. In patients with abnormal visually evoked potentials (VEPs), PERG can help differentiate between an optic nerve retinal dysfunction.[6]

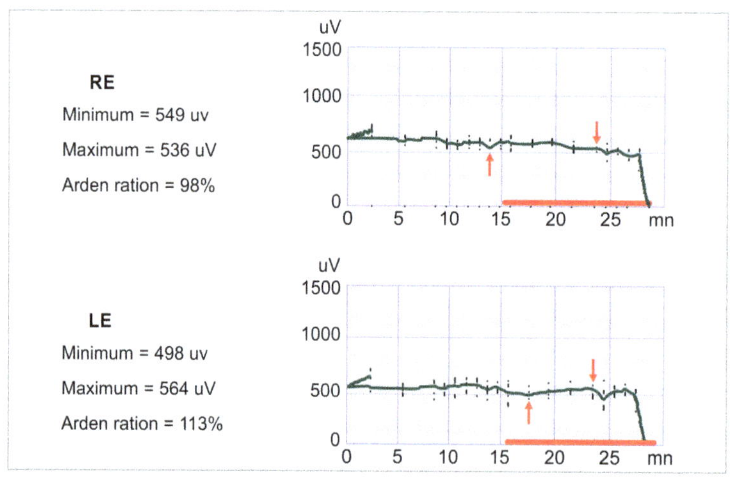

Fig. 4.5.6: Extinguishing electroretinogram (ERG). (RE: right eye; LE: left eye).

Pattern electroretinogram recording is difficult as signal strength is only 2–8 μV. The standard PERG response is called transient response, as it is almost complete before the next reversal of contrast pattern. This allows clear separation of the wave components.

The patient should be given a proper refractive correction during testing which is not necessary for ERG. Also, no mydriasis is required here. Rest of the setup is the same as standard ERG. During testing luminance of lit area should be 80 cd/m^2 and mean luminance of screen remains constant during pattern reversal. The contrast between light and dark areas should be not less than 80%. A reversal rate of 4.0 ± 0.8 reversals per second (rps) is standard.[6]

The waveform consists of following parts:

- *N35*: Negative wave; peak time at approximately 35 ms.
- *P50*: Positive wave; peak time at approximately 45–60 ms. The amplitude of P50 is measured from the trough of N35 to peak P50.
- *N95*: Large amplitude negative wave; peak time at approximately 90–100 ms. The amplitude of N95 is measured from the peak of P50 to trough of N95.

P50 and N95 amplitude and peak time are important parameters to be reported. Implicit time is defined as the time between onset of contrast reversal and peak of the wave.

Uses of Pattern Electroretinogram

- A measure of central retinal function
- Differentiation between the optic nerve and macular dysfunction
- Evaluation of ganglion cell function and early diagnosis of glaucoma[7]
- Approximate determination of visual acuity.

Multifocal Electroretinogram

Multifocal electroretinogram is first developed by Eric Sutter in 1992. It is a topographical record of the local retinal electrophysiological response. It gives the cone-driven response, recorded under light adapted condition. ISCEV (2007) has given clear guidelines to record and describe it.

Patient Preparation

Pupils should be fully dilated and 15 minutes of light adaptation under ordinary room light is required. Good central fixation is necessary and optimal refractive correction is provided. Rest of the precautions is the same as for recording ERG. Electrode placement is the same as for ERG. Recording can be done both monocularly and binocularly.

Stimulus

It consists of a display containing 61 or 103 hexagonal elements subtending an angle of 40–50° with a central fixation point. Each hexagonal element has a 50% chance of illumination every time the frame changes in a pseudorandom pattern. Also, the size of elements increases from center to periphery to compensate for reducing the concentration of cones from center to periphery. Most commonly used frame frequency is 75 Hz. Background luminance and luminance of stimulus are 30 cd/m^2 and 100 cd/m^2 respectively. There should be a contrast of 90% or greater between lighted and darkened areas of the stimulus pattern. Test duration is 4 minutes for 61 element and 8 minutes for 103 element display.[8]

Response and Interpretation

Multifocal ERG test results are represented as:

- *Trace array*: It is the basic mfERG display. It should always be taken into account while reporting. It can be displayed with a retinal or field view, which should be specified along with the breadth of trace array. A trace length of 100 ms or more is used. Trace arrays are examined for any delayed signal and abnormal waveform. They show topographic variations and quality of records.

- *Topographic 3D response density plots*: It shows an overall signal strength per unit area of the retina. A normal plot in presence of central and steady fixation has a peak corresponding to the fovea, due to high cone density in this area and an evident depression corresponding to the blind spot. They give a quick, easy to understand representation of retinal function but should never be used in isolation to trace arrays. This is because an abnormal and delayed response can also produce a normal looking 3D plot.
- *Ring and other regional averages*: A group of trace arrays from an area of interest can be averaged to compare normal and abnormal areas. This comparison can be done between quadrants, hemiretinal areas or successive rings from center to periphery. Latter is advantageous in diagnosing diseases which produce retinal dysfunction with approximate radial symmetry.

First order kernel: It is thought to represent the activity of outer retina, i.e. photoreceptors and Müller cells and is obtained by subtracting the average of all responses from when a hexagon dark from the average of responses from when it is lit. The typical waveform is biphasic, consisting of an initial negative followed by a positive deflection. A third negative deflection is usually found and the three peaks obtained are designated as N1, P1, and N2 respectively.

Second order kernel: It is thought to arise from the inner retina, especially ganglion cells and is a measure of mfERG responses to adaptation by successive flash. Its waveform consists of an initial positive (P1) followed by a negative (N1) peak.

Advantages of Multifocal Electroretinogram

- It gives a topographic representation of retinal function and help in identifying the site of disease.
- Helpful in monitoring progression of the disease.
- Distinguishing between inner and outer retinal disease.

Affected By

- The decrease in amplitude and increase in implicit time is seen with increasing age.
- The amplitude of N1 and P1 are reduced in patients with cataract.
- Reduced first and second order kernel responses with increasing refractive error and axial length.

Uses

- Toxic retinopathy—mfERG can be used in early detection of drug-induced retinopathy, for example in chloroquine, hydroxychloroquine, vigabatrin, and sildenafil.
- Differentiate diseases affecting inner (predominantly effects second-order kernel) and outer retinal layers (effects first-order kernel).
- Age-related macular degeneration (ARMD)—mfERG has been used to evaluate the extent of retinal involvement in ARMD. Significant reduction in P1 amplitude and N1 implicit time has been seen in the early foveal disease.
- Diabetic retinopathy—implicit time has been shown to be better than amplitude in detecting early diabetic retinopathy.

- Central serous retinopathy—decreased amplitudes and increased implicit time is seen.
- Macular hole—decrease in response density in the foveal region.
- Epiretinal membrane—decreased response density is seen which improves after ERM removal.
- Vascular occlusions—decreased amplitudes and increased implicit time is seen.
- It has been useful in evaluating other acquired retinopathies such as MEWDS, MFC, AMN, AZOOR, AIBSE, Purtscher-like retinopathy, MAR, CAR, etc.[9]

ELECTROOCULOGRAM

It is the measurement of the resting potential of the eye, between the cornea (positively charged) and retina (negatively charged). Like ERG, it is also a mass response and cannot be used for localized retinal conditions. Active electrodes are placed on both lateral and medial canthi, and a grounding electrode is placed on the forehead. There are three fixation lights and the right and left lights are lit alternatively to produce a saccadic movement in the eye. First baseline amplitude is recorded with stimulus lights on. A recording in dark-adapted state follows this with stimulus light off, and a recording in the light-adapted state with stimulus light on.

In dark-adapted state, resting potential decreases progressively reaching to a "dark trough" in approximately 10 minutes. The dark trough has contributions from RPE, photoreceptors and inner nuclear layer. The amplitude increases in light-adapted state and reaches a "light peak" in approximately 5 minutes. Light peak is affected by photoreceptors.

Arden ratio is calculated as the amplitude of light peak divided by the amplitude of dark trough. Its normal value is more than or equal to 180 and is considered abnormal below 165.

Clinically it has found application only in diagnosing Best vitelliform dystrophy in which Ardens ratio is less than 165, but ERG is normal. In other retinal diseases, it usually does not provide any additional information over ERG.[10]

REFERENCES

1. Vincent A, Robson AG, Holder GE. Pathognomonic (Diagnostic) ERGs: A Review and Update. Retina. 2013;33(1):5-12.
2. McCulloch DL, Marmor MF, Brigell MG, et al. ISCEV Standard for full-field clinical electroretinography (2015 update). Doc Ophthalmol. 2015;130(1):1-12.
3. NCBI. (1995). The Electroretinogram: ERG—Webvision—The Organization of the Retina and Visual System. [online]. Available from https://www.ncbi.nlm.nih.gov/books/NBK11554/ [Accessed January, 2019].
4. Wack MA, Peachey NS, Fishman GA. Electroretinographic findings in human oculocutaneous albinism. Ophthalmology. 1989;96(12):1778-85.
5. Wachtmeister L. Oscillatory potentials in the retina: what do they reveal. Prog Retin Eye Res. 1998;17(4):485-521.
6. Bach M, Brigell MG, Hawlina M, et al. ISCEV standard for clinical pattern electroretinography (PERG): 2012 update. Doc Ophthalmol. 2013;126(1):1-7.
7. Tafreshi A, Racette L, Weinreb RN, et al. Pattern electroretinogram and psychophysical tests of visual function for discriminating between healthy and glaucoma eyes. Am J Ophthalmol. 2010;149(3):488-95.
8. Hood DC, Bach M, Brigell M, et al. ISCEV standard for clinical multifocal electroretinography (mfERG) (2011 edition). Doc Ophthalmol. 2012;124(1):1-13.
9. Lai TYY, Chan WM, Lai RY, et al. The clinical applications of multifocal electroretinography: a systematic review. Surv Ophthalmol. 2007;52(1):61-96.
10. Arden GB, Constable PA. The electro-oculogram. Prog Retin Eye Res. 2006;25(2):207-48.

4.6 MULTISPOT LASER SYSTEM

Anusha Sachan, Brijesh Takkar, Amber Bhayana

INTRODUCTION

The laser was first used in ophthalmology by Meyer-Schwickerath.[1] Laser photocoagulation is one of the most commonly performed ocular procedures.[2] It is aimed at the destruction of outer retina, especially photoreceptors which have high oxygen consumption. This results in decreased retinal oxygen demand along with increased diffusion of oxygen from choroid to inner retina, which improves the inner retinal homeostasis. This leads to a decrease in the production of angiogenic factors such vascular endothelial growth factor (VEGF) and platelet-derived growth factor (PDGF) resulting in regression of neovascularization.[3]

Common indications include proliferative diabetic retinopathy, arterial and venous occlusions, and sealing breaks. Multiple types of lasers have been employed for this, including double frequency neodymium-doped yttrium aluminum garnet (Nd:YAG) laser, argon laser, and diode laser. A relatively recently developed platform for quick delivery of laser spots is the multispot laser (MSL), and a commercially available form of the same is the Pattern scanning laser (PASCAL). It was FDA approved in 2005. Systems for scanning beam technology in retinal photocoagulation were first developed at Stanford University by Blumenkranz et al. around 2006. Other similar laser systems are also now available commercially.

MULTISPOT LASER NEODYMIUM-DOPED YTTRIUM ALUMINUM GARNET

It is a semiautomatic device, which delivers ultrashort pulses of double frequency Nd:YAG laser in selected patterns.

With the PASCAL system, a maximum of 56 spots can be delivered together in 0.6 seconds. Each pulse has a duration of 10–20 ms compared with 100–200 ms of conventional laser delivery systems. Space between spots can be varied from 0.25 to 2 spot diameters. The short duration of pulses results in decreased thermal damage to surrounding structures, though laser power required may be higher. Spots can be delivered in different patterns such as square, arc or grid[4] selected by the physician by using control screen (Fig. 4.6.1).[2,4]

Fluence is defined as (power × time)/area. If the spot size remains unchanged with a burn duration of 20 ms as in MSL, the fluence is less than with a 100-ms burn typically delivered with single spot laser. Hence, reduced diffusion of heat and subsequent collateral damage occur. Multiple studies have shown better "qualitative visual aspects" with MSL in comparison to traditional laser systems. Another reason for the same is the inconsistent laser delivery typical of single spot laser systems in real-world situations.

Advantages over conventional single spot systems:

- Decreased duration of the procedure
- Decreased thermal damage
- Increased precision and uniformity (Figs. 4.6.2 to 4.6.4)
- Less pain
- Less scarring (creep phenomenon) and collateral damage
- Customized patterns for different conditions such as the macular laser, laser around holes and breaks.

A major practical utility is the ability to perform PRP for indications like PDR in a single sitting, rather than the traditional technique of 2–3 sittings. Even more useful

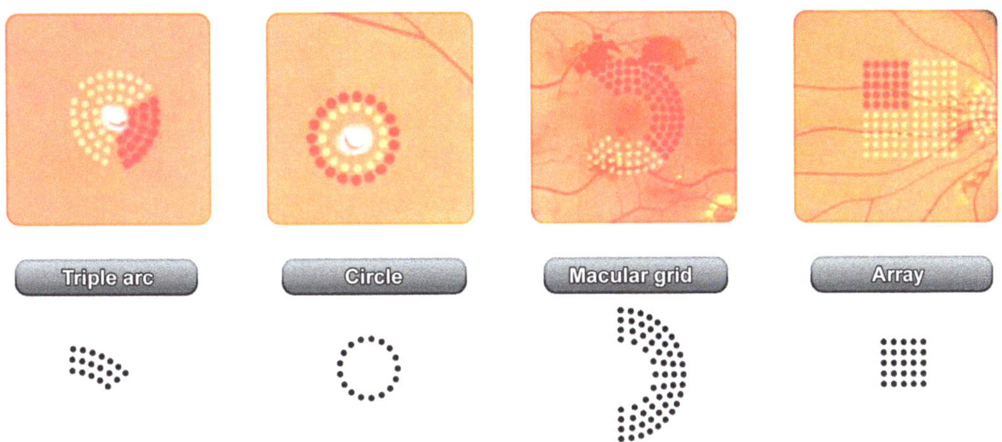

Fig. 4.6.1: Patterns of laser.

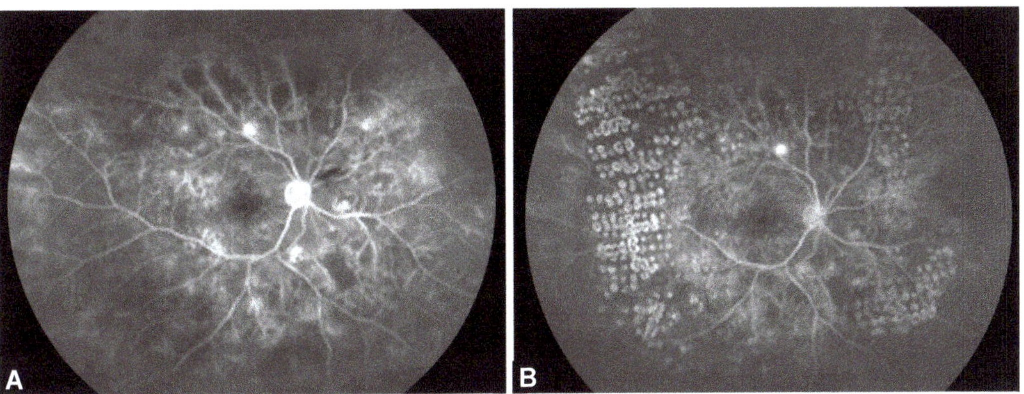

Figs. 4.6.2A and B: (A) A case of PDR; and (B) 3 months after PASCAL laser.

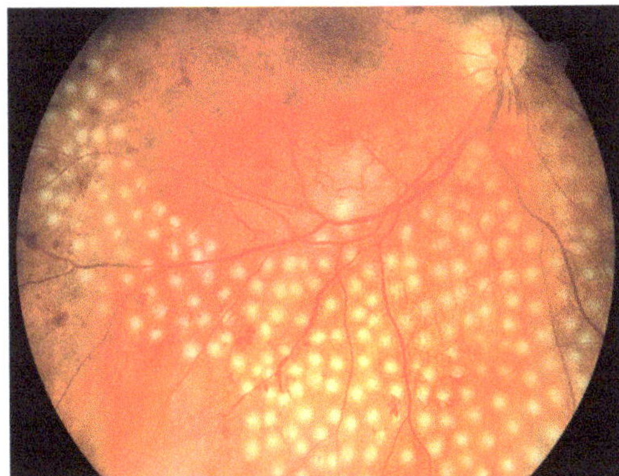

Fig. 4.6.3: Fundus image showing PASCAL laser spots in inferior retina of right eye.

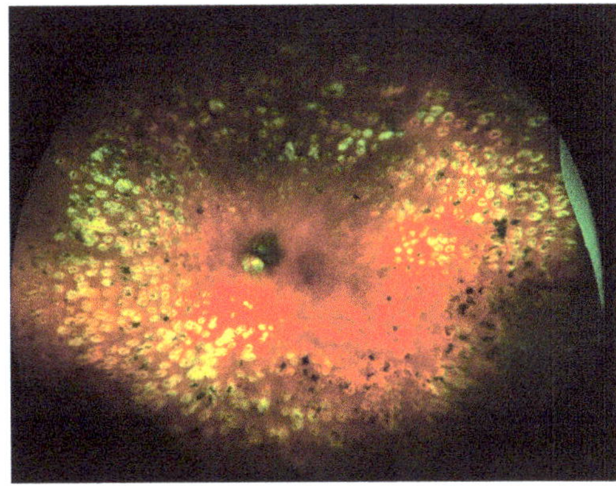

Fig. 4.6.4: Optos image depicting PASCAL laser panretinal photocoagulation in PDR.

may be the use in ROP that is considered a tedious laser, which is anecdotal as of now. A comparison between MSL and conventional systems has been drawn in.

Optical coherence tomography (OCT)-based studies have shown that damage from burns in PASCAL is confined to outer retina. More precisely, maximum damage and healing response are seen at the level of IS/OS junction and apical RPE. Also, burn marks which may not always be visible on fundus biomicroscopy are seen more clearly on FAF as hypofluorescent spots.[5] Newer MSLs offer macular photocoagulation also, along with different color modes. However, the surgeon must titrate the desired laser burn before shooting in continuity as multiple burns will be delivered in a very short interval. Titration may be done with single spots that are also available with the MSL systems.

Examples of MSL available with the PASCAL system:

- *PASCAL 577 nm laser*: Subthreshold 577 nm yellow PASCAL laser has been used to treat DME with excellent results.
- *PASCAL red laser*: Useful when photocoagulation is to be done in the presence vitreous hemorrhage.

PATTERN SCANNING LASER TRABECULOPLASTY

It makes use of 633 nm aiming and 532 or 577 nm therapeutic lasers. A gonioscopic (PSLT gonioscopic lens) lens is used to project a laser pattern on trabecular meshwork. Half or the full length of trabecular meshwork can be treated. It is applied to 180° in 16 steps and 360° in 32 steps respectively.[6] 13 spots are present in each row. Laser power is first titrated by using 10 ms pulse on the inferior segment of the eye to produce a visible blanching reaction. Once appropriate power is selected, using the same power and 5 ms pulse duration does the rest of the treatment. No visible reaction is seen. Studies have shown 20–30% reduction in IOP at a mean follow-up of 1 month.

REFERENCES

1. Meyer-Schwickerath RE, Schott K. Diabetic retinopathy and photocoagulation. Am J Ophthalmol. 1968;66(4):597-603.
2. Salman AG. Pascal laser versus conventional laser for treatment of diabetic retinopathy. Saudi J Ophthalmol. 2011;25(2):175-9.
3. Funatsu H, Hori S, Yamashita H, et al. [Effective mechanisms of laser photocoagulation for neovascularization in diabetic retinopathy]. Nippon Ganka Gakkai Zasshi. 1996;100(5):339-49.
4. TOPCON. (2018). Eye Care: Pattern Scanning Laser PASCAL Series. [online]. Available from https://www.topcon.co.jp/en/eyecare/products/product/surgical/pascal/PASCAL_s_E.html [Accessed January, 2019].
5. Joan W Miller, Szilárd Kiss. The Pattern Scanning Laser (PASCAL®) Photocoagulator for Diabetic Retinopathy. US Ophthalmic Rev. 2011;4(1):94-5.
6. IOVS. (2013). Patterned Laser Trabeculoplasty with PASCAL streamline 577. [online]. Available from http://iovs.arvojournals.org/article.aspx?articleid=2146511 [Accessed January, 2019].

4.7 ADAPTIVE OPTICS

Anusha Sachan, Divya Agarwal, Rohan Chawla

INTRODUCTION

Adaptive optics is a novel technology which compensates for the eye's optical aberrations, allowing exceptional visualization of retinal structures in the eye, including individual photoreceptors, the microvasculature, retinal nerve fiber bundles, the retinal pigment epithelium (RPE), and the lamina cribrosa (LC).[1,2] Junzhong Liang, David Williams, and Donald Miller at the University of Rochester (NY) developed the first adaptive optics (AO) fundus camera, which was able to image individual cones at multiple retinal eccentricities.[2] Retinal imaging modalities depend on the optical elements of the eye mainly the cornea and lens to produce retinal images and are therefore affected by the specific arrangement and curvatural imperfections of these optical elements known as wavefront aberrations. It can be a lower order aberration (defocus, astigmatism) which can be easily managed in imaging devices and higher order aberration (coma, trefoil) which are unstable aberrations and require complex corrections to allow excellent resolution.[3] The highest possible transverse resolution of retinal imaging is affected by the optical properties, which produces wavefront aberrations of the imaging light and degrade the quality of the image. In order to compensate or correct these wavefront aberrations and improve the image quality, a novel technology of adaptive optics has been tried. Initially, it was used for astronomy in the ground-based telescope, but now it has been integrated with many ophthalmic imaging devices like fundus photography, scanning laser ophthalmoscopy (SLO) and optical coherence tomography (OCT) for retinal imaging.[4]

PRINCIPLE

Adaptive optics retinal imaging system consists of three main components:

1. Wavefront sensor (typically Hartmann-Shack aberrometer)
2. Corrective element or adaptive optical element
3. Control system or software system.

A beam of light enters the eye, and a small part of it is reflected back into the optical system of the eye. This reflected beam of light forms a wavefront which is detected by the wavefront sensor. The deformable mirror alters reflected light for optical aberrations based on the measurements of the wavefront sensor. This integration between the sensor and deformable mirror is controlled by the control system, which is a software to process information from the sensor and provide the feedback to the deformable mirror to reduce the optical aberrations of the imaging light and provide good quality of images (Fig. 4.7.1).[1,3] By compensating for the wavefront aberrations of the eye, transverse (lateral) resolution up to 2 μm can be achieved, thereby allowing visualization of the cone mosaic and individual cone photoreceptors.

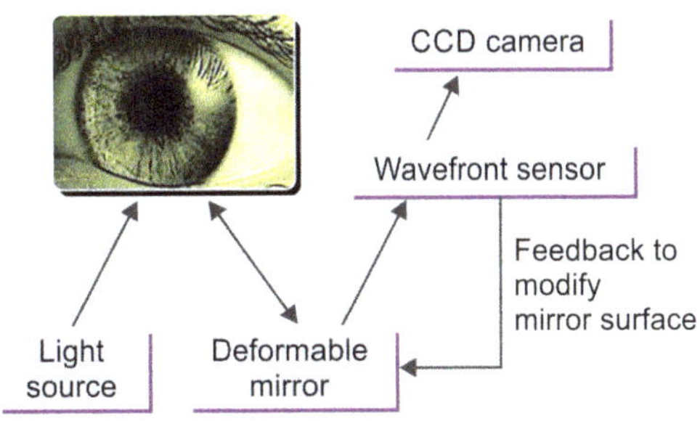

Fig. 4.7.1: Working principle of adaptive optics.

Adaptive optics integrated with optical-retinal imaging modalities provides noninvasive histology of the retinal tissue. It allows in vivo visualization of cone photoreceptors, RPE, red and white blood cells, lamina cribrosa and retinal blood vessels.[4] Imaging of rod photoreceptors is difficult due to its small diameter (less than 2 μm) and reduced wave-guiding properties as compared to cones.[5,6]

ADAPTIVE OPTICS RETINAL IMAGING SYSTEMS

Fundus Camera

- Retina illuminated by krypton arc flash lamp, Xinetics deformable mirror
- Visualize cone mosaic (cone spacing, cone bidirectionality, temporal fluctuations in cone reflectance) and loss of fixation
- Advantage—incoherent light source to reduce speckle, brief imaging exposure
- Disadvantage—effective frame rate slow, images collected one at a time.

Scanning Laser Ophthalmoscopy

- Greatly enhanced image quality through the use of a confocal pinhole to eliminate out-of-focus light.
- Continuous, high resolution, raster scanning at a faster rate than AO fundus camera.
- Eye tracking, laser modulation for stimulus delivery, multichannel imaging, and stabilized stimulus delivery for psychophysics and electrophysiology.
- Advantage—confocality increases the contrast of the final image, axial sectioning of retina and visualization of its various layers like nerve fiber layer, blood vessels, photoreceptors, and RPE.

Optical Coherence Tomography

Three-dimensional (3D) visualization of the nerve fiber layer, ganglion cells, and lamina cribrosa as well as the RPE mosaic and choriocapillaris was demonstrated using high-speed AO-OCT (120,000 scans/second).

INTERPRETATION

Adaptive optics image data from a normal individual is essential for establishing the baseline for the cone characteristics, in order to detect early pathological changes. In one of the AO prototype (rtx1, imagine eye, Orsay, France) 750 nm wavelength light is used to visualize different retinal layers. 850 nm wavelength light source capture sequential images of a 4 × 4 picture with frame rate 9.5 frames/sec (total 40 frames). The final image is formed using image J software and region of interest is analyzed for three main parameters—(1) cone packing density, (2) cone spacing, and (3) Voronoi analysis (to access the regularity of photoreceptors and hexagonal polygons percentage) (Figs. 4.7.2 and 4.7.3).

APPLICATIONS

- Functional adaptive optics imaging—high-speed AO fundus camera and AOSLO can be used to study temporal fluctuation

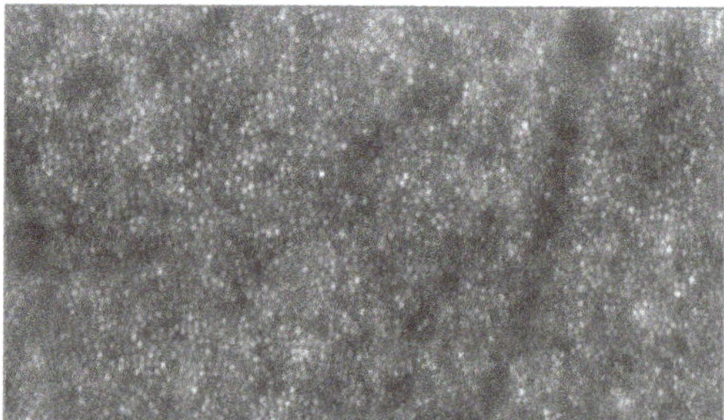

Fig. 4.7.2: White dots correspond to cone photoreceptors.

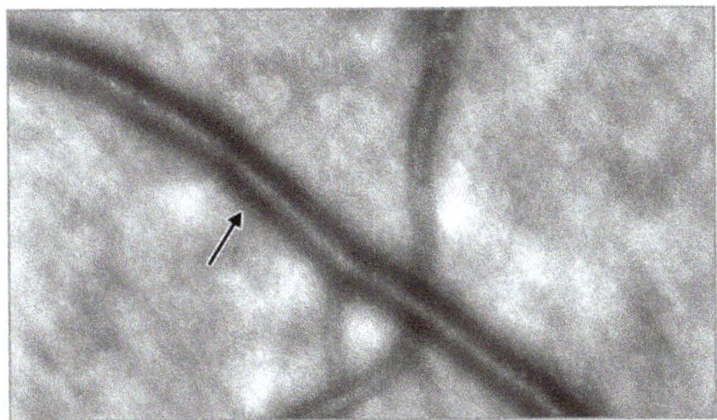

Fig. 4.7.3: The black arrow points to the vessel wall. Lumen is bright as compared to the vessel wall. The defocused retinal nerve fiber layer is in the background.

in cone reflectance. Two hypotheses are there for temporal fluctuations. Firstly, it is caused due to molecular changes within the photoreceptor during transduction; secondly, it is due to changes in the cone outer segment related to disc shedding. AO can be helpful in measuring this reflectance and providing the functional status of the normal and diseased retina. It is used in conditions like opsin mutations, AMN, and closed globe blunt trauma.[7]

- Photoreceptor density and structure in retinal diseases, e.g. Stargardt disease—abnormal cone morphology and packing.
- *To assess the prognosis of disease*: In conditions of achromatopsia, patients with some amount of retained cone structure benefit more from gene therapy than those with a complete absence of cones.
- *Monitoring treatment outcomes*: Talcott et al. tried CNTF encapsulated implants in patients with retinal degenerations and monitoring was done with AOSLO. They concluded that AOSLO provided early information on progression or treatment than conventional modalities.[8]
- *Vascular analysis*: Vascular system gives an insight into the health of the retinal tissue. Diseases like diabetes, hypertension, and dyslipidemia can cause changes in the vessel architecture and lumen size. Preclinical abnormalities can be seen in retinal vasculatures like capillary dropout areas, abnormal AV tortuosity, and subclinical FAZ enlargement.[9]

LIMITATIONS

- Difficult to perform in patients with unstable fixation, dense cataract, and opaque media. Imaging sessions are prolonged and demand excellent subject fixation, as the field of view studied is between 1° and 4°.[2]
- The system is very sensitive to media opacities, higher refractive error, and tear film deficiencies.
- Image processing and analysis are time-consuming processes that lack automated techniques.[2]
- High cost and expertise to interpret the images.

REFERENCES

1. Godara P, Dubis AM, Roorda A, et al. Adaptive optics retinal imaging: emerging clinical applications. Optom Vis Sci Off Publ Am Acad Optom. 2010;87(12):930-41.
2. Retinal Physician. (2016). Adaptive Optics Retinal Imaging: Applications and Clinical Implications. [online]. Available from https://www.retinalphysician.com/issues/2016/may-2016/adaptive-optics-retinal-imaging-applications-and [Accessed January, 2019].
3. Lombardo M, Lombardo G. Wave aberration of human eyes and new descriptors of image optical quality and visual performance. J Cataract Refract Surg. 2010;36(2):313-31.
4. Babcock HW. Adaptive optics revisited. Science. 1990;249(4966):253-7.
5. Lombardo M, Serrao S, Ducoli P, et al. Eccentricity dependent changes of density, spacing and packing arrangement of parafoveal cones. Ophthalmic Physiol Opt. 2013;33(4):516-26.

6. Alpern M, Ching CC, Kitahara K. The directional sensitivity of retinal rods. J Physiol. 1983;343:577-92.
7. Cooper RF, Dubis AM, Pavaskar A, et al. Spatial and temporal variation of rod photoreceptor reflectance in the human retina. Biomed Opt Express. 2011;2(9):2577-89.
8. Talcott KE, Ratnam K, Sundquist SM, et al. Longitudinal study of cone photoreceptors during retinal degeneration and in response to ciliary neurotrophic factor treatment. Invest Ophthalmol Vis Sci. 2011;52(5):2219-26.
9. Lombardo M, Parravano M, Serrao S, et al. Analysis of retinal capillaries in patients with type 1 diabetes and nonproliferative diabetic retinopathy using adaptive optics imaging. Retina. 2013;33(8):1630-9.

4.8 AMSLER GRID

Ankit Singh Tomar, Saurabh Verma, Atul Kumar

INTRODUCTION

In today's ever-changing healthcare environment, the best defense against disease is self-detection and monitoring. Many disease states such as diabetes and age-related macular degeneration can have long-term effects on the eyesight. Early detection of deteriorating vision is key to preventing permanent vision damage.

Marc Amsler, a Swiss ophthalmologist in 1945, developed Amsler grid. It evaluates the 20° of the visual field centered on fixation. It is principally useful in screening for and monitoring macular disease, but will also demonstrate central visual field defects originating elsewhere. Patients with a substantial risk of choroidal neovascularization (CNV) should be provided with an Amsler grid for regular use at home.

TECHNIQUE

The pupils should be undilated, and slit-lamp examination should be avoided in order to avoid the photo-stress effect on the eyes. A presbyopic refractive correction should be worn if appropriate. The chart should be well illuminated and held at a comfortable reading distance, optimally around 33 cm.[1]

The following steps are followed:

- One eye is covered.
- The patient is asked to look directly at the central dot with the uncovered eye, to keep looking at this, and to report any distortion, broken lines, blurred area, dark area or waviness of the lines on the grid.
- Remind the patient to maintain fixation on the central dot.
- The patient may be provided with a recording sheet and pen and asked to draw any anomalies.[2]

TYPES

There are seven charts, each consisting of a 10 cm outer square. The charts and the relevant points are described in Table 4.8.1.

Table 4.8.1: Types of Amsler charts and their salient features.[1]

Charts	*Characteristics*
Chart 1	I. Most often used chart II. It consists of a high contrast white grid on a black background III. The outer grid enclosing 400 smaller 5 mm squares IV. When viewed at about one-third of a meter, each small square subtends an angle of 1° V. Absolute scotoma appears as not seen at all or black area VI. Relative scotoma appears as blur
Chart 2	I. Similar to chart 1 but has diagonal lines that aid fixation for patients with a central scotoma II. If the patient still is unable to achieve or maintain fixation, a larger white central spot may be applied to center of the grid
Chart 3	I. Similar to chart 1 but has red squares II. Red-on-black design stimulates the long wavelength foveal cones III. Useful to detect subtle color scotoma and desaturation in cases such as: toxic maculopathy, nutritional amblyopia, optic neuropathy and optic tract lesions IV. Can be used to detect patients with functional vision loss in conjunction with red green glasses (grid will not be seen when viewed through green lens)
Chart 4	I. It has only white random dots distributed like stars in sky II. It is useful in differentiating scotoma from metamorphopsia (no form to be distorted)
Chart 5	I. It has horizontal lines and is useful in detecting metamorphopsia along specific meridians II. It can be rotated to any meridian to check for irregularities in a particular area III. It is of particular use in the evaluation of patients describing difficulty reading
Chart 6	I. Similar to chart 5 but has a white background and the central lines 1° above and below fixation point are closer together II. Enables evaluation that is more detailed
Chart 7	I. It has a fine central grid of area 6° × 8° in the central area II. Each square subtends an angle of a half-degree III. It is highly sensitive to early macular diseases and mild visual disturbance

INTERPRETATION

Questions asked of the patient: A set of question, as given in Table 4.8.2, is asked to the patient to interpret the results.

Uses: The various clinical conditions and their interpretations are given in Table 4.8.3. Amsler chart is extremely helpful in following diseases:[3]

- Dry age-related macular degeneration (AMD)
- Diabetic retinopathy (DR)
- Macular degenerations
- Epiretinal membrane (ERM) and other vitreomacular traction disorders
- Macular hole
- Toxic maculopathy
- Optic neuropathy[3]
- Chiasmal lesion.

VIVA QUESTIONS

1. What part of the visual field is evaluated by Amsler grid?

Ans. 20°

2. What are the indications of using the Amsler grid?

Ans. Refer to text.

3. How many types of Amsler grid are there?

Ans. Seven types (Figs. 4.8.1 to 4.8.7).

Table 4.8.2: Questions asked to the patient while interpreting Amsler chart.

1.	Can you see the central dot?	To rule out central scotoma.
2.	While looking at the central dot, can you see all four quadrants of chart simultaneously?	To rule out arcuate, altitudinal, quadrantic or hemianopic field defect as well as field constrictions
3.	Does the grid appear to have any missing or distorted area?	To rule out paracentral, cecocentral or altitudinal scotomas
4.	Any area of grid having an unusual appearance (lines appear wavy)?	To rule out metamorphopsia
5.	Any square shimmering or colored?	To rule out scintillating scotomas

Table 4.8.3: Clinical conditions and their impact on Amsler chart interpretation.

Type of disease	*Character*	*Example*
Progressive disease	Which develop significant alterations over time	Toxic maculopathy/atypical RP
Active disease	May improve or worsen in short span of time	Optic neuritis or macular neuroretinopathy
Recurrent disease	Already suffering vision loss but at a risk of reactivation of disease process	Central serous choroidopathy, toxoplasma retinochoroiditis

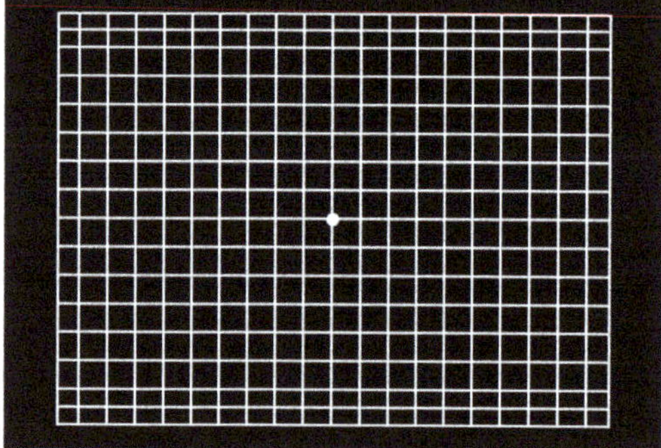

Fig. 4.8.1: Chart 1.

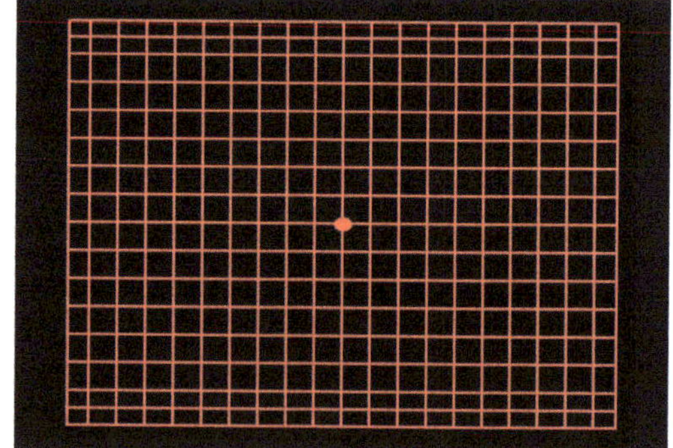

Fig. 4.8.3: Chart 3.

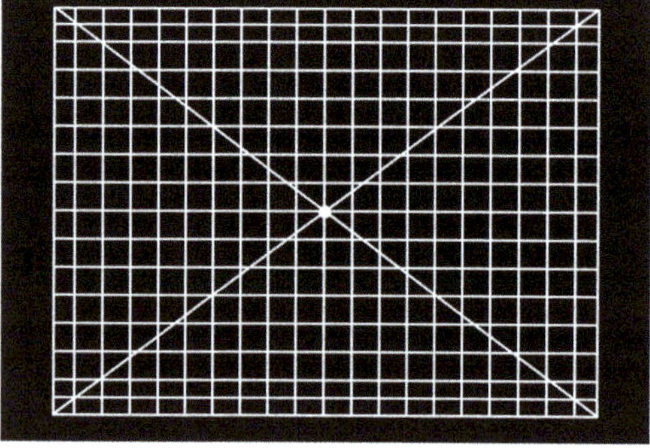

Fig. 4.8.2: Chart 2.

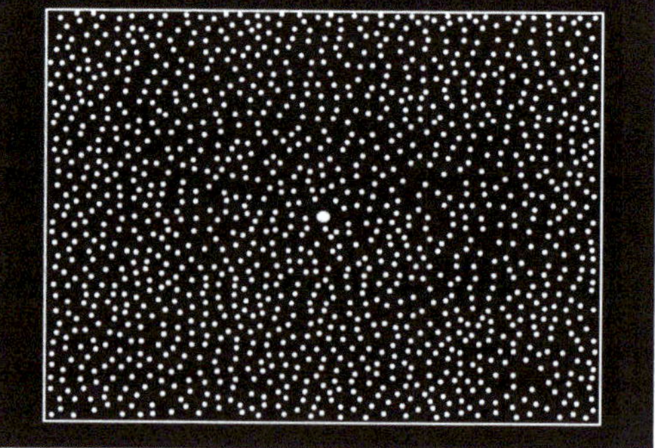

Fig. 4.8.4: Chart 4.

Fig. 4.8.5: Chart 5.

Fig. 4.8.6: Chart 6.

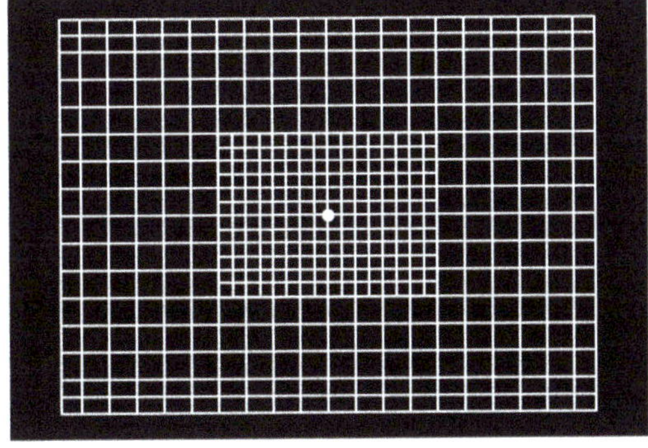

Fig. 4.8.7: Chart 7.

4. What instructions need to be given to the patients?

Ans. Refer to text.

REFERENCES

1. Mattice E, Wolfe CP. Using the Amsler grid. J Ophthalmic Nurs Technol. 1986;5(1):34.
2. Lederman ME. Demonstration of scotoma on an Amsler grid examination. Am J Ophthalmol. 1985;100(5):740.
3. Easterbrook M. The sensitivity of Amsler grid testing in early chloroquine retinopathy. Trans Ophthalmol Soc UK. 1985;104 (Pt 2):204-7.

4.9 VITREORETINAL INSTRUMENTS

Devesh Kumawat, Pranita Sahay, Anusha Sachan, Atul Kumar

TROCAR AND CANNULA

- Trocars (Fig. 4.9.1) are used to make pars plana sclerotomy entries. Trocar needle can be 20 G/23 G/25 G/27 G.
- Microcannulas made up of polyimide and are already loaded over the needle trocars.

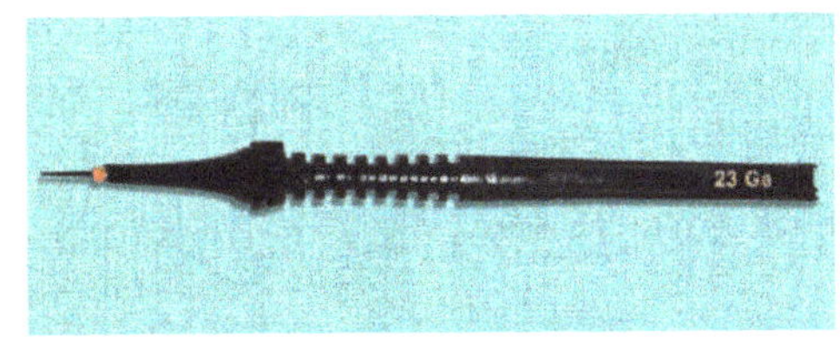

Fig. 4.9.1: Trocar.

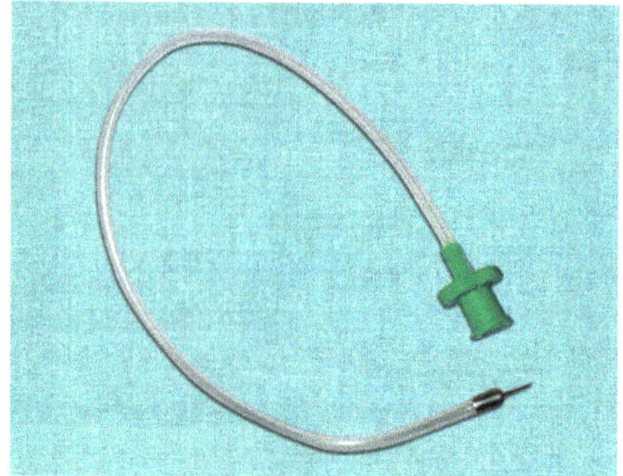

Fig. 4.9.2: Infusion cannula.

- Microcannula can be valved or nonvalved.
- Plugs usage and instrument exchanges for its removal and placement are eliminated in valved cannulas.
- Trocar needle, microcannula, and trocar handle together constitute the trocar/ cannula assembly. This system helps in instrument access from outside within eye without any obstruction and maintains entry hole between conjunctiva and sclera aligned.

INFUSION CANNULA

Self-retaining infusion cannulas (Fig. 4.9.2) of different sizes according to microcannula (20 G/23 G/25 G/27 G) are used to introduce irrigating solution into the vitreous cavity.

VITRECTOMY CUTTER

- Vitreous cutters (Fig. 4.9.3) utilize suction and inclusive shearing force to cut vitreous.
- These can be of two broad types:
  1. Electrodynamic cutters are heavy and become hot on prolonged use. It can cause fatigue and aggravate tremors.
  2. Pneumatic cutters are lighter than the electrodynamic cutters and so they cause fewer tremors. They are cheaper and of higher efficiency.

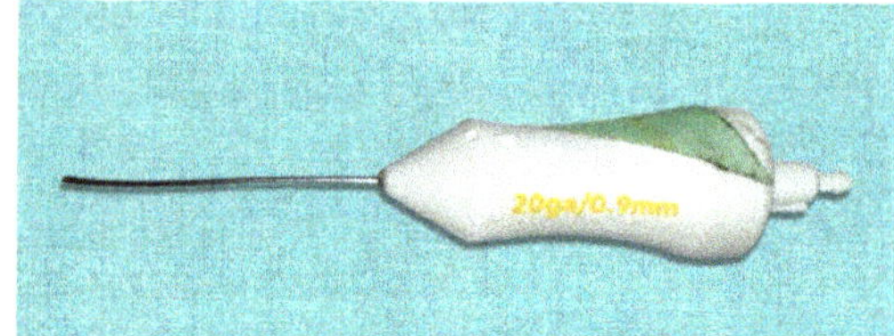

Fig. 4.9.3: Vitrectomy cutter.

- Vitrectomy cutters are of three types based on the cutting mechanism:
  1. Cutters using rotating mechanism.
  2. *Cutter using oscillating mechanism or Peyman type*: This type of cutter is more efficient and superior than rotating cutter as it produces less shearing effect on retina.
  3. *The Guillotine type cutters*: Most frequently used vitrectomy cutter. It has an outer tube which has an opening through which vitreous is aspirated. The inner tube slides across the port thus cutting the vitreous with minimal traction over retina.
- *Vitrectomy mode*: A standard high-speed vitrectomy cutter has a cutting frequency of up to 5,000 cpm and can be increased up to 7,500. High-speed cutting reduces traction on retina hence increases stability while cutting vitreous close to the retina. The vitrectomy machine supports both pneumatic and electric drive for pneumatic and electric vitrectomies when needed. It should be used in a single cut, fixed, and linear cutting control. Horizontal cutting probes have a new concept of radial reciprocating action which minimizes the traction, turbulence or fluttering of tissues (cutting blade moves from left to right across the port). Latest vitrectomy machine by Alcon "the Constellation" can cut vitreous up to a frequency of 7,000 cpm. Three different

vitrectomy modes exists in the machine, i.e. proportional vacuum, 3D (dual dynamic drive), and momentary mode. Usually proportional vacuum mode vitrectomy is done.

- *3D technology*: This allows the surgeon to change the parameters of cut rate and vacuum simultaneously as needed throughout the surgery. Vacuum can be set to start at low level and rise to max at full foot pedal depression while cutting rate can be set to start at its max setting and decreased with foot pedal is depression. It allows more cutting of vitreous while doing core vitrectomy and fine cutting without much traction when cutting near the retinal surface.

END GRASPING FORCEPS

- These forceps have jaws at the tip to hold tissues at the edge only (Fig. 4.9.4).
- The tips are fine and allow visualization of the tissue while grasping.
- These are used for epiretinal membrane peeling.

INTERNAL LIMITING MEMBRANE FORCEPS

- These have fine tips with smaller jaws which help in picking up of delicate tissues like internal limiting membrane (ILM) (Fig. 4.9.5).
- These are used for ILM peeling in macular hole surgery.

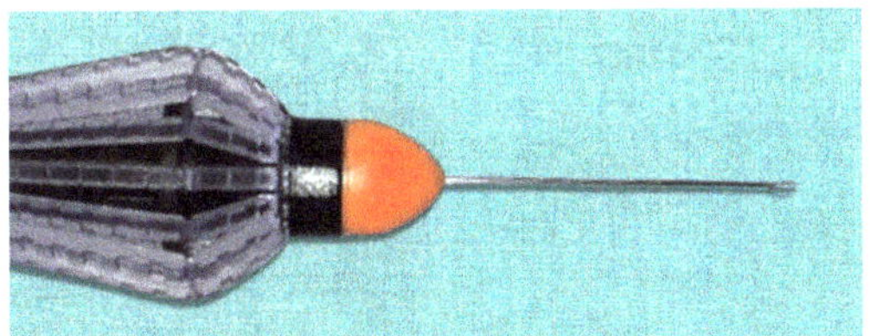

Fig. 4.9.4: End grasping forceps.

SERRATED FORCEPS

- These have large flat grasping blades without jaws (Fig. 4.9.6), which help in strong grip over tissues while managing proliferative vitreoretinopathy.
- These are used in tough epiretinal membrane peeling and retinal pucker release.

FOREIGN BODY FORCEPS

- These are large gauge forceps with serrated or diamond dusted tips for removal of intraocular foreign bodies (Fig. 4.9.7).
- These have stout jaws which help in the firm holding of the foreign body.

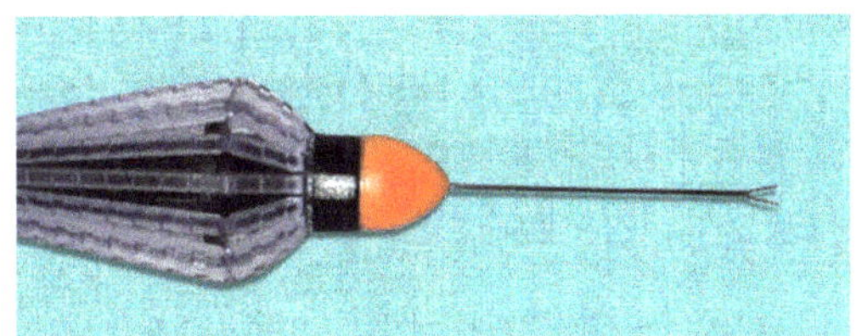

Fig. 4.9.5: Internal limiting membrane (ILM) forceps.

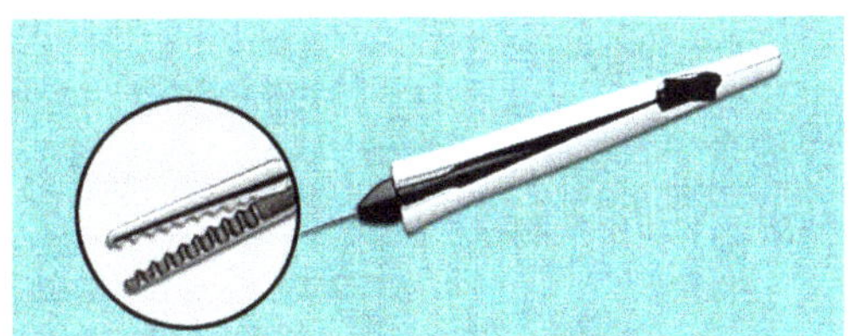

Fig. 4.9.6: Serrated forceps.

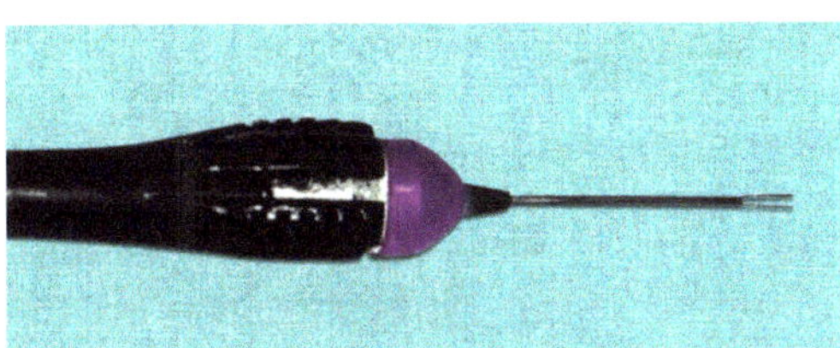

Fig. 4.9.7: Foreign body forceps.

EXTRUSION INSTRUMENTS

- *Charles flute needle*: It consists of a blunt needle attached to a detachable handle (Fig. 4.9.8).
  - It is used for controlled passive extrusion of fluid during internal drainage of subretinal fluid, removal of preretinal blood, and fluid-air exchange.
  - The internal channel leads to an exit port on the side of the handle. Egress of fluid occurs when cannula tip is in fluid, and exit port is open, driven by infusion pressure which is above the atmospheric pressure.
  - The blunt tip can be replaced with a soft silicone tip needle as well with decreased risk of iatrogenic retinal damage.
- *Backflush* (Fig. 4.9.9) is a modified flute handle with large silicone reservoir. Pressure on this reservoir leads to retrograde flushing of the fluid or accidentally aspirated/incarcerated tissues. It can also be used to disperse sedimented preretinal bleed. It can be used with either blunt or soft tip needle.

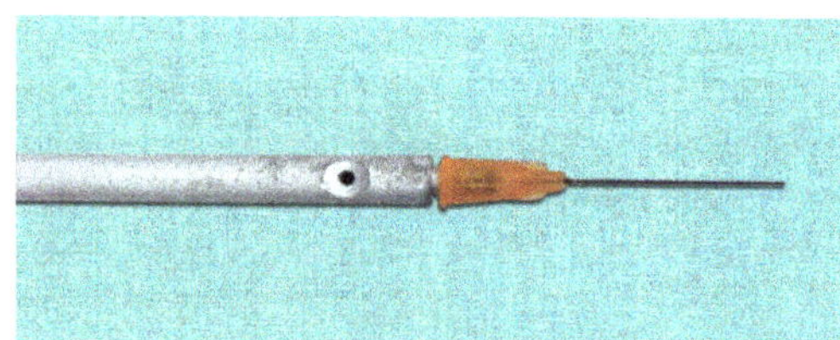

Fig. 4.9.8: Charles flute needle.

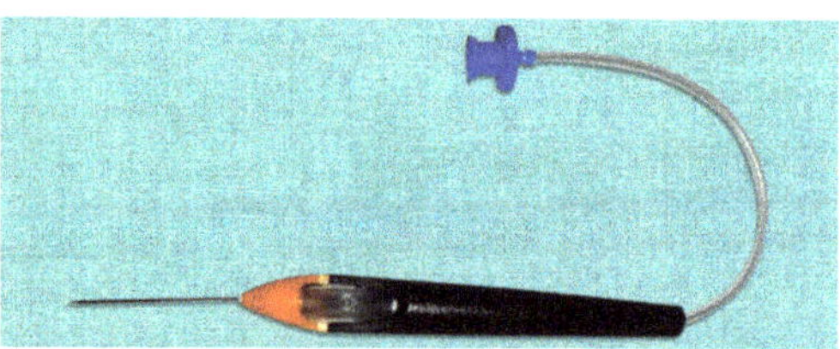

Fig. 4.9.9: Backflush.

CANNULA

Cannula tips can be of several types:

- *Silicone brush tip cannula*: It has a soft silicon brush tip (Fig. 4.9.10), which is used for gentle brushing and manipulation of the retina. These are excellent for removing blood from the retina surface.
- *Diamond dusted soft silicone tip cannula*: These are used for the removal of triamcinolone particles from the retinal surface.
- *Charles flute cannula:* Smooth, finished tip provides atraumatic entry, reduces the risk of trauma to surrounding tissue, and help to aspirate blood and debris.
- *Soft silicone tip cannula*: The soft, flexible tip on the cannula provides nontraumatic entry through retinal or macular tears or holes. These are used for fluid-fluid or fluid-air exchange in vitrectomy surgery.
- *Dual bore cannula*: Simultaneous infusion of heavy liquids like perfluorocarbon liquid (PFCL) and aspiration of intraocular fluids with dual-bore cannula helps to control and maintain a constant intraocular pressure (IOP) during the procedure.

The cannula can be connected to flute handle or backflush handle or active extrusion handle.

DIAMOND-DUSTED MEMBRANE SCRAPER

Tano diamond-dusted membrane scraper (DDMS) (Fig. 4.9.11) helps to find the edge

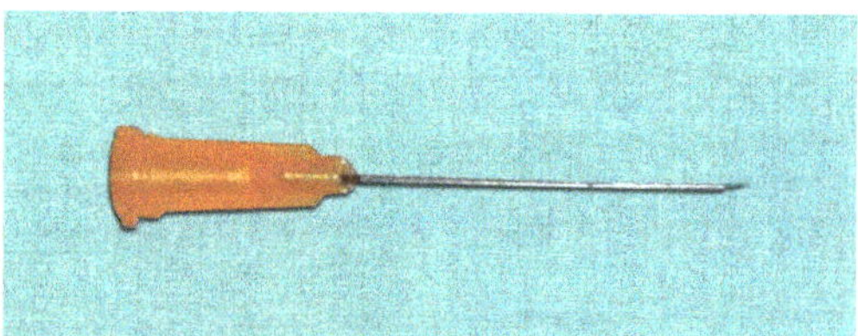

Fig. 4.9.10: Soft silicone tip cannula.

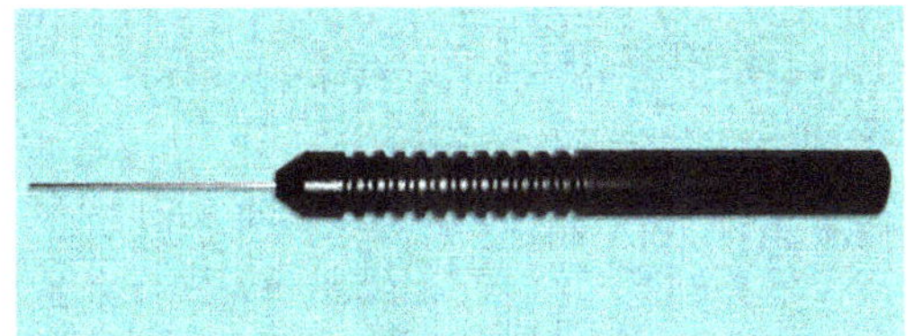

Fig. 4.9.11: Diamond-dusted membrane scraper (DDMS).

of the epiretinal membranes. It is made of tongue-shaped soft silicone with inert diamond dust. It is very helpful in ILM and epiretinal membrane removal; the diamond dusted soft silicone tip is grazed over the retinal surface to find the edge of membrane. The edge is then grasped with the ILM forceps to complete the membrane removal.

VITREORETINAL SCISSORS (FIG. 4.9.12)

- *Horizontal scissors* are used for delamination during epiretinal membrane removal. Their cutting edge moves conformal to the retinal surface. Their blades can have a gentle curve or can be straight, with an angle of 30° or 45° to the shaft.
- *Vertical scissors* have vertical blades with pointed tips that move along the axis of the shaft. Proximal blade moves down toward the fixed distal blade to cut the tissue vertically. These are used for epiretinal membrane segmentation.

GASS RETINAL DETACHMENT HOOK

Used for localization of retinal breaks onto the sclera in retinal detachment surgery (Fig. 4.9.13).

MAGNETS

These are used to remove magnetic intraocular foreign bodies (Fig. 4.9.14).

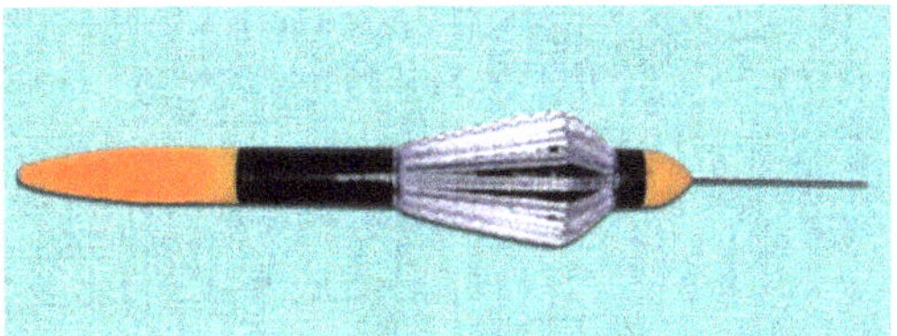

Fig. 4.9.12: Vitreoretinal scissors.

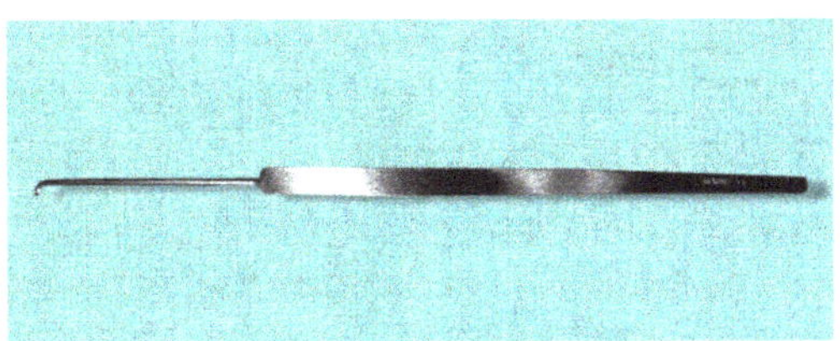

Fig. 4.9.13: Gass retinal detachment hook.

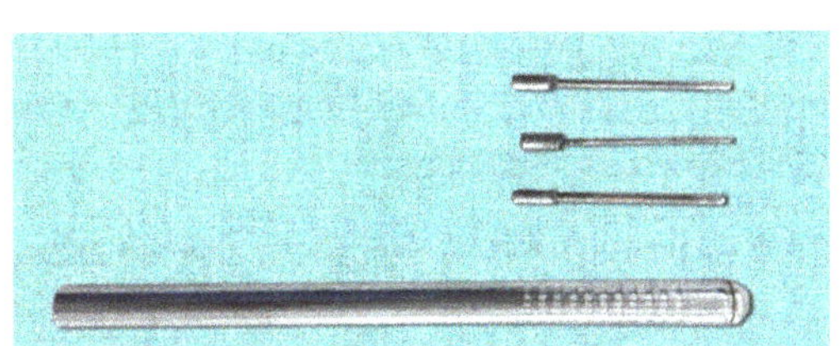

Fig. 4.9.14: Magnets.

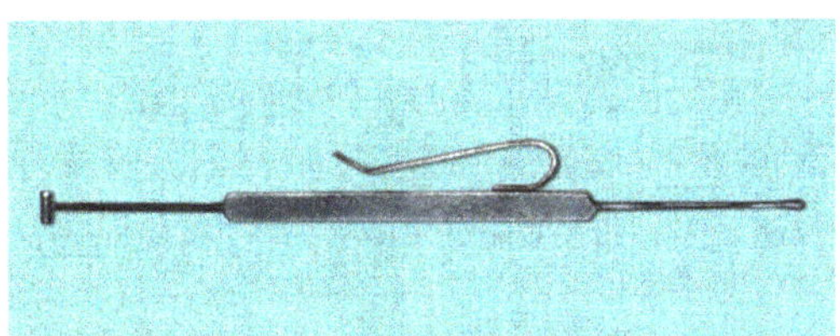

Fig. 4.9.15: Schocket scleral depressor.

Electromagnets are more powerful than rare earth magnets (REMs) and their magnetic force can be varied, but they are used only as external magnets. REMs are available for both intraocular and extraocular use.

SCHOCKET SCLERAL DEPRESSOR

It has a rounded end used for depressing sclera and curved marking end for indenting posteriorly by reaching behind the globe (Fig. 4.9.15).

Table 4.9.1: Dimension, color coding, and inventor of various trocar cannula.

Trocar cannula	*Dimension (outer diameter in mm)*	*Color*	*Scientist*
17	2.3		
19	1.1		
20	0.9	Yellow	O'Malley and Heintz
23	0.7	Orange	Eckardt
25	0.5	Blue-green	Fujji
27	0.4	Purple	Oshima

VIVA QUESTIONS

1. What is the full form of MIVS?

Ans. Microincision vitrectomy surgery (MIVS) [initially known as transconjunctival sutureless vitrectomy (TSV)].

2. What is the dimension, color coding, and inventor of various trocar cannula?

Ans. Refer to Table 4.9.1.

3. Who is the father of vitreoretinal surgery?

Ans. Robert Machemer in 1971 did first 17 G single port closed pars plana vitrectomy in an egg by making a small opening in egg shell to remove its albumin.

4. What are the advantages of MIVS?

Ans. Following are the advantages of MIVS:

- Beveled incisions made with the help of these instruments are sutureless or require only a single 7-0 Vicryl suture to close.
- Prevent herniation of retina and vitreous from port site.
- Less chances of port site dialysis or retinal detachment.
- Enhanced postoperative comfort and reduces healing time.
- Port being closer to the distal tip of the vitrectomy cutter in smaller gauge system enhances the ability to go close to the retina (0.23 mm in 25 G cutters and 0.43 in 20 G cutters).
- Small cutters can be easily navigated through the gaps between the fibrovascular membranes and to create cleavage planes for easy dissection.

5. What are the disadvantages of MIVS?

Ans. Following are the disadvantages of MIVS:

- *Intraoperative*: Increased surgical time (due to the reduction in flow and aspiration), IOP rise, cannula retraction, retinal break formation, hypotony, jamming of vitrectomy cutters, and breakage of cutter or microcannula.
- *Postoperative*: Postoperative hypotony and endophthalmitis.

6. Use of 41 G instrument system.

Ans. It is a 0.1 mm diameter port cannula system, which is used to create small retinotomy to create perimacular subretinal blebs for submacular surgeries and in introducing tissue plasminogen activator (tPA) in patients with submacular bleed. These retinotomies do not require laser delimitation.

7. The benefit of valved small gauge cannulas.

Ans. Valved cannulas help to reduce the turbulence and IOP variation in the vitreous cavity during insertion and removal of instruments through the ports during surgery.

8. How to reduce the malleability of 25 G instruments?

Ans. As we are heading towards the smaller gauge instrument systems, reducing the thickness of the probe reduces its stiffness, which results in bending and difficulty to direct the instrument in the required direction. Addition of a stiffening sleeve is done to small gauge instruments to reduce its malleability to promote good maneuverability.

9. What is bimanual vitreoretinal surgery?

Ans. When vitrectomy is done under chandelier light then it is called bimanual vitreoretinal surgery. It provides a good opportunity to the surgeon to use his both hands to dissect membranes with minimal damage in cases like diabetic retinopathy.

10. What is digitally-assisted-vitreoretinal surgery (DAVS)?

Ans. It is a novel concept of Novartis "NGENUITY" 3 D visualization system, a platform for DAVS (Fig. 4.9.16). It allows the surgeon to operate looking at a high definition 3 D screen, instead of bending their necks to look through the eyepiece of the microscope (heads-up viewing system). This microscope free design is engineered to improve the surgeon's posture and help to reduce the fatigue during the surgery.

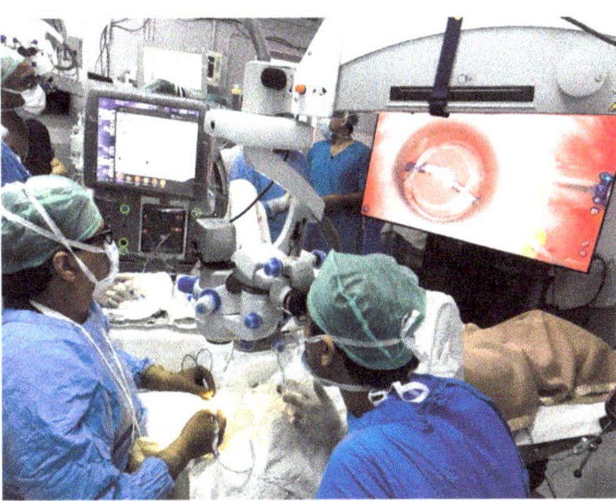

Fig. 4.9.16: "NGENUITY" 3 D visualization system.

11. What are the various modes of vitrectomy?

Ans. These are:

- Momentary
- 3 D
- Proportional.

12. What is the duty cycle in vitrectomy?

Ans. The duty cycle of a vitrectomy probe is the percentage of time the port is open measured against the entire cycle of the cutter.

13. What are the various steps of a diabetic vitrectomy surgery?

Ans. The following are the critical maneuvers while doing a diabetic vitrectomy:

- *Segmentation*: Vertical cutting of epiretinal membranes into smaller segments to release circumferential traction.
- *Delamination*: Finding the correct plane and horizontal cutting of individual neovascular frond from the retinal surface.
- *En-bloc*: Enables complete removal of all the fibrovascular tissue over the retinal surface. A small window is created in partially detached posterior hyaloid such that horizontally cutting scissor can create a plane between the epiretinal membranes and underlying retina.

14. What is the speed of vitrectomy cutters?

Ans. 750–7,500 cpm.

15. What is interface vitrectomy?

Ans. It describes the use of vitreous cutters, scissors, forceps, and other instruments at the interface between silicon oil, air, or PFCL and residual vitreous, epiretinal membrane, and retina.

5 CHAPTER Glaucoma

5.1 GONIOSCOPY

Talvir Sidhu, Abhipsa Sharma, Tanuj Dada

INTRODUCTION

The term "gonioscopy" is derived from the Greek words go-'ne- (angle) and ŏs'k - pe - (view). It is a clinical biomicroscopic technique of examining the angle of the anterior chamber of the eye with the use of a special contact lens known as the gonioscope.

Alexios Tarantas first viewed the angle in a living keratoglobus eye during indentation by finger when trying to view the ciliary body. He coined the term gonioscopy and viewed the anterior chamber angle by indenting the limbus and using high plus lenses. Maximilian Salzmann is rightly called "*the father of gonioscopy*" as he recognized total internal inflection and introduced the goniolens and described angle pathology in detail.

PRINCIPLE OF GONIOSCOPY

The anterior chamber angle situated at the attachment of iris-ciliary body complex to the sclera-corneal junction is called the irido-corneal angle. The angle structures are not visible due to *total internal reflection* of the light originating from angle at the corneal surface. *Total internal reflection* is an optical phenomenon that occurs when a ray of light traveling from denser to rarer medium (such as cornea to air) strikes the interface between two media at an angle larger than the "critical angle" for that pair of media. In this situation the light beam is completely reflected back to the denser medium. The critical angle for cornea-air interface is 46° (Fig. 5.1.1). Hence, the light coming from angle structures strikes the cornea at an angle higher than the critical angle gets reflected internally. When a goniolens is applied over the cornea, the cornea-air interface is obliterated and the light is able to exit the eye and gets reflected from the gonio mirror and angle structures become visible (Fig. 5.1.2).

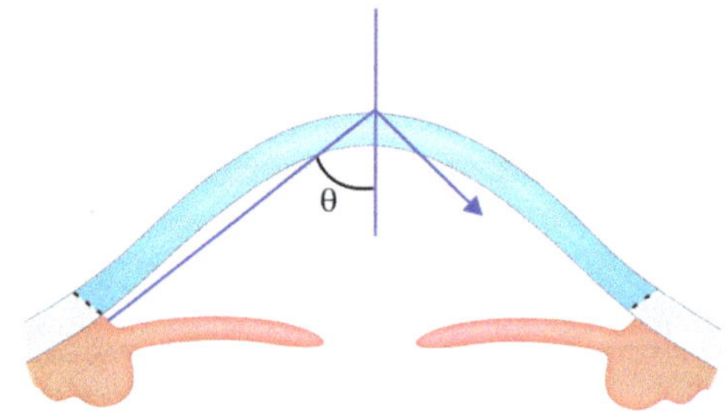

Fig. 5.1.1: Total internal reflection occurs at the cornea-air interface for light traveling from angle due to angle more than critical angle.

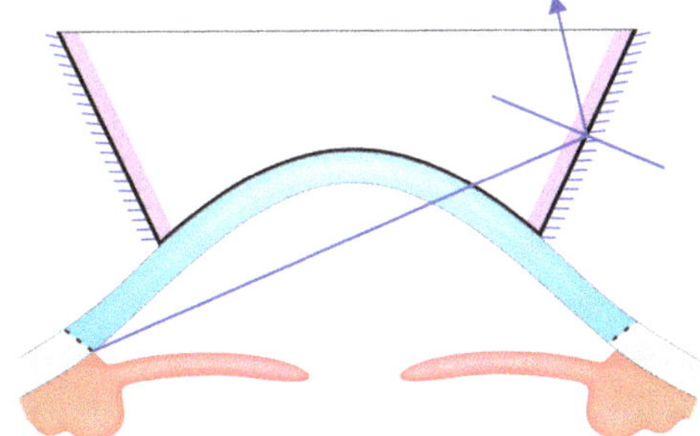

Fig. 5.1.2: A goniolens obliterates the cornea-air interface and light coming from angle can be seen as reflected from gonio mirror.

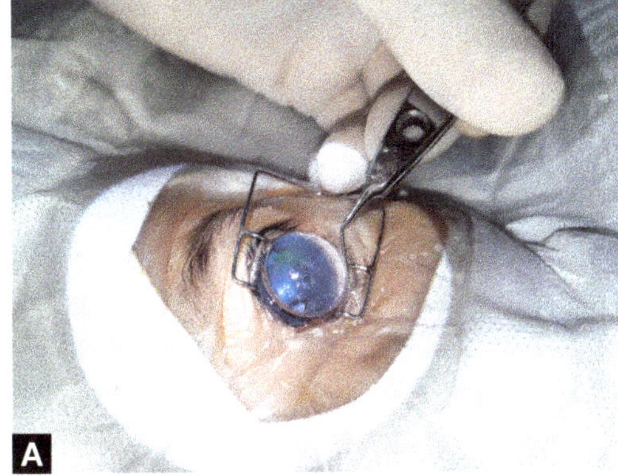

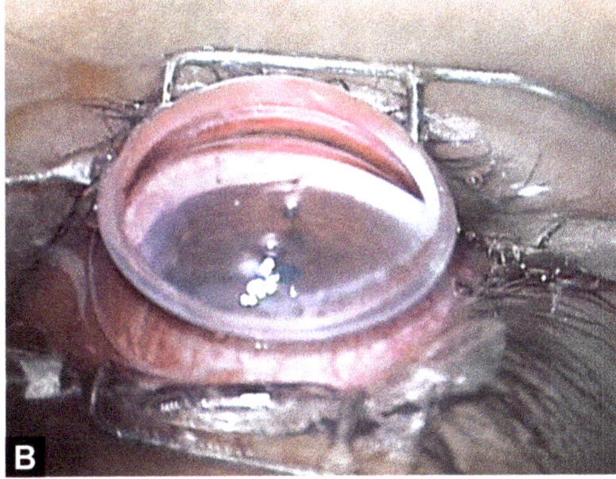

Figs. 5.1.3A and B: Koeppe's lens—dome-shaped lens placed over eye for direct gonioscopy.

INDICATIONS OF GONIOSCOPY

- To identify open versus closed angle
- To assess for risk of angle closure by identifying iris apposition to trabecular meshwork (TM)
- To grade angle closure and distinguish between apposition and synechiae
- To identify angle pathologies like abnormal angle pigmentation, angle recession, foreign body in angle, developmental anomalies, neovascularization of angle, and grade them
- Post-trabeculectomy patency of fistula/ scleral opening
- Laser procedures like selective laser trabeculoplasty (SLT)/argon laser trabeculoplasty (ALT)
- Intraoperatively to insert minimally invasive glaucoma surgery (MIGS) like iStent or perform surgery like goniosynechiolysis.

TYPES OF GONIOLENSES

Direct Goniolenses

A steeply convex domed lens obliterates the total internal reflection and allows the angle visualization. It is placed over the eye with patient lying in supine position for direct visualization of the angle by a hand-held slit lamp or operating microscope. They are mostly used for surgical procedures or examination under anesthesia in children or in bed ridden patients.

Examples: Koeppe lens (+50 D lens made of barium crown glass or plastic; prototype direct goniolens) (Figs. 5.1.3A and B); Richardson-Shaffer (Small Koeppe lens for infants); Swan-Jacob (Surgical goniolens for children) (Figs. 5.1.4A and B); Hoskins-Barkan (Prototype surgical lens); Thorpe (Surgical and diagnostic lens); Worst lens (Surgical goniolens for children).

Indirect Goniolenses

A corneal contact lens with mirrors is used to reflect the light coming from angle to obtain an inverted angle image. The lenses may have a large-sized corneal contact well which fit onto the sclera—*the scleral*

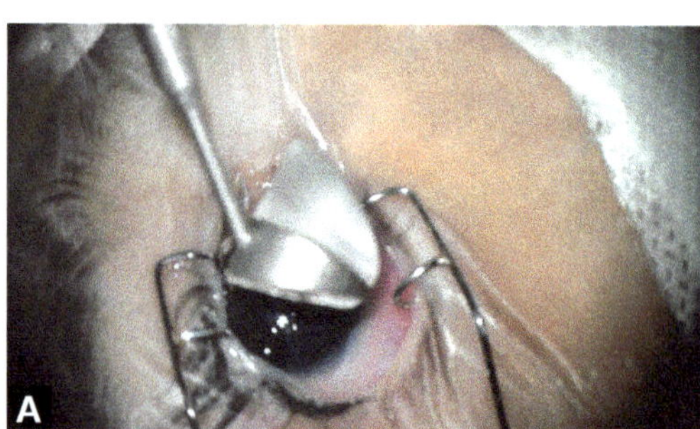

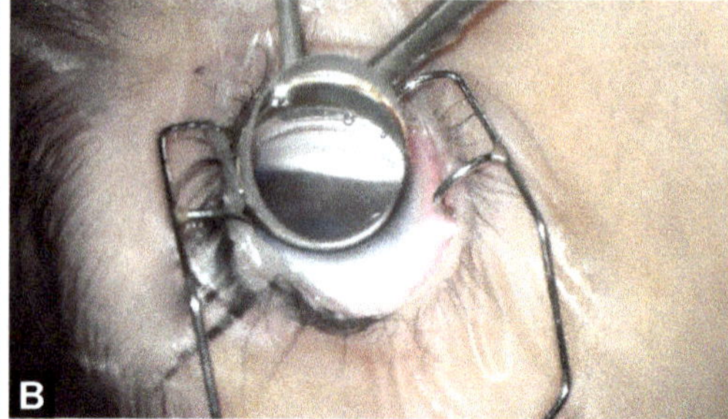

Figs. 5.1.4A and B: Swan Jacob lens used intraoperatively to see the angle.

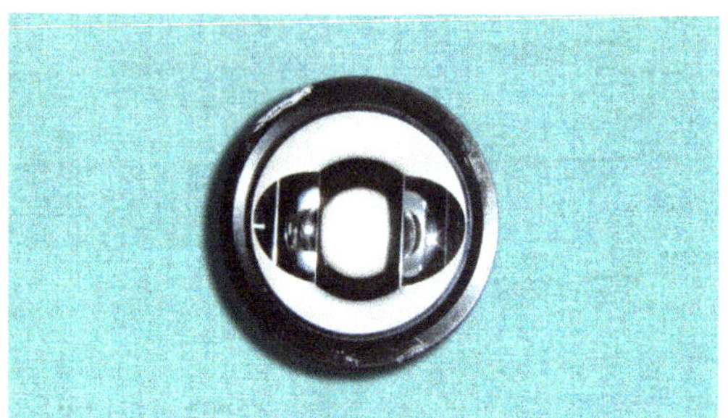

Fig. 5.1.5: Goldmann 2 mirror lens.

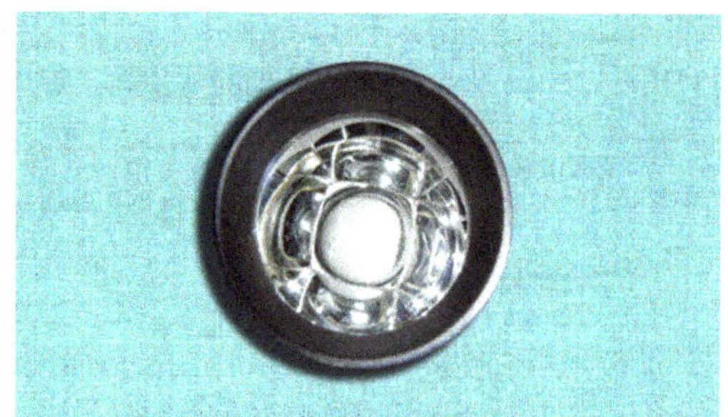

Fig. 5.1.6: Zeiss 4 mirror lens.

type lenses, e.g. Goldmann 1/2/3 mirror lens (Fig. 5.1.5) or a smaller lens contact surface which gently rests over the cornea—*the corneal type lenses*, e.g. Zeiss/Posner 4 mirror lenses (Fig. 5.1.6).

The scleral type contact lenses have a large area of contact with eye and they fit over the sclera adjacent to the limbus. They are used for *manipulation gonioscopy* in case of closed angle due to convexity of iris, where the patient is asked to look towards the mirror the observer is viewing to open the angle being viewed. Manipulation helps to visualize the angle structures hidden behind a convex iris by allowing used to get an "over the hill" view. If too much pressure is applied, they falsely close the angle because the pressure directly goes to the limbus and folds may be visible at the limbal area in gonioscope mirror. Their curvature is steeper than the cornea, therefore a coupling fluid like methyl cellulose is required to obliterate the space left between contact lens and cornea while using a two mirror gonioscope.

The corneal type goniolens have a contact lens curvature similar to cornea and therefore they do not need coupling fluid. The well diameter is smaller than cornea therefore the contact lens rests on the cornea. Any pressure applied while doing gonioscopy leads to displacement of fluid into the angle, falsely opening the angle. These lenses are used for *indentation gonioscopy*, where pressure is applied with a corneal type goniolens to push the aqueous into the angle in a convex iris to visualize the angle structures. Indentation gonioscopy can help to differentiate between appositional and synechial angle closure. Sometimes indentation gonioscopy is also used to abort the acute angle closure attack by pushing fluid into the angle as a therapeutic procedure (only in expert hands).

ADVANTAGES AND DISADVANTAGES OF DIRECT AND INDIRECT GONIOSCOPY (MANIPULATION AND INDENTATION)

Direct gonioscopy
- Erect and panoramic view
- Minimal distortion of chamber and angle
- Both eyes can be visualized simultaneously
- Less magnification

Manipulation gonioscopy
- Small learning curve
- Details are better visible
- Excellent for documentation and imaging
- Coupling fluid needed
- Can underestimate the angle if rim of lens indents at the limbus

Indentation gonioscopy
- Differentiates between appositional and synechial angle closure
- Coupling fluid not needed
- Higher learning curve
- Tendency to overestimate the angle if indentation on center of cornea

Features of Indirect Goniolenses (Table 5.1.1)

Table 5.1.1: Features of indirect goniolenses.

Type of the lens	*Goldmann 1/2 mirror*	*Goldmann 3 mirror*	*Zeiss 4 mirror*
Diameter of contact	12 mm	12 mm	9 mm
Overall diameter	15 mm	18 mm	9 mm
Mirror angulation	62°	59°	64°
Mirror height	17 mm	12 mm	12 mm
Radius of curvature	7.4 mm	7.4 mm	7.8 mm
Coupling fluid	Required	Required	Not required
Dynamic gonioscopy	Manipulation	Manipulation	Indentation

HOW TO PERFORM INDIRECT GONIOSCOPY

Application of a Goniolens

Patient is positioned at the slit lamp in a dim lit room as bright light can cause miosis and open up an "occludable angle". The gonioscope surface is cleaned and disinfected. Topical anesthetic is instilled in both the eyes (4% xylocaine or 0.5% proparacaine eye drops).

Scleral Type Lens

The concave well is filled with artificial tears or viscoelastic. Air bubbles should be avoided in the solution. The patient is asked to look up and the eyelids are parted with two fingers or the lower lid may be retracted with a swab stick. The gonioscope is placed near the lower limbus and quickly rotated into the eye to avoid spillage of the coupling fluid. The patient is asked to look straight and gonioscope is stabilized with the left hand and right hand is used to move the slit lamp into position to visualize the angle. The thumb, index, and middle fingers hold the lens, while the other two fingers stabilize the head of the patient.

Corneal Type Lens

The patient is asked to look straight and the lens is gently laced over the center of the cornea. Two fingers hold the lens and others take support on the patient's forehead or cheek. The mirrors should be placed in the 12, 6, 3, and 9'o clock positions.

Minimal contact is maintained just to eliminate the air underneath the lens surface and avoid formation of Descemet's folds, which indicate too much pressure. If air bubbles form underneath lens surface, they can be easily removed by gently rocking the lens.

Angle Viewing

The slit lamp beam height should be adjusted to 2 mm to 3 mm in height and it should be a thin beam. The slit lamp should be put on while the beam is directed only into the angle without crossing the pupil. It is important to remember that image formed in the gonio mirror is of the opposite angle but it is not laterally inverted. The inferior angle is usually the widest and pigmented, and should be viewed first, followed by superior angle. The beam can be turned horizontal for viewing the temporal and nasal angle.

For manipulation, the patient is asked to look towards the examining mirror and angle is viewed over a steep iris. Indentation (or compression) gonioscopy can be performed by pressing a corneal type lens to push the aqueous into angle in eyes with primary angle closure glaucoma to differentiate an appositional from synechial angle closure. Examine each quadrant and note the findings.

GONIOSCOPY GRADING SYSTEMS

Shaffer's System

Shaffer's system describes the angle between trabecular meshwork and iris (Table 5.1.2). Angles greater than 20° are considered to be wide open and incapable of closure. The angle is not actually measured in degree, it is only a rough estimation of the angle width (Fig. 5.1.7).

Spaeth System

The *Spaeth* system grades four aspects of angle anatomy (Table 5.1.3):

1. Level of iris insertion
2. Angular width of angle recess
3. Iris configuration
4. Angle pigmentation.

RPC CLASSIFICATION

This is the classification routinely used at our institute for grading the angle with the patient in primary position. Grade 3 or less is considered as a narrow angle.

Grade 0: Closed, no dipping of the slit lamp beam

Grade 1: Dipping of the beam

Grade 2: Schwalbe's line and anterior third of TM seen

Grade 3: Posterior two-third of TM is seen

Grade 4: Scleral spur is seen

Grade 5: Ciliary body band is seen

Grade 6: Last roll of iris seen.

Table 5.1.2: Shaffer's system.

Grade number	*Angle width*	*Comments*
4	35–45°	Wide open—closure impossible
3	20–35°	Wide open—closure impossible
2	20°	Narrow—closure possible
1	≤ 10°	Extremely narrow—closure probable
Slit	Slit	Narrowed to slit—closure probable
0	0°	Closed

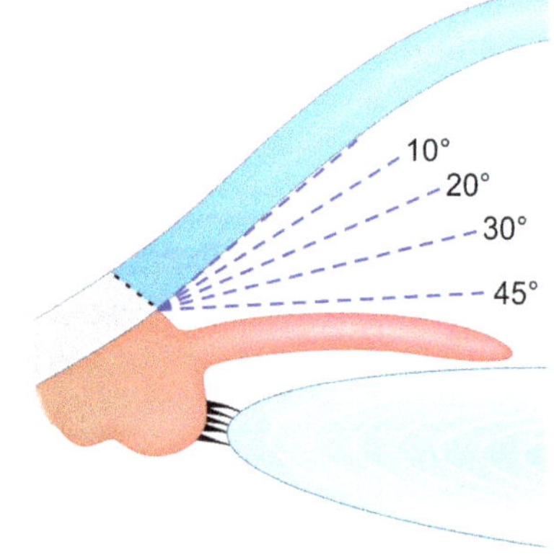

Fig. 5.1.7: Shaffer angle width determination.

Table 5.1.3: The *Spaeth* system.	
Insertion of iris root (Fig. 5.1.8)	• *Anterior*: Iris inserts anterior to the Schwalbe's line • *Behind Schwalbe's line*: Anterior to posterior limit of trabecular meshwork • *Centered on Sclera*: On the scleral spur • *Deep to Scleral spur*: Behind the scleral spur • *Extremely deep*: On the ciliary band
Angular width slit (Fig. 5.1.9)	10° Narrow 20° 30° Wide 40°
Configuration of the peripheral iris (Fig. 5.1.10)	s = steep, anteriorly convex r = regular or flat q = queer, anteriorly concave
Angle pigmentation (Fig. 5.1.11)	*0*: None *1*: Minimal *2*: Mild *3*: Moderate *4*: Intense

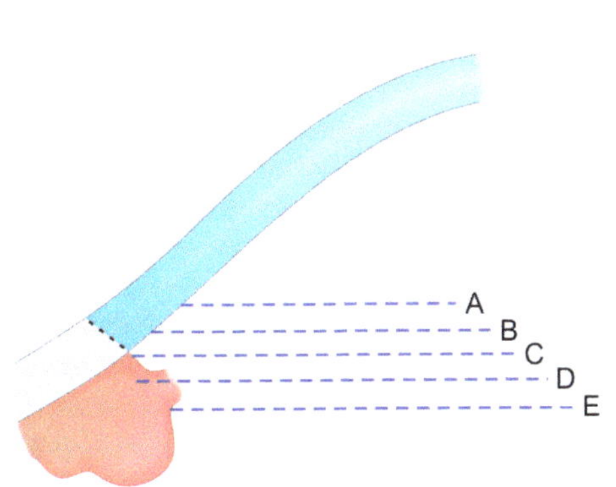

Fig. 5.1.8: Spaeth grading of site of iris insertion.

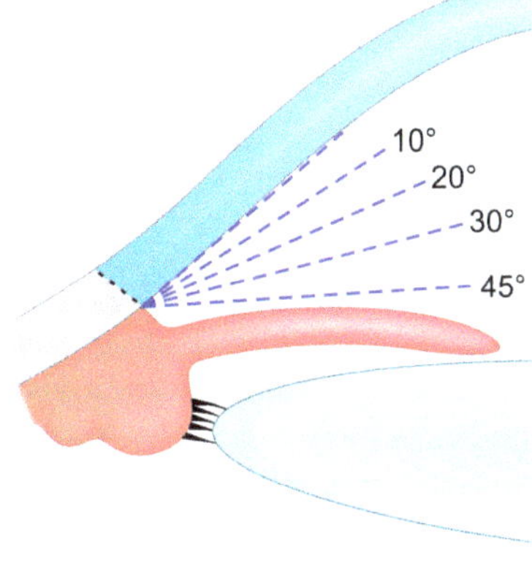

Fig. 5.1.9: Spaeth grading of angle width.

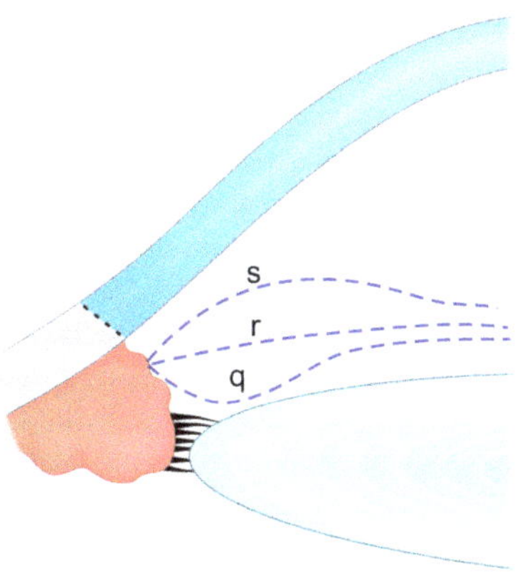

Fig. 5.1.10: Spaeth grading of peripheral iris curvature.

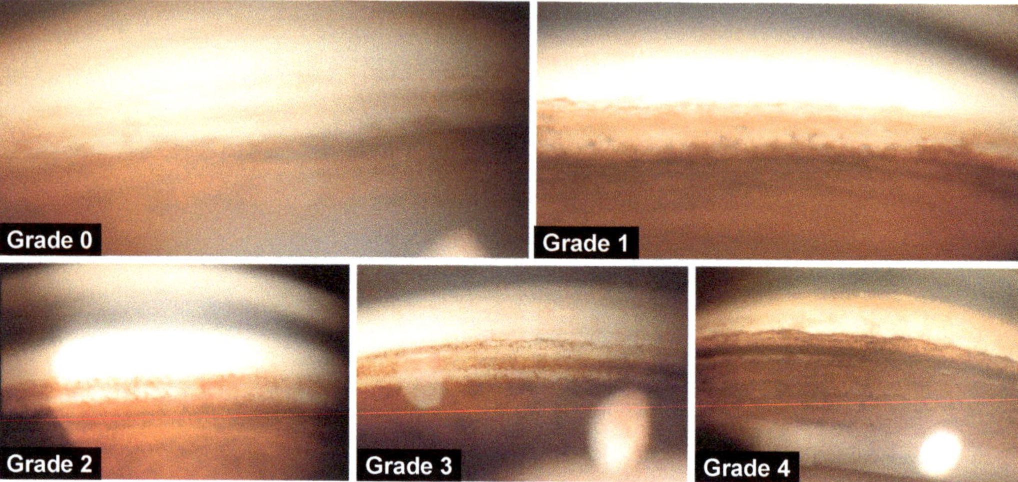

Fig. 5.1.11: Spaeth grading of angle pigmentation.

The angle is written as:

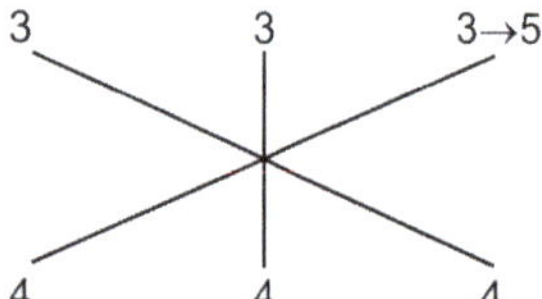

This denotes the superior and inferior angle and the most posterior structure seen (3 = posterior trabecular meshwork visible in superior angle, 4 = scleral spur visible in inferior angle). The arrow 3→5 indicates the actual angle structure visible in primary gaze (in this case the trabecular meshwork = 3) and the structure which becomes visible after doing manipulative gonioscopy (in this case the ciliary body band = 5).

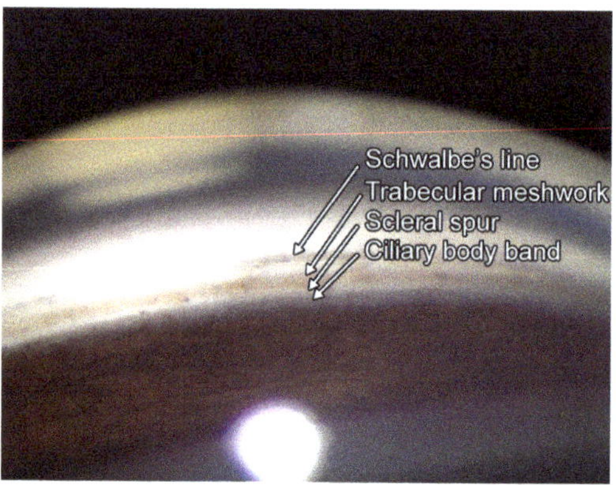

Fig. 5.1.12: Angle structures in a normal eye.

NORMAL ANGLE STRUCTURES VISIBLE ON GONIOSCOPY

Gonioscopy helps us to determine the angle anatomy of a patient based on recognition of landmarks (Fig. 5.1.12).

- *Schwalbe's line and corneal wedge*: Corneal wedge is used to locate the Schwalbe's line (Figs. 5.1.12 and 5.1.13). It is formed by the meeting of the reflections

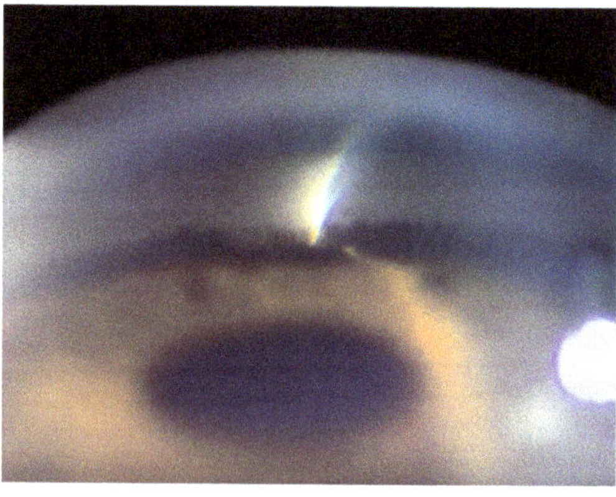
Fig. 5.1.13: Corneal wedge formation.

of light from internal and external surface of cornea into one single light beam at the point where the cornea merges into sclera and loses its transparency. This is the point where the Descemet membrane terminates. It marks the starting of angle structures. Sometimes pigmentation may lie anterior to the Schwalbe's line leading to confusion with trabecular meshwork, where corneal wedge helps in identification of angle structures. Trabecular meshwork lies behind the corneal wedge and Schwalbe's line. It is visualized by projecting a thin and sharp beam at the angle. The pigmentation anterior to Schwalbe's line may be seen in pseudoexfoliation (PXF) called the Sampolesi's line, may be confused with trabecular meshwork. Corneal wedge is used to identify its location. A prominent Schwalbe's line may be seen in Axenfeld anomaly called a posterior embryotoxon.

- *Trabecular meshwork*: It starts right behind the Schwalbe's line. It is divided into anterior non-pigmented non-functional part and posterior functional pigmented part. The pigmentation of trabecular meshwork may vary from none to dark and is graded accordingly. Inferior TM tends to be more pigmented due to gravity and aqueous currents. The pigmentation may become especially heavy in pigment dispersion syndrome, PXF, uveitis.
- Scleral spur is a white band like structure behind the trabecular meshwork, which gives attachment to the ciliary body. Visibility of scleral spur in primary position denotes an open angle.
- *Ciliary body band*: The greyish portion of ciliary body visible behind the scleral spur is the ciliary body band. It may get abnormally widened after trauma—angle recession (Fig. 5.1.14) which is a sign of significant trauma to the eye. Ciliary body band may be wide in myopes and narrower in hyperopes.

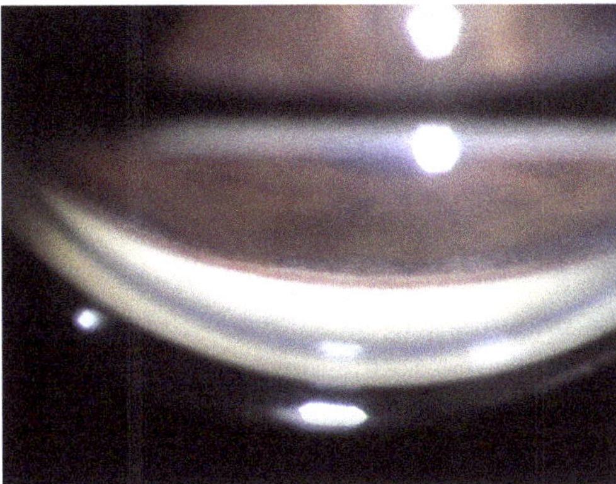

Fig. 5.1.14: Abnormal widening of ciliary body band-angle recession.

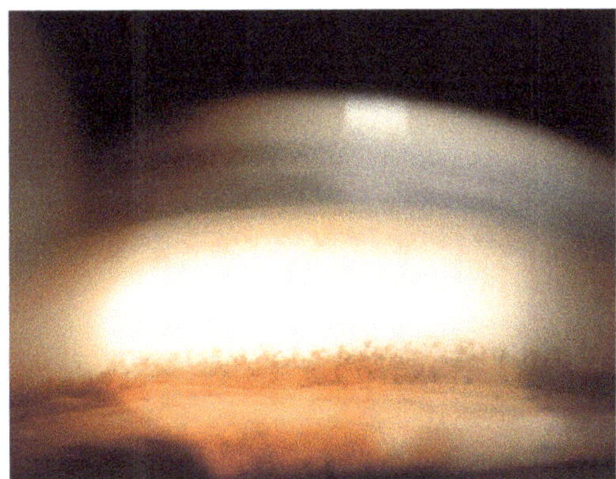

Fig. 5.1.15: Iris processes.

- *Normal blood vessels*: They are usually visible in thin/blue-grey eyes and rarely in brown or black eyes. They can be seen as loops of vessels near root of iris that radially run towards the center of pupil. They never cross the scleral spur. Any vessel crossing the scleral spur is abnormal.
- Iris processes are finger like extensions arising from the iris and attaching in the angle at variable positions generally not crossing the trabecular meshwork. They follow the concavity of the iris and allow free movement of iris posterior during indentation. They may be confused with synechiae (Fig. 5.1.15).

DOCUMENTATION OF GONIOSCOPY/RECORDING—GONIOGRAM

- Posterior most structure visible in primary gaze with thin short slit beam
- Posterior most structure on indentation or manipulation
- Angle recess—degree
- Iris configuration—concave, regular or steep
- Any specific angle abnormality:
  - Goniosynechiae
  - Pigmentation
  - Angle recession
  - Anterior insertion of iris
  - Iridodialysis/cyclodialysis
- Record any anomalies in the appropriate quadrant in a goniogram (Fig. 5.1.16).

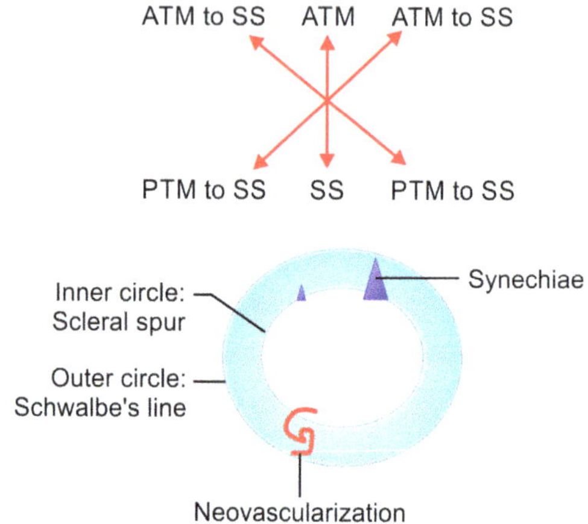

Fig. 5.1.16: Goniogram for easy recording of angle configuration.

STERILIZATION OF GONIOSCOPES

Gonioscopy being an invasive procedure, infections can spread through infected gonioscopes. Hence, sterilization and disinfection of gonioscopes between uses is imperative.

A goniolens should be immediately rinsed with clean cold water with mild soap or detergent, after removing the lens from the patient's eye. After cleaning, the lens is disinfected. Disinfection may be done using either glutaraldehyde or bleaching powder. The lens is soaked in 2% glutaraldehyde for at least 20 minutes or a 10% bleach solution (sodium hypochlorite) at 1 part bleach to 9 parts water for 10 minutes. The lens is then thoroughly rinsed with clean water and air dried. The gonioscope can also be wiped for 10 seconds with a sterile swab soaked in 70% isopropyl alcohol or cleaned with 1:1000 merthiolate solution. Sterilization follows disinfection which is achieved by ethylene oxide (ETO) exposure. The sterilization of direct gonioscopes (Koeppe, Swan Jacob, etc.) used during surgery can be done with ethylene oxide gas sterilization. ETO is achieved by exposure at 56°C (130°F) for 1 hour.

Steam autoclave or soaking in alcohol should not be done.

5.2 TONOMETRY

Jyoti Shakrawal, Shahnaz Anjum

INTRODUCTION

Intraocular pressure (IOP) is the only modifiable risk factor in glaucoma. The regular monitoring of IOP is an important parameter in follow-up cases of glaucoma. Therefore, the knowledge of practical application of IOP measurement is essential for every general ophthalmologist. The accuracy and precision in IOP measurement are of clinical significance.

TYPES OF TONOMETRY

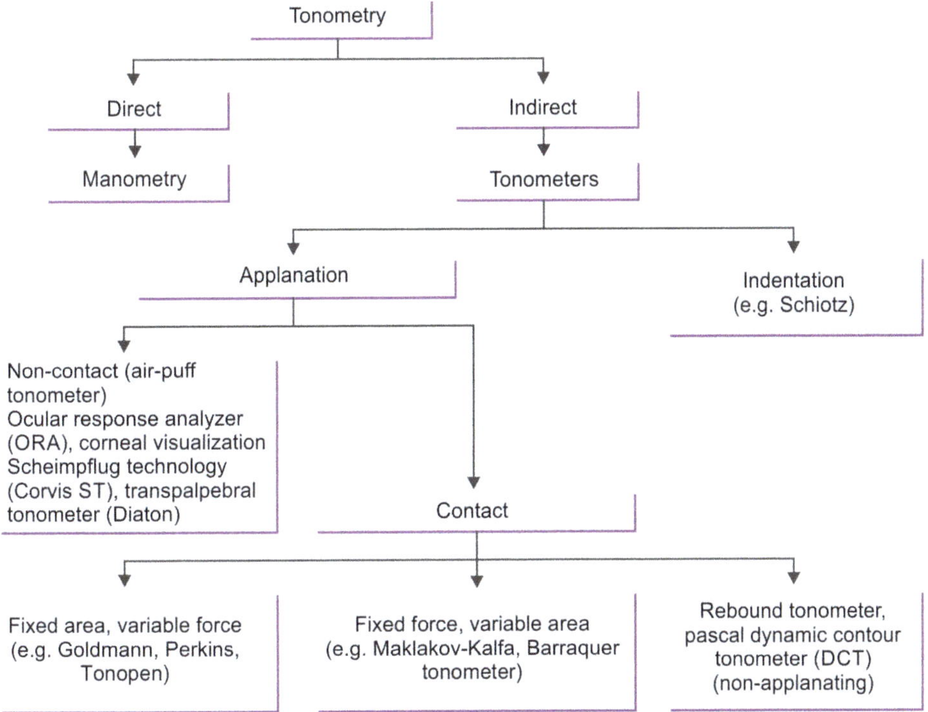

PROTOTYPES

1. Schiotz tonometer (indentation tonometer)
2. Goldmann applanation tonometer/GAT (introduced by Hans Goldmann and Theo Schmidt).

Schiotz Tonometer

Principles

- *Imbert-Fick's law*: This law states that the force (W) required to deform a perfectly dry, thin, and flexible sphere is equals to product of area (A) deformed and pressure (P_t) inside that sphere (Fig. 5.2.1):

$$W = P_t \times A$$

- *Modified Imbert-Fick's law*: As the cornea is neither perfect sphere nor absolutely dry, above equation needs some modification. The new equation considered surface tension due to tear meniscus and corneal resistance to applanation into account (Fig. 5.2.2):

$$W + S = (P_t \times A_1) + B$$

where, W is force of tonometer, P_t is intraocular pressure, and A_1 is applanation area. The surface tension (S) and force required to bend the cornea (B) balance each other, whenever, the internal area of applanation is 7.35 mm^2, i.e. diameter of external applanated surface is 3.06 mm.

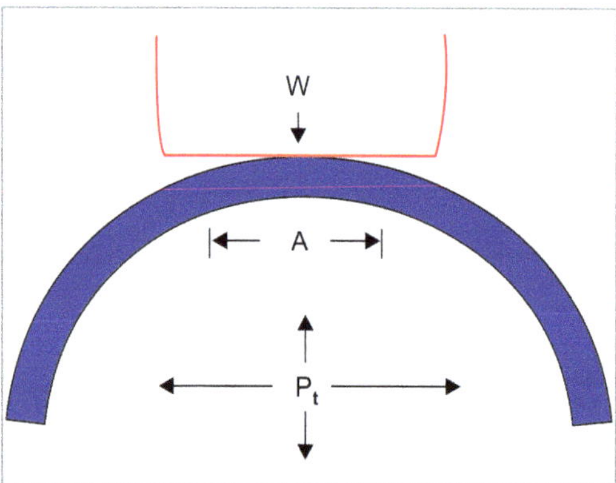

Fig. 5.2.1: The Imbert-Fick's law for the cornea ($W = P_t \times A$).

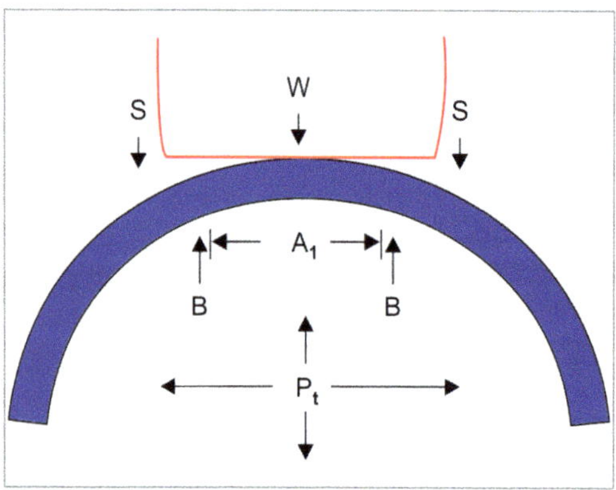

Fig. 5.2.2: Modification of Imbert-Fick's law for the cornea [$W + S = (P_t \times A_1) + B$].

Goldmann Applanation Tonometer

Parts

The different parts of GAT are as follows (Fig. 5.2.3):

- Measuring prism
- Feeler arm
- Weight insert
- Housing
- Revolving knob with measuring drum.

Calibration

Following points are important for calibration of GAT:

- Ideally, should be done every monthly for verification of accuracy.
- It is done at dial positions 0, 2, and 6, which is equivalent to 0, 20, and 60 mm Hg.
- The dial position 2 and 6 are checked by using check weight. While, dial position 0 is checked without check weight.

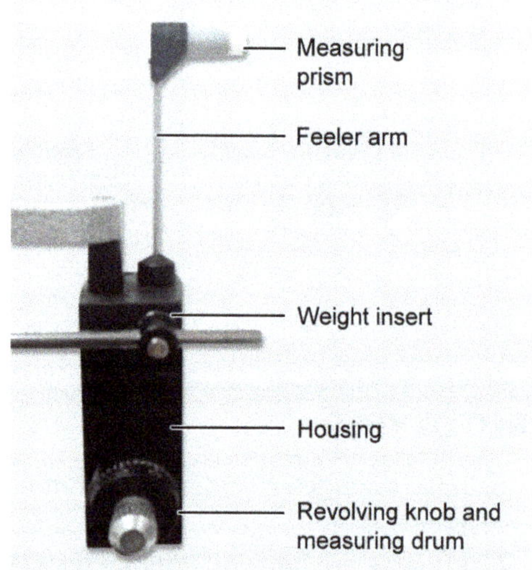

Fig. 5.2.3: Basic parts of Goldmann-type applanation tonometer.

- The check weight is a bar-shaped rod with five markings engraved on it. The middle one represents 0, with two markings on either side representing 2 and 6, respectively (Fig. 5.2.4).
- Check the alignment of adjustable holder with respective marking on check weight, with longer end facing towards the examiner.
- On turning the dial backwards (position equivalent to 0.05 less than 2 or 6), the feeler arm should move towards the examiner. Similarly, on moving the dial forwards (position equivalent to 0.05 more than 2 or 6), the feeler arm should move towards the patient.

Procedure

The GAT is performed in following manner:
- Topical anesthetic agent (proparacaine 0.5%) and fluorescein into conjunctival sac.
- 60° angle between illumination beam and viewing beam, and place cobalt blue filter.

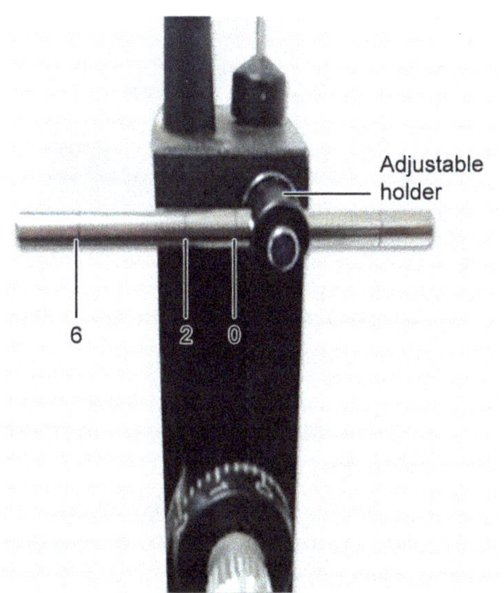

Fig. 5.2.4: Housing of Goldmann applanation tonometer with a bar-shaped check weight with five markings engraved on it (6,2,0,2,6).

- Prism with tonometer should fix in the notch.
- Keep the dial at low settings; approximately 1 (10 mm Hg).
- Obtain contact, observe cornea via viewing beam.
- Two semicircular, green color mires should be seen. When overlapping contact between inner edges of two semicircles visible, end point is reached. (Fig. 5.2.5).
- Regular pulsations of two semi-circular rings of equal size confirmed correct position of tonometer (mire thickness should be 1/10th of total diameter of applanated area).
- Doubling prism is used to applanate the cornea which optically splits circular area of contact with cornea into two horizontal semicircles by inducing horizontal shift.

Sources of Error

The different sources of error have been summarized in Table 5.2.1.[1,2]

Cleaning of Prism

- Sodium hypochlorite (1:10 household bleach)
- Isopropyl alcohol 70%
- Hydrogen peroxide 3%
- Soap and water wash.

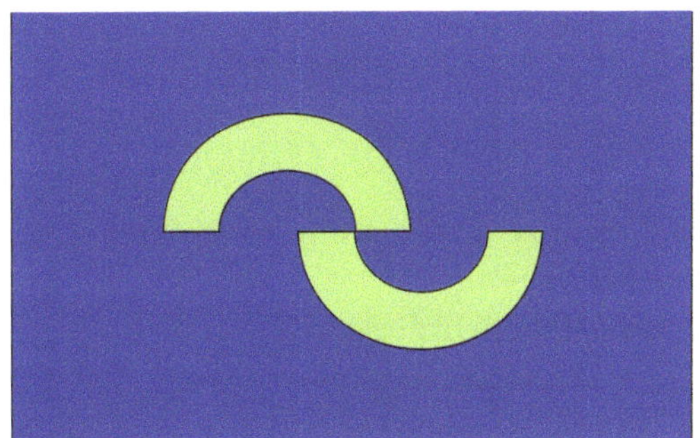

Fig. 5.2.5: Slit-lamp view of correct alignment of Goldmann mires.

Table 5.2.1: Sources of error in Goldmann applanation tonometer (GAT).

Central corneal thickness (CCT) and corneal curvature	• Thicker cornea—overestimation • Thinner cornea—underestimation • (For every 10 microns, change of 0.7 mm Hg) • Steeper cornea—overestimation[2]
Corneal edema	Underestimation
Width of mires	• Thick mires—overestimation • Thin mires—underestimation
Astigmatism	With-the-rule astigmatism—underestimation Against-the-rule astigmatism— overestimation (If more than 3 dioptres, take average reading of two perpendicular axis, or align the minus cylindrical axis to red indicator of tonometer housing)
Repeated readings in short duration	Slight underestimation due to massaging effect on the globe
Incorrect calibration	Should be checked at least once in a month

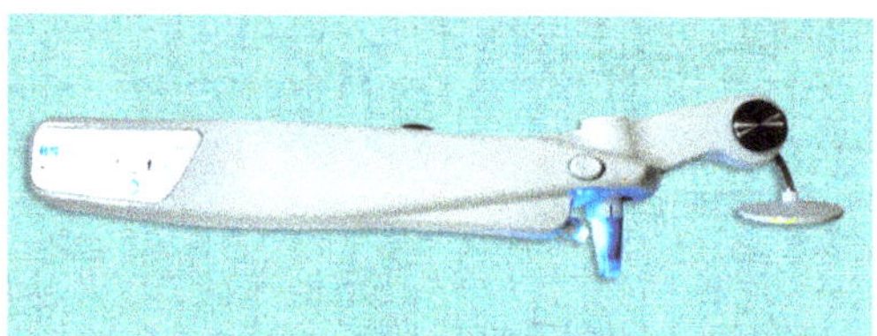

Fig. 5.2.6: Perkins applanation tonometer.

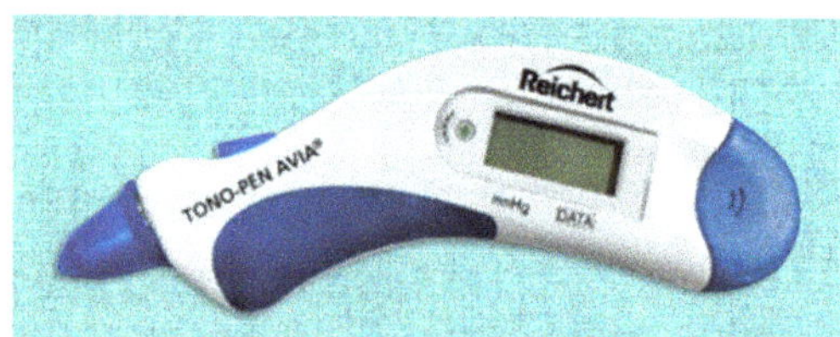

Fig. 5.2.7: Tonopen.

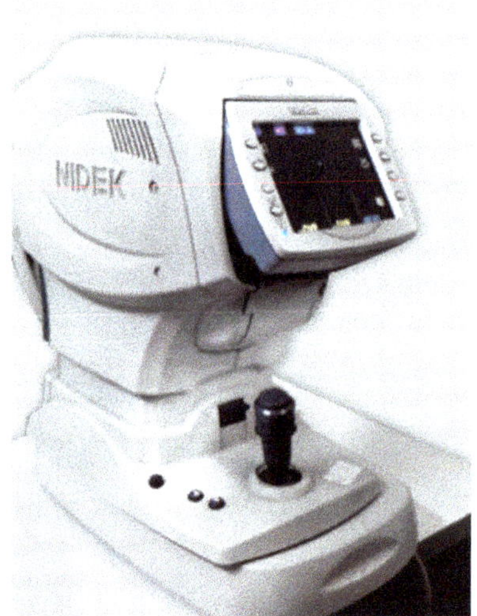

Fig. 5.2.8: Non-contact tonometer.

Limitation

- Irregular corneal surface
- Over bandage contact lens.

OTHER TYPES OF TONOMETER

- **Perkins applanation tonometer (Fig. 5.2.6)**
  - Handheld device
  - Portable
  - Used in sitting or supine position, both.
- **Tonopen (Fig. 5.2.7)**
  - Mackay-Marg type
  - A central plunger of diameter 1.02 mm is surrounded by a footplate
  - Can be used in children, irregular corneal surface, after photorefractive surgeries.
- **Non-contact tonometer (Fig. 5.2.8)**
  - Uses a rapid air pulse to applanate the cornea of known area
  - Reflected light from the cornea is aligned by an electro-optical system
  - Fair agreement with GAT (± 3 mm Hg)

- Overestimate the IOP for pressures lower than 10 mm Hg
- Underestimate the IOP for pressures more than 19 mm Hg
- Limited role in poor corneal surface or poor fixation.

- **Pascal dynamic contour tonometer**[3]
  - Non-applanating type, slit lamp mounted
  - With a disposable silicone cover
  - Measures IOP 100 times per second dynamically
  - Independent of central corneal thickness (CCT), corneal edema or rigidity
  - Overestimate IOP by 2.3–3.4 mm Hg approximately
  - Good agreement between dynamic contour tonometer (DCT) and GAT when CCT is 540 mm to 545 mm[4]
  - Difference between tonometers also increase, as CCT and IOP increases.
- **Ocular response analyzer (ORA) (Reichert, Depew, NY, USA) (Fig. 5.2.9)**
  - Measures the biomechanical properties (corneal hydration or bioelasticity) of cornea, which influences IOP readings.[5]
  - *Parameters measured are*: Goldmann-correlated IOP, corneal-compensated IOP, corneal resistance factor (CRF), corneal hysteresis (CH).
  - Important for taking IOP in various conditions of cornea like after refractive surgeries or keratoconus.
- **Corneal visualization Scheimpflug technology (Corvis ST) (Fig. 5.2.10)**
  - Non-contact type
  - Similar to ocular response analyzer, working on the principle of consideration of biomechanical properties of cornea.
- **Rebound tonometer (Icare Finland, Helsinki)**[6] **(Fig. 5.2.11)**
  - No need for anesthesia
  - Less discomfort to patient
  - A very light weight plastic probe is used, which make momentary contact and rebounds back from the cornea.
- **Indentation tonometer (Schiotz) (Fig. 5.2.12).**
  - Portable device
  - A plunger of known weight is used to measure the extent of corneal indentation.

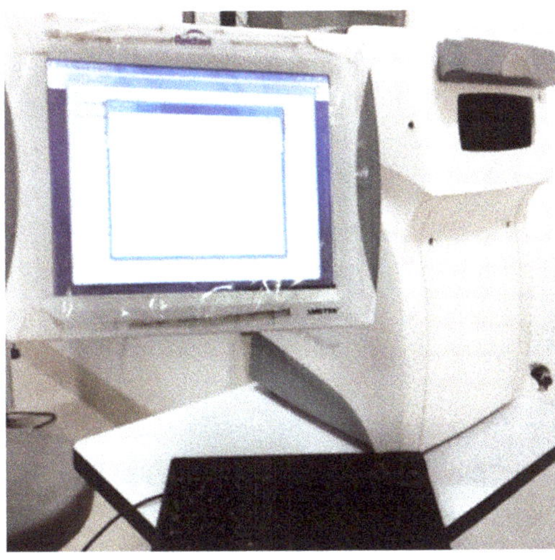

Fig. 5.2.9: Ocular response analyzer (ORA) (Reichert, Depew, NY, USA).

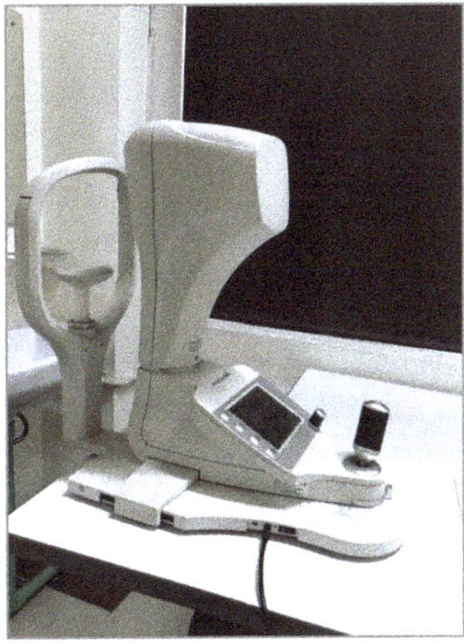

Fig. 5.2.10: Corneal visualization Scheimpflug technology (Corvis ST).

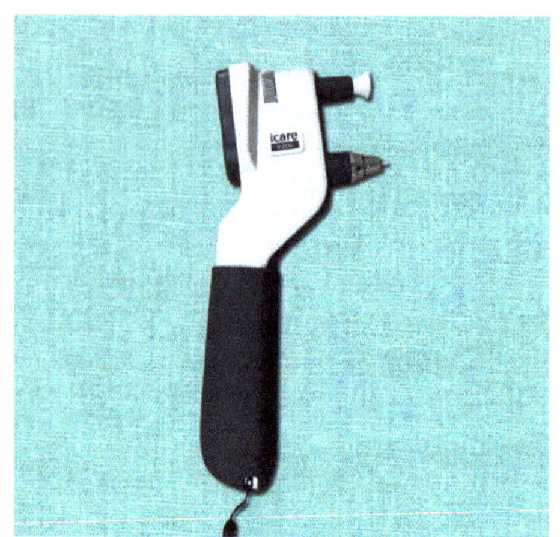

Fig. 5.2.11: Rebound tonometer (Icare Finland, Helsinki).

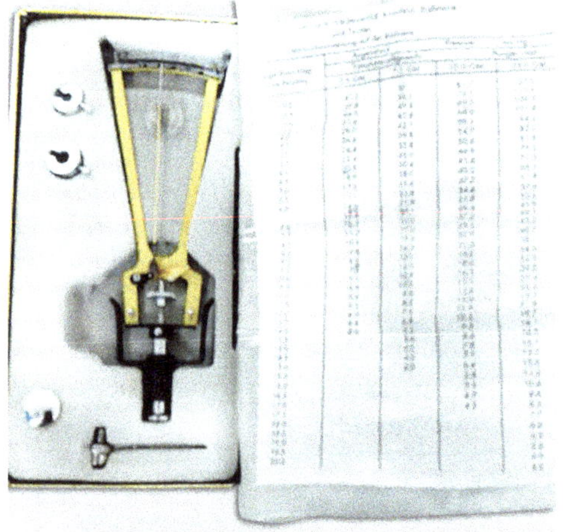

Fig. 5.2.12: Schiotz indentation tonometer.

- **Transpalpebral tonometer (Diaton)**
  - Measures IOP through the eyelid
  - Moderate correlation with applanation tonometry
  - Can be used in presence of allergic conditions, viral infections.
- **Contact lens sensor (Sensimed, Lausanne, Switzerland) (Fig. 5.2.13)**

DIURNAL PHASING

Intraocular pressure is subject to cyclic fluctuations in whole day. Therefore, increase

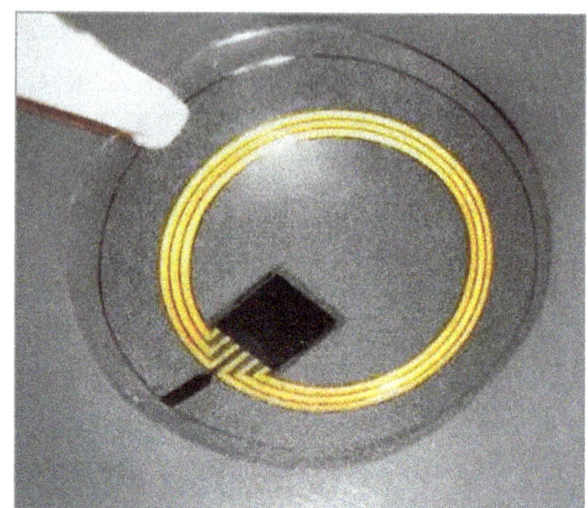

Fig. 5.2.13: Contact lens sensor (Sensimed, Lausanne, Switzerland).

chances of missing peak IOP with one single reading. Normal variation is 3-6 mm Hg in normal eyes, which can increase up to 10 mm Hg in glaucoma patients before starting treatment. The *World Glaucoma Association (WGA)* guidelines advocate a minimum of IOP measurements at 8 am, 12 pm, 4 pm, and 8 pm to assess its diurnal variation.

- Indications:
  - Normal tension glaucoma
  - Ocular hypertension
  - Progression despite adequate IOP during day time
  - Advanced glaucoma patients at high-risk of progression.
  - After doing a peripheral iridotomy.

CONCLUSION

- Both, indentation and applanation tonometry measure the intraocular pressure indirectly by some degree of globe deformation and converting it into the ocular pressure.
- Intraocular pressure is affected by diurnal, environmental, and physiological factors.
- Establish a target IOP according to grade of glaucomatous damage, with minimal fluctuation during 24 hours IOP measurement.

VIVA QUESTIONS

1. Summarize different types of tonometers.

Ans. Refer to text.

2. What is the principle of applanation tonometry?

Ans. Refer to text.

3. How to calibrate a Goldmann applanation tonometer?

Ans. Refer to text.

4. What are the different ways of cleaning a Goldmann applanation prism?

Ans. Refer to text.

5. What are the factors related in establishing a target IOP?

Ans. Refer to text.

6. What is the best method to record IOP in following circumstances: corneal opacity; corneal edema; post-lasik eyes; post-keratoplasty?

Ans. No single tonometer or method works best to gauge IOP across various corneal configurations; however, clinicians often prefer one type of device to another, depending on the circumstances. Goldmann applanation tonometry (GAT) remains the gold standard, but it is susceptible to error due to variations in corneal biomechanics. However, in general, tonometry based on the principle of Mackay-Marg is considered the best.

Corneal opacity: Tono-Pen may be useful to take the measurement in an area of the cornea that is clear.

Corneal edema: Tono-Pen in the peripheral part of the cornea.

Post-lasik eyes: Both GAT and Tono-Pen are suitable for these eyes, but underestimation to be kept in mind.

Post-keratoplasty: In eyes that have undergone penetrating keratoplasty, GAT pressure measurements are significantly lower than those obtained with the Tono-Pen. However, not proven which tonometer more accurately reflects the true IOP in such eyes.

7. What is scleral tonometry?

Ans. Measuring the IOP on the sclera can be an alternative to conventional corneal measurement in eyes with scarred corneas/ keratoprosthesis. Tono-Pen is used to measure IOP at limbal and scleral area.

8. How to record IOP in GAT in presence of astigmatism?

Ans. In eyes with high astigmatism, two GAT readings should be obtained: one with the prism-oriented horizontally and the other with the prism-oriented vertically. "The mean of those two measurements is a better estimate of true IOP". Tono-Pen can also be used, as it is not influenced by the shape of the cornea in high astigmatism.

It is important to remember following facts:

- If the patient has less than 3.00 D of astigmatism, the prism is placed so that the patient's minus cylinder axis is aligned with the white line on the prism holder.
- If the patient has greater than 3.00 D of astigmatism the prism is placed in the prism holder so that the patient's minus cylinder axis is aligned with the red line on the prism holder.
- It is important to remember that, as the prism is rotated according to the cylinder axis the mires will tilt with the direction of axis and the alignment has to be dome accordingly.

9. What is the normal range of IOP in infants, children, and adults?

Ans. In Indian eyes approximately

- Infants 8–10 mm Hg
- Children 10–14 mm Hg
- Adults 16–18 mm Hg.

10. What is the time period for IOP spike following cataract surgery?

Ans. Most of the patients may experience an IOP greater than 26-30 mm Hg following phacoemulsification, but most pressures will return to normal by 24 hours postoperatively. The peaks most commonly occur 8-12 hours after surgery.

11. What is the time period for IOP spike following laser peripheral iridotomy (LPI) and yttrium aluminum garnet (YAG) capsulotomy?

Ans. Usually IOP spike is seen, 4-6 hours after the procedure.

12. What is the importance of sleep time IOP recording?

Ans. IOP is subject to cyclic fluctuations through the day. Diurnal variation in glaucoma was first reported in 1898. Duke-Elder and others reported high IOP on awakening. There is therefore a chance of missing a pressure elevation with single readings. Across sleep stages, IOP is highest during REM sleep and progressively decreases as NREM sleep deepens.

REFERENCES

1. Whitacre MM, Stein R. Sources of error with use of Goldmann-type tonometers. Surv Ophthalmol. 1993;38(1):1-30.
2. Doughty MJ, Zaman ML. Human corneal thickness and its impact on intraocular pressure measures: a review and meta-analysis approach. Surv ophthalmol. 2000;44(5):367-408.
3. Glaucoma Today. (2004) Robert L. Dynamic contour tonometry. [online] Available from http://glaucomatoday.com/pdfs/0304_10.pdf [Accessed January, 2019].
4. Kaufmann C, Bachmann LM, Thiel MA. Comparison of dynamic contour tonometry with Goldmann applanation tonometry. Invest Ophthalmol Vis Sci. 2004;45(9):3118-21.
5. Congdon NG, Broman AT, Bandeen-Roche K, et al. Central corneal thickness and corneal hysteresis associated with glaucoma damage. Am J Ophthalmol. 2006;141(5):868-75.
6. Kontiola A, Puska P. Measuring intraocular pressure with the Pulsair 3000 and Rebound tonometers in elderly patients without an anesthetic. Graefes Arch Clin Exp Ophthalmol. 2004;242(1):3-7.

5.3 HUMPHREY VISUAL FIELD

Jyoti Shakrawal, Harika Regani, Tanuj Dada

INTRODUCTION

The Humphrey visual field (HVF) is a standard method of automated static perimetry. Therefore, it is also known as standard automated perimetry (SAP), with the protocol of "white-on-white" stimuli.

It has several advantages over Goldmann visual field (GVF) such as:

- Less perimetrist subjectivity
- Maintain the uniformity and reproducibility of visual fields
- Random presentation of targets is possible
- Calculate the patient's reliability Statistical calculation of data at various levels
- Faster.

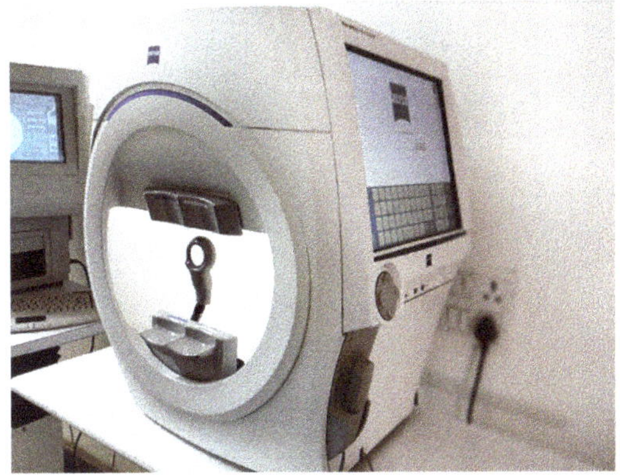

Fig. 5.3.1: Exclusive gaze tracker of Humphrey field analyzer 3 (HFA3).

PRINCIPLE

It detects differential light sensitivity (DLS), which is the ability to detect a difference in contrast, between two areas of different contrast (background vs stimulus). Each point is examined by projecting a stationary stimulus of increasing intensity until the threshold is reached.

Fixation is monitored during the examination by:

- Heijl-Krakau method—by checking the patient's response by projecting stimulus on the previously detected blind spot.
- Light reflex monitoring by corneal reflex.
- Gaze monitoring by gaze tracker (Fig. 5.3.1).

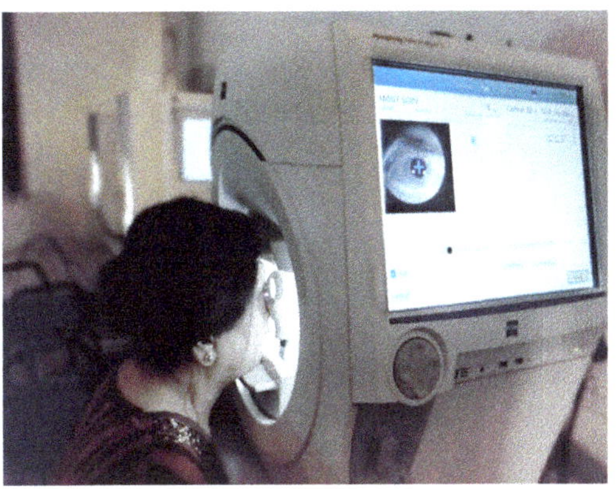

Fig. 5.3.2: Humphrey field analyzer 3 (Carl Zeiss HFA3).

EXAMINATION METHODS

Components of Humphrey Visual Field (Figs. 5.3.2 and 5.3.3)

- *Perimetric unit*: Consist of a bowl-shaped screen. The targets are projected onto it. The background illumination is 31.6 apostilbs.
- *Control unit*: Consist of a computer, dialog screen, keyboard, and printer. Controls the interaction between the operator and the system to evaluate the patient's response. Lastly, give us a printout after data processing. The hard copy consists of symbols and numerical values. The information is also stored in the computer for future need.

Stimuli

- Spots of white light are projected on white background. The size and intensity combination of the stimuli is fixed for a test

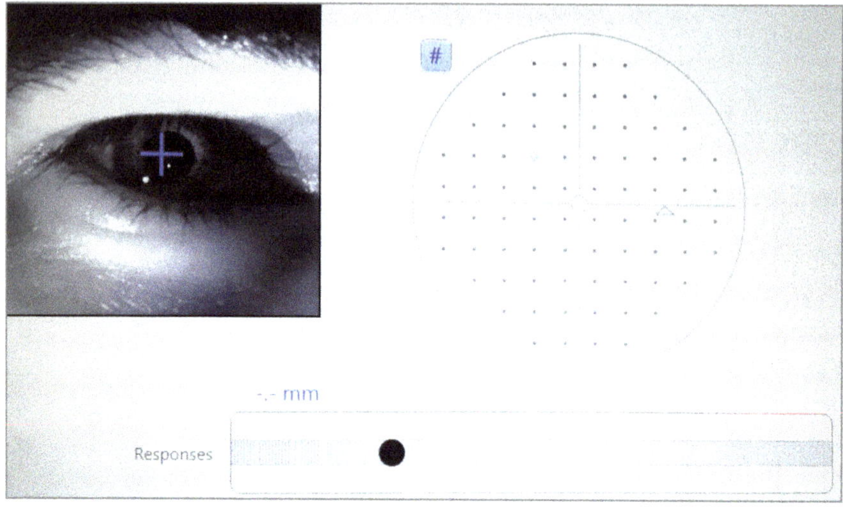

Fig. 5.3.3: Humphrey field analyzer examination for right eye of the patient with near correction given, after covering the left eye.

- Measured light intensity (logarithmic unit) is decibels (dB) = 0.1 log apostilbs
- Brightest target = 0 dB
- Dimmest target = 50 dB (10^5 times dimmer than 0 dB)
- *Threshold stimulus*: Target which is bright enough to be seen 50% of the time at a given set of test parameters at a given retinal location.

Parameters of the Test

- *Background luminance*: 31.6 apostilb
- *Background color*: White
- *Stimulus size*: Goldmann size III (4 mm^2)
- *Stimulus color*: White
- *Exposure time*: 0.2 seconds.

Testing Strategy

- *Suprathreshold strategy*: A similar intensity bright stimulus is used across the entire visual field, and the patient's responses are recorded as seen or not seen. Therefore, used for a rapid screening like the motor vehicle driving tests.[1]
- *Threshold strategy*: Visual sensitivity at a point is estimated by using a stimulus approximately 4–5 dB brighter than the normal level for that point. Here, the stimulus brightness is different for different test locations. This is not used in clinical practice routinely.[2]
- *Full threshold strategy*: Visual sensitivity is estimated at each point by a staircase or bracketing strategy. Used for monitoring glaucoma progression and worsening.
- *Threshold strategy and bracketing*: First, the threshold is determined at four primary locations which are symmetrically placed 9° from both, horizontal and vertical meridian. The threshold for each point is then determined in 4 dB up step and 2 dB down steps.
- Strategies for Humphrey visual field are:
  - Full threshold
  - Swedish interactive threshold algorithm (SITA)
  - Swedish interactive threshold algorithm fast.

Table 5.3.1: Commonly used programs for Humphrey visual field (HVF).

Commonly used programs	
30–2	Central 30° tested, 76 points, 6° apart
24–2	Central 24° tested, 54 points, 6° apart
10–2	Central 10° tested, 68 points, 2° apart
5–2	Central 5° tested, 16 points, 2° apart
Pattern	1: Along vertical and horizontal meridian
	2: Grid of points 6º apart, which are 3° on either side of meridian.

Swedish Interactive Threshold Algorithm

- An updated version of a patient's forecast visual field is estimated from whatever information of the patient is available. The machine itself modifies the questions to the patient after seeing their responses during the test (visual field modeling).
- Reaction time assessment and post processing.
- Time efficient.
- More accuracy.
- Increases patient acceptance.

Programs Used

Refer to Table 5.3.1.

INTERPRETATION OF RESULTS (FIG. 5.3.4)

- *Patient details*: It which includes name, age, ID number, eye examined, pupil diameter, visual acuity.
  Near correction should be given.
- *Test information*: Test name, strategy, stimulus, and background.
- *Reliability indices*:
  - *Fixation losses*: Unreliable field if fixation losses of greater than 15%.
  - *False positive errors*: Patient responds even when the target is not presented. They are "trigger happy" patients. Unreliable field if greater than 33%. This results in Swiss cheese pattern of the field.
  - *False negative errors*: Patient does not respond to the maximum intensity stimulus on which he had responded previously. It indicates an inattentive patient. Unreliable field if greater than 33%. This results in Cloverleaf pattern of the field.
- *Numeric data*: It shows the measured light sensitivity in dB at a particular test location.
- *Gray scale*: It is calculated from the numeric data itself. Represents the general impression of the visual field. Threshold sensitivities are combined into a group of 5 dB each (range 1-40 dB/eight levels of gray).
- *Total deviation and pattern deviation*: Total deviation is the difference between the measured light threshold of the patient and the age-matched normative data for every point tested. Pattern deviation is derived from total deviation. Represents an average of 17 worst test locations of total deviation plot. Adjusts for generalized depression due to cataract which exposes localized scotoma.
- *Total and pattern deviation probability plot*: It is represented by symbols, which represent the probability of a given value within the age-matched normal population. Helpful in depicting the overall field loss. Pattern deviation probability plot depicts the pattern deviation plot in symbols. Helpful in identifying small glaucomatous defects also.
- *Glaucoma hemifield test*:[3,4] Comparison of five zones in corresponding areas of the superior and inferior quadrants/mirror images of each other. Threshold values are compared and depicted as:

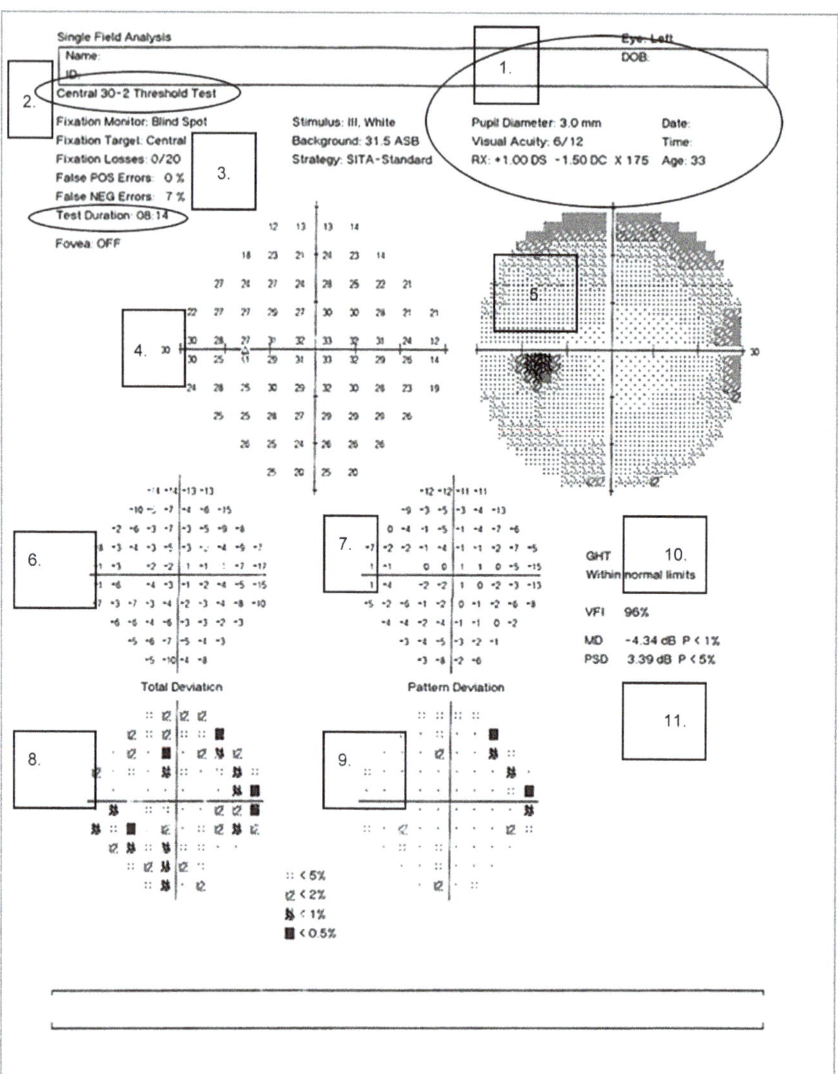

Fig. 5.3.4: Humphrey visual field (HVF) 30-2 showing: 1. Patient's details, 2. Test details, 3. Reliability index, 4. Raw data numerically, 5. Gray scale, 6. Total deviation, 7. Pattern deviation, 8. Total deviation probability plot, 9. Pattern deviation probability plot, 10. Glaucoma hemifield test (GHT), 11. Global indices.

- Within normal limits
- Borderline
- Outside normal limits
- General reduction of sensitivity
- Abnormally high sensitivity.

- *Global indices*: Used for staging and follow-up.
  - *Mean deviation (MD)*: It is the average of total deviation values. Ideally, it should be zero. Negative value shows worsening of the field.
  - *Pattern standard deviation (PSD)*: It shows the grade by which the total deviation plot values differ from each other.
  - *Visual field index (VFI)*: Percentage of the normal visual field after adjusting for age-matched.[5]

Table 5.3.2: Hodapp-Parrish-Anderson classification.

Parameters	*Mild*	*Moderate*	*Severe*
Mean deviation	< –6 dB	< –12 dB	> –12 dB
Points depressed below the 5% probability level	< 18	< 37	> 37
Points depressed below the 10% probability level	< 10	< 20	> 20
Central 5°	No point with sensitivity < 15 dB	• No absolute deficit • Only one hemifield with sensitivity < 15 dB	• Absolute deficit (0 dB) • Both hemifields with sensitivity < 15 dB

- Abnormality of the report?
  Anderson's criteria for scotoma—Any two out of the three features:
  1. The localized defects should be a cluster of at least three or more points which have sensitivities occurring in less than 5% of the population and one of which has a sensitivity occurring in less than 1% of the population. Test locations surrounding the blind spot are to be ignored in this analysis.
  2. The PSD has a value that occurs in less than 5% of the population
  3. The Glaucoma hemifield test is abnormal.
- Always correlate clinically.
- *Hodapp-Parrish-Anderson classification*: Refer to Table 5.3.2.
- Visual field progression:
  - Development of a new defect
  - Enlargement/Deepening of a pre-existing defect
  - Diffuse loss of sensitivity.

Frequency of visual field:

- Baseline
- At least six visual field examination in the first 2 years
- After that, once or twice yearly if stable
- In case, a progression is noted proceed with another confirmatory test.

CLINICAL EXAMPLES

Figures 5.3.5 to 5.3.11 give examples of HVF.

CASE

Reading the printout and interpretation—Figure 5.3.12 is showing:

- Single field analysis of patient named ...., 61 years old.
- By using central 30-2 SITA—fast strategy for the right eye with near correction given.
- The visual field is reliable.
- Total deviation plot shows a defect in the superior arcuate area.
- Pattern deviation plot also shows a similar defect suggesting localized damage.
- Global indices are abnormal.
- Glaucoma hemifield test is outside normal limits.
- Anderson's criteria will be met with if these defects are reproducible on consecutive visual fields.
- Therefore, given visual field shows a superior arcuate scotoma breaking into the periphery, suggestive of glaucomatous damage. Clinical correlation is needed.

CONCLUSION

- Standard automated perimetry, being the more sensitive, is the most commonly used method for assessing visual field defects in glaucoma.
- Always establish a baseline after first few tests, as there is a learning curve in a patient undergoing visual field testing.

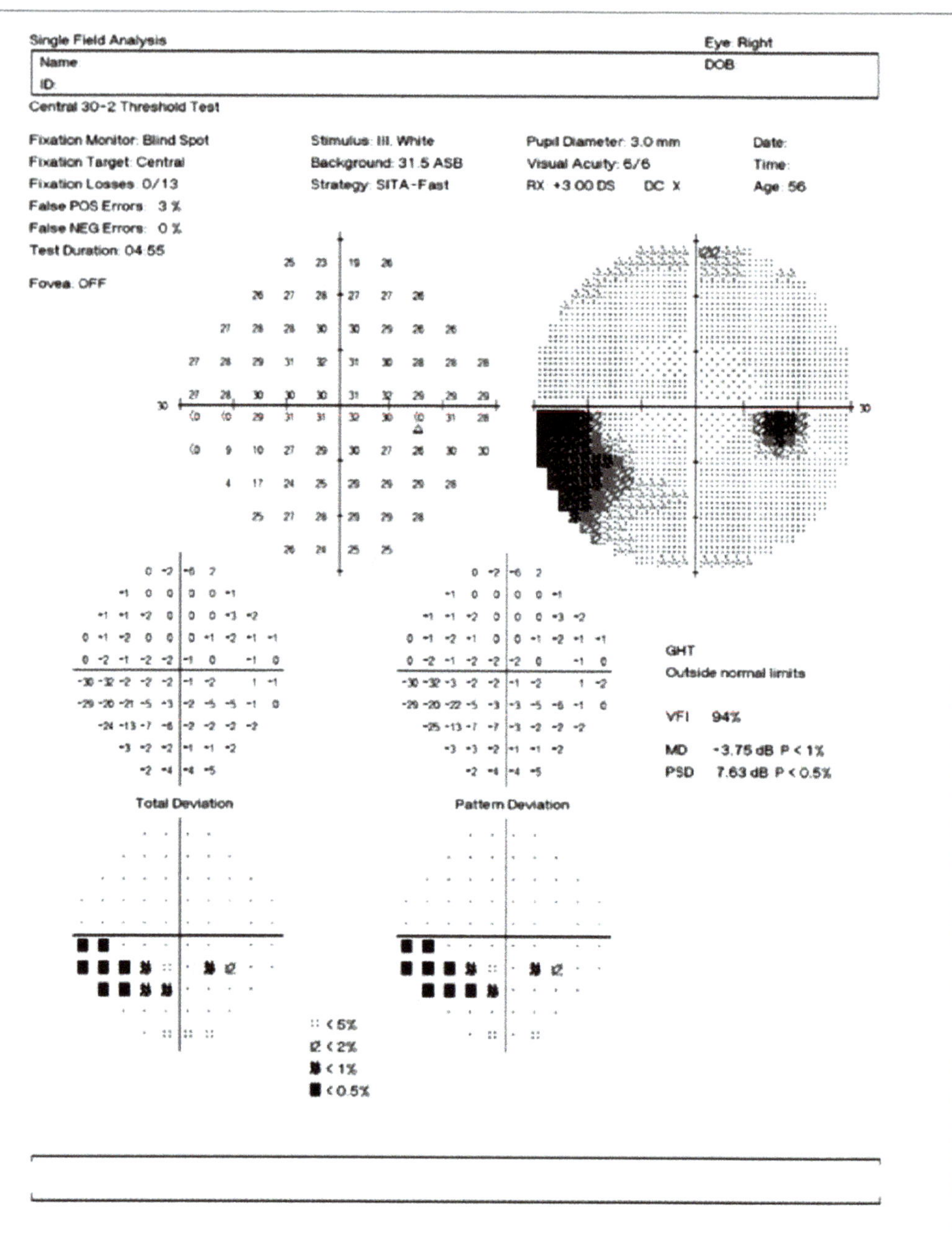

Fig. 5.3.5: Humphrey visual field (HVF) 30-2 of right eye of a patient showing inferior nasal step.

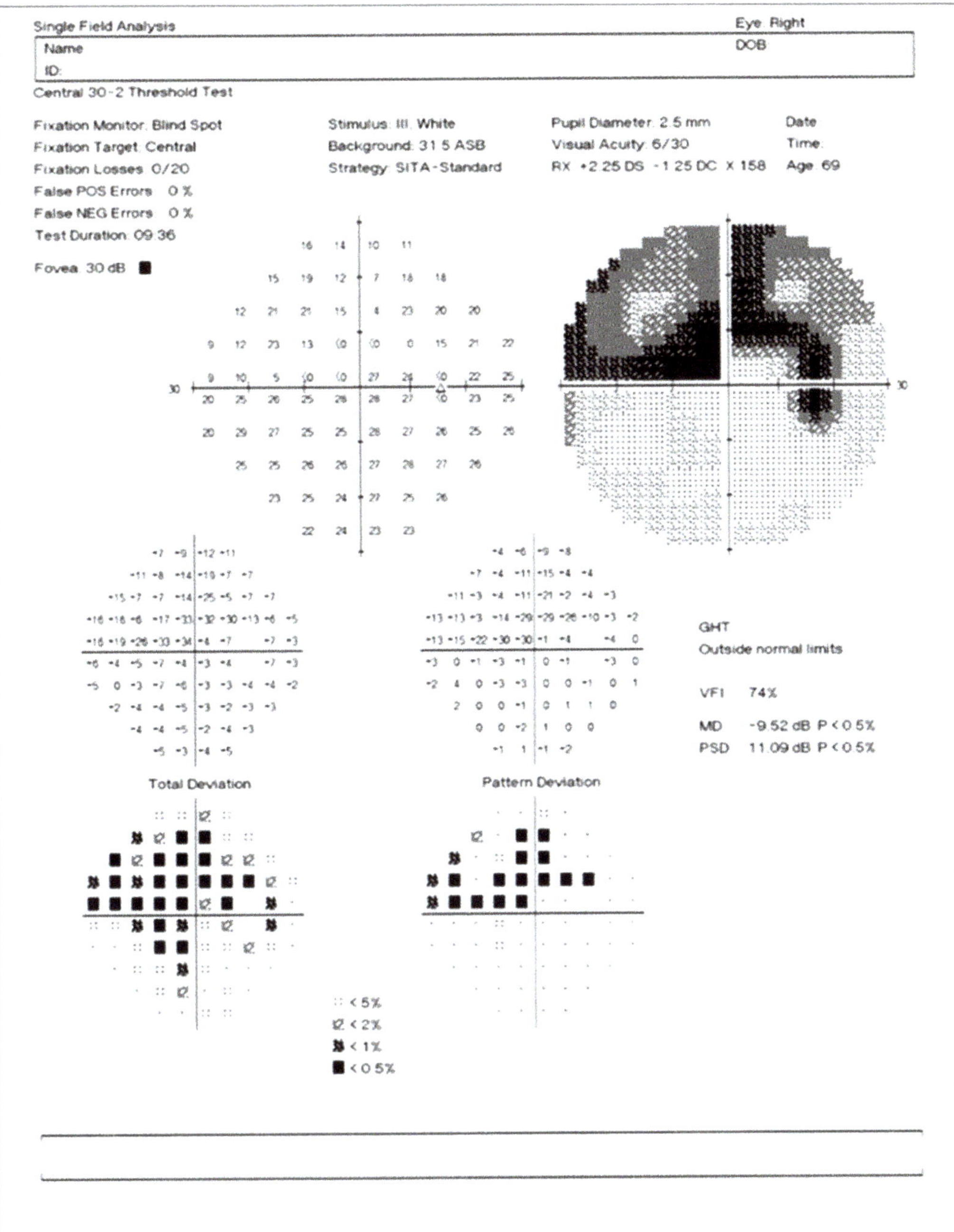

Fig. 5.3.6: Humphrey visual field (HVF) 30-2 of right eye of a patient showing superior nasal step extending further to the blind spot.

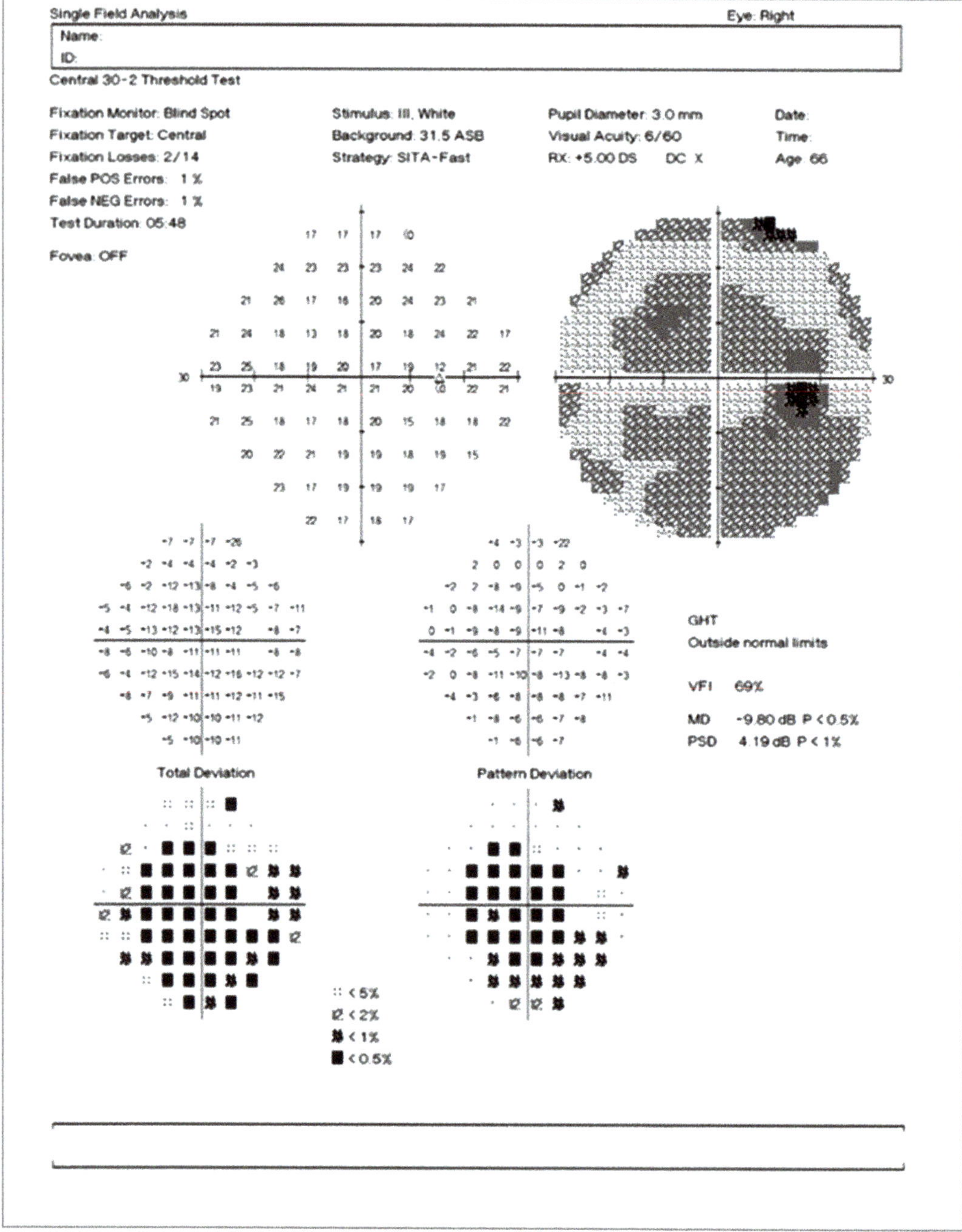

Fig. 5.3.7: Humphrey visual field (HVF) 30-2 of a patient showing inferior arcuate and superior nasal step extending further into the blind spot.

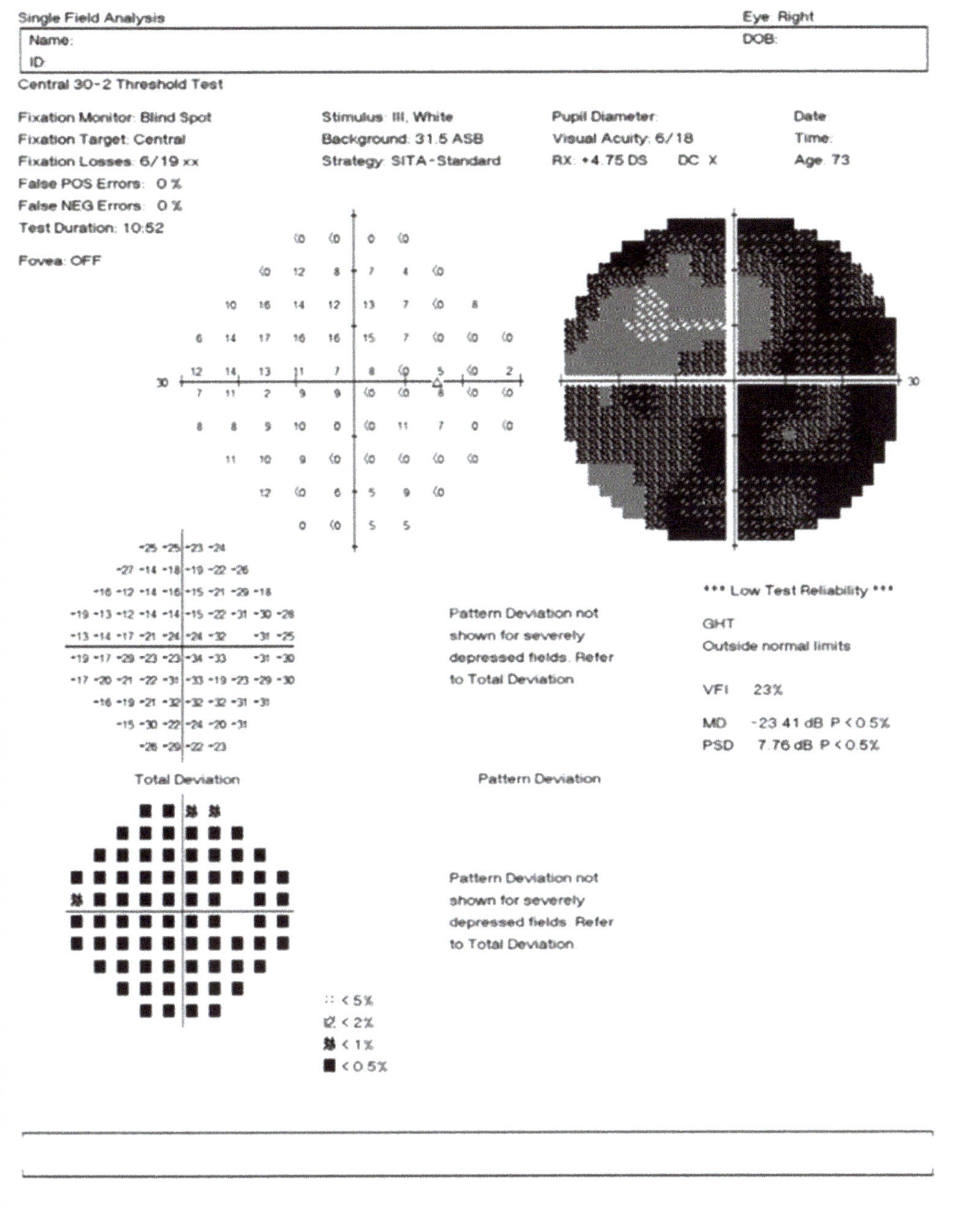

Fig. 5.3.8: Humphrey visual field (HVF) 30-2 of right eye of a patient showing severely depressed fields.

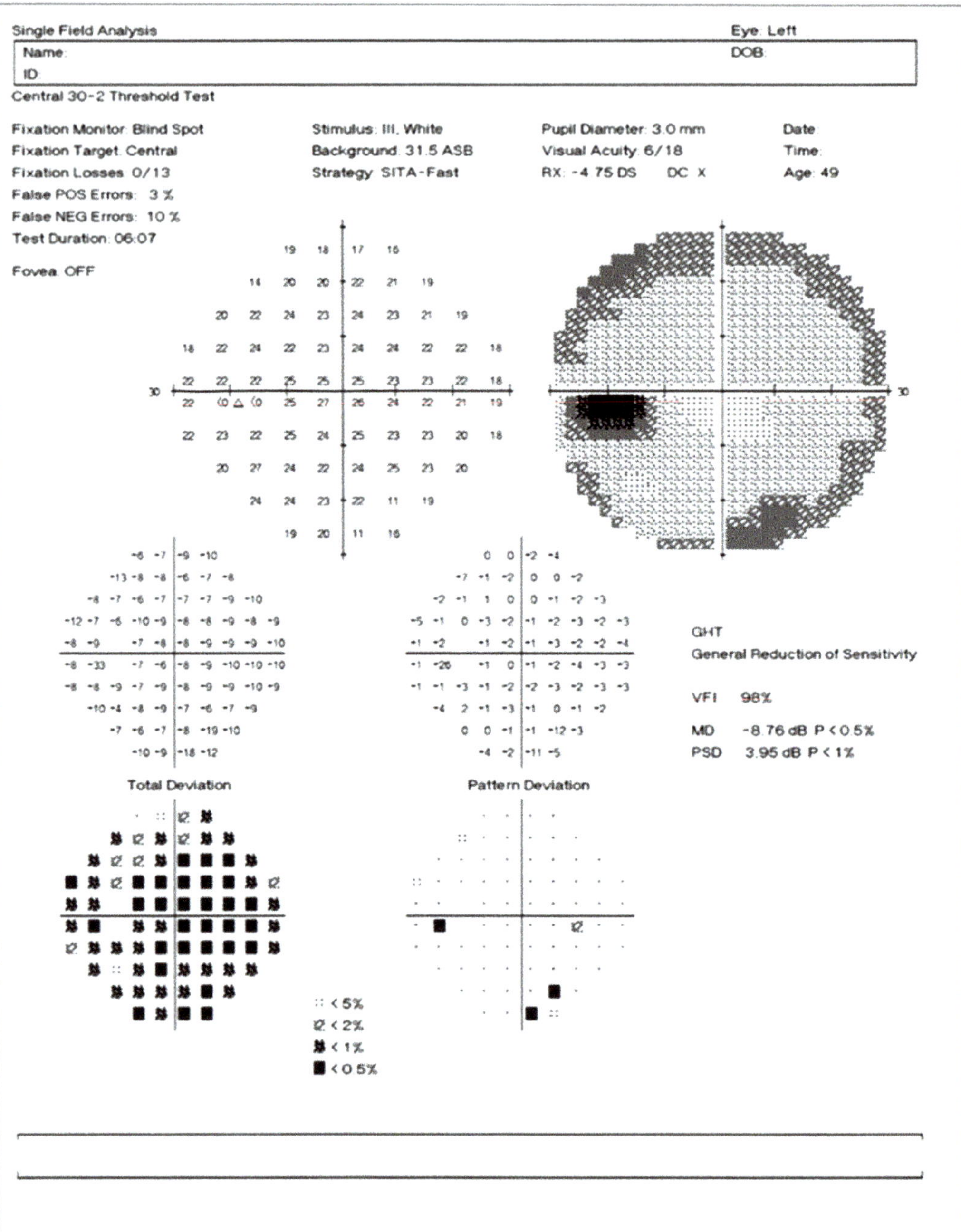

Fig. 5.3.9: Humphrey visual field (HVF) 30-2 of left eye of a patient showing generalized depression in total deviation probability plot which is not present in pattern deviation probability plot, suggestive of non-glaucomatous defect like cataract.

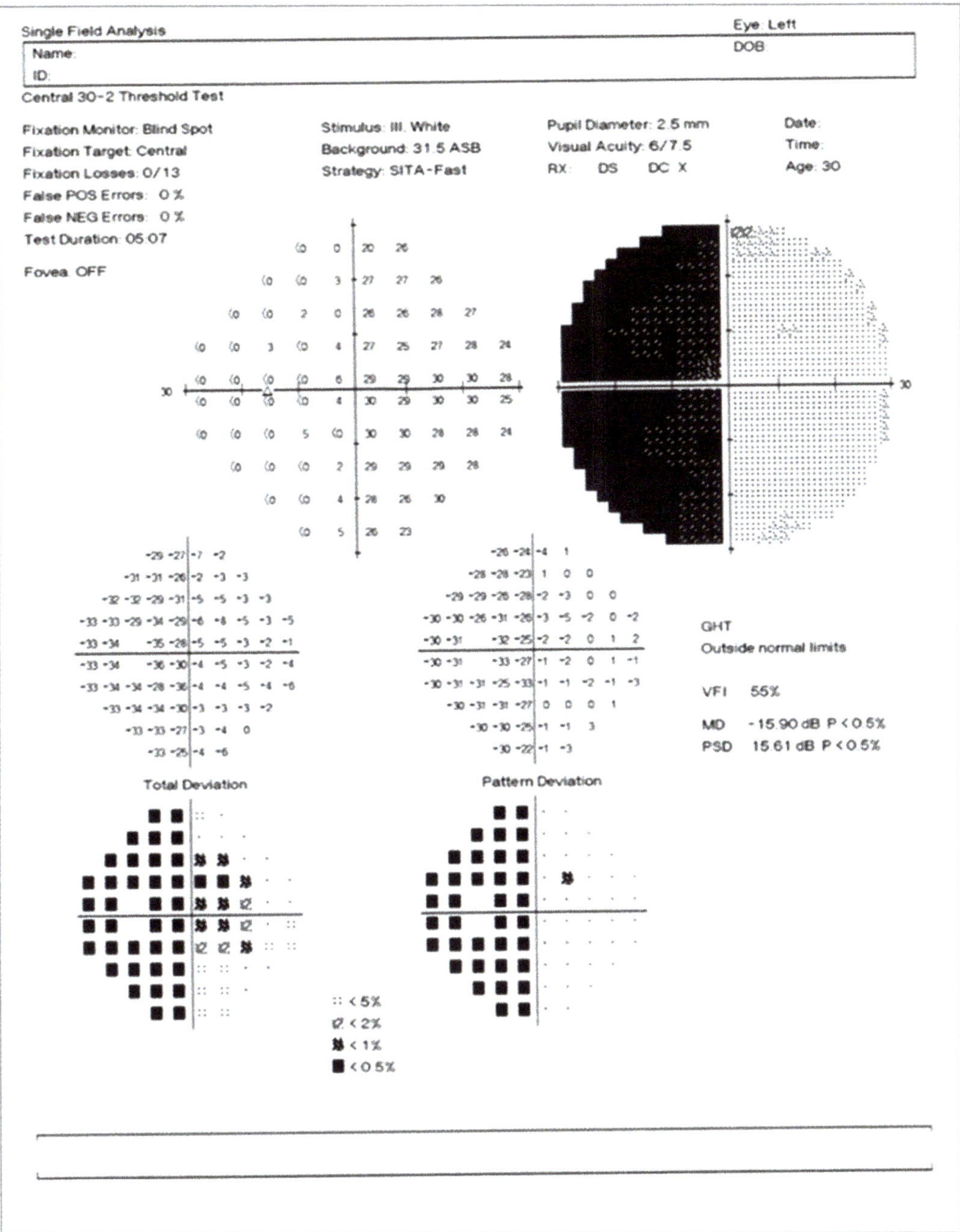

Fig. 5.3.10: Humphrey visual field (HVF) 30-2 of right eye of a patient showing complete bitemporal hemianopia secondary to pituitary adenoma.

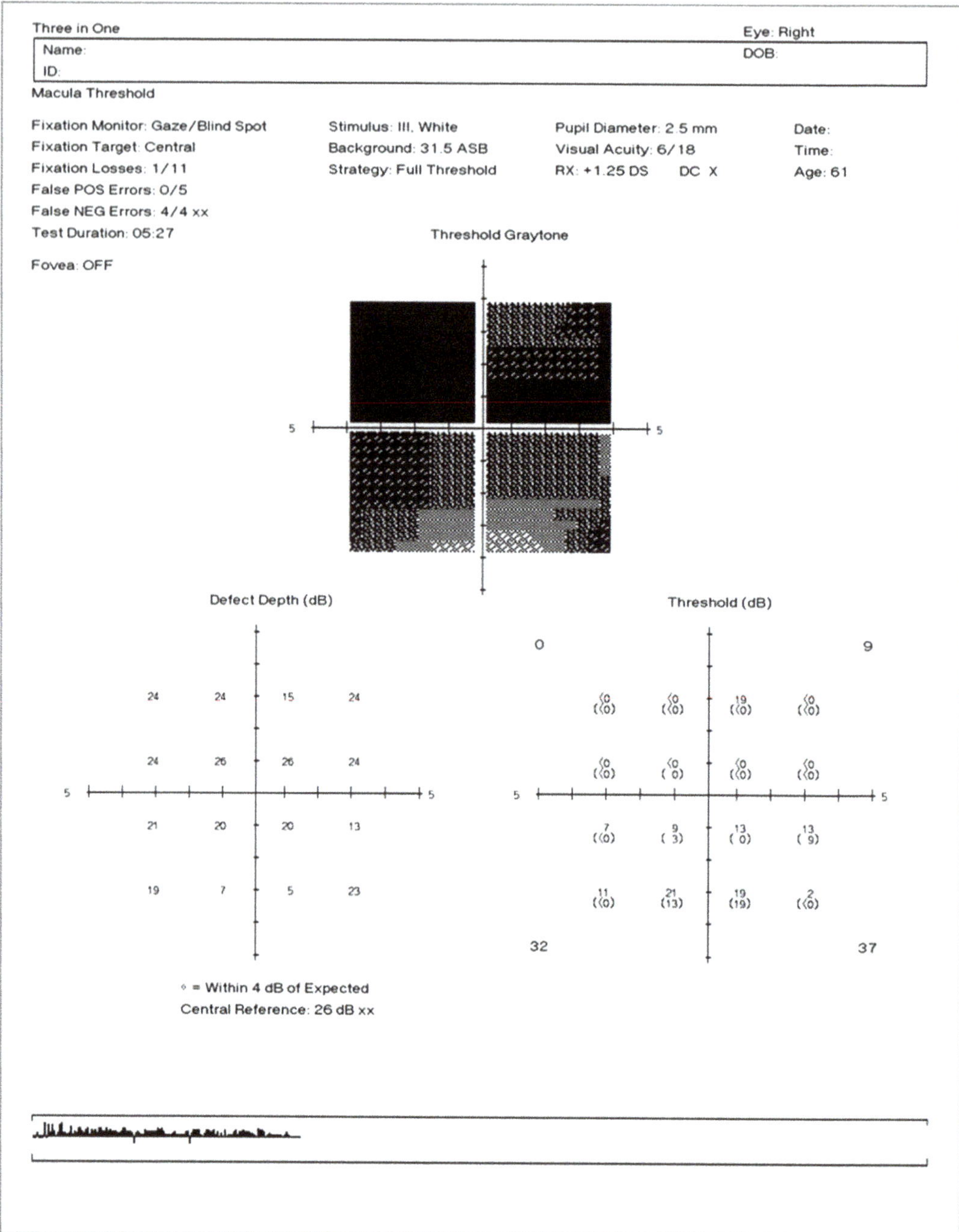

Fig. 5.3.11: Macular threshold test.

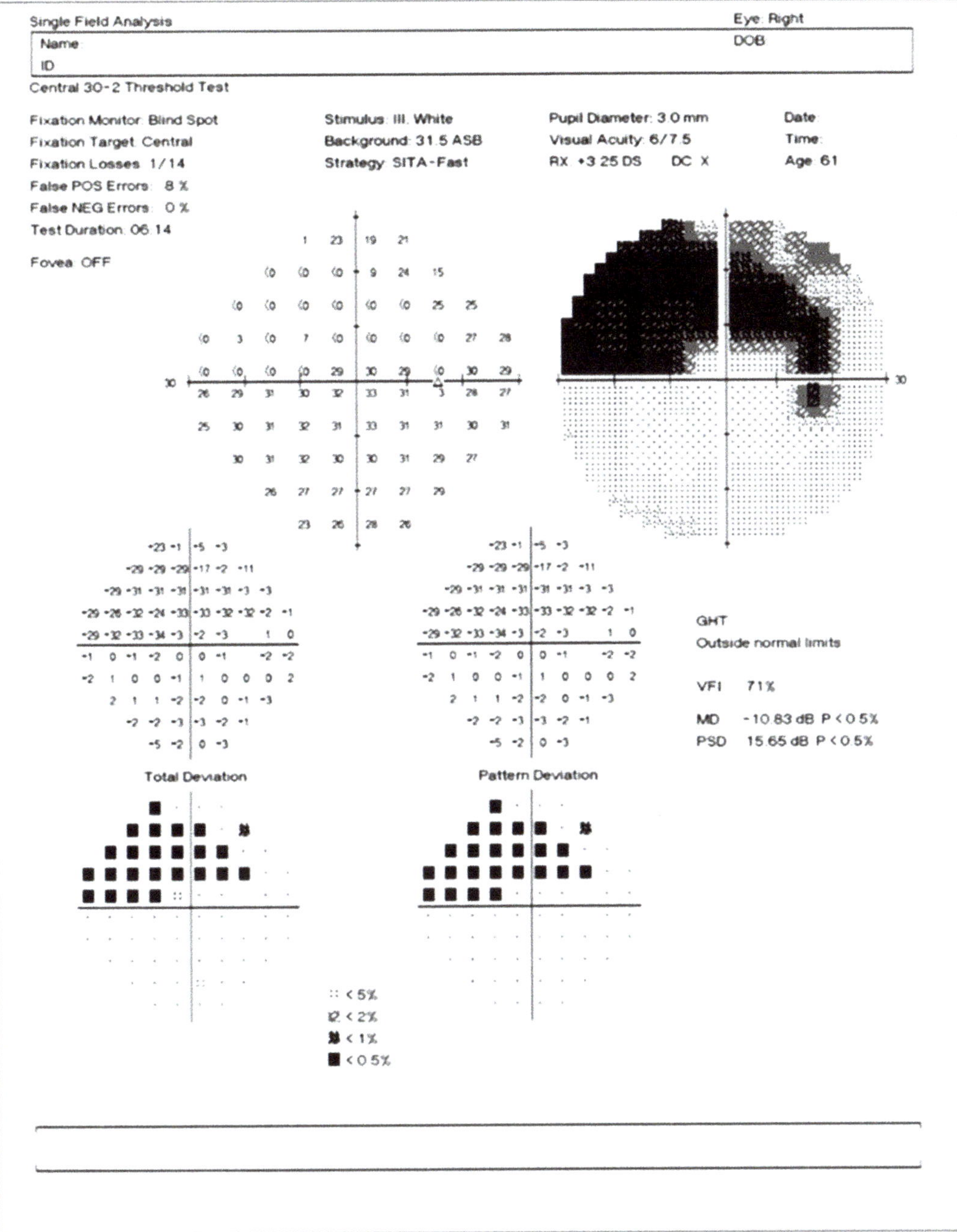

Fig. 5.3.12: Humphrey visual field (HVF) 30-2 of right eye of a patient showing superior arcuate breaking into periphery.

- Unexplained visual field defects always raise suspicion of other causes like neurological causes.

VIVA QUESTIONS

1. What is a scotoma?
Ans. Refer to text.

2. What is threshold value and how to estimate it?
Ans. Refer to text.

3. What is Swedish interactive threshold algorithm (SITA)?
Ans. Refer to text.

4. How to read Humphrey's visual field print out?
Ans. Refer to text.

5. How is reliability estimated?
Ans. Refer to text.

6. What is Anderson's criteria?
Ans. Refer to text.

REFERENCES

1. Henson DB, Artes PH. New developments in supra-threshold perimetry. Ophthalmic Physiol Opt. 2002;22(5):463-8.
2. Stewart WC, Shields MB, Ollie AR. Full threshold versus quantification of defects for visual field testing in glaucoma. Graefes Arch Clin Exp Ophthalmol. 1989;227(1):51-4.
3. Asman P, Heijl A. Glaucoma Hemifield Test. Automated visual field evaluation. Arch Ophthalmol. 1992;110(6):812-9.
4. Duggan C, Sommer A, Auer C, et al. Automated differential threshold perimetry for detecting glaucomatous visual field loss. Am J Ophthalmol. 1985;100(3):420-3.
5. Bengtsson, B. and A. Heijl. A visual field index for calculation of glaucoma rate of progression. Am J Ophthalmol. 2008;145(2):343-53.

5.4 GOLDMANN VISUAL FIELD

Jyoti Shakrawal, Nikita Gupta

INTRODUCTION

Normal Visual Field

An island of vision (the hill) with a central peak in the sea of darkness.[1] Extends normally as:

- Superiorly—60°
- Nasally—60°
- Inferiorly—75°
- Temporally—90-100°

Visual sensitivity of a given point is related well with the altitude of island. The physiological blind spot represents as a pit/ well in the island.

Types of Perimetry (Fig. 5.4.1)

Following types of perimeter are available currently:

- *Static perimetry*:
  - More sensitive
  - *Target*: Static, size usually constant for a test, stimulus intensity varies
  - *Axis*: Tests in *z*-axis also
  - *Print out*: Computerized
  - 3-dimensional, threshold based test
  - *Examples*: Humphrey visual field, Octopus, white noise campimetry
- *Kinetic perimetry*:
  - More fast

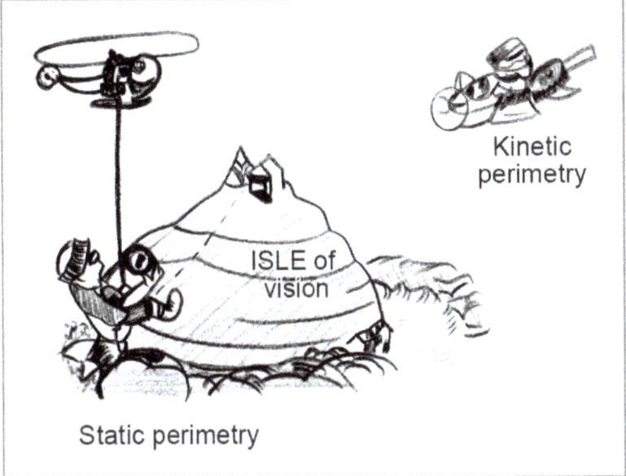

Fig. 5.4.1: The normal hill of vision with comparison of kinetic versus static perimetry.

- *Target*: Mobile, size and intensity of stimulus can be altered
- *Axis*: Tests in *x* and *y*-axis
- *Print out*: Manual (isopter maps)
- 2-dimensional
- *Examples*: Goldmann, confrontation, Tangent screen, Lister

- Combined perimetry:
  - Both, sensitive and fast
  - For central visual field-static
  - For peripheral visual field and scotoma-kinetic
  - Usually manual perimetry.

PRINCIPLE

The principle of Goldmann visual field (GVF) involves following points:

- An isopter is plotted, by moving the test target from the non-seeing area (at the rate of 2° per second approximately) to seeing area, kinetically
- At the end, an isopter is formed by joining the series of points obtained respective to the stimulus used
- Size or brightness of the stimulus can be increased or decreased to plot different isopter
- By using sequential stimuli, reproducibility of the test can be increased[2]
- For defining a scotoma, the stimulus is placed in the scotoma and move outward until the observer perceives it. It is repeated in all directions to get all edges of the scotoma.

The edges of scotoma might be:

- *Sloping edge:* Brighter stimulus describes a smaller scotoma. Dimmer stimulus describes a large scotoma.
- *Steep edge*: Size of scotoma varies slightly with stimulus.

EXAMINATION METHOD

Indications of Goldmann Visual Field

- Poor vision is less than 6/18
- Poor performance on automated testing
- Defects outside central 30° of visual field
- Residual islands of vision
- Functional visual loss.

Target

Three alphanumeric digits represent the target (Table 5.4.1).

- *Size*: By the first *Roman numeral* (0, I, II, III, IV, V). 0 is the smallest; V is the largest.
- Brightness: By *Arabic number* (1, 2, 3, 4). 1 is the dimmest, 4 is the brightest in 5 dB steps (Fig. 5.4.2).

Table 5.4.1: Different sizes of targets used in Goldmann visual field represented by various Roman numeral.

Target	*Size*
0	1/16 mm^2
I	1/4 mm^2
II	1 mm^2
III	4 mm^2
IV	16 mm^2
V	64 mm^2

- Luminance finer calibration: By *alphabetical letter* (a, b, c, d, e). a is the dimmest, e is the brightest in 1 dB steps.
- Background illumination, V1e; 31.5 apostilbs.
- Isopter is represented as (Roman numeral; Arabic number; letter)/(0-V; 1-4; a-e)
- *V4e*: maximum outline of the field; absolute scotoma.
- *I4e*: far periphery.
- *I2e*: central.
- *Maximum stimulus, V4e*: 1,000 apostilbs.

Technique

Goldmann visual field is performed in following way.

Patient Preparation

- Appropriate refractive correction should be inserted in the lens holder.
- Pupil should not be dilated or pilocarpinized.
- In comfortable position with chin and forehead firmly against the support.
- Should be instructed properly regarding the procedure.

Examination (Figs. 5.4.3A to C)

- Done uniocularly.
- Working distance = 33 cm, with examiner sitting opposite viewing via the eyepiece. Examiner should ensure good fixation of the patient during the test (Fig. 5.4.4).
- Illuminated white target is projected from non-seeing (periphery) to seeing area (center). The patient is instructed to press the buzzer, as they see the target.
- Same maneuver is done at every 15° interval around 360° visual field.
- Plot blind spot with at least 8 points (oval, around 10° in diameter, 12–15° temporal to fixation point; 5° below horizontal). Patient will press the buzzer, as they first see the target moving from blind area to seeing area.

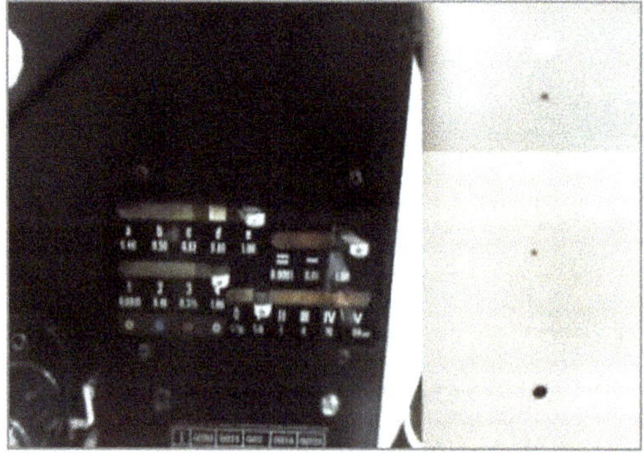

Fig. 5.4.2: Controls for target size and intensity in Goldmann perimetry.

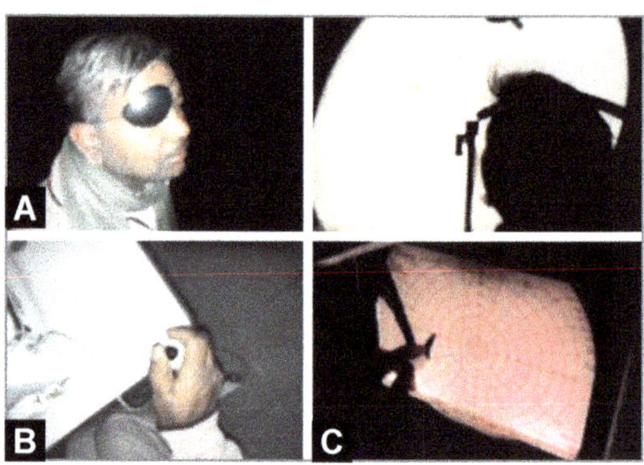

Figs. 5.4.3A to C: (A) Cover the other eye of the patient; (B) Patient pressing the buzzer as the target first comes in seeing area; and (C) After patient's response, examiner marks the location of that point on a printout.

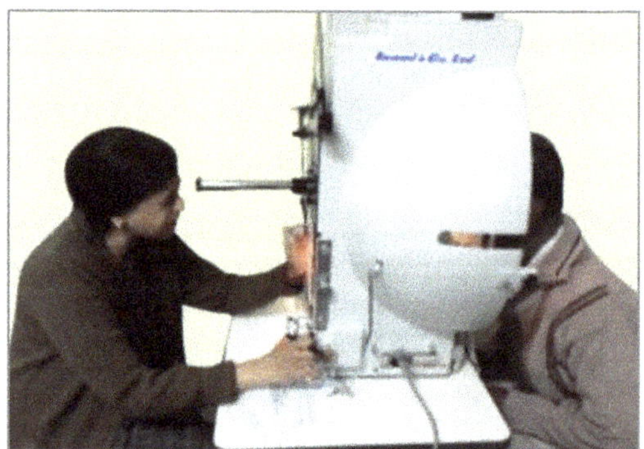

Fig. 5.4.4: During the test, examiner should ensure good fixation of the patient by viewing through an eyepiece.

- Static testing of central field:
  - Static target, shown for 1 second
  - Starts at 2.5° centrally: 5, 10, 15°
  - Circle all points missed
  - Second reading still missed, mark an X in the circle
  - Check all 76 points
  - Kinetically plot out scotoma moving from centre to outside in 8 directions or more
  - Ask to fixate on centre, move target within scotoma isopter to look for additional non seeing points
  - Recheck X points with increasing intensities (relative/absolute scotoma).

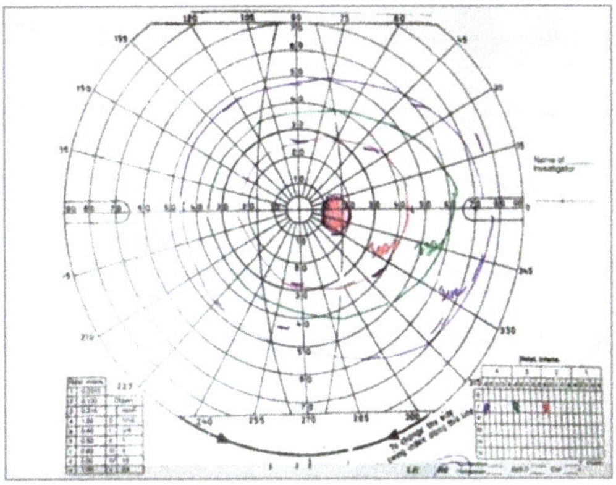

Fig. 5.4.5: Interpreting the normal Goldmann visual field.

INTERPRETATION

Following points are important while interpreting GVF:

- Patient name and age, the date of test and the eye tested?
- Look for the largest peripheral field, topographic map; with target V4e.
- Response affected by the age of patient.
- Any distortion in the "contours":
  - The smaller isopters, respective to smaller or dimmer stimulus are known as contours.
  - Check the:
    - *Margins of contours*: Smooth or irregular?
    - *Restriction*: For example, nasal step in papilledema.
    - *Spacing between the isopters*: 2 isopters should not cross each other. Functional overlay is denoted by a very small central field with stacked (close) isopters. Seen in patients with striate cortex lesions.[3]
    - Scotomas present or not?
- *Blind spot:* Enlarged?
- *Central field*: Static testing done or not?
- *Compare both eye fields*: Monocular or binocular defect? If binocular, homonymous or heteronymous?
- Comments regarding fixation.

Interpretation of Normal Goldmann Visual Field (Fig. 5.4.5)

- Patient details, date of test
- The largest peripheral isopter (violet color)
- Other isopters are with smooth margins (green and red color). No scotoma present in between
- Blind spot
- Central vision.

CLINICAL EXAMPLES

Figures 5.4.6 to 5.4.13 give examples of GVF.

CASE (FIG. 5.4.14)

This figure is showing GVF of right eye of a patient named Mahender aged 84 years, done on October 2014. The largest isopter done by using stimulus V4e is showing generalized constriction of visual field. The blind spot is normal in location and size.

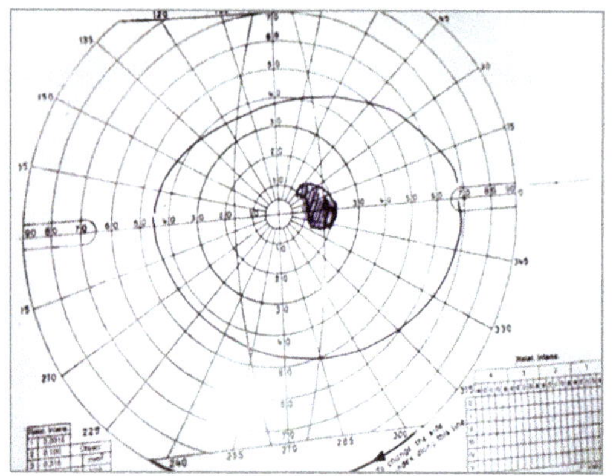

Fig. 5.4.6: Goldmann visual field of a glaucoma patient showing "siedels scotoma".

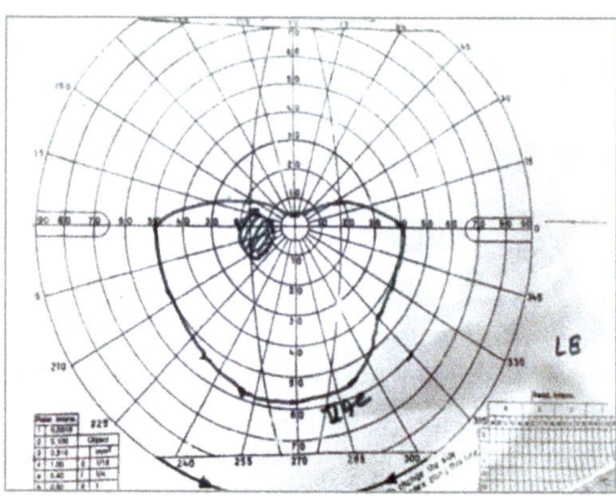

Fig. 5.4.9: Goldmann visual field in advanced glaucoma showing superior field defect with inferior nasal step.

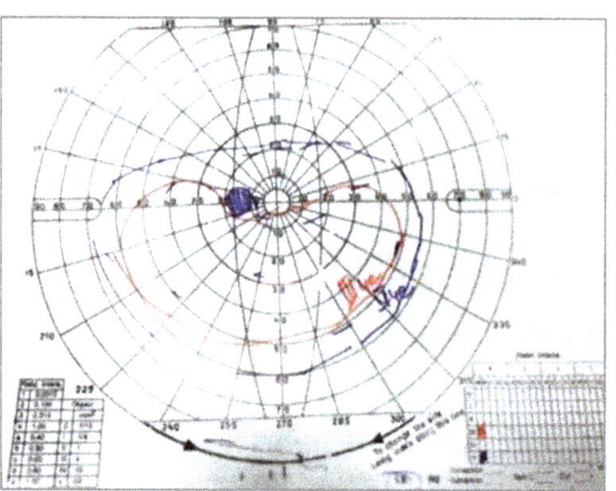

Fig. 5.4.7: Goldmann visual field of glaucoma patient showing baring of blind spot with superior arcuate.

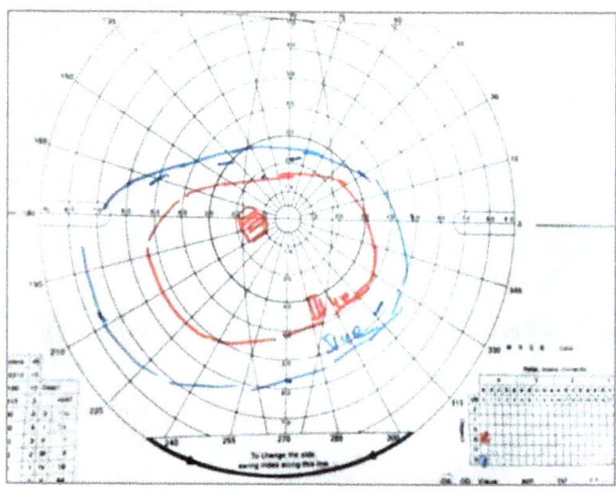

Fig. 5.4.10: Goldmann visual field of a patient with ptosis showing superior field defect.

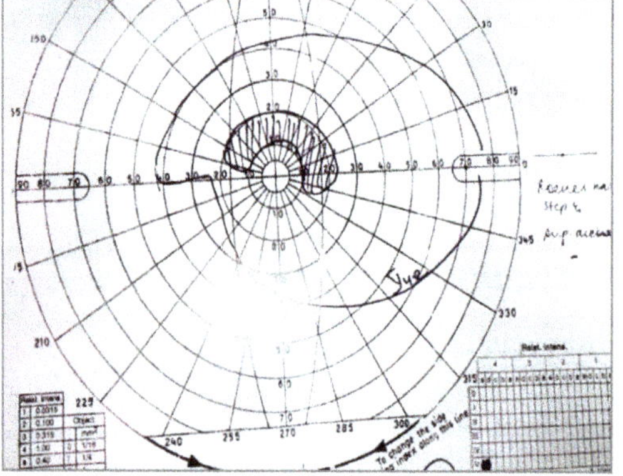

Fig. 5.4.8: Goldmann visual field of glaucoma patient showing Roennes nasal step and Bjerrum's scotoma.

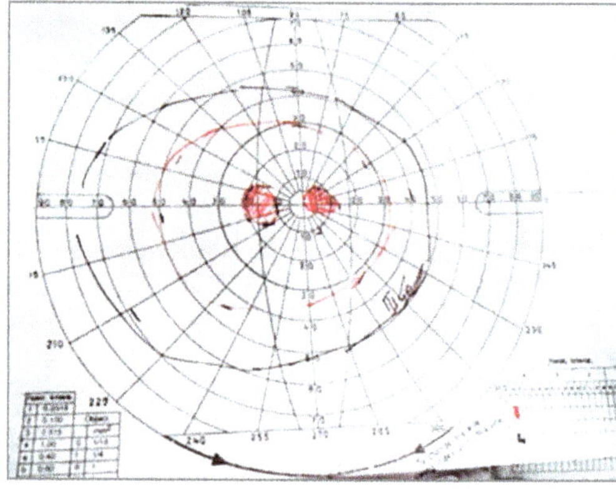

Fig. 5.4.11: Goldmann visual field of a patient with macular drusen.

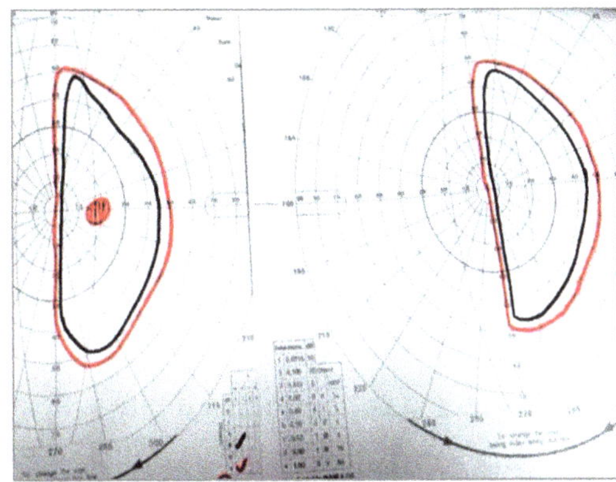

Fig. 5.4.12: Goldmann visual field from pituitary adenoma patient (optic chiasma lesion), showing left side hemianopia.

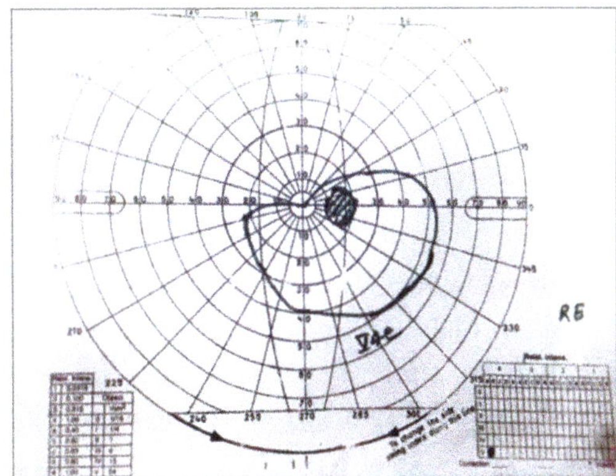

Fig. 5.4.14: Goldmann visual field of glaucoma patient showing generalized constriction of visual field.

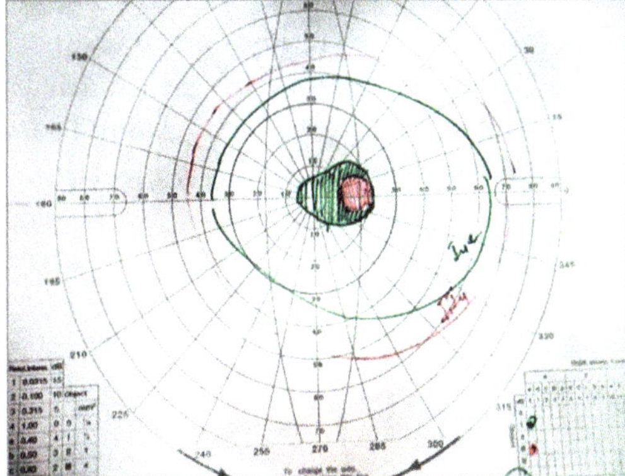

Fig. 5.4.13: Goldmann visual field from optic neuritis, showing Centrocecal scotoma.

CONCLUSION

- Goldmann visual field gives an alphanumeric digits coded print out of patients "hill of vision". Always consider the normal hill in thoughts while interpreting these results.
- Always correlate the results of visual field with clinical examination.
- Goldmann visual field is also helpful in representing neurological conditions, in addition to glaucomatous field defects.
- Therefore, perimetry not only helps in diagnosis of disease, also to look for progression of disease and monitoring the therapy.

VIVA QUESTIONS

1. Difference between kinetic and static perimetry:

Ans: Refer to text.

2. Indications of Goldmann visual field.

Ans: Refer to text.

3. How to read a print out of Goldmann visual field?

Ans: Refer to text.

4. How to elaborate the alphanumerical representation of target size?

Ans: Refer to text.

REFERENCES

1. Harrington DO, Drake MV. The visual fields: a textbook and atlas of clinical perimetry, 6th edition. St Louis: Mosby; 1990.
2. Gandolfo E, Capris P, Corallo G, et al. Effects of random presentation on kinetic threshold, Doc Ophthalmol Proc Series. 1985;42:539.
3. Hickman SJ. Neurological visual field defects. Neuro-ophthalmology. 2011;35:242-50.

5.5. ULTRASOUND BIOMICROSCOPY

Saurabh Verma, Talvir Sidhu, Tanuj Dada

INTRODUCTION

Ultrasound biomicroscopy (UBM) was first developed by Pavlin and associates as a method to obtain high resolution images of anterior segment in situ.[1] They used 50–100 MHz frequency probe to demonstrate its ability to determine relationship between cornea, angle, iris, zonules, and lens. With time, it has emerged as a useful imaging modality to study other conditions such as adnexal pathology, assessment of trauma, lens position, iris cysts, corneal changes with refractive surgeries, etc.

PRINCIPLE

Ultrasound biomicroscopy (Fig. 5.5.1) makes use of a transducer capable of producing very high frequency ultrasound. Conventional ophthalmic ultrasound uses around 10 MHz frequencies. UBM uses frequency between 35–100 MHz. This increases resolution of images but at the expense of depth of penetration and smaller angular field. An axial and lateral resolution up to 25 and 50 microns respectively can be achieved. An image up to ciliary zonules and anterior part of lens can be obtained.

TECHNIQUE

After explaining the procedure to the patient in detail, topical anesthesia is given with 0.5% proparacaine or 4% xylocaine. Patient is made to lie in supine position and an eye cup made up silicon or plastic (Fig. 5.5.2), of sufficient size is applied. Then it is filled with water to create a small water bath. Scanning is performed with ultrasound transducer dipped in water bath. The transducer is held in such a way that the scanning beam strikes the target tissue as perpendicularly as possible.[2] It is difficult to perform if palpebral aperture is small.

USES

- *Glaucoma:* Ultrasound biomicroscopy can be used for following in glaucoma[3]:
  - *Anterior chamber biometry*: Corneal thickness, anterior chamber depth,

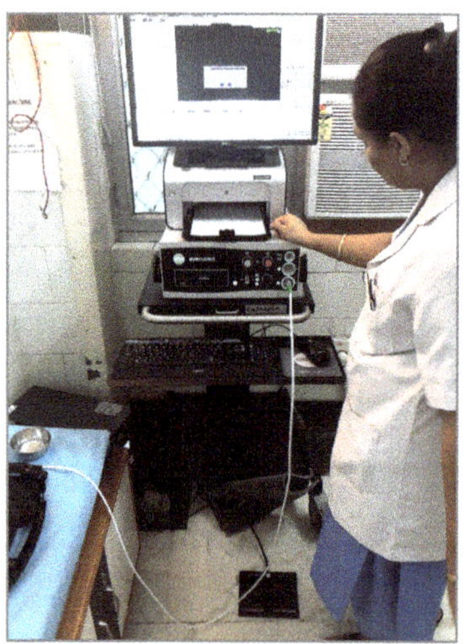

Fig. 5.5.1: Ultrasound biomicroscopy (UBM).

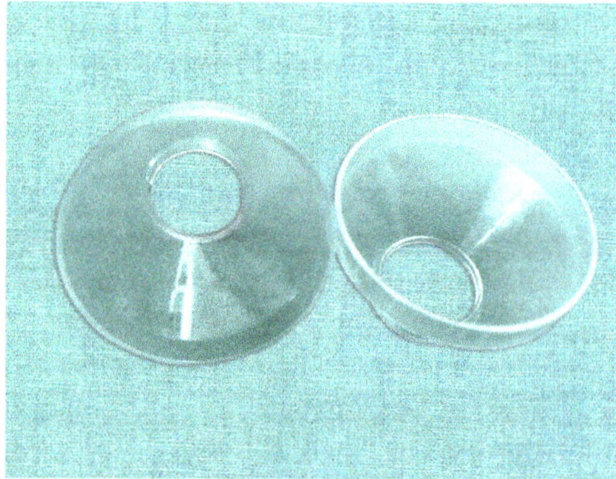

Fig. 5.5.2: Eye cup made up silicon or plastic.

posterior chamber depth, intraocular lens (IOL)/lens thickness, scleral thickness, iris thickness, etc. (Fig. 5.5.3).

- To examine angle structures and their mutual relationship. Scleral spur can easily be identified and is used as a landmark for interpretation of images.
- *Plateau iris syndrome*: It is characterized by presence of anteriorly directed ciliary processes with obliteration of the iridociliary sulcus and steeply rising root of iris followed by flat iris profile. This is seen "sine wave configuration" of iris on indentation gonioscopy (Fig. 5.5.4).
- *Pigment dispersion syndrome*: It is characterized by posterior bowing of mid peripheral iris called "s-shaped" configuration (Fig. 5.5.5).
- *To determine occludability of angle*: UBM is better than dark room gonioscopy because it can be better standardized (Figs. 5.5.6 and 5.5.7).
- To determine patency of iridotomy
- *To determine functional status of filtering surgery*: UBM can be used to show patency of sclerotomy and peripheral

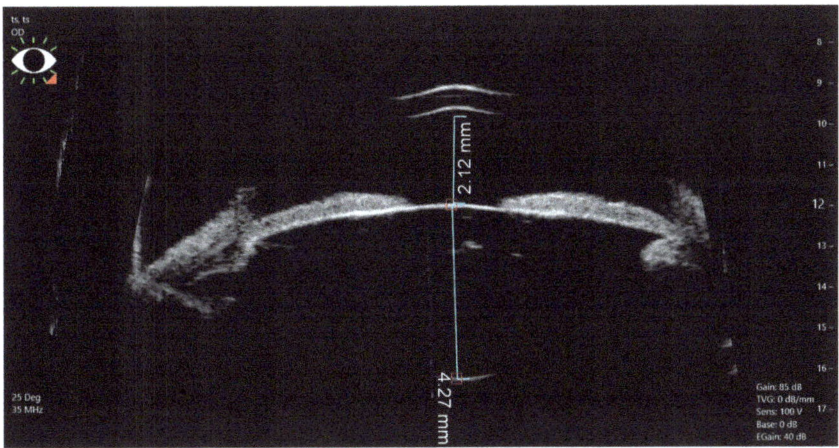

Fig. 5.5.3: Biometry using UBM.

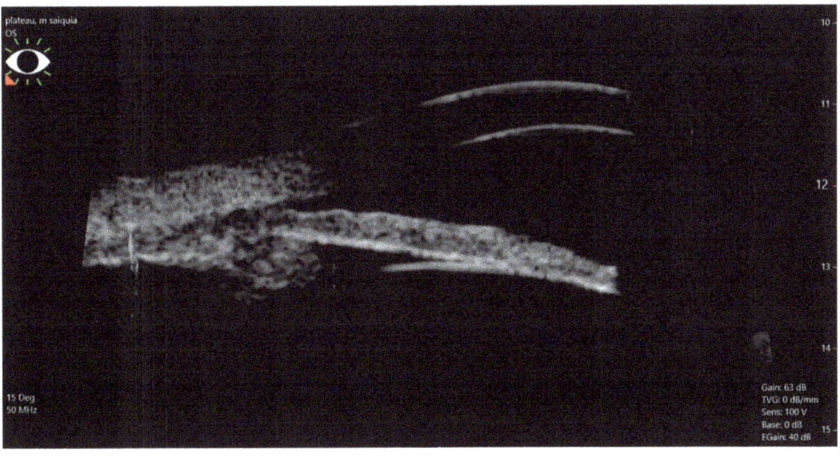

Fig. 5.5.4: Obliteration of iridociliary cleft in plateau iris.

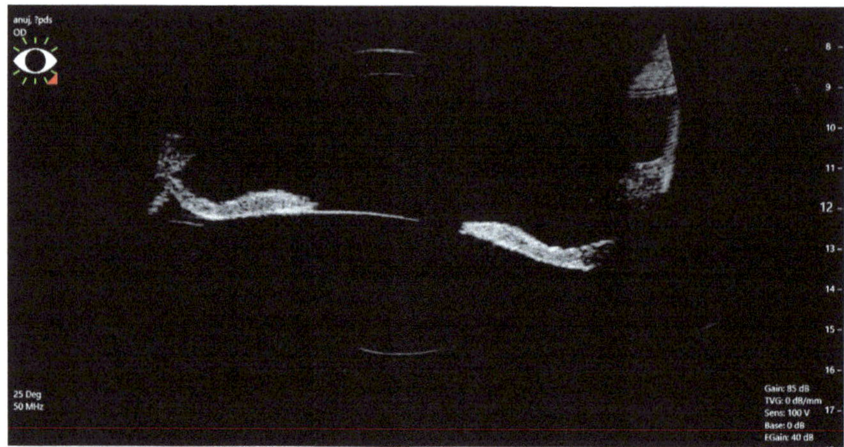

Fig. 5.5.5: Pigment dispersion syndrome showing posterior bowing of the mid-peripheral iris causing s-shaped iris configuration.

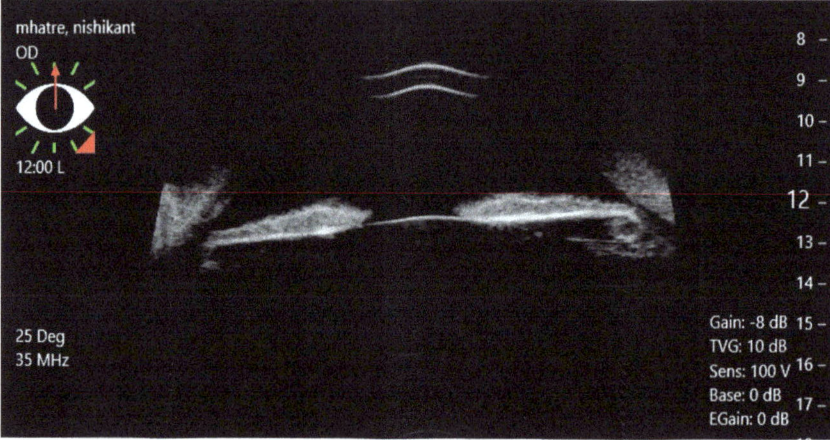

Fig. 5.5.6: Flat iris configuration in a wide open angle.

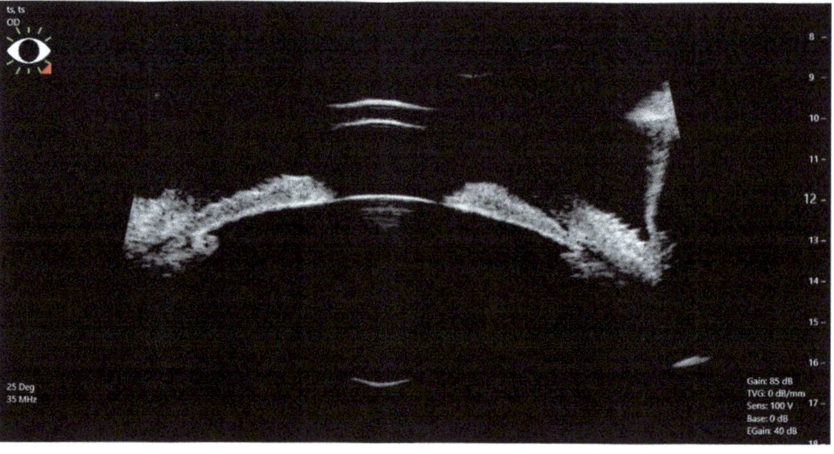

Fig. 5.5.7: UBM done in mesopic conditions in a patient with thick lens showing relative pupillary block.

iridotomy. It has been used to study characteristics of blebs based on their height and reflectivity.

- It can be used to study glaucoma secondary to solid tumors, cysts, lens, anterior push of lens on iris, etc.
- It is a very good procedure for determining presence and extent of shallow choroidal detachments and cyclodialysis clefts (Fig. 5.5.8).

- To evaluate cysts and tumors of iris, ciliary body and angle. It can be used to determine exact location, dimension, thickness of wall and internal characteristics of cysts and tumors[4] (Fig. 5.5.9).
- *To evaluate tumors of ocular surface*: It is a very useful tool for evaluating dimensions and intraocular extension of ocular surface tumors.
- *To evaluate eyelid lesions*: It is a useful tool to determine tissue characteristics depth of eyelid lesions.[5,6]
- *To evaluate aponeurotic ptosis*: It can be used for measuring thickness of levator palpebrae aponeurosis which is thinned out in aponeurotic ptosis.[7]
- *To evaluate corneal conditions*: It has been used to examine sclerocornea, corneal dystrophy, limbal dermoids, etc.[8,9]

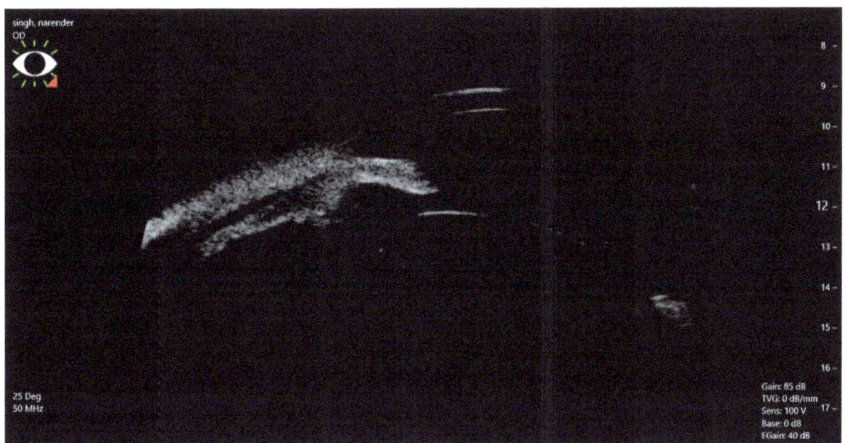

Fig. 5.5.8: UBM showing shallow CD.

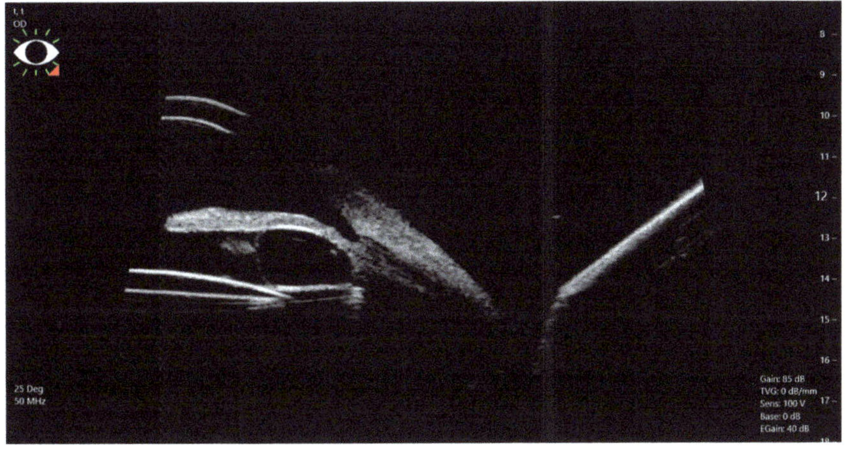

Fig. 5.5.9: Iris cyst causing localized shallowing of anterior chamber.

- To evaluate eyes with retinoblastoma: UBM is a sensitive method for studying ciliary region, anterior retina and anterior segment in eyes with retinoblastoma. It is useful for better staging of advanced disease.[10]
- To evaluate extent of anterior proliferative vitreretinopathy (PVR) in cases with retinal detachment.
- To determine capsular support in patients with dropped IOL or lens.
- To examine any foreign body impacted in the region of ciliary body.
- To study anterior segment details in patients with corneal opacity.
- To rule out cases with lens subluxation in non-dilating pupil.
- To study stability of sulcus fixated IOL.
- To study capsular defects in patients with posterior polar cataract.

LIMITATIONS

- It is contact procedure.
- Cannot be done in eyes with perforations and open globe injuries.
- Application of cup may distort angle structures during examination.

VIVA QUESTIONS

1. What is the role of UBM in Limbal dermoid?

Ans. Limbal dermoid is choristoma more commonly seen in the temporal quadrant. It involves variable thickness of corneal stroma and may even extend into anterior chamber. It is difficult ascertain depth of involvement with slit lamp because of opaque nature of lesion. Surgical management varies according to on size and depth of lesion. A superficial lesion can be managed with shave excision or lamellar keratoplasty where as a deep lesion might require penetrating keratoplasty. Sometimes it can be associated with disorganization of internal structures, which is a relative contraindication for any surgery. UBM can help in accurate measurement of depth and dimensions of dermoid thus helping in proper management of dermoid.[11]

2. What is the role of UBM in corneal hydrops?

Ans. Ultrasound biomicrosopy has been used in qualitative and quantitative evaluation of morphology of corneal hydrops.[12] Descemet membrane tear can be visualized and its edges and length can be quantified. After intracameral air or gas injection, UBM can also be used to visualize Descemet memberane (DM) apposition, apposition of gas bubble to tear edges and resolution of corneal edema and cysts. UBM based studies have shown significant correlation between length of DM tear and corneal thickness in corneal hydrops.

3. Difference between UBM and ASOCT?

Ans.

UBM	*Anterior segment optical coherence tomography (ASOCT)*
Makes use of 35–100 MHz ultrasound to visualize eye structures	Based on optical principle and makes use 1310 nm wavelength
Can visualize beyond iris. Ciliary body and processes can be seen	Cannot visualize beyond anterior limiting membrane of iris
Image quality is worse than ASOCT	Better quality image
Contact procedure	Non contact procedure
Axial resolution: 25 microns Lateral resolution: 50 microns	Axial resolution: 5 microns Lateral resolution: 15 microns

4. Role of UBM in evaluation of filtering Bleb.

Ans. Ultrasound biomicroscopy has been used for evaluating function and morphology of subconjunctival filtering bleb. It has shown to predict a functioning or a non-functioning bleb in 66 and 75% cases respectively.[13] However, ASOCT has proven to be superior in evaluating bleb function. MacWhae et al. classified bleb functioning as good, fair and poor based on presence of a patent pathway and presence or absence of cavities in bleb.

UBM has also been used to study bleb status after laser suture lysis.

5. Role of UBM in PVR.

Ans. Ultrasound biomicroscopy can be used to evaluate anterior PVR. Different patterns which can be identified are dots and cords, echo augmentation and central displacement of retina along with circumferential contraction.[14]

6. What is pseudoplateau iris (PPI)?

Ans. Pseudoplateau iris is a rare cause of glaucoma and is difficult to be differentiated from plateau iris clinically. In PPI, presence of a single large or multiple small iridociliary sulcus cysts result in narrowing of angle. Clinically s-shaped configuration of iris can be seen in both. Bumpy appearance of peripheral iris on slit lamp or gonioscopic examination points towards PPI but is not always evident. UBM is very useful in diagnosing PPI as cysts can be easily visualized with it. Rupturing the cysts with Nd:YAG laser or needle is an effective treatment.[15]

7. Features of malignant glaucoma in UBM.

Ans. Ultrasound biomicroscopy of eyes during malignant glaucoma shows anterior rotation of ciliary processes. They press against periphery of lens in phakic patients or anterior hyaloid phase in aphakic patients thus preventing anterior flow of aqueous. UBM based studies have also shown that lens size in such patients is often smaller than normal which allows for easy anterior movement.[16]

REFERENCES

1. Pavlin CJ, Harasiewicz K, Sherar MD, et al. Clinical use of ultrasound biomicroscopy. Ophthalmology. 1991;98(3):287-95.
2. Ishikawa H, Schuman J. Anterior segment imaging: ultrasound biomicroscopy. Ophthalmol. Clin N Am. 2004;17(1):7-20.
3. Dada T, Gadia R, Sharma A, et al. Ultrasound biomicroscopy in glaucoma. Surv Ophthalmol. 2011;56(5):433-50.
4. Conway RM. Ultrasound biomicroscopy: role in diagnosis and management in 130 consecutive patients evaluated for anterior segment tumours. Br J Ophthalmol. 2005; 89(8):950-5.
5. Kikkawa DO, Ochabski R, Weinreb RN. Ultrasound biomicroscopy of eyelid lesions. Ophthalmologica. 2003;217(1):20-3.
6. Smyth CJ, Möllby R, Wadström T. Phenomenon of hot-cold hemolysis: chelator-induced lysis of sphingomyelinase-treated erythrocytes. Infect Immun. 1975;12(5):1104-11.
7. Hoşal BM, Ayer NG, Zilelioğlu G, et al. Ultrasound biomicroscopy of the levator aponeurosis in congenital and aponeurotic blepharoptosis. Ophthal Plast Reconstr Surg. 2004;20(4):308-11.
8. Kim T, Cohen EJ, Schnall BM, et al. Ultrasound biomicroscopy and histopathology of sclerocornea. Cornea. 1998;17(4):443-5.
9. Castelo Branco B, Chalita MRC, Casanova FH et al. Posterior amorphous corneal dystrophy: ultrasound biomicroscopy findings in two cases. Cornea. 2002;21(2):220-2.
10. Vasquez LM, Giuliari GP, Halliday W, et al. Ultrasound biomicroscopy in the management of retinoblastoma. Eye. 2011; 25(2):141-7.
11. Lanzl IM, Augsburger JJ, Hertle RW, et al. The role of ultrasound biomicroscopy in surgical planning for limbal dermoids. Cornea. 1998; 17(6):604-6.
12. Sharma N, Mannan R, Jhanji V, et al. Ultrasound biomicroscopy-guided assessment of acute corneal hydrops. Ophthalmology. 2011;118(11):2166-71.
13. Wu Q, Zhang Y, Song B, et al. [Evaluation of the bleb morphology and the function of post filtration surgery using slit-lamp adapted optical coherence tomography and ultrasound biomicroscopy in glaucoma patients]. Zhonghua Yan Ke Za Zhi Chin J Ophthalmol. 2008;44(5):402-7.
14. Liu W, Wu Q, Huang S. [Examination of anterior proliferative vitreoretinopathy with ultrasound biomicroscopy]. Zhonghua Yan Ke Za Zhi Chin J Ophthalmol. 1998;34(4): 264-6, 17.
15. Shukla S, Damji KF, Harasymowycz P, et al. Clinical features distinguishing angle closure from pseudoplateau versus plateau iris. Br J Ophthalmol. 2008;92(3):340-4.
16. Shahid H, Salmon JF. Malignant Glaucoma: A Review of the Modern Literature. J Ophthalmol. 2012; 2012:1-6.

5.6 RETINAL NERVE FIBER LAYER OPTICAL COHERENCE TOMOGRAPHY INTERPRETATION

Jyoti Shakrawal, Ritu Nagpal

INTRODUCTION

Optical coherence tomography (OCT) is a noninvasive tool for preperimetric glaucoma detection. Besides, quantitative parameters provided by it are useful for monitoring disease progression.[1] The details of OCT, its principle, and uses have been discussed elsewhere (chapter on ASOCT). Spectral-domain (SD) OCT, capable of taking up to 20,000 A-scans, has almost replaced time-domain OCT. This chapter will discuss a few examples of retinal nerve fiber layer (RNFL) OCT analysis.[2]

SPECTRAL-DOMAIN OPTICAL COHERENCE TOMOGRAPHY PARAMETERS

Following parameters are extremely useful for glaucoma diagnosis and management.

- *Retinal nerve fiber layer parameters*: RNFL measurements are sensitivity as well as specific in differentiating glaucomatous from normal subjects. Following parameters are measured:
  - Temporal-superior-nasal-inferior-temporal (TSNIT) curves
  - Average RNFL thickness
  - Sectoral RNFL thickness.

  Inferior RNFL thickness, along with the mean RNFL thickness are cautiously examined in any glaucoma suspect patients.[1,2]
- *Optic nerve parameters*: Following parameters are measured:
  - Disc size
  - Rim area
  - Rim volume
  - Cup volume.

  The significance of these parameters is still not well defined.
- *Macular thickness*: Following parameters are measured:
  - Ganglion cell complex
  - Inner retina
  - Total macular thickness.

  The average macular thickness in glaucoma eyes is less than those of normal eyes. However, it must be remembered that the measurement of macular thickness is less sensitive RNFL measurements in detecting glaucoma.[2,3]

IMAGE ACQUISITION

Two types of scans can be obtained, a line scan for optic nerve head (ONH) protocols or a circle scan for RNFL protocols. A reliable OCT scan should have signal strength of more than 6.

EXAMPLES

- *Retinal nerve fiber layer thickness (Figs. 5.6.1A to E)*: Following points must be remembered:
  - The first map is color coded RNFL thickness map.
  - Below to it is RNFL deviation map which compares the RNFL thickness with an age-matched normal data.[2]
  - The thicker superior and inferior RNFL around the ONH gives a "double hump" appearance of the RNFL graph in a normal individual.
  - The different color codes suggest:
    - *White*: 5% of the normal population fall within this band
    - *Green*: 5–95% of the normal population fall within this band
    - *Yellow*: 1–5% fall within this band
    - *Red*: 1% of the normal population fall within this band (outside normal limits).
- *Optic disc analysis (Figs. 5.6.2A to E):* The reference plane is used to delineate the

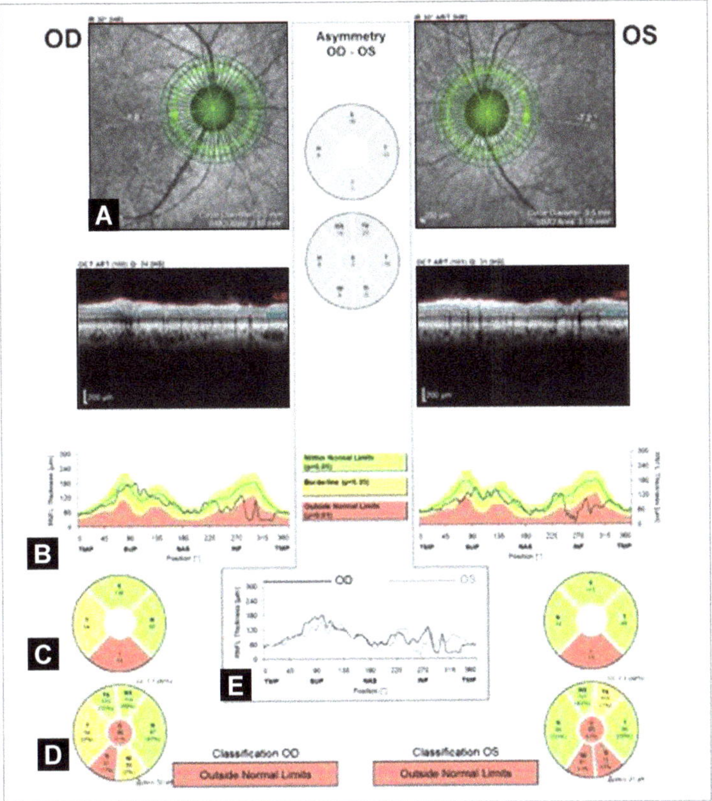

Figs. 5.6.1A to E: Retinal nerve fiber layer (RNFL) optical coherence tomography (OCT) average thickness analysis printout. (A) Fundus photo showing the placement of scan along with an OCT scan inferior to it; (B) Color-coded RNFL thickness graph is indicated by: Within normal limits = Green; Borderline = Yellow; Outside normal limits = Red; (C) Color-coded quadrant thickness map; (D) Color-coded clock-hour thickness map; (E) Blanket RNFL thickness graph of the two eyes together.

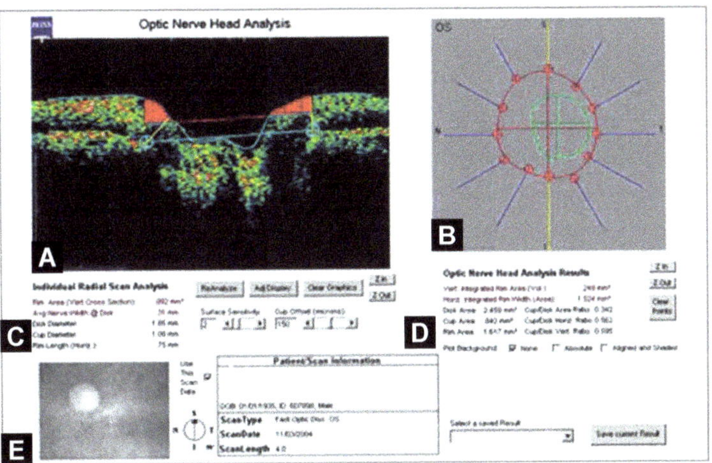

Figs. 5.6.2A to E: Optic disc analysis. (A) Single optical coherence tomography (OCT) image; (B) Radial scans plot, the axis is denoted by a yellow line; (C) Single scan analysis parameters; (D) Overall analysis parameters; (E) Fundus picture showing scan alignment.

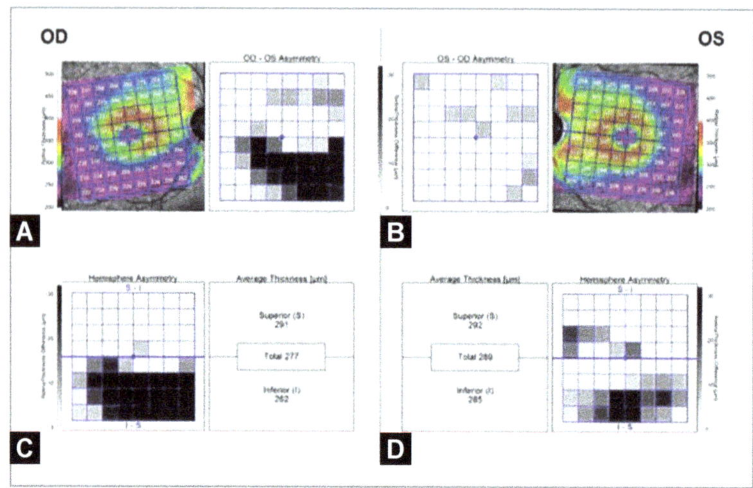

Figs. 5.6.3A to D: Ganglion cell analysis showing inferotemporal thinning. (A) Thickness map showing posterior pole retinal thickness in an 8 × 8 mm grid; (B) OD-OS asymmetry map showing asymmetry in the thickness, between the two eyes (Color scale—the large difference is indicated by darker gray color); (C) Hemisphere asymmetry analysis map showing asymmetry between the two hemispheres; (D) Average thickness, along with superior and inferior hemisphere mean thickness.

cup and neuroretinal rim (NRR) of ONH. The reference plane is set as 150 μ above the line joining both edges of retinal pigment epithelium (RPE).[4]

- *Macular thickness map (Figs. 5.6.3A to D)*: The upper map shows the color-coded retinal thickness, while the inferior map shows the mean retinal thickness of all areas.

REFERENCES

1. Guedes V, Schuman JS, Hertzmark E, et al. Optical coherence tomography measurement of macular and nerve fiber layer thickness in normal and glaucomatous human eyes. Ophthalmology. 2003;110(1):177-89.
2. Stephen V, Chakrabarti A, Rani S, et al. OCT in Glaucoma. Kerala J Ophthalmol. 2007;19(2):183-90.
3. Zangwill LM, Bowd C. Retinal nerve fiber layer analysis in the diagnosis of glaucoma. Curr Opin Ophthalmol. 2006;17(2): 120-31.
4. Bussel II, Wollstein G, Schuman JS. OCT for glaucoma diagnosis, screening, and detection of glaucoma progression. Br J Ophthalmol. 2014;98 (Suppl 2):ii15-9.

5.7 HEIDELBERG RETINA TOMOGRAPH

Gaurav Garg, Jyoti Shakrawal

INTRODUCTION

With the recent advances, diagnosis of glaucoma which was previously just based on clinical assessment is shifting to newer modalities such as visual field (VF) testing for progression, various imaging methods for retinal nerve fiber layer (RNFL) and optic disc characteristics. Optic disc evaluation is always a subjective finding. Heidelberg retina tomograph (HRT, Heidelberg Engineering, Heidelberg Germany) is an imaging technique for topographical assessment of optic disc (Fig. 5.7.1). HRT gives us an objective and reproducible method of documentation. It is based on confocal scanning laser ophthalmoscopy (CSLO) principle for 3 D acquisition of optic disc.[1]

PRINCIPLE

In CSLO-HRT, uses a 670 nm diode-laser light beam for the quantitative imaging of the following:

- Optic disc
- The retinal nerve fiber layer
- Posterior pole.

The procedure does not require dilatation of pupil and take less than a minute to image an eye. The periodic laser beam is deflected by the oscillating mirrors and reflected light is detected by the light-sensitive detector (Fig. 5.7.2). Based on the intensity of reflected light, sequentially scan of optic disc are obtained.

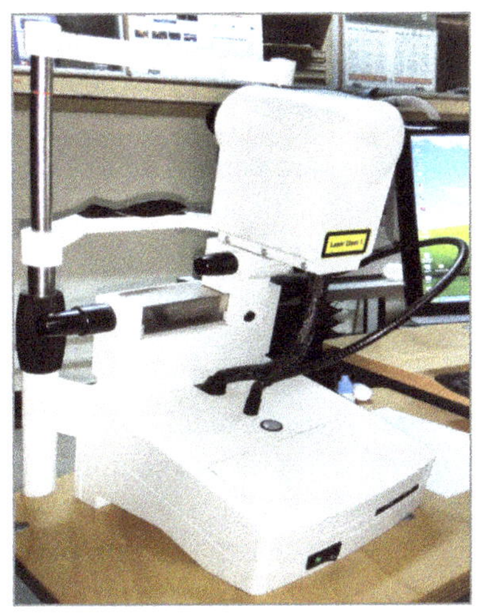

Fig. 5.7.1: Heidelberg retina tomograph 3 (HRT3).

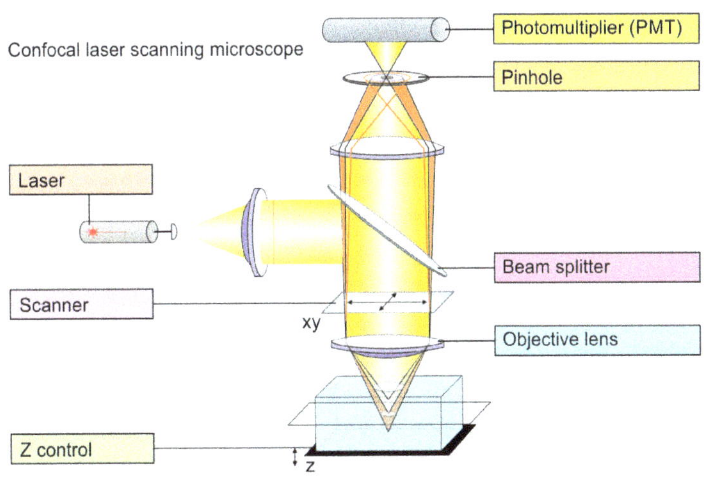

Fig. 5.7.2: Optics of confocal scanning laser ophthalmoscopy (CSLO).

Table 5.7.1: Comparison between HRT II vs HRT III.

S. No.	*Parameters*	*HRT II*	*HRT III*
1.	Normative data for morefield regression analysis (MRA)	110 subjects	733 Caucasian, 215 African American and 100 Asian Indians
2.	Contour line	Manual	Automated
3.	Subjective variation	Present	Absent
4.	Glaucoma probability score (GPS)	Absent	Present
5.	Confocal images acquired	32	64

SCANS

- Successive 2 D scans of optic disc are acquired.
- The depth of 4.0 mm, with approximately 16–64 reflectance images.
- Each consecutive scan is about 0.0625 deeper.
- These scans are combined to give a 3 D contour map of the optic disc.
- $15 \times 15°$ is imaged in a scan.
- Lateral resolution is 10 µm.
- After image acquisition, the contour line is drawn at the scleral ring inner border, either manually as in HRT II, which gives a subjective variation[2] or automated as in HRT III (Table 5.7.1)
- A reference plane is automatically generated as the contour line is drawn, which is parallel and 50 µm below the retinal surface (Fig. 5.7.3). The reference plane helps in dividing the optic disc into rim and cup area. The color-coded images are used as:
  - Green—Rim
  - Blur—Rim slope
  - Red—Cup.

EXAMINATION

- The patient is allowed to sit in front of the machine.
- No mydriasis is required.
- Internal fixation target is given.
- Refractive error of more than 1 diopter cylinder is corrected.

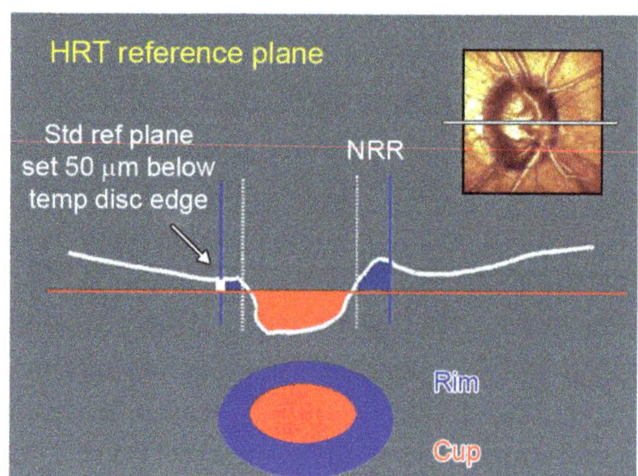

Fig. 5.7.3: Reference plane is located 50 µm below the mean height of the surface along the contour line.

- The diode laser is aimed via the pinhole onto the retina.
- Smaller the aperture size, higher will be the resolution.

INTERPRETATION OF PRINTOUT

A standard deviation (SD) value is obtained in each scan, which gives the idea of image quality of the scan. SD value:

- ≤20 µm: excellent
- 20–30 µm: good
- 30–40 µm: acceptable

Patient Data (Fig. 5.7.4)

- Provides information on exam type as baseline or follow-up.
- Demographic information (patient name, age, gender, date of birth etc.).
- Information including image quality score, and focus position.

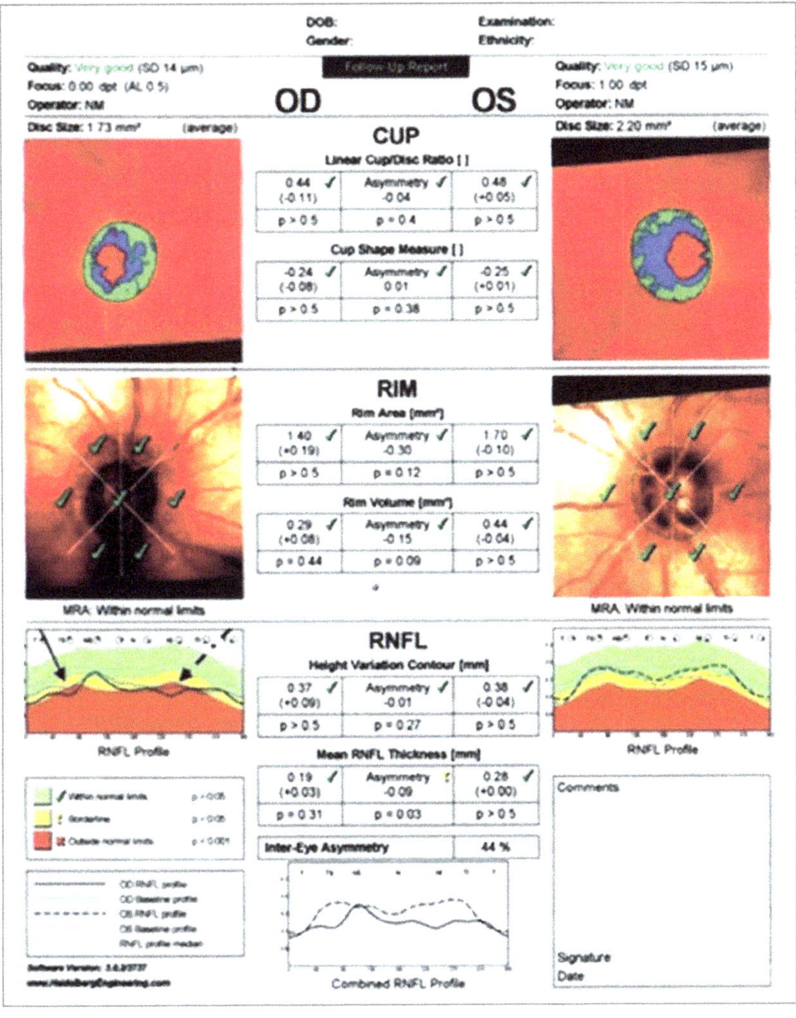

Fig. 5.7.4: Normal heidelberg retina tomograph print out.

Topography Image

- Pseudocolor image.
- Gives disc size, shape, and location of the cup.
- Neuroretinal rim (NRR) appears green, sloping NRR appears blue, and cup appears red.

Reflectance Image

- Pseudocolor image.
- The optic disc is divided into 6 sectors and is compared to a standard database.
- All sectors are then classified with Moorefield regression analysis (MRA), as within:
  - Normal limits (✓)
  - Borderline (!)
  - Outside normal limits (×).

Retinal Nerve Fiber Layer Graph

- The color coded graph in which reference plane is indicated by the red line and retinal surface height by the green line.

- The profile starts 0 as temporal and moves superior, nasal and inferior to temporal again.
- It provides a calculation of the thickness of the nerve fiber layer (NFL).
- Normally, the appearance is "Double Hump Appearance."

Stereometric Analysis of Optic Disc (Table 5.7.2)

- About 75–90% sensitivity
- About 80–97% specificity.

A. *Optic disc*
  - *Area (mm²):* It is the area bounded by the contour line.

B. *Optic cup*
  - *Area (mm²):* It is the area bounded by the contour line, which is located below the reference plane.
  - *Volume (mm³):* It is the volume bounded by the contour line, which is located below the reference plane.

C. *Neuroretinal rim*
  - *Area (mm²):* It is the area bounded by the contour line and located above the reference plane.
  - *Volume (mm²):* It is the volume bounded by the contour line and located above the reference plane.

D. *Cup/disc area ratio:* The ratio between the cup area to disc area.

E. *Linear cup/disc ratio:* The square root of the ratio between cup area to disc area.

F. *Cup-shaped measure:* It is the measure of the overall 3 D shape of optic disc cup. Independent of the reference plane and optic disc size.

G. *Height variation contour:* It is the height difference between the maximum elevated and maximum depressed point of the contour line.

H. *Mean RNFL thickness:* Mean thickness of RNFL along the contour line.

Moorfield's Regression Analysis

- Histogram representation (Fig. 5.7.5).
- Depends on the reference plane, disc area.
- Compares the patient's data (global and local rim area) with an age matched normative data.
- Rim area is coded as green and cup area as red.

Table 5.7.2: Normative stereometric parameter.[3]

S. No.	*Parameters*	*Normal*	*Early defect*	*Moderate defect*	*Advanced defect*
1.	Disc area (mm²)	2.257 ± 0.563	2.345 ± 0.569	2.310 ± 0.554	2.261 ± 0.461
2.	Cup area (mm²)	0.768 ± 0.505	0.953 ± 0.594	1.051 ± 0.647	1.445 ± 0.562
3.	Rim area (mm²)	1.489 ± 0.291	1.393 ± 0.340	1.260 ± 0.415	0.817 ± 0.334
4.	Cup volume (mm³)	0.240 ± 0.245	0.294 ± 0.270	0.334 ± 0.318	0.543 ± 0.425
5.	Rim volume (mm³)	0.362 ± 0.124	0.323 ± 0.156	0.262 ± 0.139	0.128 ± 0.096
6.	Cup/disc ratio	0.314 ± 0.152	0.380 ± 0.179	0.430 ± 0.203	0.621 ± 0.189
7.	Mean cup depth (mm)	0.262 ± 0.118	0.279 ± 0.115	0.289 ± 0.130	0.366 ± 0.182
8.	Maximum cup depth (mm)	0.679 ± 0.223	0.680 ± 0.210	0.674 ± 0.249	0.720 ± 0.276
9.	Cup shape measure	–0.181 ± 0.092	-0.147 ± 0.098	–0.122 ± 0.095	–0.036 ± 0.096
10.	Height variation contour (mm)	0.384 ± 0.087	0.364 ± 0.100	0.330 ± 0.108	0.256 ± 0.090
11.	Mean RNFL thickness (mm)	0.384 ± 0.063	0.217 ± 0.076	0.182 ± 0.086	0.013 ± 0.061
12.	RNFL cross sectional area (mm²)	1.282 ± 0.328	1.155 ± 0.396	0.957 ± 0.440	0.679 ± 0.302

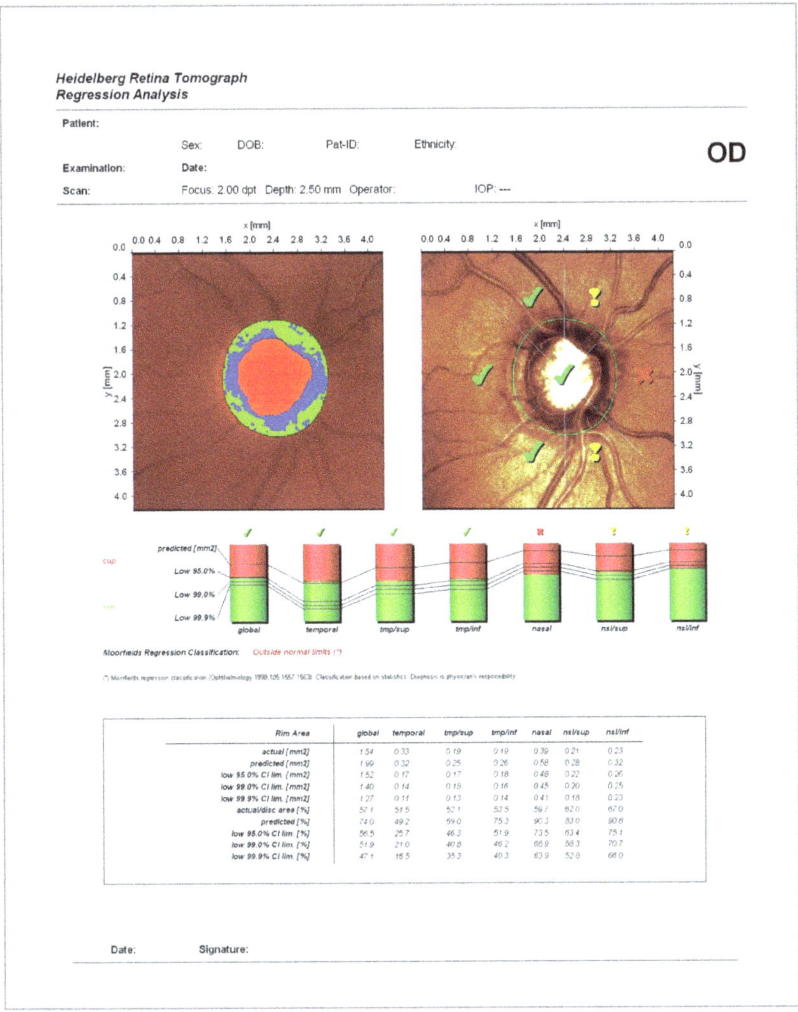

Rim Area	global	temporal	tmp/sup	tmp/inf	nasal	nsl/sup	nsl/inf
actual [mm2]	1.54	0.33	0.19	0.19	0.39	0.21	0.23
predicted [mm2]	1.99	0.32	0.25	0.26	0.58	0.28	0.32
low 95.0% CI lim. [mm2]	1.52	0.17	0.17	0.18	0.48	0.22	0.26
low 99.0% CI lim. [mm2]	1.40	0.14	0.15	0.16	0.45	0.20	0.25
low 99.9% CI lim. [mm2]	1.27	0.11	0.13	0.14	0.41	0.18	0.23
actual/disc area [%]	57.1	51.5	52.1	53.5	59.7	62.0	67.0
predicted [%]	74.0	49.2	69.0	75.3	90.3	83.0	90.8
low 95.0% CI lim. [%]	56.5	25.7	46.3	51.9	73.5	63.4	75.1
low 99.0% CI lim. [%]	51.9	21.0	40.8	46.2	68.9	58.3	70.7
low 99.9% CI lim. [%]	47.1	16.5	35.3	40.3	63.9	52.0	66.0

Fig. 5.7.5: Moorefield's regression analysis.

- Four white lines represents 50%, 95%, 99% and 99.9% prediction interval.

Glaucoma Probability Score

- *Based on five parameters*: Cup size, cup depth, optic nerve rim steepness, horizontal RNFL, and vertical RNFL curvature.
- Does not depend on the reference plane.
- All sectors are then classified same as in MRA as, within normal limits, borderline and outside normal limits (Fig. 5.7.6).

MONITORING THE PROGRESSION

Progression can be measured by comparing ONH stereometric parameters of different scans done on follow-ups.

Progression Analysis with Change Probability Map

- *Top row:* Sequential topographic images
- *Second row:* Sequential reflectance images

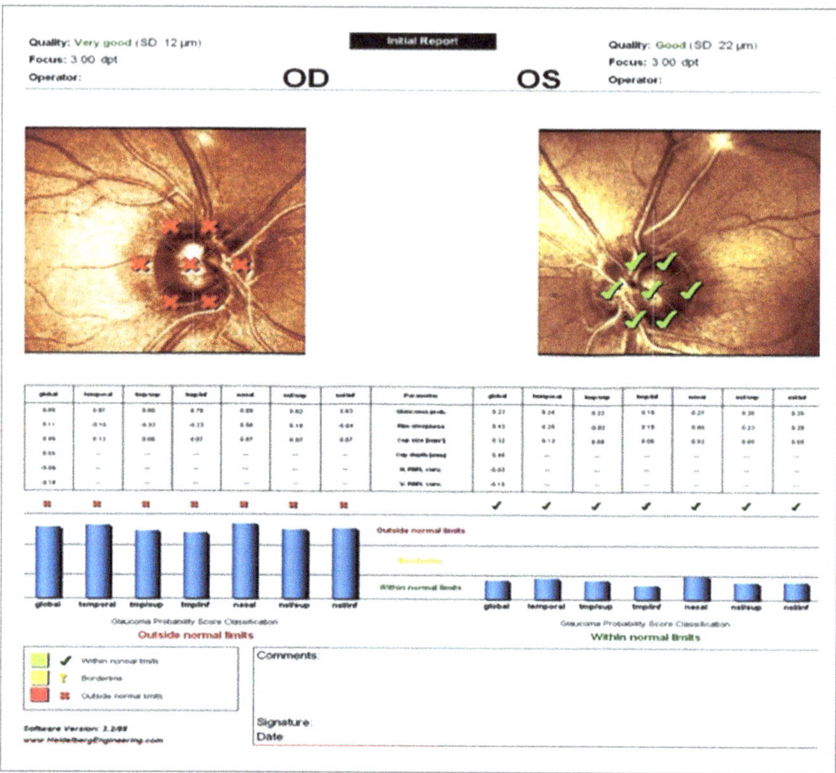

Fig. 5.7.6: Glaucoma probability score (GPS).

- *Third row:* Appears after capturing 4th follow-up scan which starts flagging significance level if the same area is showing a similar change in at least 2 consecutive examinations progression is suspected, and if in 3 consecutive examinations progression is confirmed (Fig. 5.7.7).

CASE (FIG. 5.7.8)

This is a HRT, "OU report" print out of patient named........., age.......

- The quality of the scan is very good with 0.00 dpt focus. This gives us information on both eyes of a glaucoma patient on a single paper.
- The OD disc is larger, whereas the OS disc is average size.
- The linear cup/disc ratio is 0.87 and 0.82 in both eyes, with a cup shape measure of -0.01 and -0.05. The neuro-retinal rim area is 0.81 mm^2 each with the volume of 0.09 mm^3. The RNFL height variation contour shows 0.23 mm variation for both eyes with mean RNFL thickness of 0.04 mm and 0.09 mm in OD and OS.
- For all these parameters, classification as within normal limits (green mark), borderline (yellow mark), outside normal limits (red mark) and the degree of asymmetry is also written. For both the eyes, neuro-retinal rim area and volume are below normal limits. In most of the sectors, MRA results are outside normal limits.
- This HRT concludes inferotemporal RNFL defect of RE, as seen in stereophotograph of RE similarly.

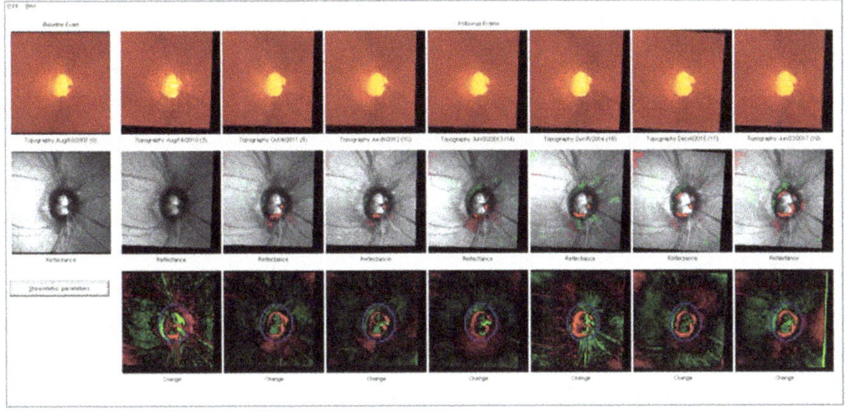

Fig. 5.7.7: Progression analysis with change probability map.

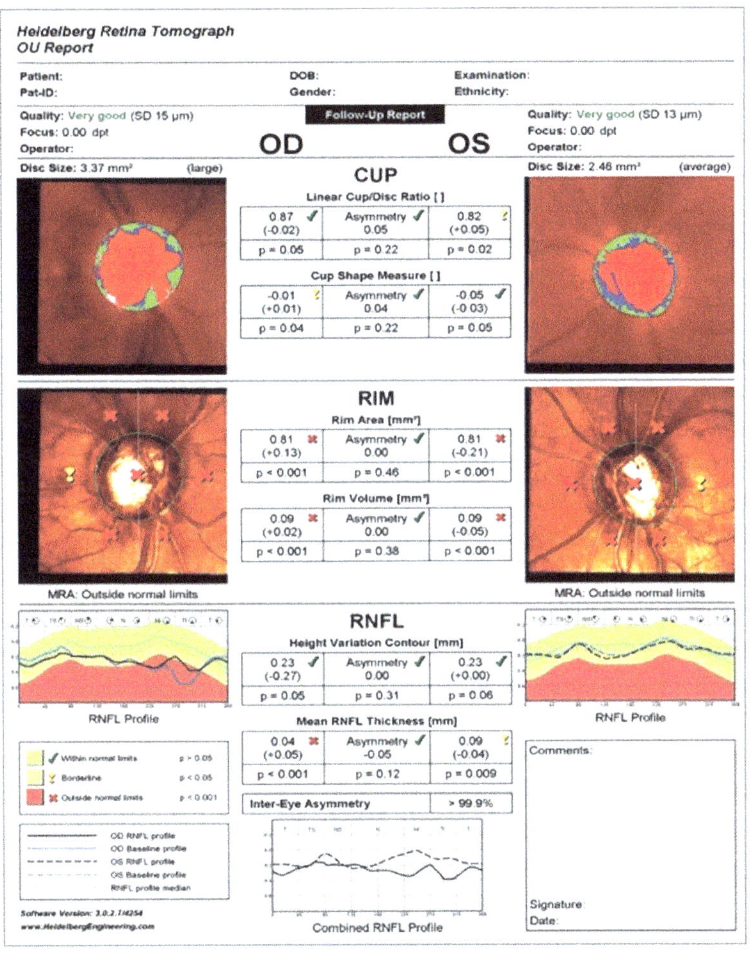

Fig. 5.7.8: Glaucoma probability score (GPS) report.

CONCLUSION

Heidelberg retina tomography provides quick and noninvasive reproducible, objective measurements of the optic disc and RNFL. It helps both in detecting early glaucomatous changes and its progression.

VIVA QUESTIONS

1. What is the principle of HRT?
Ans: Refer to text.

2. How to read a HRT printout?
Ans: Refer to text.

3. What is the significance of green, yellow and red color coding?
Ans: Refer to text.

REFERENCES

1. Quigley HA, Katz J, Derick RJ, et al. An evaluation of optic disc and nerve fiber layer examinations in monitoring progression of early glaucoma damage. Ophthalmology. 1992;99(1):19-28.
2. Miglior S, Albé E, Guareschi M, et al. Intraobserver and interobserver reproducibility in the evaluation of optic disc stereometric parameters by Heidelberg Retina Tomograph. Ophthalmology. 2002;109(6):1072-7.
3. Burk R. Laser Scanning Tomographie: Interpretation der Ausdrucke des Heidelberg Retina Tomographen HRT II. Z prakt Augenheilkd. 2001;22:183-90.

5.8 INSTRUMENTS USED IN GLAUCOMA SURGERIES

Vatsalya Venkatraman, Pranita Sahay, Jyoti Shakrawal

INTRODUCTION

Surgical intervention for glaucoma includes chiefly trabeculectomy and trabeculotomy.

Most instruments required for this procedure are routine except for a few additional ones. The following details will give you a comprehensive idea regarding the appearance and use of each instrument required during the procedure.

WIRE SPECULUM

This instrument is an essential need for almost all ophthalmologic surgeries. It aids to keep the lids apart so one can get a clear field of the area where the surgical procedure needs to be performed. It keeps the eyelashes away from operating field (Fig. 5.8.1).

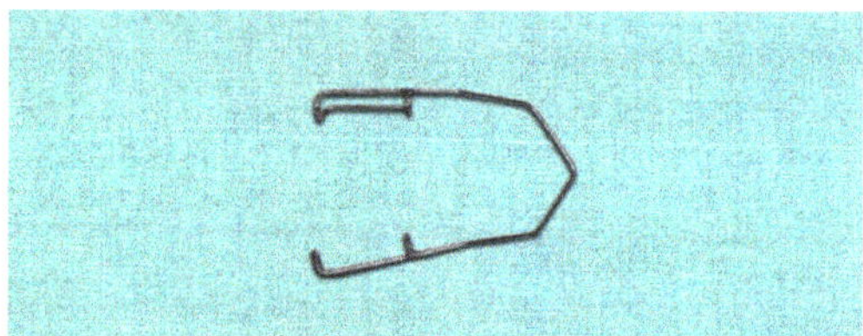

Fig. 5.8.1: Wire speculum.

PLAIN FORCEPS

It is a blunt forceps without any tooth. Its tip has serrations (Fig. 5.8.2).

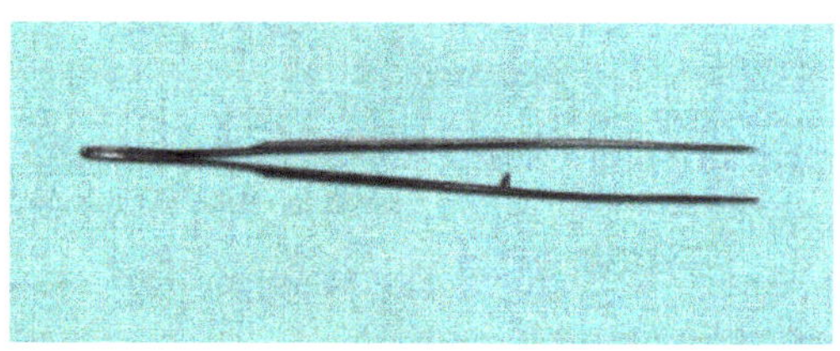

Fig. 5.8.2: Plain forceps.

Uses

- For holding conjunctiva, scleral flap or skin
- For holding sutures while tying.

SUPERIOR RECTUS HOLDING FORCEPS

It is a toothed S-shaped forceps specially designed to fit into the orbit while trying to grasp the muscle belly while passing the bridle suture (Fig. 5.8.3).

LIM FORCEPS

It is also a toothed forceps to hold the limbus or scleral flap or sutures (Fig. 5.8.4).

ARTERY (HEMOSTATIC) FORCEPS

It is a blunt tipped forceps with multiple serrations near the tip and a locking mechanism on the other end. It is available in various sizes (Fig. 5.8.5).

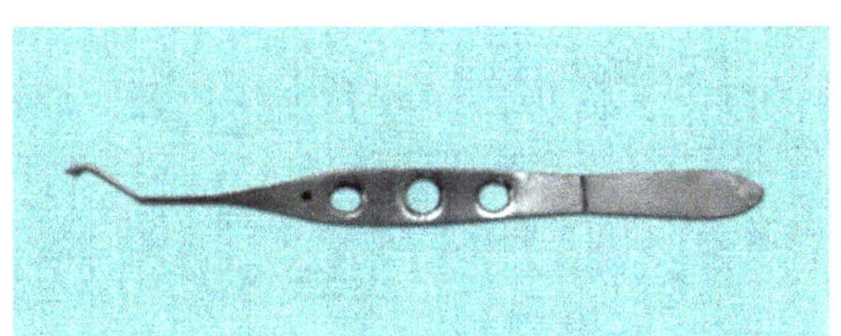

Fig. 5.8.3: Superior rectus holding forceps.

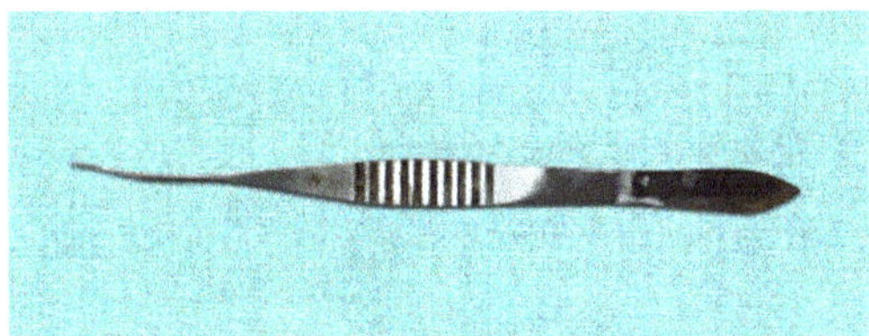

Fig. 5.8.4: Lim forceps.

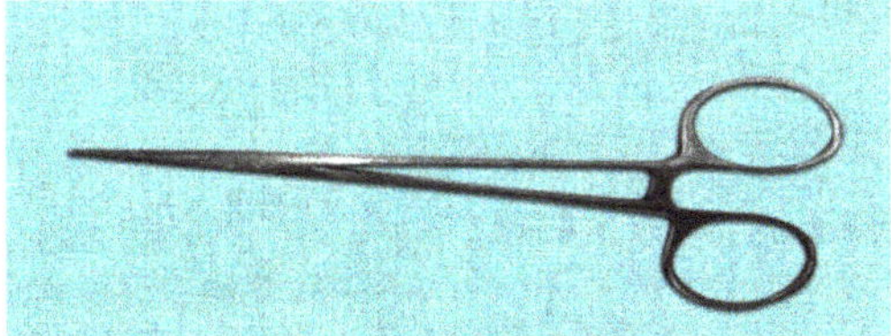

Fig. 5.8.5: Artery (hemostatic) forceps.

Uses

- To hold the bleeders during the surgery
- To tie the fixation suture.

BARRAQUER NEEDLE HOLDER

It is a needle holder with fine serrations at the jaw for better grip while passing sutures through the conjunctiva, cornea and sclera (Fig. 5.8.6).

ARRUGA NEEDLE HOLDER

It is a large needle holder with one end being flat for placement of the surgeon's thumb and the other end having serrations for better grip of the suture. In glaucoma surgery, it is used to pass the superior rectus bridle suture (Fig. 5.8.7).

GLOBE HOLDING FORCEPS

The tip of this forceps is toothed for better grip while holding conjunctiva and episcleral tissue near the limbus. It can also be used while mitomycin application (Fig. 5.8.8).

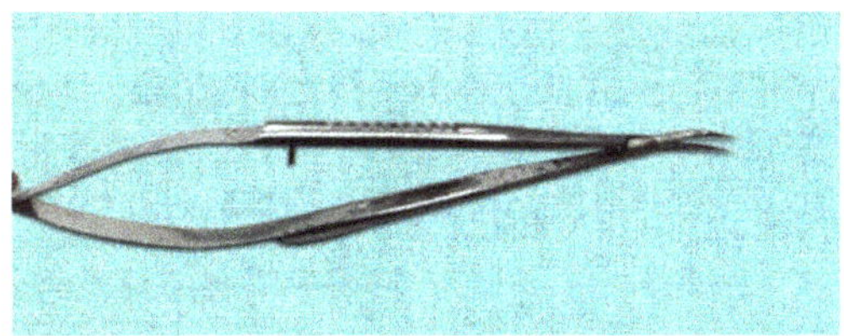

Fig. 5.8.6: Barraquer needle holder.

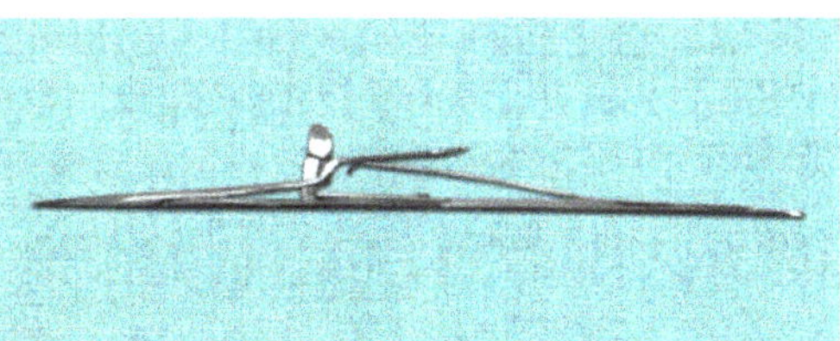

Fig. 5.8.7: Arruga needle holder.

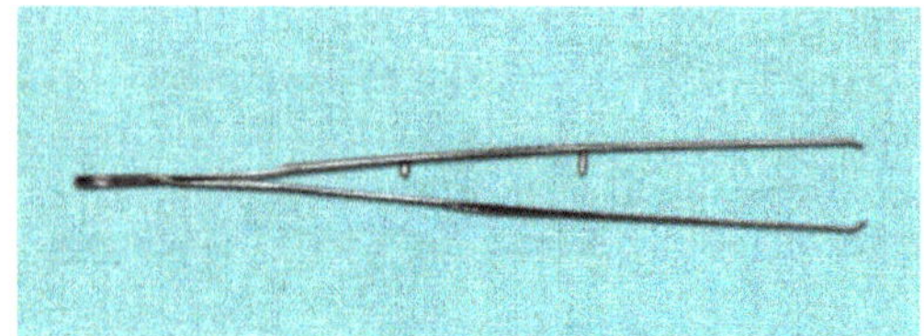

Fig. 5.8.8: Globe holding forceps.

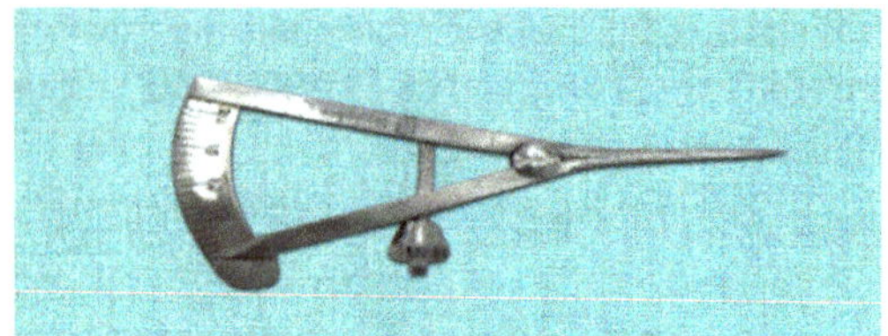

Fig. 5.8.9: Castroviejo caliper.

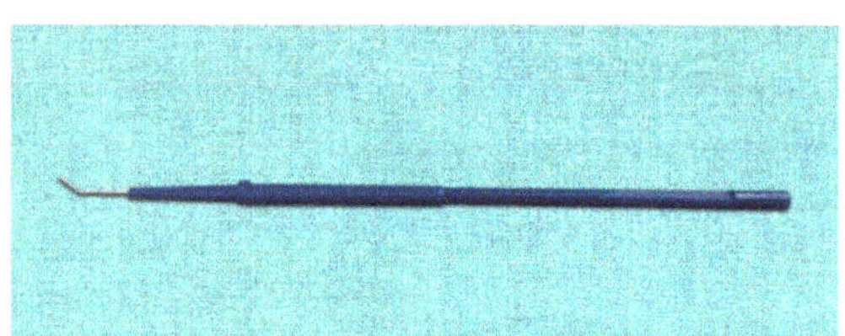

Fig. 5.8.10: Crescent blade.

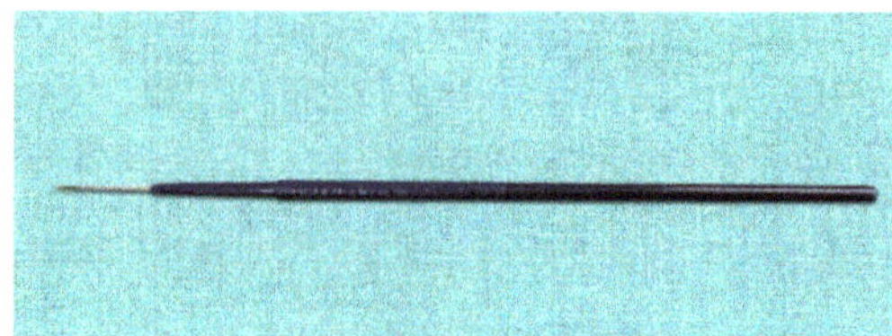

Fig. 5.8.11: Microvitreoretinal (MVR) blade.

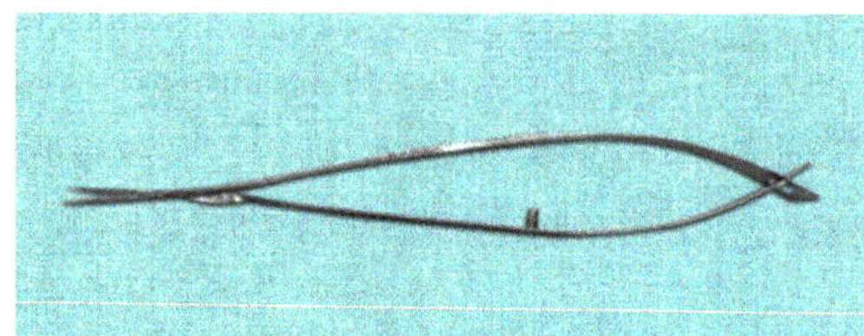

Fig. 5.8.12: Vanas scissors.

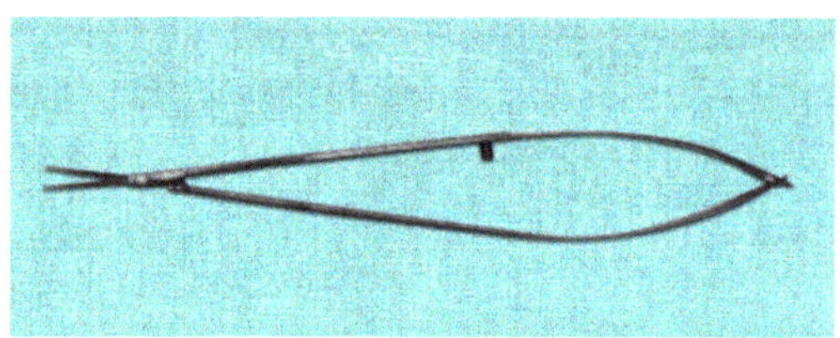

Fig. 5.8.13: Castroviejo corneoscleral scissors.

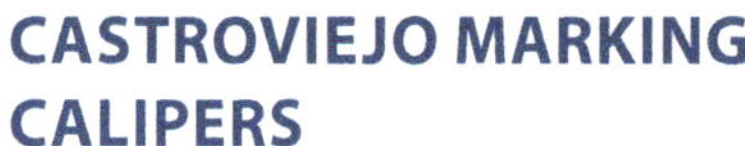

CASTROVIEJO MARKING CALIPERS

It measures from 0 mm to 15 mm in 0.25 increments. It consists of a standard caliper handle and an adjustable screw in the center. The center of the tips measures the size of the objects that needs to be measured. In trabeculectomy, this instrument is used to measure the size of scleral flap (Fig. 5.8.9).

CRESCENT BLADE

It is a blunt tipped instrument with beveled edges and having cut-splitting action on both the sides. It is used for faster dissection of the scleral flap in trabeculectomy (Fig. 5.8.10).

MICROVITREORETINAL BLADE

It is a fine straight instrument with triangular knife at its distal end having cutting edge on both the sides. It is used to make side port entry at the limbus. Also, used while making ostium (Fig. 5.8.11).

VANAS SCISSORS

It is a fine scissor working on spring action used for cutting fine sutures. Also, for cutting tissue while making ostium (Fig. 5.8.12).

CASTROVIEJO CORNEO-SCLERAL SCISSORS

It is a fine curved scissor working on spring action used to cut the scleral tissue flap or for conjunctival dissection (Fig. 5.8.13).

KELLY'S PUNCH

This instrument is used to perform the sclerotomy to drain the excess fluid from the anterior chamber. It has a serrated squeeze handle for precise control. The advantage

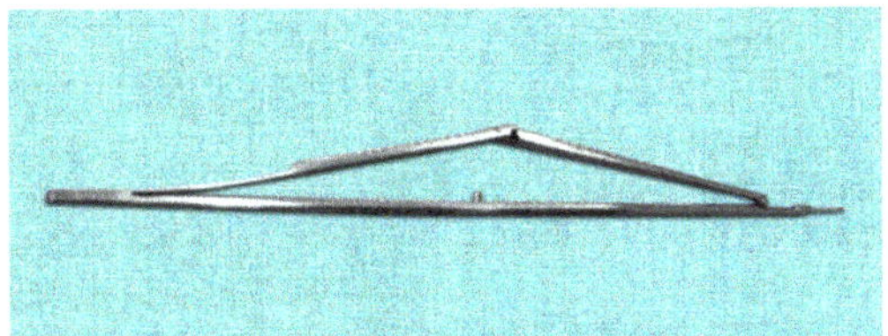
Fig. 5.8.14: Kelly's punch.

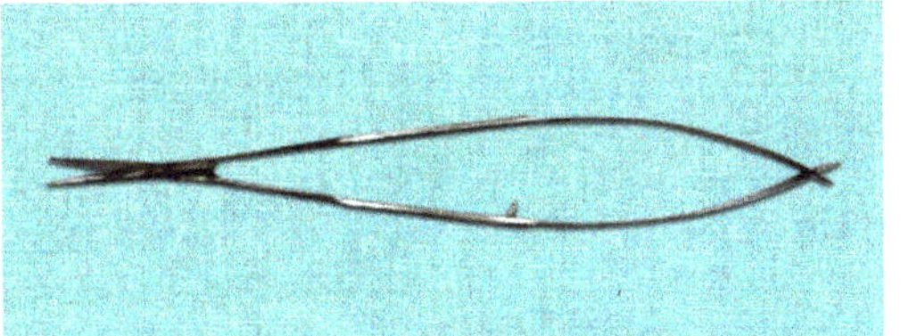
Fig. 5.8.15: Westcott conjunctival scissors.

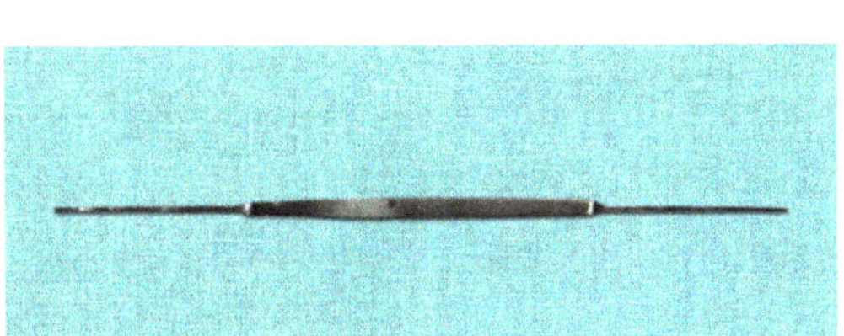
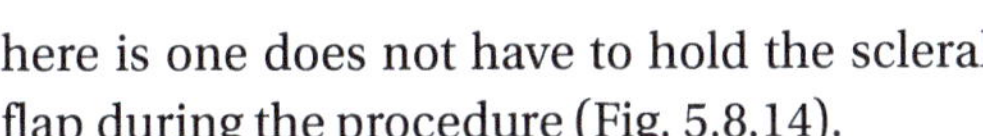
Fig. 5.8.16: Dastoor iris repositor.

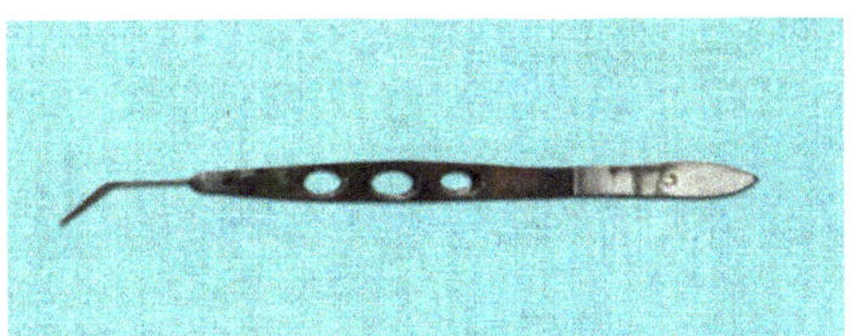
Fig. 5.8.17: McPherson's forceps.

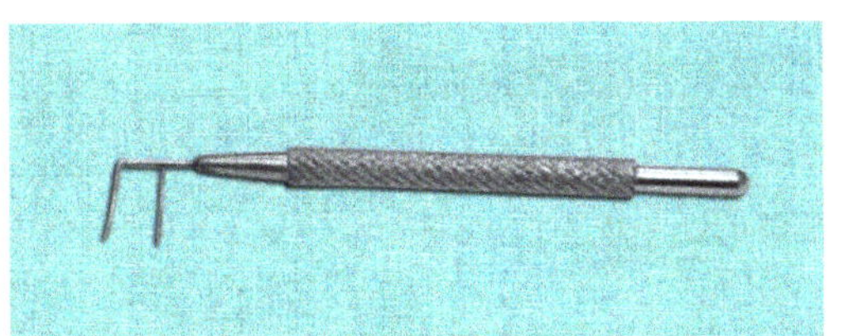
Fig. 5.8.18: Trabeculotome.

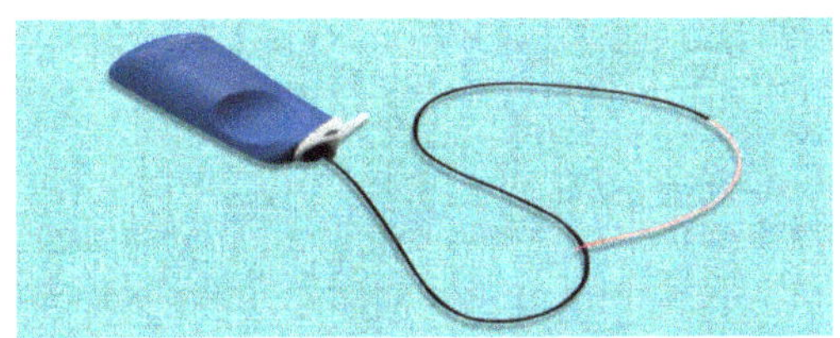
Fig. 5.8.19: Illuminated microcatheter.

here is one does not have to hold the scleral flap during the procedure (Fig. 5.8.14).

WESTCOTT CONJUNCTIVAL SCISSORS

It is a stout scissor with straight/curved blades for conjunctival dissection (Fig. 5.8.15).

DASTOOR IRIS REPOSITOR

It is a flat and straight/curved blade with blunt edges used for repositioning the iris back in the anterior chamber. In trabeculectomy, it can be used to send the iris back after iridotomy to prevent ostium from block (Fig. 5.8.16).

KELMAN-MCPHERSON FORCEPS

It is a fine sharp tipped non-toothed forceps with angulation to hold sutures while tying. Also, can be used for mitomycin application or holding conjunctiva (Fig. 5.8.17).

HARMS TRABECULOTOME

It is of both sides, right sided and left sided. This instrument is used to manually catheterize the Schlemm's canal for about 120° approximately (trabeculotomy) along with trabeculectomy (Fig. 5.8.18).

ILLUMINATED MICROCATHETER

It is used for 360° catheterization of the Schlemm's canal. It has an atraumatic tip for smooth passage along with an illumination source at the tip, which acts as a guide through the canal (Fig. 5.8.19).

6 CHAPTER

Squint and Neuro-ophthalmology

6.1 HESS CHART/LEES SCREEN

Ritu Nagpal, Mousumi Bannerjee, Anin Sethi, Pallavi Singh

INTRODUCTION

A Hess chart is plotted to aid in the diagnosis and monitoring of a patient with incomitant strabismus, such as an extraocular muscle palsy (e.g. third, fourth or sixth nerve paresis) or a mechanical or myopathic limitation (e.g., thyroid ophthalmopathy, blow-out fracture or myasthenia gravis).[1]

The chart is commonly prepared using either the Lees or Hess screen, which facilitate plotting of the dissociated ocular position as a measure of extraocular muscle action.

Information provided by the Hess chart should be regarded in the context of other investigations such as the field of binocular single vision.

Following points must be remembered:

- *Principle*: It is based on the haploscopic. Here two targets are projected, examiner points one target and the subject is asked to superimpose it with the point (Fig. 6.1.1).
- Both Hering's law of equal innervation and Sherrington's law of reciprocal innervation are utilized in this test[2]:
  - *Hering's law of equal innervation*: An equal and simultaneous innervation flows from the brain to the pair of muscles of both eyes (yoke muscle) which contract simultaneously in different binocular movements.
  - Sherrington's law of reciprocal innervation states that "When a muscle contracts, its direct antagonist relaxes to an equal extent allowing smooth movement".
- Dissociation of two eyes is through colors.
- *Prerequisites for testing*: Patient should have the following:
  - A proper understanding of the procedure
  - Patients visual acuity must be good
  - Patient must have a central fixation
  - NRC (Normal retinal correspondence).

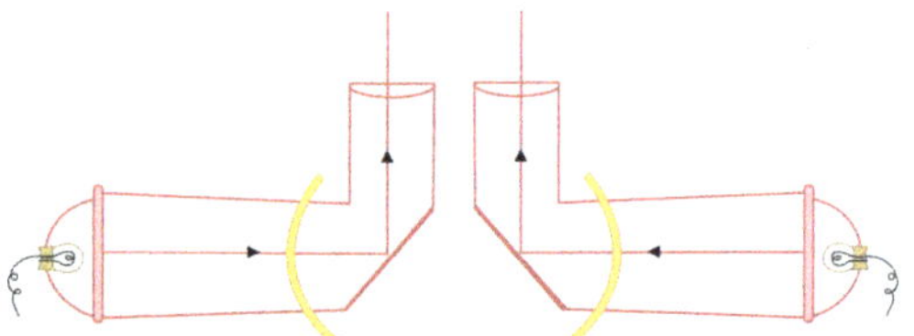

Fig. 6.1.1: Haploscopic principle.

HESS SCREEN

- The Hess screen (Fig. 6.1.2) contains a tangent pattern displayed on a dark gray background.

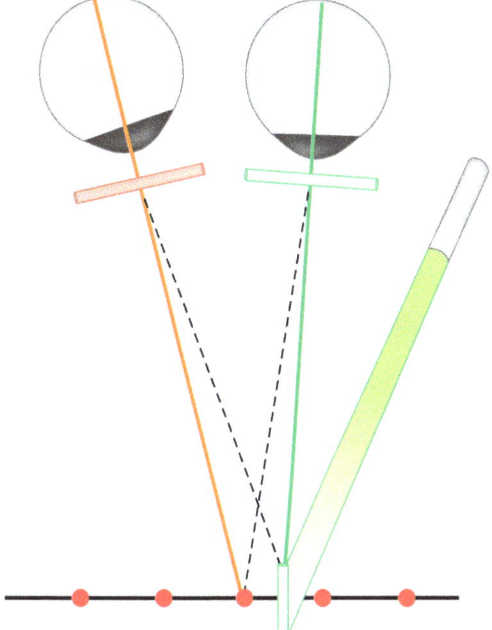

Fig. 6.1.2: Hess charting.

- The cardinal positions are indicated by use of red lights that can be illuminated through a control panel.
- The cardinal positions are illuminated both in the central (which is 15° from the primary position) as well as the peripheral field (30°).
- Within the screen, each square represents 5° of ocular rotation.
- The testing procedure includes:
  - The test is performed with each eye fixating in turn.
  - It is done at 50 cm.
  - The patient wears red and green glasses. The eyes are dissociated by the use of reversible goggles incorporating a red and a green lens, the red lens in front of the fixating eye and the green lens the nonfixating eye.
  - Green glass is placed over the eye to be tested.
  - The chart has electronically operated board with small red lights.
  - Next, the goggles are changed.
  - Red points of lights are illuminated at selected positions on the screen.
  - The patient is instructed to match these points using a green pointer.
  - If the patient is orthophoric the red and green lights superimpose in all the positions of gaze.
  - The goggles are then reversed and the procedure repeated.

LEES SCREEN

- It consists of 2 opalescent glass screens positioned at 90° to each other. Dissociation of the eyes is achieved by a two-sided plane mirror that bisects these two screens (Figs. 6.1.3A to C).
- Each of the eyes can see only one of the two screens.
- Each screen has a tangent pattern which is revealed only when the screen is illuminated.
- The patient faces the nonilluminated screen.
- The chin positioned over the chin rest.
- Using a pointer, the examiner indicates a target point on the illuminated tangent pattern and the patient places the pointer on the nonilluminated screen, at a position supposed to be superimposed on the spot pointed by the examiner.
- The nonilluminated screen is briefly illuminated by the examiner using a footswitch to facilitate recording of the dot indicated by the patient.
- When the procedure has been completed for one eye, the patient is rotated through 90° to face the previously illuminated screen and the procedure repeated.

INTERPRETATION

- The eye with paretic muscle is represented by the smaller chart (Figs. 6.1.4 to 6.1.8),

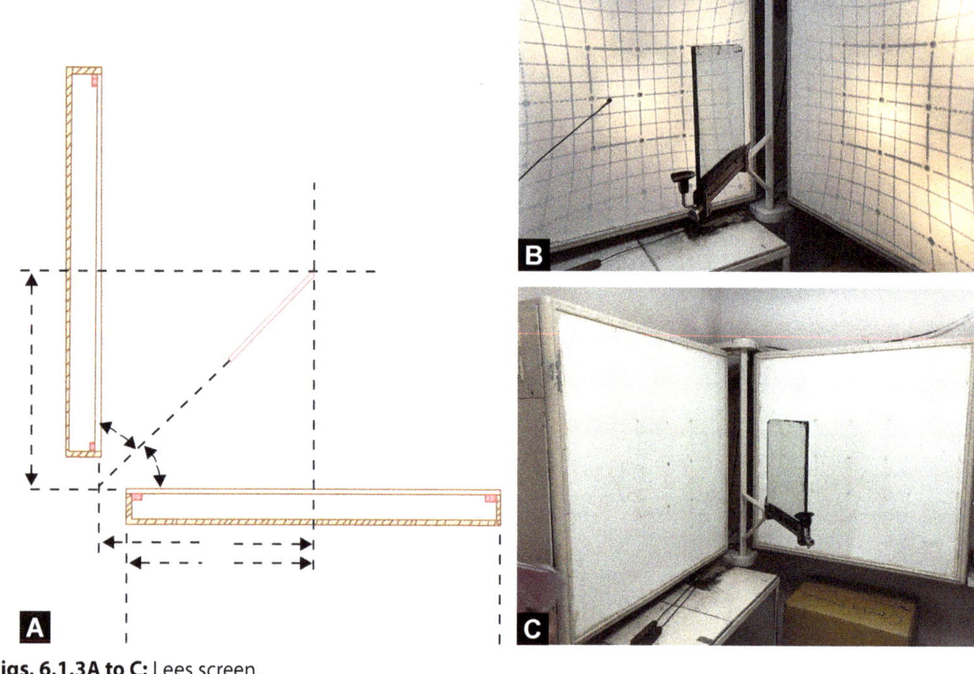

Figs. 6.1.3A to C: Lees screen.

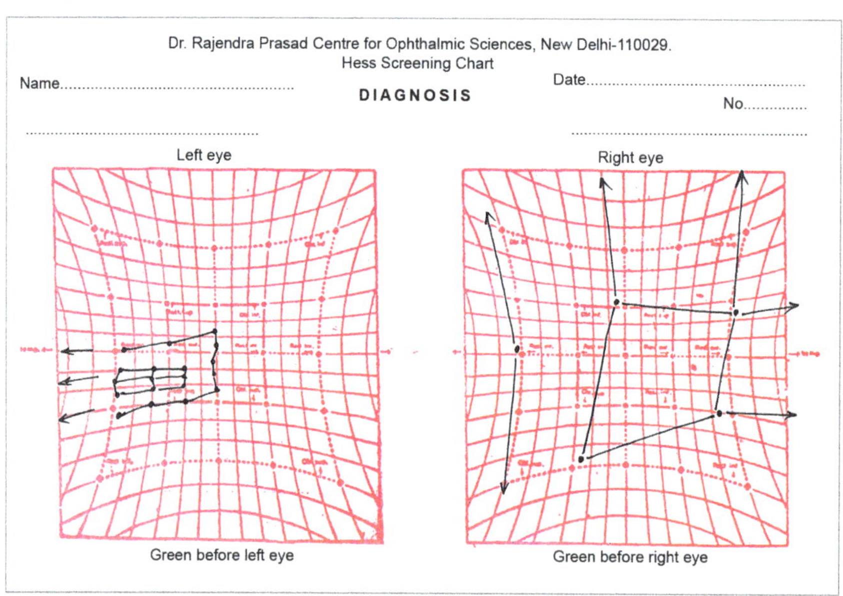

Fig. 6.1.4: Hess chart of 3rd nerve palsy.

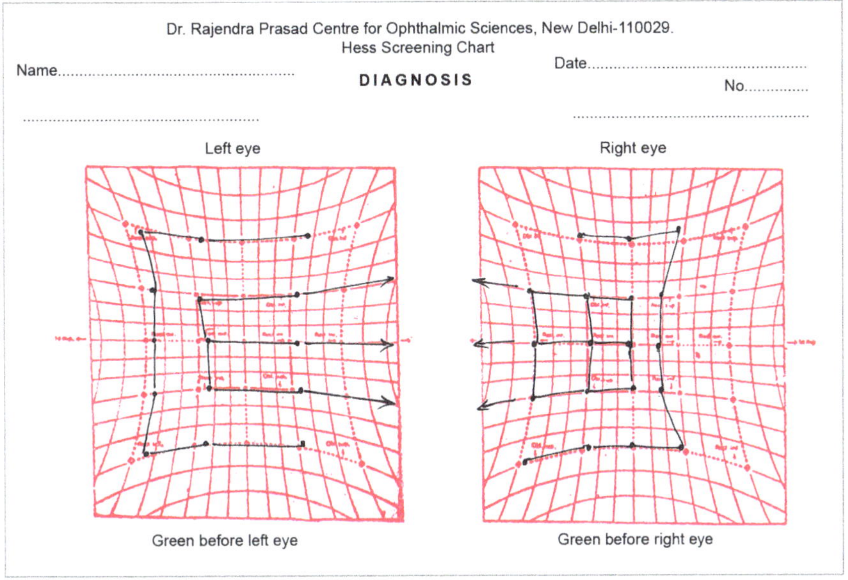

Fig. 6.1.5: Hess chart of 6th nerve palsy.

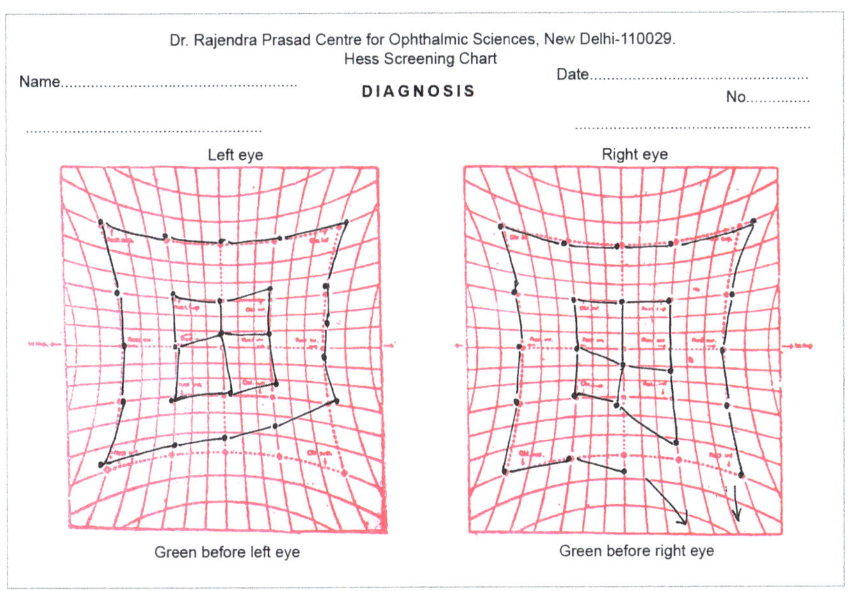

Fig. 6.1.6: Hess chart of superior oblique palsy.

while the eye with overacting yoke muscle is represented by the larger chart.

- The maximum restriction will be seen in the smaller chart along the direction of action of the paretic muscle while maximum expansion will be seen in the larger chart along action of the yoke muscle.
- In comitant deviation, the fields are of similar size and shape while in case of incomitant deviation it varies in shape and size.

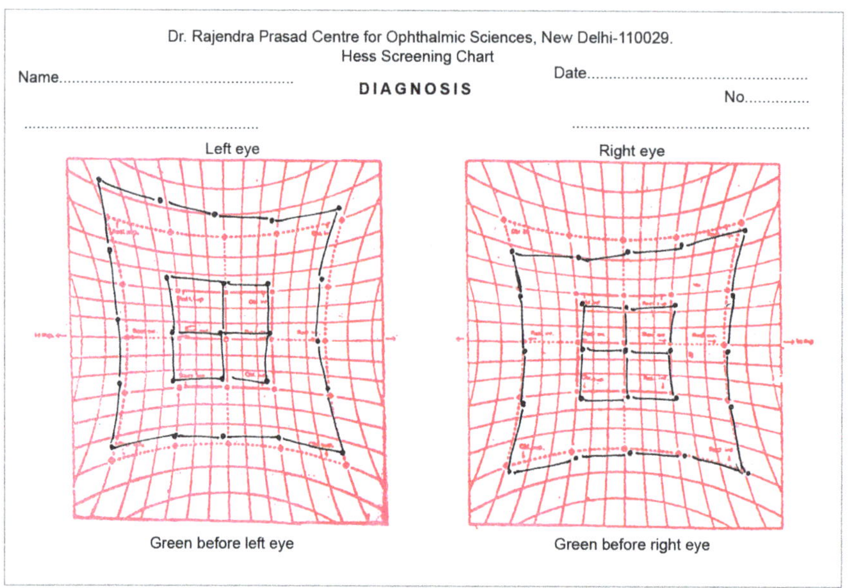

Fig. 6.1.7: Hess chart of Brown's syndrome.

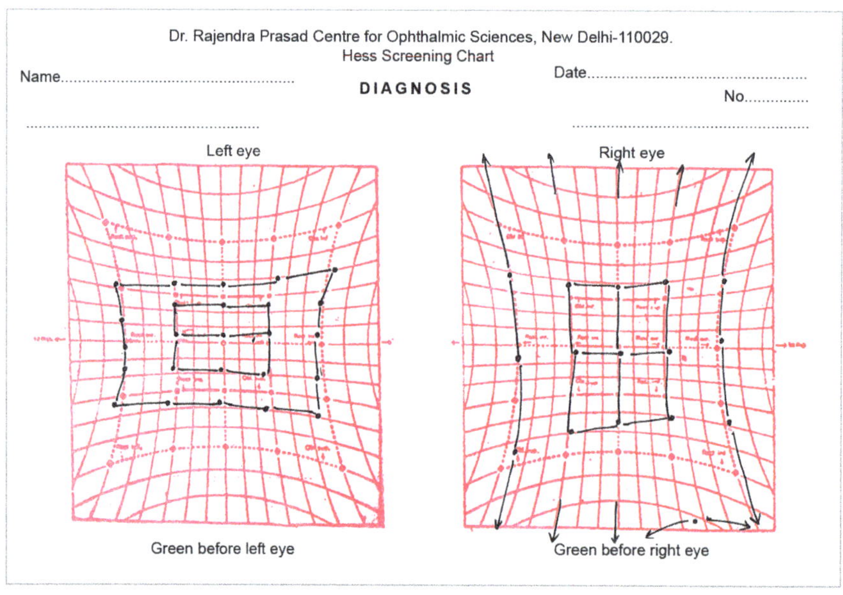

Fig. 6.1.8: Hess chart of orbital flow fracture.

- *If compressed, consider mechanical causes.*
- The angle of deviation is measured by the difference between the plotted point and the template in any position of gaze.

VIVA QUESTIONS

1. Can the Hess/Lees chart be used in all types of strabismus?

Ans. It is useful in incomitant strabismus only.

2. What is the difference between Hess screen and Lees screen?

Ans. See text, the fundamental difference is in the method of dissociation. While in Hess chart the dissociation is achieved by using color glasses, in case of Lees screen it is achieved by the use of a bisecting two-sided plane mirror bisecting the two opalescent glass screens placed at right angles to each other, bisected by a two-sided plane mirror.

3. What are the uses of Hess chart?

Ans. The uses of Hess chart are:

- To monitor progress
- Treatment plan
- Evaluating the results of incomitant strabismus.

4. Is Hess chart alone useful for assessing incomitant strabismus?

Ans. No, it has to be interpreted along with other tests.

5. What are the prerequisites for using the Hess charts?

Ans. Refer to text.

6. What does the shape of the Hess chart indicate?

Ans. A charts with sloping edges points to A or V pattern.

7. What happens to Hess chart over time?

Ans. It becomes uniform.

8. What is a compressed chart suggests?

Ans. Mechanical cause.

9. How can the amount of deviation be measured with Hess chart?

Ans. The amount of deviation can be calculated by measuring the gap between the pointer and the dot, taking into consideration that each small square subtends an angle of 5°. The torsional measurements can be calculated by using a specially adapted linear pointer.

10. What is the clinical significance of the outer field?

Ans. The outer field is useful in the detection of a small amount of incomitant strabismus where the central field can be normal.

11. Original Hess chart.

Ans. The original Hess chart consisted of a black cloth of 80 × 80 cm with the tangent coordinates stitched as red embroidered dots. The pointer was 50 cm long with a green arrow at its end.[1]

12. Interpret Figure 6.1.4.

Ans. Steps to interpretation:

- Smaller chart indicates the eye with the paretic muscle—left eye.
- Larger chart indicates the eye with overacting yoke muscle—right eye.
- Smaller chart shows a greater limitation in the main direction of muscle: In this case the medial rectus, superior rectus, inferior rectus, and inferior oblique of the left eye show underaction (can be noted by inward displacement of dots, therefore the whole curve).
- An overaction of the left lateral rectus is seen (outward displacement of the dots).
- In the larger field of right eye, maximum displacement can be seen in the primary direction of action of the contralateral synergist. Hence overaction of the all muscles can be seen except the right medial rectus and inferior rectus ("yokes" of spared muscles).
- This is a case of left third nerve palsy.

13. Interpret Figure 6.1.5.

Ans. Steps to interpretation:

- Both fields are similar in size this denotes that either it is a comitant squint or both eyes may be involved. The chart as mentioned above shows incomitance; hence probably both eyes are involved.

- In both eyes, overaction of the medial rectus is seen, and underaction of lateral rectus is seen (more apparent in the outer field).
- Also the right eye shows more underaction of the lateral rectus than the left eye.
- This is a case of bilateral asymmetric sixth nerve palsy.

14. Interpret Figure 6.1.6.

Ans. Steps to interpretation:

- The smaller field of the left eye denotes that the affected eye is left eye.
- Underaction of the left eye superior oblique is noted.
- Overaction of the ipsilateral antagonist the left inferior oblique is noted.
- The right field shows the larger secondary deviation—right hypotropia (Hering's law) and the greatest enlargement is in the field of action of the right inferior rectus (contralateral synergist—Sherrington's law).
- This is a case of left superior oblique palsy.

15. Interpret Figure 6.1.7.

Ans. Steps to interpretation:

- Hypotropia of the right eye can be seen.
- The right eye shows impairment of elevation in adduction whereas elevation is normal in the abduction.
- An increase in exotropia is seen in upgaze with the same amount of deviation in primary position and downgaze denoting a Y pattern.
- This is a case of right eye Brown's syndrome.

16. Interpret Figure 6.1.8.

Ans. Steps to interpretation:

- The smaller field of the left eye denotes that the affected eye is the left eye.
- Left eye denotes a hypotropia with a limitation of elevation.
- The amount of deviation increases in the upgaze or downgaze.
- This denotes an entrapment of the left inferior rectus at the equator postorbital floor fracture of the left eye.

REFERENCES

1. Roper-Hall G. The Hess screen test. Am Orthopt J. 2006;56:166-74.
2. The Principles of Hess Chart. [online] Available from http://www.mrcophth.com/commonhesschart/principlesofhesschart.html [Accessed January 2019].

6.2 SYNOPTOPHORE

Pallavi Singh, Vatika Jain, Pranita Sahay

INTRODUCTION

Synoptophore, derived from the Greek language (syn = with, ops = eye, phoros = bearing), is an orthoptic instrument used for both motor and sensory evaluation of strabismus. It is also used for the nonsurgical treatment of strabismus in the form of orthoptic exercises.

PRINCIPLE

It is based on the haploscopic principle, which states that *there is a division of physical space into two separate areas of visual space, each of which is visible to one eye only.*

HISTORY

In 1838, the first stereoscope was constructed by Sir Charles Wheatstone. Subsequently, Claud Worth made the amblyoscope, to evaluate and stimulate binocular vision. The slides used in these earlier devices for determining the extent of simultaneous perception and measuring the area of suppression were developed by MC Maddox. Nowadays, Clement Clarke's major synoptophore is the most commonly used version.

Older versions include Moorfields synoptophore, Lyle-Major amblyoscope, and Curpax-Major amblyoscope.

DESIGN

The instrument has a base that contains the electrical components and controls (Fig. 6.2.1). Attached to the base are scales for measuring vergence movements. Supported at the base are two optical tubes that contain a light source; high intensity light for after image test and Haidinger's brushes and a low intensity light; a slide carrier; various scales and control knobs for measuring horizontal, vertical and torsional deviations; a reflecting mirror and an eyepiece with a +6.5 D convex lens. Plus lenses in the eyepiece ensure relaxation of patient's accommodation and the image appears to come from the distance. Accommodation can be induced by placing –3 D lenses in the lens holder placed in front of the eyepiece. Degrees and prism dioptres (Δ) are used as scales on the synoptophore to measure displacement.

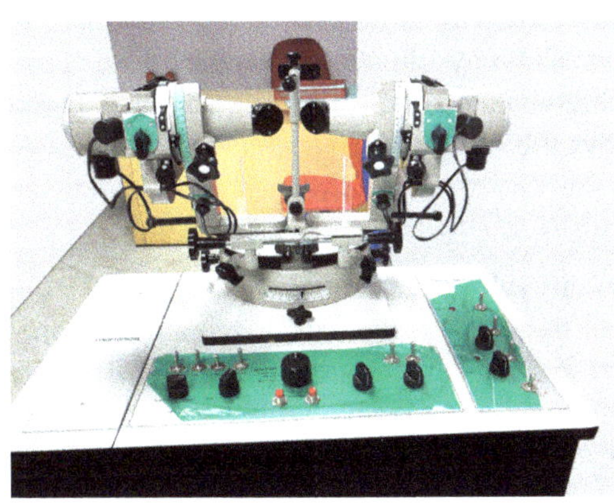

Fig. 6.2.1: Synoptophore.

USES

Diagnostic Uses

- To measure interpupillary distance (IPD).
- To measure the angle of deviation, primary and secondary deviations.
- To assess anomalous retinal correspondence (ARC).
- To measure angle kappa (K), accommodative convergence/accommodation (AC/A) ratio.
- To assess various grades and anomalies of binocular vision.
- To measure fusional reserve.
- To assess special functions such as adaptability to function in aniseikonia with the help of special slides, appreciation of entopic phenomenon (visual effects whose source is within the eye itself) with Haidinger's brushes.
- After image testing.

Therapeutic Uses

- For various orthoptic exercises.
- To treat convergence insufficiency.
- To improve fusional reserve.
- To combat suppression and ARC.

TYPES OF SLIDES

A wide variety of slides are used as summarized in Table 6.2.1. The size of each slide has been calculated to subtend a different angle at the nodal point of the eye (Table 6.2.2).

Table 6.2.1: Different types of slides in synoptophore.		
Series	*Use*	*Binding*
A	Maddox test	White
D	Stereoscopic vision	Yellow
F	Fusion	Green
G and H	Simultaneous perception	Red
S	Automatic flashing, after images, Haidinger brushes	Blue
Mayou series of 8	Simultaneous perception	Orange

Note: The strict following of color codes for different types of slides are rarely followed nowadays.

Table 6.2.2: Angle subtended by different slides in synoptophore.	
Slide size	*Angle subtended*
Foveal	1°
Macular	1–3°
Paramacular	3–5°
Peripheral	>5°

MEASUREMENTS

Interpupillary Distance Measurement

This is the first step before starting any measurement of strabismus. Set all the scales to zero, put the slides of foveal fixation and ask the patient to look into the right picture with his right eye and then align the corneal reflection with the white line on the top of the tube by closing your right eye. Repeat similarly for the left eye of the subject, note down the IPD and lock it for further measurements.

Angle of Deviation

Objective Angle of Deviation

It can be measured based on the principles of either the Hirschberg's test or the alternate cover test. The patient should be sitting comfortably and in the correct position in front of the instrument. The interpupillary distance is then adjusted, and the first-grade targets are inserted. In the Hirschberg's test, the patient looks at the center of the target slides, and the angle of slide carrier is adjusted to make corneal reflection symmetrical (in the center of the pupillary area in both eyes), and the deviation is measured. For measuring the angle of deviation by the alternate cover test the lion or car is placed in front of the fixing eye and the cage or gate in front of the non-fixing eye. The arms are set to zero, and the patient is fixing at the center of the slide; when the fixing light in front of the fixing eye is turned off, the non-fixing eye will immediately take fixation. It will move either inwards (in exotropia), outwards (in esotropia), upwards or downwards to take fixation. If the non-fixing eye moves out to take fixation, the arm is moved into a more convergent or less divergent position and so on for other deviations as well. The alternate flashing is continued and the tube adjusted until there is no movement in either eye on fixation. The reading on the horizontal scale and vertical scale in front of the nonfixing arm represents the objective angle of deviation.

Subjective Angle of Deviation

First measure the objective angle of deviation, if the patient sees superimposition (the lion in the cage) at the objective angle, it is the same as the subjective angle. If this is not the case, the patient is asked to superimpose the two slides by adjusting the angle between two slides by the handle. Reading on the scale will give the subjective angle of deviation.

Angle of Anomaly

- If subjective and objective angles of deviation are same, it is called normal retinal correspondence, and if they are different, it is called ARC.
- The difference between the subjective and objective angle of deviation is the angle of anomaly is. For instance, if a patient has

an objective angle of deviation of 25Δ base out (BO) and a subjective angle of 10ΔBO, his angle of anomaly is 15Δ.

- If the objective angle is equal to the angle of anomaly, i.e. subjective angle is zero, it is called a harmonious ARC.
- If objective angle exceeds the angle of anomaly, it is known as unharmonious ARC.

Measurement of Cyclodeviation

It can only be measured subjectively. Simultaneous perception slides (Fig. 6.2.2) are used, the patient is asked to look at each slide in turn and is asked whether the cage appears level or tilted. A cyclodeviation is present if the image appears to be tilted. If with the right eye focusing, the cage's right-hand side is lower than the left-hand side, incyclophoria or tropia is present. It is important to note that the tilt of the image is in the direction opposite to the tilt of the eye. The deviation is corrected with the torsional deviation screw and the amount of deviation is measured from the scale.

Grades of Binocular Single Vision

There are three grades (Fig. 6.2.3) of binocular single vision (BSV):

1. *The first grade of BSV*: Simultaneous perception (usually red slides).
2. *The second grade of BSV*: Binocular fusion (usually green slides).
3. *The third grade of BSV*: Stereopsis (usually yellow slides).

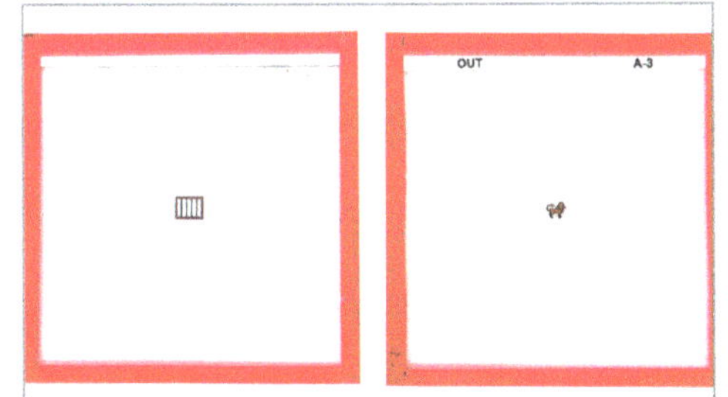

Fig. 6.2.2: Simultaneous perception slides.

Simultaneous Perception

It is the ability to perceive two images, one formed on each retina simultaneously. The smaller picture, i.e. the lion, is kept in the slide holder in front of the fixing eye, while the bigger picture is kept in front of the fellow eye. The slides (Fig. 6.2.4) are designed so that the patient puts something into something, e.g. a lion in a cage. Either parafoveal, foveal, or macular slides may be used. If the patient sees the lion in the cage, he is using each eye simultaneously and has a grade 1 binocular vision.

Binocular Fusion

Sensory fusion is the ability to fuse two slightly dissimilar images and perceive them as one. These consist of targets which are mainly the same, but each has a different control on it (Fig. 6.2.5). A grade 2 target will show a picture of a

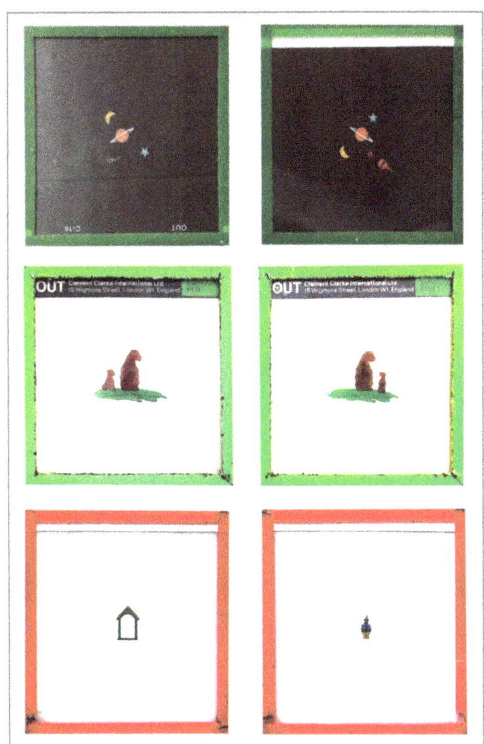

Fig. 6.2.3: Slides used for testing different grades of binocular single vision.

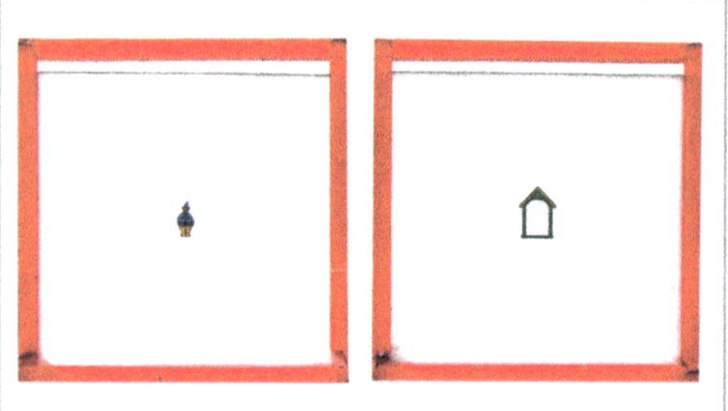

Fig. 6.2.4: Slides used for testing simultaneous perception.

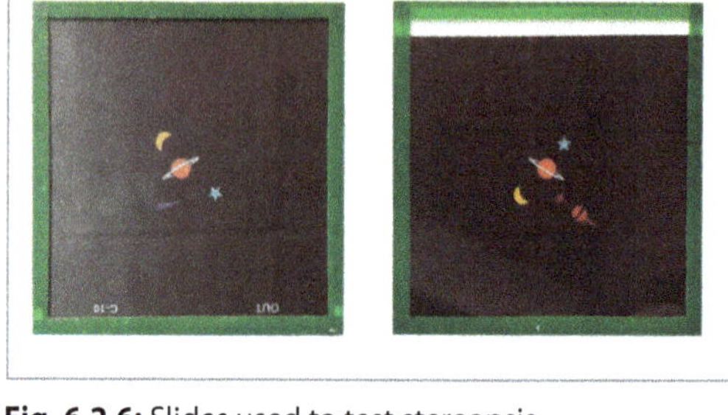

Fig. 6.2.6: Slides used to test stereopsis.

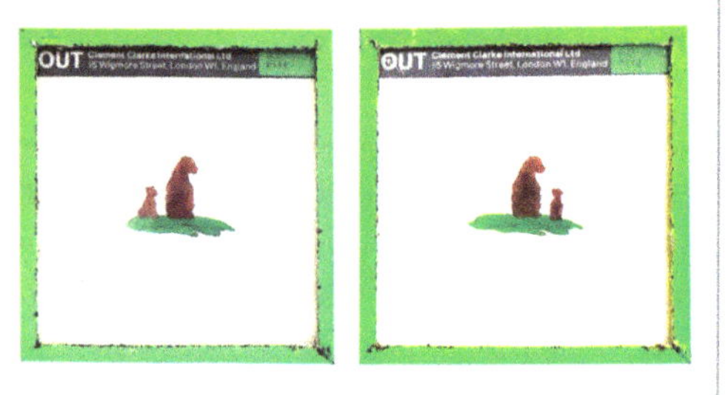

Fig. 6.2.5: Slides for testing binocular fusion.

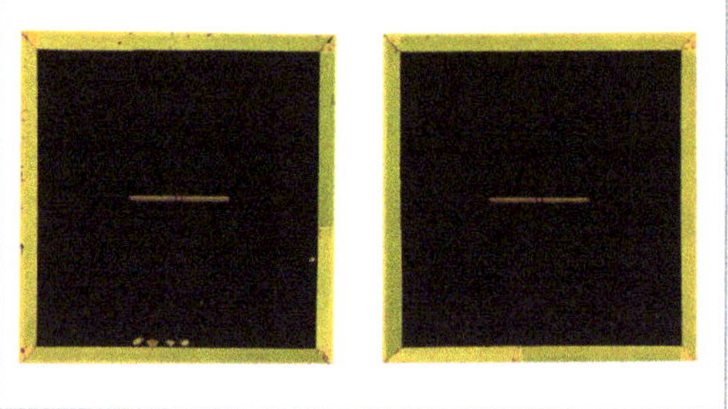

Fig. 6.2.7: Slides used for after-image testing.

rabbit with no tail and clutching flowers to one eye, and the other eye will see a picture of the same rabbit, but it would have a tail, and held in its hand would be a stem without flowers. The patient has a grade 2 binocular vision if he fuses these images and confirms seeing a tailed rabbit clutching a bunch of flowers by a stem.

Stereopsis

It is the perception of depth based on binocular image disparity. Images of the same object are hypothetically taken from slightly different angles, to denote depth perception. These slides (Fig. 6.2.6) have slightly disparate targets; the fusion of these minutely dissimilar images by the brain creates the perception of depth or stereopsis. If fused correctly, a three-dimensional image is perceived.

Torsion

Maddox slides (white binding) help in the assessment of 9 positions of gaze. Horizontal and vertical deviations are assessed by the usual method. However, the torsional control is rotated until the patient is satisfied that it superimposes in the center of the green surroundings and all lines should run parallel.

After Image Test

It is a fovea-to-fovea sensory test used to measure ARC. Special slides (Fig. 6.2.7) that present the retina with a linear strobe of light (one vertical and one horizontal) are used. The center of the linear strobe light is masked to spare the fovea; thus, the afterimage line has a break in the middle. Stronger 12 V lamps are used to stimulate the fovea for fixation in dense amblyopia.

Determination of Fusional Amplitudes

After determining the objective angle and presence of first and second grades of binocular vision, the examiner blocks the arms at the objective angle (divided equally between both arms). Utilizing the horizontal vergence controls, both arms are first diverged/converged (depending on whether divergence or convergence fusional amplitude is being measured) and the point of fusion breakage is noted. The arms are then reversed to a less divergent/converged position, and the point of fusion recovery is noted. The recovery point is usually 2–4 ΔD below breakpoint. Fusional amplitude should be tested slowly as vergence movements are slow and tonic.

Orthoptic Exercises

Orthoptics is the training process of an individual to obtain the best possible binocular interaction in the form of BSV. For the treatment of convergence/divergence insufficiency, fusional reserve and all grades of binocular single vision are first assessed. Stereoscopic slides are used as they are the strongest stimulation for fusion. The patient first fuses the slides; tubes are then converged until the patient can sustain fusion; when diplopia occurs, the patient is asked to try to fuse the images. This exercise is continued for 5 minutes at each weekly visit, and the patient is given a home exercise in the form of pencil convergence exercise and physiological diplopia exercise (stereogram card) before he comes for the next visit.

VIVA QUESTIONS

1. Grades of binocularity and their age of development.

Ans. Refer to text.

2. Principle of synoptophore.

Ans. Refer to Text.

3. Amblyopia therapy on synoptophore.

Ans. Amblyopia therapy is performed on synoptophore using Haidinger brushes.

4. What is "instrument convergence"?

Ans. Even though targets are placed at optical infinity in the synoptophore by using +6.0 D or +6.5 D lenses in the eyepiece, proximal convergence comes into play while measuring deviations (especially horizontal) and fusional vergences. This might distort the values obtained for the said measurements.

5. Different angles.

Ans.

- *Angle alpha*: The angle between the optical axis and the visual axis. A positive angle, (corneal reflection placed nasally) leads to pseudo divergent squint; negative angle (corneal reflections placed temporally) leads to pseudoconvergent squint.
- *Angle gamma*: The angle between the axis and the fixation axis.
- *Angle kappa*: The angle between the mid-pupillary line and visual axis.

6.3 TESTS FOR STEREOPSIS

Pallavi Singh, Shreya Nayak, Pranita Sahay

DEFINITION

Stereopsis is defined as the relative positioning of visual objects in depth, i.e. in the third dimension.

PHYSIOLOGIC BASIS OF STEREOPSIS

Wheatstone in 1838 was the first to understand that stereopsis occurs when horizontally disparate retinal elements are stimulated simultaneously and the fused image lies within the Panum's area of single binocular vision. Vertical displacement produces no stereopsis.

Stereopsis is lacking in infants less than 3 months of age, and develops to adult levels by about the 6th month of life.

PRINCIPLE OF TESTS FOR STEREOPSIS

As a principle, all tests for stereopsis provide disparate images to each eye. They fundamentally differ in their methodology of dissociating the two images. The commonly used dissociation methodologies are described below:

- *Haploscopic principle*: Used in synoptophore where the dissociation occurs by placing angled mirrors in front of both eyes so that the right eye sees the right temporal field while the left eye sees the left temporal field.
- *Anaglyph principle*: Dissociation is produced by using colors. It consists of stereograms in which the half images have been overlaid and are present in complementary colors. Used in The Netherlands Organization (TNO).
- *Vectographic principle*: It dissociates the eyes optically. A vectograph consists of Polaroid material on which two stereo-paired images are etched in such a way that each target is polarized 90° with reference to the other. Used in titmus fly test and Randot stereopsis test. It avoids the color tint annoyance as seen in anaglyph.
- *Panographic principle*: At times, children do not comply with wearing Polaroid or red-green glasses, and it is needed to observe the position of the eyes while the patient is being tested. To overcome this, Lang reported a real-time stereogram where a different image is provided to each eye through cylindrical lamination/gratings on the surface of stereoscopic random dot plates used in Lang test.

TESTS FOR NEAR STEREOACUITY

The Netherlands Organization Test

- Based on anaglyph principle[1]
- *Equipment*: 7 plates booklet (Fig. 6.3.1) and red-green spectacles (Fig. 6.3.2)

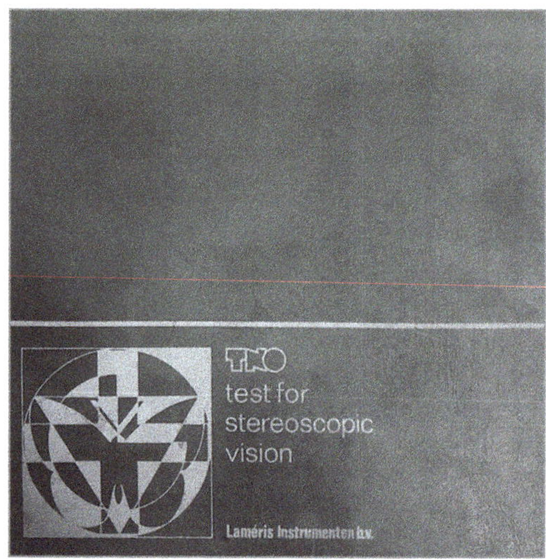

Fig. 6.3.1: The Netherlands Organization (TNO) test, 7 plates booklet.

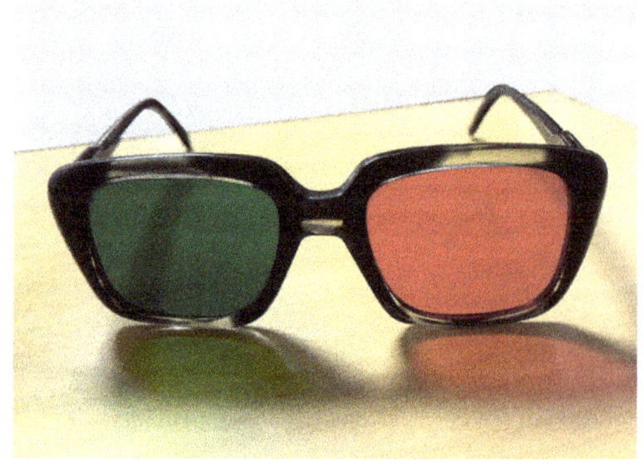

Fig. 6.3.2: Red-green spectacles.

- Seven plates with test figures:[2]
  - *Plates I–III*, screening plates, to establish gross stereopsis, tells if stereopsis is present or not (Figs. 6.3.3 to 6.3.5)
  - *Plate IV* is a suppression test (Fig. 6.3.6)
  - *Plates V–VII* are for quantitative examination for exact determination of stereoacuity (Figs. 6.3.7A to C)
- *Method*: Plates are presented at 40 cm from the subject, well-lit room
- *Advantage*:
  - Can be used in children (2.5–5 years)
- *Disadvantages*:
  - Tests only near stereoacuity
  - Color tint annoyance.

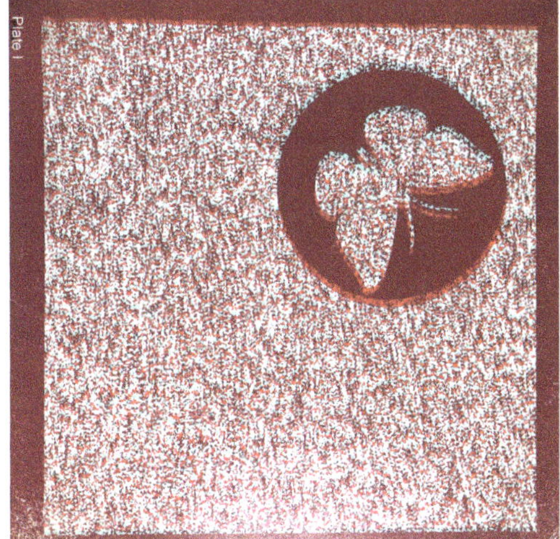

Fig. 6.3.3: The Netherlands Organization (TNO) plate I—two butterflies are present, one can be seen monocularly and the other is only seen in stereopsis.

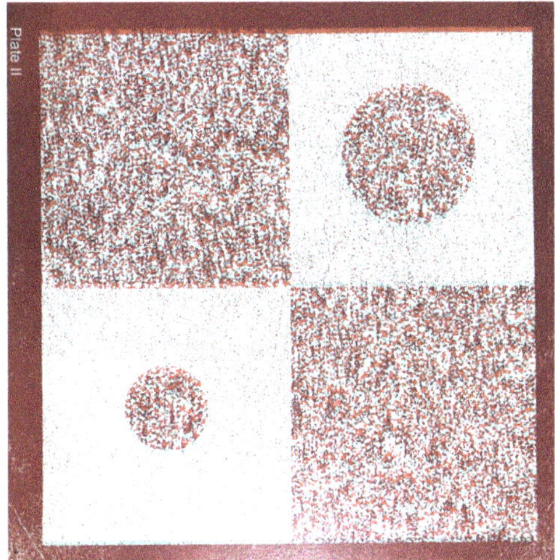

Fig. 6.3.4: The Netherlands Organization (TNO) plate II—four discs, two are seen monocularly and two require stereopsis.

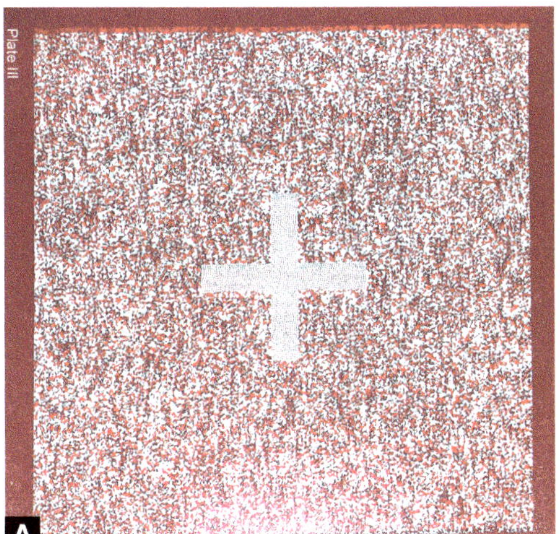

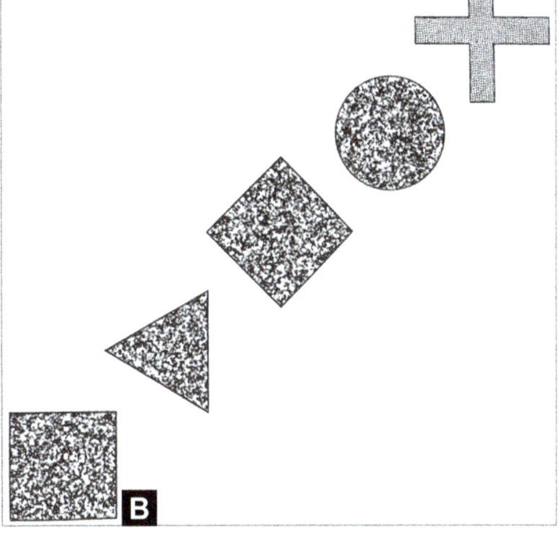

Figs. 6.3.5A and B: The Netherlands Organization (TNO) plate III—four hidden shapes (O, □, Δ, ∨) are arranged around a centrally placed cross. The child is first asked to look at one of the example in the opposite page (B) and find the corresponding one in the test plate (A).

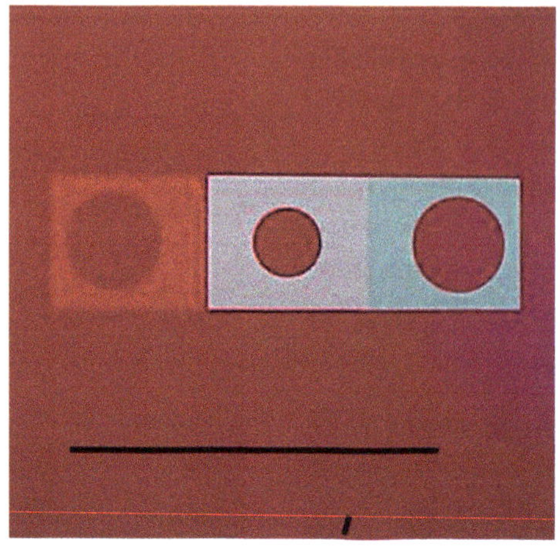

Fig. 6.3.6: The Netherlands Organization (TNO) plate IV—this is a suppression test. There are three discs, one seen by the right eye, one by the left, and one is seen binocularly.

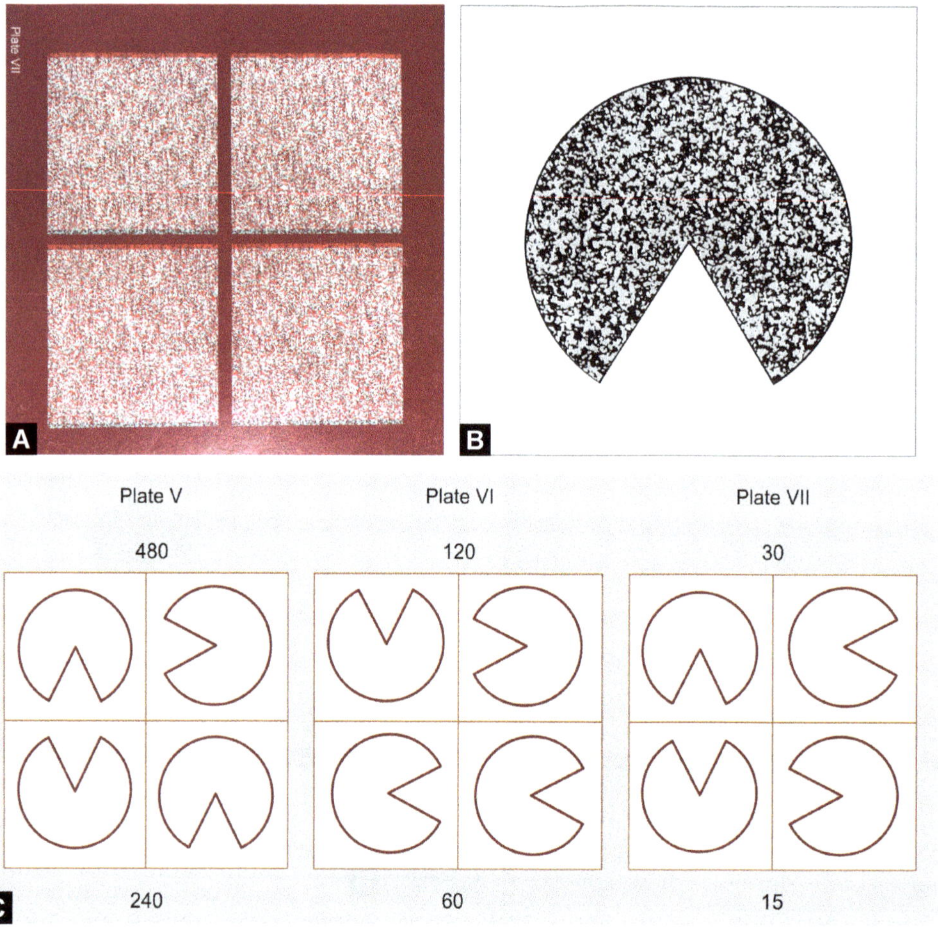

Plate VII

A

B

Plate V
480

Plate VI
120

Plate VII
30

C
240
60
15

Figs. 6.3.7A to C: Plate V-VII here the test items (Pac-man shapes) are presented at six different disparities ranging from 15 to 480 seconds of arc.

Titmus Stereotest

- Based on vectographic principle, that uses crossed polarized filters located at the axis of 45° and 135° in front of either eye.
- *Equipment*: Stereo housefly card or circles or animal test plates, and polarized glasses.
- Children can be asked to touch the wings of the fly.
- *Uses*: For screening and fine depth perception in strabismus.
- *Advantages*:
  - Used in children above 3 years
  - Offers no monocular clues.
- *Disadvantages*:
  - Patients might choose the correct animal/circle without seeing stereoscopically. To overcome this they are asked to see it monocularly and asked for difference or, one can turn the plate vertically by 90° which would block the stereoscopic effect.
  - Only tests for near stereoacuity.

Stereo Butterfly Test

Equipment: Like titmus fly test but it has a hidden configuration of a butterfly.

Randot Stereotest

- Randot stereotest (Fig. 6.3.8) is based on vectographic principle. The arrangement of dots eliminates monocular cues for stereopsis. However, the introduction of shapes and form in the random dots facilitates global stereopsis. This allows for elimination of false results, which can be produced by correspondence of ambiguous localized areas within the Panum's area.
- It evaluates the depth perception by requiring patients to identify six geometric forms from random dot backgrounds (500–20 seconds of arc) (Figs. 6.3.9A and B).[3]

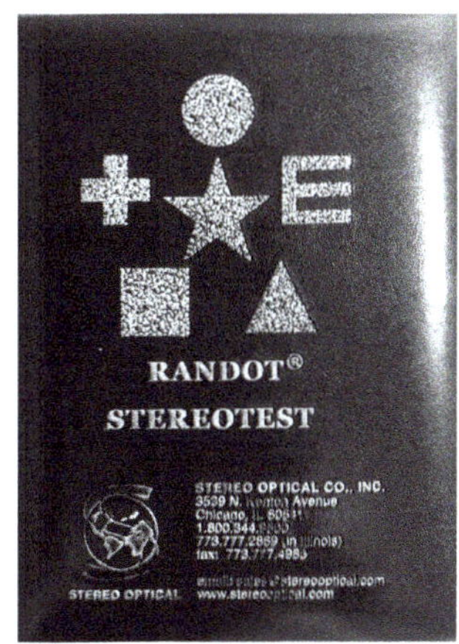

Fig. 6.3.8: Randot stereotest for near.

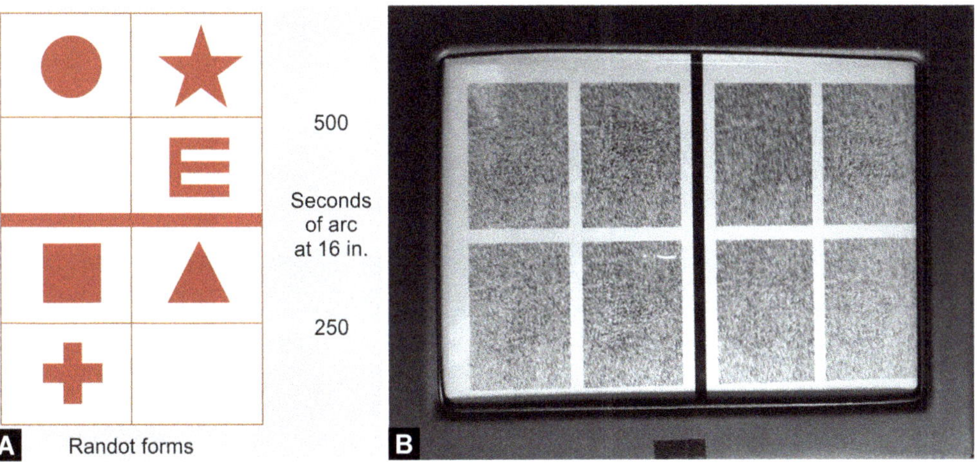

Figs. 6.3.9A and B: Identify six geometric forms (A) from background dots; and (B) in Randot stereotest.

- Random dot patterns necessitate the person to recognize images from a background. The distance between the image and background in question does not affect the judgment of the individual, as both are in immediate juxtaposition.
- The test images can be recognized only with polarized three-dimensional (3 D) viewing glasses (Fig. 6.3.10).
- It consists of the graded circle test (400–20 seconds of arc) and animal test for children (400 to 100 seconds of arc) (Fig. 6.3.11; Tables 6.3.1 and 6.3.2).
- *Equipment*: Plates with random dot stereograms.

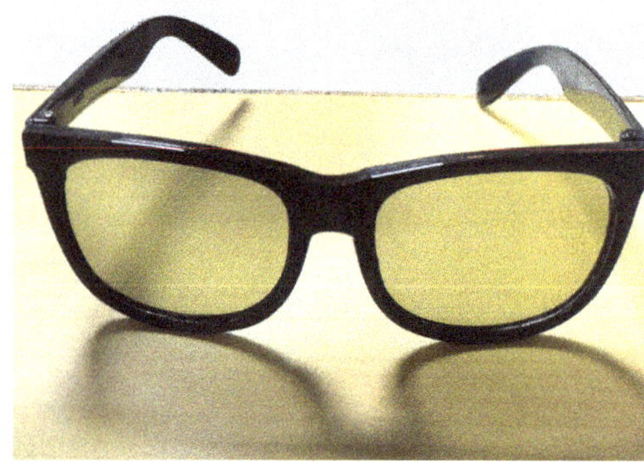

Fig. 6.3.10: Polarized three-dimensional viewing glasses for Randot stereotest.

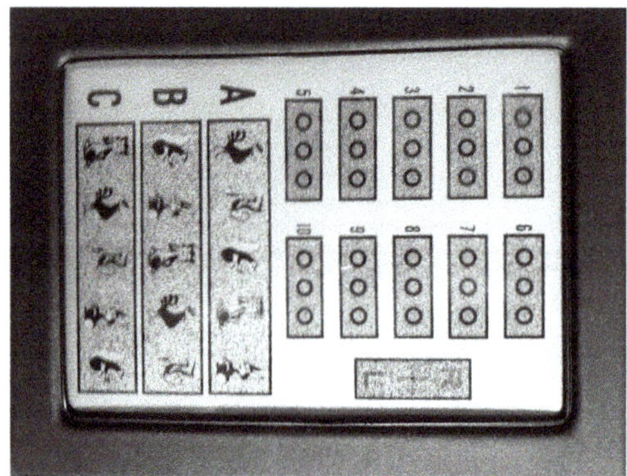

Fig. 6.3.11: Graded circle and animals of Randot stereotest.

- *Uses*: Screening and fine depth perception in strabismus.
- *Advantages*:
  - Used in children above 3 years of age
  - Offers no monocular clues.
- *Disadvantage*: Only tests near stereoacuity.

Lang Test

- Based on panographic presentation of a plate on random dot pattern.
- Two types have been described:
  1. Lang stereotest I with a star, a cat, and a car (Fig. 6.3.12). Children as young as 6 months of age can be tested, as the child looks at a particular form helping us to draw the inference.
  2. Lang stereotest II is performed with a moon, a truck, and an elephant.

Lang Two-pencil Test

No equipment is needed in this test. The patient is asked to hold a pencil in his hand

Table 6.3.1: Graded circle interpretation of Randot stereotest.

Scoring key		*Seconds of arc at 16 in.*
1	L	400
2	R	200
3	L	140
4	M	100
5	R	70
6	M	50
7	L	40
8	R	30
9	M	25
10	R	20

Table 6.3.2: Animal test interpretation of Randot stereotest.

Scoring key		*Seconds of arc at 16 in.*	*Shepard percentage*	*Verhoff distance*
A	Cat	400	15%	0.1
B	Rabbit	200	30%	0.2
C	Monkey	100	50%	0.3

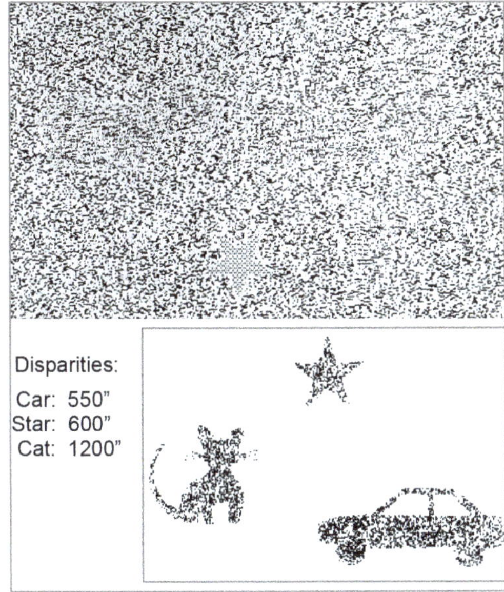

Fig. 6.3.12: Lang's stereotest I consisting of a card with pictures of a cat, a star, and a car.

and asked to touch the pencil tip-to-tip in the examiner's hand rapidly. This test has 100% sensitivity. It is frequently used as a screening test for gross stereopsis detection.

TESTS FOR DISTANCE STEREOACUITY

Two types of stereo tests were available in older days, the first one being AO vectograph stereotest, which was dissociating because of the need to wear polarized glasses. The latter one being the Mentor Binocular Visual Acuity Testing (BVAT) system, which was a computerized system, which contained a liquid crystal shutter aperture for each eye and presented disparate images alternating at 60 Hz.

Both these tests have become obsolete now. Currently used tests include (Tables 6.3.3 and 6.3.4):

- *Frisby-Davis distance test*:
  - This is a test to evaluate real depth in a free space and was designed by JP Frisby and H Davis.

Table 6.3.3: Grade of stereopsis in different tests.

Test	*Grade of stereopsis (unit-second of arc)*
Titmus fly test	*Fly*: 3,500 *Graded circle test*: 800-40 *Animal test*: 400, 200, 100
TNO test	15–480
Stereo Butterfly test	*Upper wings*: 2,000 *Lower wings*: 1,150 *Abdomen*: 700
Random dot test	400–20
Lang stereo I	*Car*: 550 *Star*: 600 *Cat*: 1,200
Lang stereo II	*Moon*: 200 *Truck*: 400 *Elephant*: 600
Lang two-pencil	3,000–5,000
Synoptophore	720–90

(TNO: The Netherlands Organization)

Table 6.3.4: Grade of stereopsis for distance.

Test	*Grade of stereopsis (unit-second of arc)*
Frisby-Davis distance stereotest	5–50 sec at 6 m
Distance Randot test	400–60

  - *Equipment*: Box containing four back illuminated various plastic objects mounted on rods pointing towards the observer. They are all translucent but also opaque enough to cover the rods giving the shapes a free-floating appearance (Fig. 6.3.13).
  - *Advantages*:
    - Can be used in children 3 years and above.
    - Repeated testing possible without the patient guessing.
    - Possible to teach the patients before the test.
    - Not using stereograms or any polarized/tinted glasses, which may break fusion.

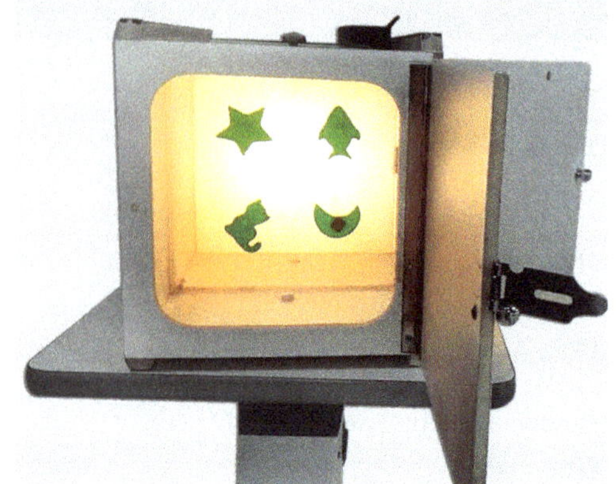

Fig. 6.3.13: Frisby-Davis stereoacuity test for distance.

- *Distance Randot test*:
  - Similar to near vectographic Randot test.
  - *Advantages*:
    - Gives no monocular clues
    - Worsening of distance stereoacuity in patients with intermittent exotropia is an indicator of poor control and necessitates early surgery.

NEWER ADVANCES IN STEREOACUITY TESTS

Three-dimensional Testing

Computer-based 3 D images are shown both at near and at a distance, in front (conventional) and behind (proposed) the background image on a 3 D monitor. It was also combined with liquid-crystal display (LCD) type shutter glasses to separate the stereoscopic images.

REFERENCES

1. Om Tao (2018). TNO Anaglyph Stereo Test. [online] Available from http://www.omtao.in/product/tno-anaglyph-stereo-test/ [Last Accessed February, 2019].
2. Good-Lite. TNO Anaglyph Stereo Test. [online] Available from https://www.good-lite.com/cw3/Assets/documents/884-TNO%20Instructions-web.pdf [Last accessed February 2019].
3. Stereo Optical (2018). Randot® Stereotest. [online] Available from https://www.stereooptical.com/products/stereotests-color-tests/randot/ [Last accessed February, 2019].

6.4 INSTRUMENTS FOR SQUINT SURGERY

Pranita Sahay, Devesh Kumawat, Divya Agarwal, Karthika Bhaskaran

SELF-RETAINING BARRAQUER EYE SPECULUM (FIG. 6.4.1)

This lid speculum has a screw that helps in giving desired exposure of the surgical site which can be changed as per the surgery or surgeon's choice.

The disadvantage is that the screw increases pressure over the eyeball and thereby increases the intraocular pressure. Hence it is not advisable in perforated cases.

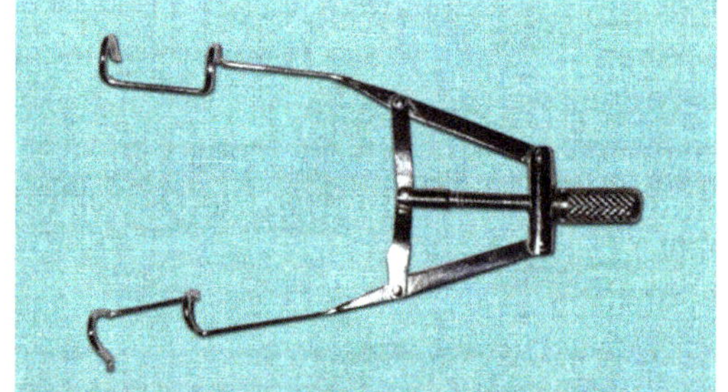

Fig. 6.4.1: Self-retaining Barraquer eye speculum.

Uses

- All intraocular surgeries such as cataract surgery, glaucoma surgery, keratoplasty, buckling and other vitreoretinal surgery.
- Extraocular surgeries such as squint surgery and pterygium removal.
- Removal of conjunctival and corneal foreign body.
- Examination of children and patients with severe blepharospasm.

ARTERY (HEMOSTATIC) FORCEPS (FIG. 6.4.2)

It is a blunt tipped forceps with multiple serrations near the tip and a locking mechanism near the other end. It is available in various sizes small, medium and large. The small sized forceps are called mosquito forceps and are the most commonly used variety in ophthalmic surgeries.

Uses

- Holding the bleeders during surgery
- To crush the muscle before cutting in squint surgery.

GREEN'S HOOK (FIG. 6.4.3)

It has a straight shaft with flat ended hooked tip. It is used for hooking the muscle during squint or enucleation surgery.

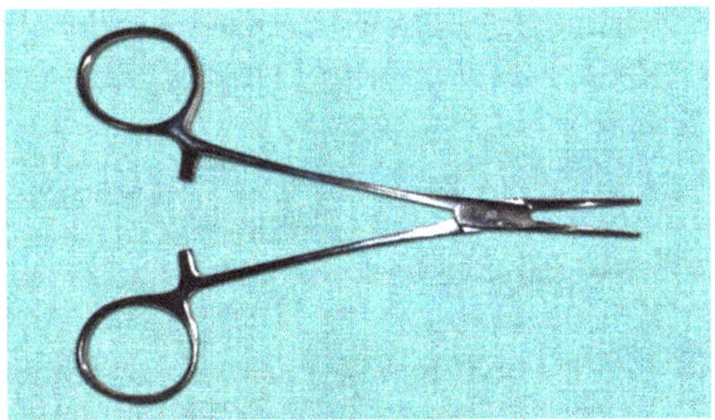

Fig. 6.4.2: Artery (hemostatic) forceps.

JAMESON'S HOOK (FIG. 6.4.4)

It has a straight shaft with flat hooked end and paddle shaped tip. It is used for retrieving the rectus muscles at their insertion site during squint or enucleation surgery.

PLAIN STRAIGHT SCISSORS/ PLAIN CURVED SCISSORS/ STEVENS TENOTOMY SCISSORS (FIG. 6.4.5)

It is a plain scissors with blunt end and comes in two designs: Straight and curved.

Uses

- For cutting the muscle
- For blunt dissection of the soft tissue in squint and oculoplasty procedures.

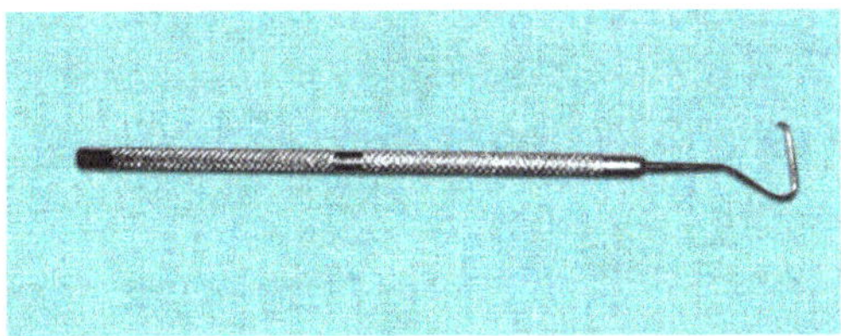

Fig. 6.4.3: Green's hook.

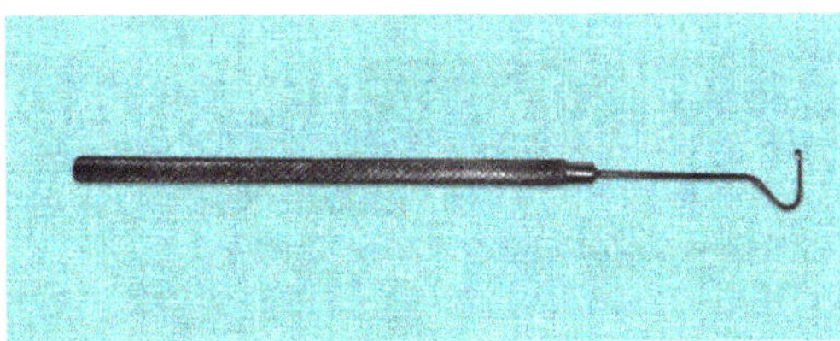

Fig. 6.4.4: Jameson's hook.

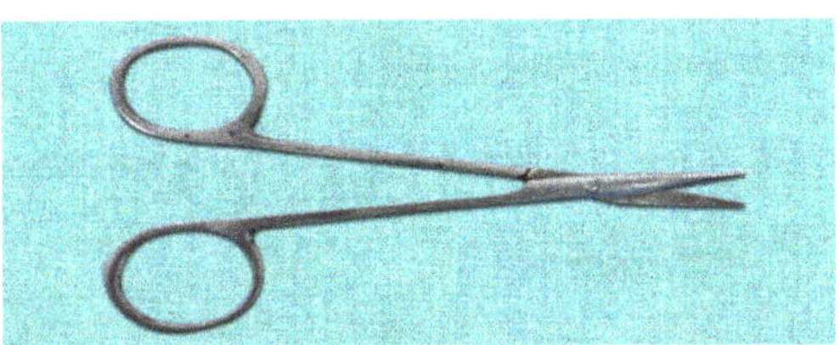

Fig. 6.4.5: Stevens tenotomy scissors.

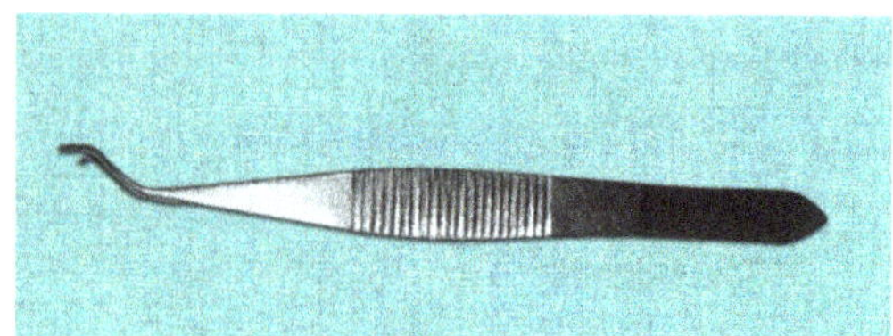
Fig. 6.4.6: Superior rectus holding forceps.

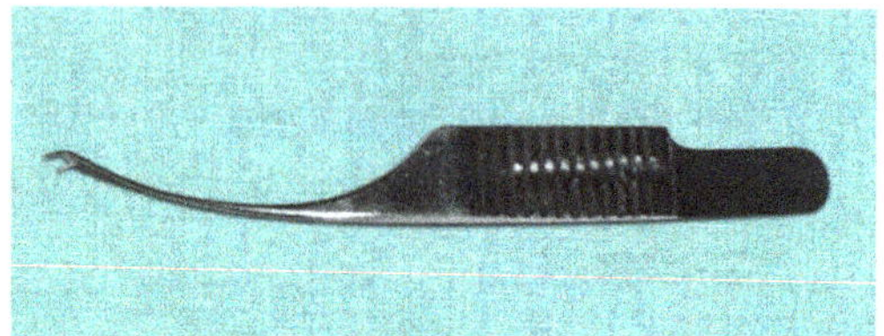
Fig. 6.4.7: Colibri forceps.

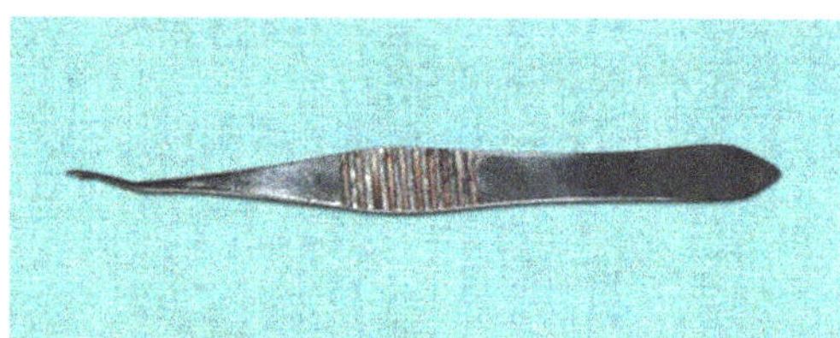
Fig. 6.4.8: Lim's forceps.

SUPERIOR RECTUS HOLDING FORCEPS (FIG. 6.4.6)

It is a toothed forceps with "S" shaped curve specially designed to fit into the orbit while trying to grasp the muscle belly.

COLIBRI FORCEPS (FIG. 6.4.7)

It is a fine toothed forceps for holding flaps of cornea or sclera and rarely the iris.

LIM'S FORCEPS (FIG. 6.4.8)

It is also a toothed forceps for holding the cornea or sclera and rarely the iris.

JAMESON MUSCLE FORCEPS (FIG. 6.4.9)

It has a flat, serrated handle with a side lock, and four teeth in one jaw that fit into holes in the opposing jaw. It is used to clamp the muscle before resection.

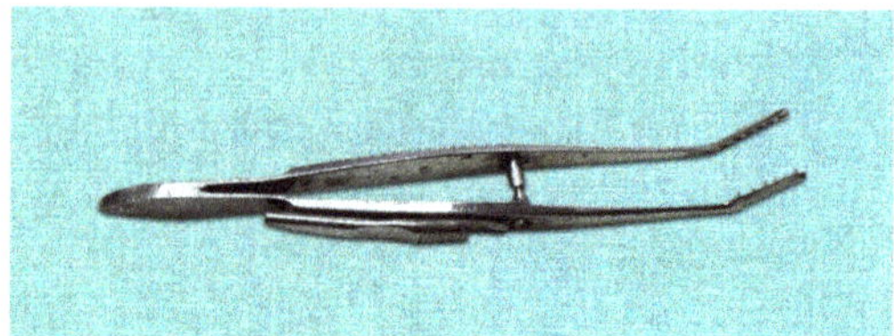
Fig. 6.4.9: Jameson muscle forceps.

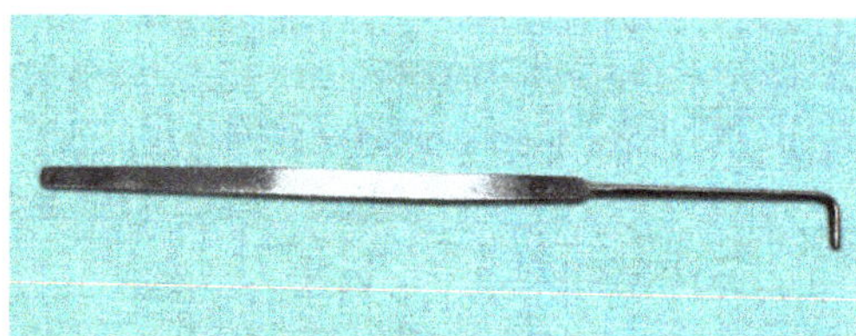
Fig. 6.4.10: Von Graefe hook.

VON GRAEFE HOOK/LENS HOOK (FIG. 6.4.10)

It is used as an alternative to muscle hook or to retract the conjunctiva during squint surgery.

VIVA QUESTIONS

1. What are the complications of squint surgery?

Ans.

Intraoperative:
- Intraoperative bleed
- Scleral perforation
- Splitting of muscle fibers
- Lost muscle/slipped muscle
- Oculocardiac reflex.

Postoperative:
- Diplopia
- Anterior segment ischemia
- Postoperative endophthalmitis/sub conjunctival abscess
- Foreign body granuloma at the suture site
- Conjunctival inclusion cyst
- Conjunctival scarring

- Fat adherence can be caused by a violation of Tenon's capsule with prolapse of orbital fat. This causes a fibro-fatty scar leading to a restrictive strabismus
- Corneal/scleral dellen
- Eyelid retraction or ptosis after surgery on vertical recti
- A lost muscle occurs when the muscle slips free of the sutures
- Residual/consecutive strabismus.

2. What are the normal insertions of recti muscles from the limbus?

Ans.

- *Medial rectus*: 5.3 mm (3.6–7.0)
- *Inferior rectus*: 6.8 mm (4.8–8.5)
- *Lateral rectus*: 6.9 mm (5.4–8.5)
- *Superior rectus*: 7.9 mm (6.2–9.2)

3. What are the types of inferior oblique (IO) weakening procedures?

Ans.

- Fink's recession
- Parks recession
- Elliot and Nankin procedure
- Modified Elliot and Nankin procedure
- Pure anteropositioning
- Total anterior positioning
- Anterior nasal transposition (Stager's)
- Myectomy
- Extirpation
- Disinsertion
- Denervation.

4. What are the types of IO strengthening procedures?

Ans.

- IO resection
- IO advancement.

5. What are the types of superior oblique (SO) weakening procedures?

Ans.

- Tenotomy
- Tenectomy
- Silicon expander lengthening
- Loop tenotomy
- Chicken suture
- Recession
- Translational recession
- Split-tendon lengthening.

6. What are the types of SO strengthening procedures?

Ans.

- SO tuck
- Harada-Ito procedure.

7. What are the various weakening procedures on recti?

Ans.

- Conventional recession
- Hang-back recession
- Slanting recession
- Adjustable recession
- Marginal myotomy
- Faden procedure
- Myectomy
- Disinsertion.

8. What are the various strengthening procedures on recti?

Ans.

- Resection
- Advancement
- Plication
- Transposition of adjacent muscles.

9. What is oculocardiac reflex?

Ans. Bradycardia associated with stretching of extraocular muscles during strabismus surgery, or compression of the eye ball is called the oculocardiac reflex. The reflex is mediated by nerve connections between the ophthalmic branch of the trigeminal nerve via the ciliary ganglion, and the vagus nerve of the parasympathetic nervous system.

10. What are the common causes of residual/recurrent strabismus?

Ans.

Preoperative:

- Very large deviation

- Difficulty in measuring deviation of very young children and uncooperative patients.

Intraoperative:

- Faulty marking during surgery
- Splitting of muscle fibers during surgery

Postoperative:

- Scar stretch.

11. What are the common causes of consecutive strabismus?

Ans.

Preoperative:

- Difficulty in measuring deviation of very young children and uncooperative patients.

Intraoperative:

- Faulty marking during surgery
- Lost muscle.

Postoperative:

- Slipped/lost muscle
- Scar stretch.

12. What is Knapp procedure?

Ans.

- Full tendon width transposition of the horizontal recti to the superior rectus. It is done in cases of monocular elevation deficit.
- Inverse Knapp is the full tendon width transposition of the horizontal recti to the inferior rectus. It is done in double depressor palsy or inferior rectus palsy.

13. What is forced duction test?

Ans. Forced duction test (FDT) assesses passive movement of the globe. This test helps in differentiating between neurogenic and mechanical limitation of ocular movements. After topical/general anesthesia, the eye is held at the limbus with forceps. Patient is asked to look in the direction of the movement limitation (to relax the muscle and prevent false positive results). The globe is then passively moved away from the direction of the muscle to be tested. If resistance is encountered, FDT is positive and the cause is mechanical. If no restriction is felt, a neurogenic cause is considered.

14. What is active force generation test?

Ans. Active force generation test (AFGT) assesses active movement of the globe. In a case of known mechanical limitation of eye movement, it helps assess whether the muscle acting in the field of limitation is paretic or normal. After topical/general anesthesia, the eye is held at the limbus with forceps. Patient is asked to look in the direction of the movement limitation. A normal muscle produces a tug on the globe which can be felt by the examiner.

2

SECTION

BASIC SCIENCES

7

CHAPTER

Pathology Basics

Seema Kashyap, Siddhi Goel, Suman Dhanda, Prafulla Kumar Maharana

INTRODUCTION

Histopathological examination of the tissue specimen is vital to know the disease process affecting the different ocular structures. It is essential to be aware of the basic histopathology of the essential structures of the eye. It is often an essential component of postgraduate and fellowship examinations.

This chapter deals with a few fundamental aspects of ocular histopathology and examples of common clinical conditions where histopathology plays a vital role in diagnosis, management, and prognostication of cases.

COMMON FINDINGS IN PATHOLOGY

The following components are typically seen in the presence of any disease process:[1]

Polymorphonuclear Leukocytes

Polymorphonuclear leukocytes are characterized by:

- A typical multilobulated nucleus
- Abundant eosinophilic cytoplasm
- Occasionally, intracytoplasmic granules which are nothing but proteolytic enzymes.

Mast Cells

Mast cells are characterized by:

- Single nucleus
- Bigger than the polymorphonuclear leukocytes
- Intracytoplasmic pink and red granules (characteristic)
- These granules contain heparin, histamine, and prostaglandins
- Important mediators of allergic conjunctivitis reactions.

Lymphocytes

Lymphocytes are characterized by:

- A very large dark staining nucleus with scanty cytoplasm
- Condensed coarse chromatin
- Play an important role in chronic inflammation and autoimmune disorders.

Plasma Cells

Plasma cells are characterized by:

- These are modified altered B-lymphocytes
- These are oval in shape
- The nucleus is eccentric with a cartwheel or "clock face arrangement" (nucleus is at one pole of the cell)
- Abundant amphophilic cytoplasm
- A paranuclear pale area is characteristic
- Produce antibodies.

GRANULOMATOUS REACTION

A granulomatous reaction usually occurs in response to some chronic low-grade infections (such as tuberculosis or aspergillosis) or a foreign body or chronic uveitis (Sarcoidosis). The inflammatory cells primarily consist of macrophages, lymphocytes and plasma cells. One of the characteristic features is the formation of epithelioid cell granulomas along with multinucleated giant cells.[1]

PYOGENIC GRANULOMA

- Clinically a pyogenic granuloma is characterized by a fleshy, granular, red mass primarily in the conjunctiva. Unlike the name suggests, it does not contain any pus, hence a misnomer.
- On histopathologically, it is a lobulated lesion with a rich vascular network within a loose fibrous connective tissue along with inflammatory cells. Surface is often ulcerated.[1]

NEOPLASIA

The different types of changes seen are:[1]

- *Hypertrophy*: Increase in size of cells.
- *Hyperplasia*: Increase in the number of cells.
- *Hyperkeratosis*: Hyperkeratosis, generally, refers to a thickening of the keratin-containing outer layer of the skin. In the eye, there is thickening of the conjunctiva.
- *Parakeratosis*: Retention of the nucleus in superficial layers of skin or conjunctiva.
- *Metaplasia*: It is the transformation of one cell type to another cell type.
  Examples:
  - *Keratinization of ocular surface*: In Stevens-Johnson syndrome (SJS), ocular cicatricial pemphigoid (OCP) and severe dry eye, the columnar epithelium of conjunctiva is transformed into the stratified squamous keratinized epithelium.
  - Metaplasia of retinal pigment epithelium (RPE) in proliferative vitreoretinopathy (PVR).
  - Metaplasia of lens epithelium in after cataract or posterior capsular opacification (PCO).
- *Dysplasia*: It is an abnormal proliferation of atypical squamous epithelial cells of the conjunctiva. They are classified as mild, moderate or severe dysplasia depending on the thickness involved. When it involves the entire thickness of the epithelium without any breach in the underlying basement membrane, it is called as carcinoma-in-situ.
- *Mitotic figures*: Instead of a nucleus, the chromosomes are visible as tangled, dark-staining threads called mitotic figures which are generally present in malignant tumors.
- *Atrophy*: It means a decrease in the size of a body part, tissue or an individual cell. It can occur following any disease or loss of trophic support due to another disease. It can be physiological (e.g. atrophy of lacrimal gland with increasing age) or it can be pathological [RPE atrophy in age-related macular degeneration (ARMD)].
- *Apoptosis*: Apoptosis is programed cell death that occurs in healthy tissue. Examples include loss of tissue/organs during embryogenesis.
- *Necrosis*: It is the death of cells in an organ or tissue due to disease, injury, or failure of blood supply. Inflammation is always there. Examples include aseptic necrosis in retinoblastoma when tumor growth exceeds the blood supply.

SPECIMENS USED IN OCULAR PATHOLOGY

- *Eyeball*: Evisceration, enucleation, exenteration
- *Eyelid*: Biopsy
- *Lacrimal gland*: Biopsy

- *Conjunctiva*: Biopsy, excised lesion, impression cytology
- *Cornea*: Lamellar keratoplasty (LK), full thickness (penetrating keratoplasty), impression cytology, and corneal biopsy in keratitis
- *Optic nerve*: Enucleation
- *Temporal artery biopsy*: Giant cell arteritis
- *Aqueous tap*: In NHL cases
- *Vitreous tap*: Vitrectomy in endophthalmitis
- *Retinal*: Rare as in retinal tumors, or retinitis.

TISSUE PREPARATION

Fixatives Used

- *Formalin*: 10% buffered formalin is the most commonly used fixative. The advantage of formalin is that it has prolonged chemical stability.[1]
- *Glutaraldehyde*: It is used for scanning electron microscopy (SEM) and transmission electron microscopy (TEM).

Preparation of Tissue

- *Paraffin embedding*: It is the most commonly used method. The tissue is embedded in paraffin wax. The wax serves two purposes; firstly, it allows the sample to adhere to the slide and secondly, it stabilizes the tissue during sectioning. Paraffin prepared blocks can be stored indefinitely.[1]
- *Fresh/frozen sections*: In frozen section, fresh tissue is immediately transported in saline to the laboratory, frozen and embedded in a special medium, and multiple sections are taken using a cryostat. Sections are stained and report is given within 20-30 minutes while the patient is still under anethesia. It is extremely useful in cases when immediate histopathology report is required as in Mohs' micrographic surgery, to know whether the margins are involved in eyelid tumor surgery in the evaluation of intracellular fat as seen in sebaceous carcinoma, and for immunohistochemical studies.[1]
- *Plastic embedding*: The tissue is embedded in a epoxy resin such as araldite. It is used in transmission electron microscopy.[1]

GROSS EXAMINATION (MACROSCOPIC EXAMINATION)

Dimensions: It is the first step. The specimen is measured and its description regarding its shape, size, texture, external and cut surface characteristics are noted.

Usually, the following things are recorded (e.g. in case of an enucleated globe) (Fig. 7.1):[1]

- The maximum dimensions are measured:
  - Anteroposterior (normal 22-24 mm)
  - Horizontal (normal 23.5 mm)
  - Vertical (normal 23 mm).

Transillumination: For this, light is projected from behind the globe to look for the location of mass lesions within the globe.

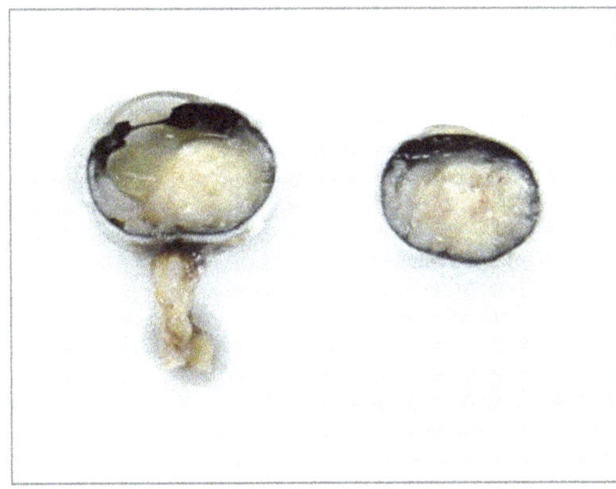

Fig. 7.1: Retinoblastoma—enucleation specimen showing an intraocular retinoblastoma with optic nerve infiltration.

The eye is then cut in a way revealing the most prominent tumor areas that include the pupil as well as the optic nerve. This half of the globe along with optic nerve is submitted for the routine examination and is termed as the pupillary-optic disc portion (PO). The remaining cut portions of the globe are called calottes, as they resemble the shape of caps. Each calotte is cut serially to maximize the tissue examined.

Commonly used stains and their uses are depicted in Table 7.1.

Example: Macular corneal dystrophy (MCD) is characterized by deposit of mucopolysaccharides in the stroma, in the keratocytes, beneath the epithelium and endothelium in advanced cases. The stains commonly used are colloidal iron or Alcian blue, both of which stain the mucopolysaccharides blue.[1]

Silver methenamine stains fungal hyphae black in color (Fig. 7.2)

IMMUNOHISTOCHEMISTRY

Immunohistochemistry involves accurate identification of cells by using an antigen-specific antibody against the antigens present within/on the cells. Specific stains are used

Table 7.1: Special stains in ocular histopathology.

Stain	*Target*	*Color*	*Diagnostic use*
Alcian blue	Mucopolysaccharides	Blue	Macular corneal dystrophy Thyroid eye disease (muscle)
Colloidal iron	Mucopolysaccharides	Blue	Macular corneal dystrophy (Fig. 7.3) Thyroid eye disease (muscle)
Alizarin red	Chelates calcium	Red	Detects calcification like in band-shaped keratopathy
Von Kossa	Calcium	Black or brown black	Calcific band keratopathy
Bodian	Axons	Black	Optic atrophy
Loyez	Myelin	Black	Demyelinating diseases (Multiple sclerosis), optic atrophy
Masson trichrome	Connective tissue hyaline material	Red	Granular corneal dystrophy (Fig. 7.4)
Periodic acid–Schiff (PAS)	Basement membranes	Bright pink	• *Cornea*: Epithelial basement membrane, Descemet's membrane • *Lens*: Capsule • *Retina*: Internal limiting membrane (ILM) • Fungal elements
Congo red with polarized light	Amyloid	Apple green birefringence	Lattice corneal dystrophy (Fig. 7.5)
Perl's Prussian blue	Iron	Dark blue	• Intraocular foreign body • Fleischer ring keratoconus
Van Gieson	Elastic fibers	Gray	Elastic tissue like in giant cell arteritis
Ziehl–Neelsen	Acid fast bacilli	Pink	Detects *Mycobacterium, Nocardia* species in inflammatory tissue and in granulomatous lesions
Oil red O	Lipid	Red	Fat within cells, sebaceous carcinoma
Fontana Masson	Melanin and argentaffin cells	Black	Melanin pigments in malignant melanoma and carcinoid tumor

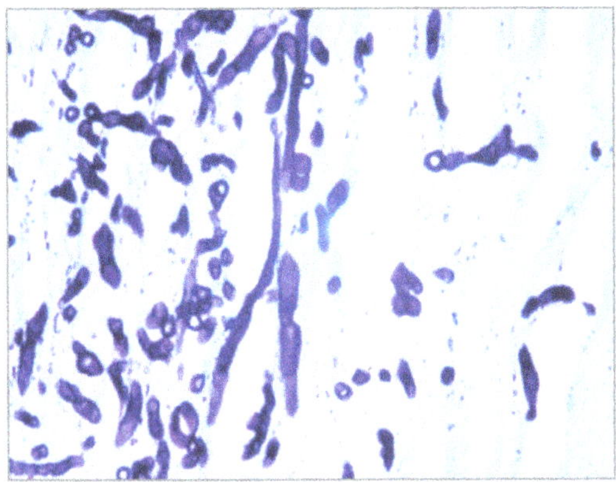

Fig. 7.2: Silver methenamine stain reveals black colored septate fungal hyphae with acute angle branching as seen in mycotic keratitis.

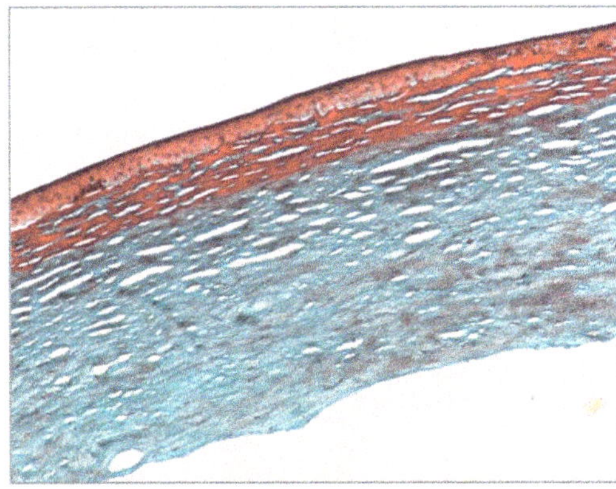

Fig. 7.4: Granular dystrophy—the granules take up a brilliant red color on Masson's trichrome stain.

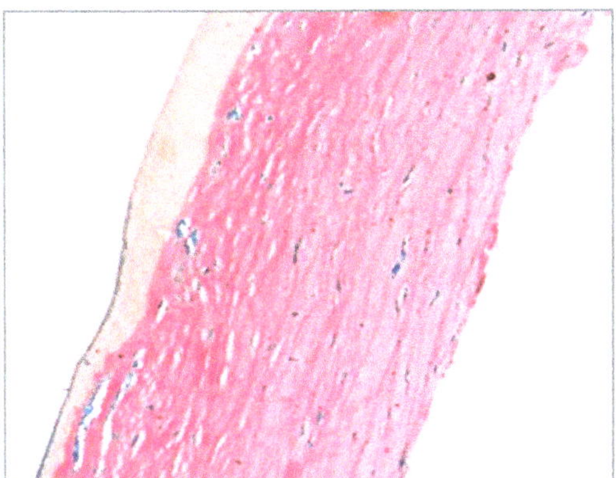

Fig. 7.3: Macular dystrophy—acid mucopolysaccharides are seen in the keratocytes and take up a Prussian blue color by colloidal iron stain.

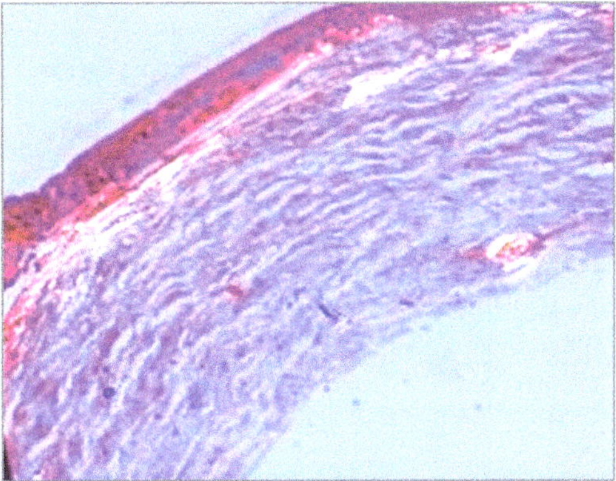

Fig. 7.5: Lattice dystrophy—apple green birefringence is demonstrated on Congo red stain in polarized light in the corneal stroma.

to label the antibody and visualize under a fluorescence microscope. The commonly used antibodies are summarized in Table 7.2.[1]

Electron Microscopy

Transmission electron microscopy (TEM) is useful in identifying cell organelles and viral particles at a very high magnification of up to 100,000X. Scanning electron microscope (SEM) is useful for the evaluation of structures like corneal endothelium.[1]

Polymerase Chain Reaction

Polymerase chain reaction (PCR) identifies DNA or RNA sequences specific to particular pathogenic organisms or cellular components. The most significant advantage of PCR is that it requires a tiny amount of sample. The nuclear chromatin is lyzed into individual sequences, and the desired sequence is amplified followed by its rapid detection using various electrophoresis methods.[1]

Table 7.2: Summary of immunohistochemistry antibodies.

Antibody	*Antigen*	*Diagnostic use*	*Ocular example*
Antiactin/myoglobin	Contractile filaments in smooth and striated muscle	Muscle derived tumors	Rhabdomyosarcoma
Desmin	Intermediate filaments in smooth and striated muscle	Muscle derived tumors	Rhabdomyosarcoma
Cytokeratin (CK 7)	High molecular weight glycoprotein epithelial cells	Metastatic adenocarcinomas, adnexal skin tumors	Sebaceous carcinoma
LCA, B cell (CD20), CD3 (T cell), Macrophage (CD68)	Components of T and B cells, macrophages	Hematological	Lymphomas
Cytokeratin/CAM 5.2/ AE1/AE3	Intermediate filaments in epithelial cells	Carcinomas derived from epidermis	Squamous cell carcinoma
Epithelial membrane antigen (EMA)	Epithelial cells and carcinomas	Carcinomas derived from epidermis	Sebaceous cell carcinoma meningioma
Factor VIII-related antigen	Endothelial cell	Vascular tumors and neovascularization	Ocular angiosarcoma
Glial fibrillar acidic protein (GFAP)	Glial cell constituents	Glial cells and astrocytes origin tumors	Astrocytic glioma of optic nerve
HMB45/Melan-A	Intracytoplasmic antigen in melanocytes	Tumors of melanocytic origin	Malignant melanomas
S-100	Neural crest cells	Peripheral nerve tumors	Schwannomas, melanocytic tumors
Vimentin smooth muscle antigen (SMA)	• Intermediate filaments • Cells of mesenchymal origin	Spindle cell tumors	Leiomyoma Fibrous histiocytoma
GLUT 1	Microvascular endothelium	Tumors of vascular origin	Infantile hemangioma

(GLUT-1: glucose transporter 1)

In Situ Hybridization

Similar to PCR the nuclear chromatin is segregated into fragments, which are detected by immunohistochemical techniques in routine light microscopy. Using this, the exact location of the protein fragments can be visualized within the tissue.[1]

Flow Cytometry[1]

Flow cytometry is useful in identification of various cell types such as B and T cells. Fluorescent antibodies specific to the antigens of different cell types are used for identification.[1]

COMMON HISTOPATHOLOGICAL SPECIMENS IN OPHTHALMOLOGY

Dermoid Cyst (Fig. 7.6)

- These are benign teratomas present since birth.
- Clinically most commonly seen in superotemporal quadrant of the eye, followed by superonasal quadrant.
- *Histologically*: It is lined by the epidermis and contains adnexal structures such as sebaceous glands and hair follicles. The lumen may contain pultaceous material, hair shafts, thyroid, bone, tooth, and other epidermal derived structures.

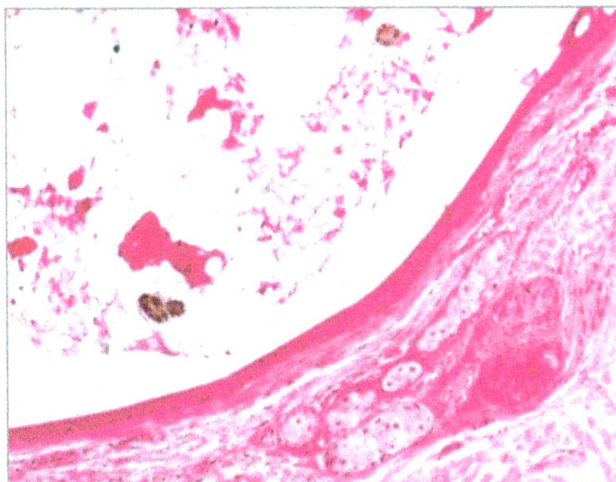

Fig. 7.6: Dermoid cyst—the cyst wall is lined by stratified squamous epithelium with hair follicle and epidermal appendages in its wall with desquamated keratin in its lumen.

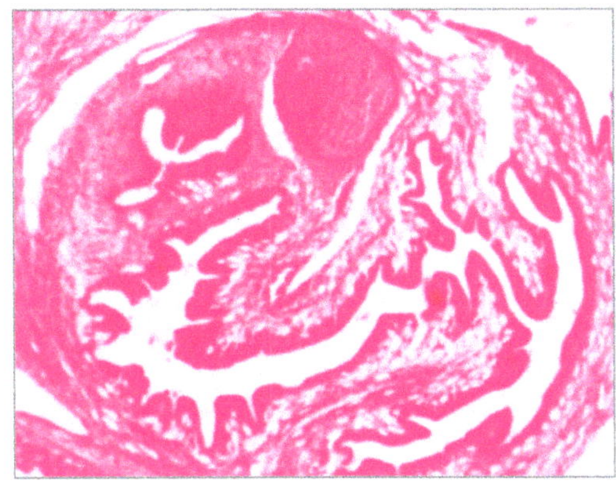

Fig. 7.7: Cysticercosis—body of a cysticercus larvae with multiple papillary infoldings.

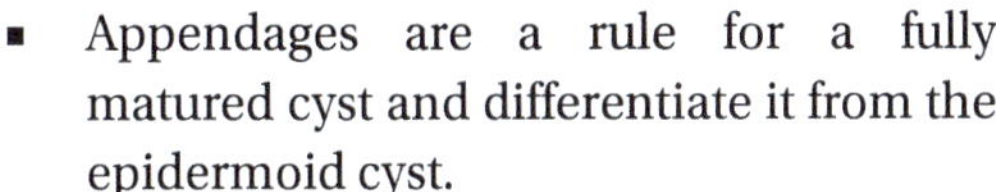

- Appendages are a rule for a fully matured cyst and differentiate it from the epidermoid cyst.
- Rupture of cyst during removal provokes a foreign body giant cell reaction and thus in toto removal of cyst should be done.

Pigmented Tumors

Benign tumors of nevus cells are called melanocytic nevi. These can be of the following types.

- *Intradermal nevus:*
  - It is the most common type of nevus.
  - Presents as an elevated mass, brown to black.
  - Histologically, nevus cells are arranged in the form of nests and cords and are located entirely in the dermis. Cells contain a moderate amount of cytoplasm and melanin. The nuclei mature as they go deeper in the dermis and cells become smaller, with less cytoplasm and less melanin and lie in a well-defined mass. Still lower down the nevus cells appear spindle-shaped. Maturation is regarded as an evidence of benignity. There is no malignant potential.
- *Congenital nevus*:
  - Larger in size than acquired nevus
  - Differentiated from acquired nevus on the basis of histology
  - Presence of nevus cells in lower reticular dermis/subcutaneous fat.
- *Compound nevus*:
  - Both intradermal and junctional component
  - Malignant potential is related to the junctional component.
- *Nevus of Ota*:
  - Bluish gray discoloration of periorbital skin with the sclera
  - Heterochromia or choroidal nevi may be present
  - Fusiform, bipolar, heavily pigmented melanocyte in the dermis.
- *Junctional nevus*:
  - Nevus cells are at the junction of epithelium and dermis
  - Low malignant potential.

Cysticercosis (Fig. 7.7)

Cysticercosis is caused by the larvae of the pork tapeworm, *Taenia solium, Cysticercus cellulosae*. The preferred tissues by the larvae are subcutaneous tissue, skeletal muscles, brain, and eye. Microscopically the scolex consists of a sucker and multiple papillary infoldings of tegument. The larvae contain a perioral double row of hooklets.[1]

The wall of the cyst shows characteristic histologic appearance, with three distinct layers:

i. *Outer layer/cuticular layer*: Corrugated containing multiple microtrichia, which are nothing but hair-like protrusions. This layer remains in contact with the host surface.
ii. Middle layer which is very thin and cellular.
iii. Inner layer which is thick and contains a network of multiple small canaliculi.

Chalazion (Fig. 7.8)

A chalazion is a chronic lipogranulomatous inflammation of the sebaceous glands (Zeis and Meibomian glands), resulting in a hard painless eyelid nodule. Microscopically, the essential lesion is the formation of focal granuloma centered around clear spaces (lipid vacuoles) discharged from sebaceous glands.

The lipid deposits can be stained using oil Red O Stain on frozen section. The granuloma contains giant cells, epithelioid cells, plasma cells, and lymphocytes.[1]

Differential diagnosis:

- Tuberculosis
- Sarcoidosis.
- Fungal infections
- Parasitic infections.

Basal Cell Carcinoma (Fig. 7.9)

Basal cell carcinoma (BCC) is the most common malignant eyelid tumor. It usually occurs in elderly patients. However, it occurs in equal frequency to squamous cell CA and sebaceous cell CA in India (33% of each). Most frequently involves the lower lid followed by upper lid, inner canthus, and lateral canthus. Clinically nodulo-ulcerative, pigmented, sclerosing or morphea types are described. The tumor tends to be locally invasive and almost never metastasize. Prognosis is good with complete excision.

Microscopically BCC shows small, moderate or large-sized groups of basaloid cells in papillary dermis with peripheral palisading. Pleomorphism and mitotic

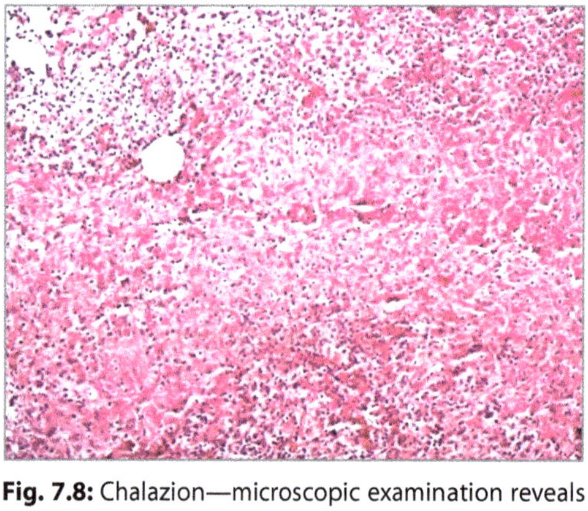

Fig. 7.8: Chalazion—microscopic examination reveals lipogranulomatous inflammation comprising of plasma cells, lymphocytes, histiocytes, giant cells and ill-defined epithelioid cell granuloma. Lipid dissolved during processing is shown as a large vacuolated area.

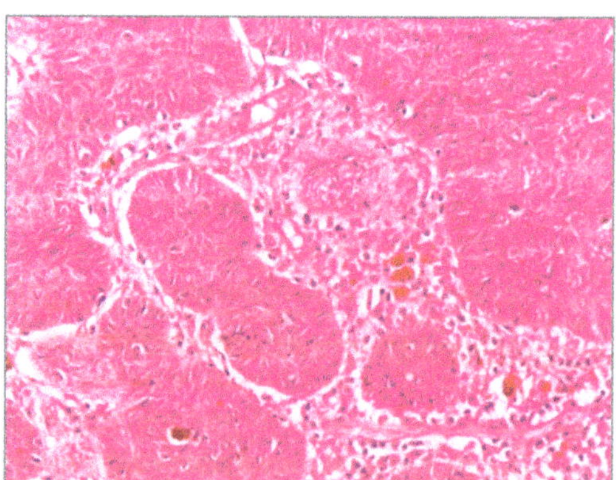

Fig. 7.9: Basal cell carcinoma—irregular islands of basophilic tumor cells arising from basal layer of the epidermis with characteristic peripheral palisading of tumor cells.

figures are often found in these cells. The surrounding and intervening dermis undergoes desmoplasia, fibroblasts become large, bizarre, and the mesenchymal tissue becomes loose and juicy.

Microscopic variants of basal cell carcinoma: Depending on the differentiation pattern, the tumor may be keratotic with parakeratotic cells and horn cysts; cystic basal cell carcinoma with cystic spaces within tumors lobules; adenoid basal cell carcinoma shows the formation of tubular, gland-like structures. The cells are arranged in a lace-like pattern. The morphea or sclerosing pattern shows elongated strands of basaloid cells embedded in a fibrous stroma.[1]

Retinoblastoma

It is the most common intraocular tumor seen in the pediatric age group. It arises from the nucleated retinal layers. The average age of presentation is 13 months. Six percent may be familial and 50% of these may be bilateral. Around 94% of the retinoblastomas are sporadic.

- *Endophytic retinoblastoma*: This form grows from the inner surface of the retina, and can be easily seen with ophthalmoscopy.
- *Exophytic retinoblastoma*: This form grows from the outer surface of retina toward the choroid.
- *Mixed, endo-exophytic*: Most common type.
- *Diffuse infiltrating retinoblastoma*: It is a rare (1-2%) histologic form of RB characterized by diffuse infiltration of the retina without a tumor mass.

Histology reveals cells with a large basophilic nucleus of variable size and shape and scanty cytoplasm. Mitotic figures are numerous (Figs. 7.10A to C). Rosettes are highly characteristic of retinoblastomas seen in well differentiated retinoblastomas. Flexner-Winter Steiner rosette is formed by cuboidal cells which are lined up around an empty central lumen. Special stains reveal acid mucopoly-

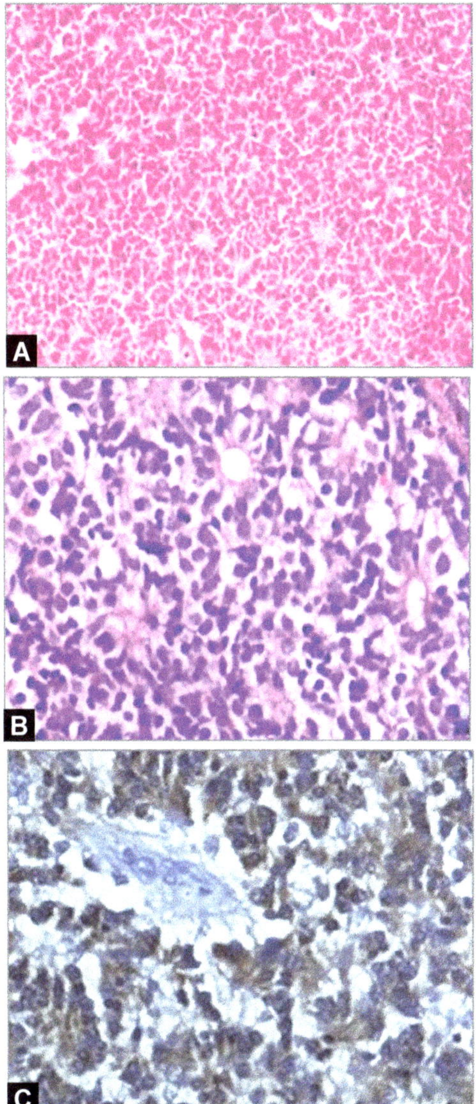

Figs. 7.10A to C: (A) Retinoblastoma—histologic section from a well differentiated retinoblastoma showing numerous Homer Wright rosettes. In these rosettes the pink material in the center represents tangle of processes of tumor cells; (B) Retinoblastoma—section shows Flexner-Wintersteiner rosettes with a central lumen; (C) Immunohistochemical stain synaptophysin shows cytoplasmic positivity in the tumor cells.

saccharides in the lumen. Homer-Wright rosettes are less common, and cells are not arranged around a lumen. The cells send out cytoplasmic processes and are lined up around cobweb-like material. Well-differentiated retinoblastoma has a better prognosis.[1]

Endophytic retinoblastomas tend to spread anteriorly by seeding into vitreous and aqueous. Aqueous seeding may stimulate a hypopyon. Deposits may appear on iris and in anterior chamber angle, and produce secondary angle closure glaucoma. Anterior uveal invasion leads to hematogenous disease or regional lymphatic spread.

Poorly differentiated retinoblastoma is composed of cells with a large basophilic nucleus of variable size and shape and scanty cytoplasm. No rossetes are identified. Mitotic figures are numerous. Necrotic retinoblastomas result in liberation of DNA from tumor nuclei. This DNA is preferentially absorbed by blood vessels.

Retinoblastoma, extraocular spread: Extraocular spread may occur to orbit and brain. All retinoblastomas show a striking tendency to invade the optic disc. Optic nerve involvement increases the mortality to 15% when the invasion is up to lamina cribrosa. This increases up to 65% when the resected margin is involved. Once in the nerve, the tumor can reach chiasma through nerve bundles or subarachnoid space through the pia. The access to subarachnoid space can occur via central retinal vessels. Histopathological high risk factors like massive choroidal invasion, optic nerve retrolaminar region and cut end involvement, iris and ciliary body involvement, scleral and extrascleral invasion should be looked for in the histopathology sections for adjuvant chemotherapy.[1]

Melanoma

Malignant melanoma of the eyelid is rare. It may originate from a long-standing nevus, acquired melanosis, or de novo. The prognosis is poor with early metastasis (bloodstream or lymphatics). Microscopically great variability can be observed. The cell size varies from small as in lymphomas to large as in soft tissue sarcoma. The cytoplasm can be basophilic, eosinophilic or completely clear. Melanin may be scanty, abundant or absent (amelanotic melanoma). The overlying epithelium and underlying dermis are invaded. The component cells of neoplasm are atypical with high nuclear-cytoplasmic ratio and mitotic figures occasionally.[1]

Squamous Cell Carcinoma

Keratoacanthoma

It is a benign tumor characterized by rapid growth (months) and hyperkeratosis. It is of an ovoid-shaped with a central keratin core. Spontaneous resolution can occur, but surgical excision is effective. Gross appearance includes a well-defined nodule with central umbilication containing keratinized core and a smooth rounded peripheral surface.[1]

Premalignant Lesions

Actinic/Solar/Senile keratosis: Precancerous changes in the epidermis follow overexposure to sunlight. The characteristic clinical appearance consists of a nonelevated, variable-sized plaque with irregular margins. The management consists of excision.[1]

Squamous Cell Carcinoma

Squamous cell carcinoma (SCC) can occur due to chronic sun exposure, exposure to ionizing radiation, chronic irritation, and infection by human papillomavirus (HPV).

Clinically, the most common presentation is as a nodule, which may ulcerate.

Grossly, the tumor appears as a heavily keratinized or ulcerated mass with irregular edges (Fig. 7.11).

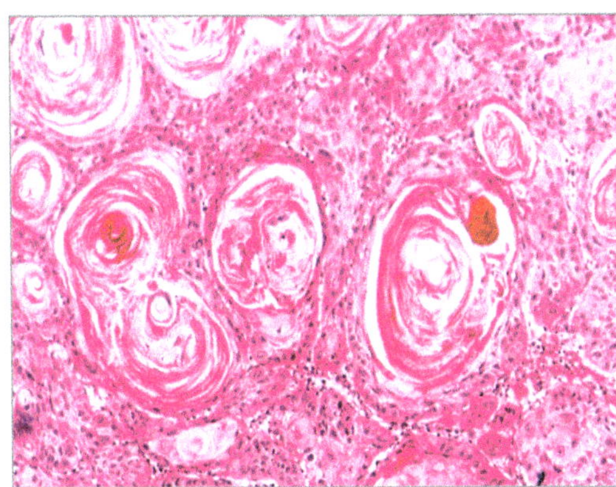

Fig. 7.11: Squamous cell carcinoma—numerous pearls seen in a well differentiated squamous cell carcinoma.

Microscopically, the appearance depends upon the grade of differentiation. A well-differentiated tumor has the formation of characteristic keratin pearls along with features of metaplasia. Keratin pearl is a focus of central keratinization within concentric layers of abnormal squamous cells around it. In doubtful cases, immunohistochemistry to identify cytokeratins such as CAM 5.2, AE1, and AE3 helps in diagnosis. In poorly differentiated type, nest-like squamous differentiation is lost, but intercellular bridges are still identified. Spindle cell type carries the worst prognosis among all types.[1]

Sebaceous Cell Carcinoma

It usually arises from pilosebaceous follicles and sebaceous glands (Meibomian and Zeiss). Clinically it presents as a yellow nodule, which may be ulcerated, along with the presence of telangiectatic blood vessels. The other mode of the presentation includes plaque-like lesion, chronic blepharoconjunctivitis, and recurrent eyelid inflammation. Lymph node and distant metastasis can occur in advanced cases.

Sebaceous carcinomas are usually nodular in form and are unilateral, but an ability to spread within the epidermis simulates a chronic blepharoconjunctivitis (masquerade syndrome).

Clinically presents as a yellow nodule that may or may not be ulcerated, if the diagnosis is delayed. It is more common in the elderly, females, and the upper lid.[1]

For special stain Oil Red O, frozen section is preferred as normal tissue preparation which removes fat, an important finding for the diagnosis. Grossly, the tumor appears as a pale yellow nodular lesion. Microscopically characterized by the presence of lobule, surrounded by a single cuboidal basal layer. The center of the lobule contains foamy cells. These cells have characteristic lipid-laden foamy cytoplasm and a small nucleus. In the neck of the follicle, the cells fragment to release lipid into the ducts (holocrine secretion) (Figs. 7.12A and B).

In a well-differentiated sebaceous gland carcinoma, the morphology is lobular, and the center of the lobule contains foamy cells. The basal cells may fail to differentiate into foamy cells and the lobules are filled with small basophilic cells.

In less well-differentiated tumors, the basal cells predominate and the cytoplasm contains small circular spaces which represent the lipid globules which were removed during paraffin processing.

In completely differentiated tumors, lipid spaces are rare and are seen only in thin sections at high magnification.

In advanced cases, the tumor infiltrates the eyelids extensively.[1]

Rhinosporidiosis

It is a granulomatous disease caused by aquatic protistan parasite *Rhinosporidium seeberi*. It primarily affects the mucous membrane including conjunctiva. The nasal form is the most common clinical type accounting for 70% of the cases.[1]

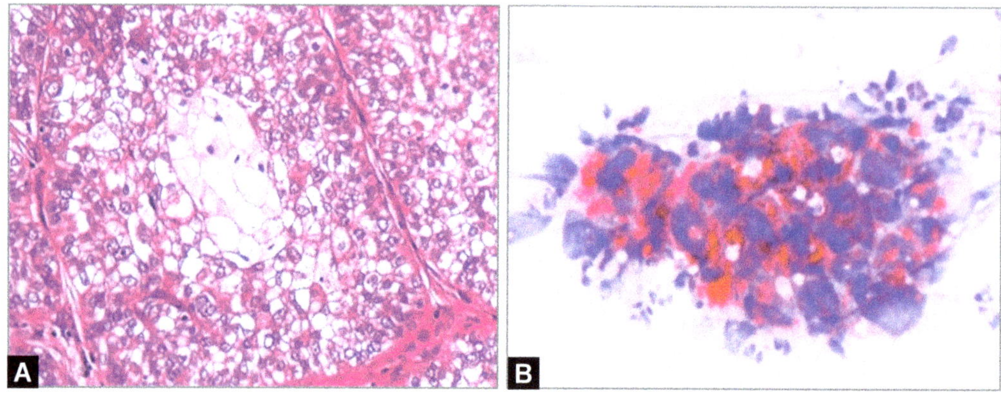

Figs. 7.12A and B: (A) Sebaceous cell carcinoma—well differentiated sebaceous cell carcinoma showing sebaceous differentiation in the center of a tumor island; (B) Aspirate from a lid mass shows orange colored intracytoplasmic lipids as seen on Oil Red O stain.

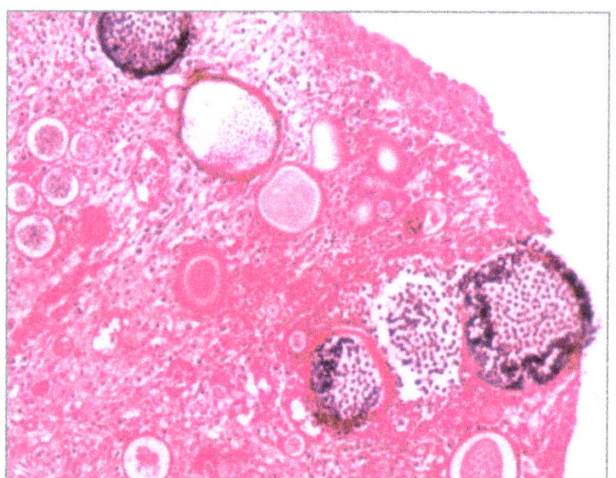

Fig. 7.13: Rhinosporidiosis—numerous sporangia of rhinosporidiosis seeberi are seen in the conjunctival stroma.

Infection of the palpebral conjunctiva occurs in around 15% of the cases. In conjunctiva and lid, it leads to the formation of a solitary, friable mass lesion.

Histologic Examination (Fig. 7.13)

Histologic examination demonstrates thick-walled sacs or sporangia. The sporangium contains numerous spores (size of an erythrocyte). A granulomatous response may be seen. Spores and sporangia can be seen on conventional sections and are highlighted by PAS or methenamine silver stain. Usually, surgery is required as there is no response to antibiotics.[1]

Lacrimal Gland Tumor

The tumor can arise from either the acinar (adenocarcinoma) or the ductal (pleomorphic adenomas/adenocarcinomas) part of the lacrimal gland.

Pleomorphic Adenoma

It is the most common lacrimal gland tumor. It accounts for 50% of the epithelial tumors of the lacrimal gland. The term pleomorphic is used as it contains cells arising from epithelium as well as mesenchyme. It is also called as mixed tumor because of this mixed cells of origin.[1]

Macroscopic examination (Fig. 7.14): Grossly, it appears as a single solid mass, gray-white in color, with a bosselated surface. On cut section, mucoid cystic spaces and hemorrhage can be seen.

Microscopic examination: Microscopically, the tissues show two different components as described below:

- *Epithelial component*: Characterized by the formation of a glandular pattern with cords and ducts. The ducts may contain

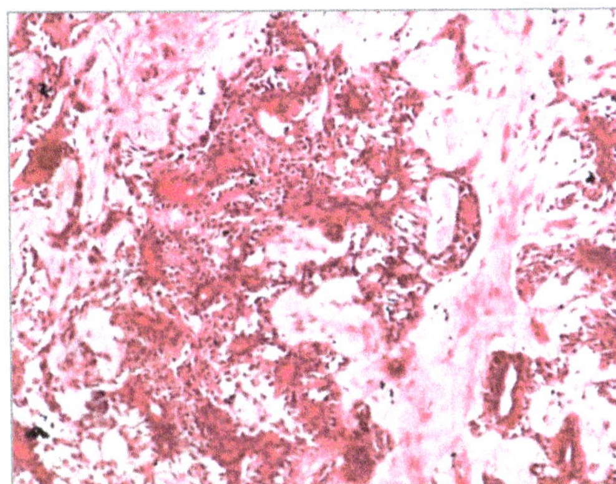

Fig. 7.14: Pleomorphic adenoma—histology shows a characteristic biphasic pattern consisting of a pale myomatous stroma and cellular area containing epithelial element.

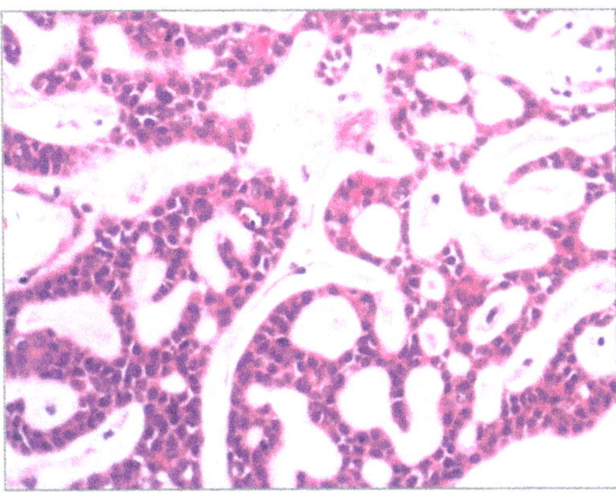

Fig. 7.15: Adenoid cystic carcinoma—characteristic swiss cheese pattern or cribriform appearance of the tumor on microscopic examination.

eosinophilic proteinaceous material within the lumen.

- *Stromal component*: Characterized by the formation of connective tissue components such as fibrous with myxoid areas, and rarely fat and cartilage within the tumor. The mass is usually surrounded by a pseudocapsule, formed due to fibrous condensation around the mass as it grows over a while.[1]

Malignant Lacrimal Gland Tumor

Malignant lesions are characterized by rapid onset, rapid progression, and presence of pain in contrast to a benign tumor.

Adenoid cystic carcinoma (ACC): ACC is the most common malignant tumor of the lacrimal gland.

Macroscopic examination: It appears as a pale-gray mass.

Microscopic examination: It may form a cribriform, solid or tubular pattern depending upon the arrangement of ducts and myxoid material. Cribriform is the most common variant. The pathognomonic appearance is called *"Swiss cheese"* appearance (Fig. 7.15). This appearance is caused by the presence of solid cords of hyperchromatic cuboidal cells with a high mitotic rate surrounding cystic spaces containing myxoid material which are PAS positive.[1] The other characteristic findings include peripheral perineurial invasion, no squamous differentiation, and no extensive necrosis. It can be graded into three grades depending upon the proportion of the solid component.

- *Grade 1*: Primarily tubular or cribriform with an occasional solid component.
- *Grade 2*: Primarily cribriform or mixed with solid component less than 50%.
- *Grade 3*: Solid component more than 50%.[1]

Adenocarcinoma: Similar to ACC, but the pattern is that of solid masses of tumor tissue.

REFERENCE

1. Sehu KW, Lee WR. Ophthalmic Pathology: An Illustrated Guide for Clinicians. New Jersey: Wiley; 2008. p. 290.

8

CHAPTER

Ocular Microbiology

Siddhi Goel, Nishat Hussain Ahmed, Geeta Satpathy

INTRODUCTION

Microbiology has an invaluable role in the management of ocular infection. Several terms are essential to understanding the basic concepts of ocular microbiology. These are described below:

- *Primary infection*: When the organism infects the eye for the first time.
- *Secondary infection*: When the infection by a microorganism occurs in an already infected eye with a different microorganism. The example includes bacterial infection over and above in a case of mycotic keratitis. The most common pattern seen in the eye is a superadded fungal infection in a patient with bacterial keratitis.
- *Reinfection*: When the same organism causes the infection again.
- *Reactivation*: When the organism remains dormant for a variable period in any of the organs and causes infection by reactivation under various conditions of stress. Recurrent herpes simplex keratitis is the best example of such reactivation.
- *Latent period*: The time gap between infection to infectiousness.
- *Incubation period*: The period between infection and onset of the disease.
- *Nosocomial infection*: When a patient acquires an infection during the hospital stay. The infection may be acquired from slit lamp, applanation tonometer, hands of hospital staff, prosthesis, tap water, etc.
- *Iatrogenic infection*: It is a physician-induced infection due to therapy; a typical example is hepatitis B infection or human immunodeficiency virus (HIV) following blood transfusion.
- *Carriers*: They are persons who harbor the pathogenic organism without actually manifesting the disease; however, they can transmit the infection to others.

ROLE OF MICROBIOLOGY IN OPHTHALMOLOGY

The normal ocular surface flora consists of a wide range of organisms mainly due to the nutrient rich nature of it. The microorganisms can either be saprophytes or commensals; both the group of organisms do not produce disease in the immunocompetent host. The eye is exposed to the atmosphere throughout the waking hours and their proximity with skin, nasopharynx, and paranasal sinuses make them vulnerable to contamination.

Ocular infections can be self-limiting requiring only symptomatic treatment while some may be mild which can be managed with empirical therapy and there may be some which are potentially blinding infections which need urgent attention and systemic antimicrobial therapy based on antimicrobial sensitivity.

Infections of the lid and adnexa are common and caused by the proliferation of the local flora or infection by a virulent organism. However, infection of the globe requires a breach of the natural barriers, either by trauma, surgery or other risk factors. Sometimes, the infection may be endogenous, which come from other parts of the body through the bloodstream or lymphatic system. The best example of endogenous infection is metastatic endophthalmitis.

There are multiple barriers to ocular infections (Table 8.1).[1] For ocular infections to occur, a breach in these defense mechanisms is essential. Various infectious diseases of the eye include:[2]

- Conjunctivitis
- Infective keratitis
- Endophthalmitis
- Panophthalmitis
- Infectious uveitis
- Orbital cellulitis
- Infections of the lacrimal system like dacryocystitis and dacryoadenitis
- Adnexal infections like blepharitis, meibomitis, etc.
- Iatrogenic infections (postsurgery).

The various organisms implicated in ocular infections can be classified as prokaryotes or eukaryotes (Table 8.2). Prokaryotic cells are primitive cells that lack any nucleus or membrane-bound organelles, in contrast, eukaryotic cells contain nucleus as well as membrane-bound organelles.

Table 8.1: Barriers to ocular infections.

Anatomical	• Bony orbit • Eyelids • Eyelashes • Epithelial barrier of cornea and conjunctiva
Mechanical	• Blink reflex • Lacrimal drainage system • Tear film lipid layer
Antimicrobial defense	• Tear film constituents like mucin, immunoglobulin A (IgA), complement proteins, lactoferrin, lysozyme, beta-lysin and ceruloplasmin • Conjunctiva-associated lymphoid tissue (CALT) consisting of both B and T lymphocytes • IgA and glycocalyx cross links on anterior surface of cornea

Table 8.2: Classification of microorganisms causing ocular infections.

Prokaryotes	*Eukaryotes*
Bacteria **Gram-positive cocci** *Staphylococcus aureus* *Staphylococcus epidermidis* *Streptococcus pneumoniae* *Streptococcus pyogenes* *Streptococcus viridans* *Enterococcus* species *Peptostreptococcus* species **Gram-positive bacilli** *Corynebacterium diphtheriae* *Clostridium* species *Bacillus* species **Gram-negative cocci/ coccobacilli** *Neisseria gonorrhoeae* *Moraxella* species *Acinetobacter* species **Gram-negative bacilli** *Pseudomonas aeruginosa* *Escherichia coli* *Klebsiella* species *Proteus* species *Serratia marcescens* **Filamentous bacteria** *Actinomyces* *Nocardia* *Mycobacterium* *Streptomyces* **Spirochetes** *Treponema pallidum* *Borrelia* *Leptospira* **Mycoplasma** **Rickettsiae and chlamydia**	***Fungi*** *Fusarium* species *Candida* species *Aspergillus* species *Acremonium* species *Alternaria* species *Penicillium* species *Bipolaris* species **Parasites** *Acanthamoeba* species *Microsporidia* *Onchocerca volvulus* *Leishmania brasiliensis* *Trypanosoma* species *Toxoplasma*

MICROBIOLOGY METHODS

The various methods used to identify the causative organism include various stains to identify the morphology of the organism and culture media to grow these organisms.

Sample Collection and Transport

Appropriate collection and transport of specimen is the first important step in diagnosing ocular infections. Since the specimens available from ocular infection are very small and the load of infectious organisms is less, extra care should be taken while obtaining samples. It is recommended to obtain dual swabs, one for smear examination and one for culture. The commonly used specimens in ocular infections are:

- A swab from the lids
- Conjunctival swab
- Corneal scraping
- Aqueous tap
- Vitreous tap/biopsy
- Explanted intraocular lens (IOL)
- Infected scleral bands, buckle, etc.
- Contact lens solution and case
- Infected corneal button
- Regurgitated material from canaliculi/sac
- Discharge from orbital and lacrimal sinuses/fistula or nasal cavity.

In cases where patient-side inoculation is not possible, transport media are used. Example of such transport media include Amies transport medium without charcoal that allows the sample to be stored for about 24 hours. For transport of specimens in suspected viral infection the sample must be transferred in ice, more so when a significant delay is expected.

Microscopy

The various methods of microscopy used to identify organisms included potassium hydroxide (KOH) wet mount preparation, Gram's stain, Giemsa stain, and special stains such as Ziehl-Neelsen (acid-fast stain) and modified Grocott-Gomori methenamine-silver nitrate stain.[3] Microscopy which is done directly from the clinical specimen is called primary microscopy whereas secondary microscopy is smear examination done on the growth obtained upon culture.

Gram's Staining

Gram staining is a differential staining technique named after Danish bacteriologist Hans Christian Gram,[4] who developed the technique. Depending on the cell wall properties the bacteria are categorized into two groups, i.e. Gram-positive or Gram-negative.

Procedure

- Take a clean glass slide
- Make a thin smear and allow it to air dry
- Heat fixation is done by passing the slide over the flame several times so that the heat is unbearable by touching the slide on the dorsum of the hand
- Pour crystal violet (primary dye) on the smear and wait for 1 minute
- Wash under running tap water
- Stain with Gram's iodine for 1 minute
- Wash under running tap water
- Decolorize with acetone for 2–4 seconds
- Wash the slide and apply safranin (counterstain) for 1–2 minutes
- Blot dry and observe under 100X (oil immersion) objective of the microscope.

Principle and Interpretation

Thicker peptidoglycan layer and acidic protoplasm of the Gram-positive bacteria allows them to retain the basic primary dye against decolorization, whereas thinner peptidoglycan layer and labile outer membrane in Gram-negative bacteria permit decolorization. Thus, a Gram-positive bacteria will appear blue as it will retain the gentian violet-iodine complex. In contrast, a Gram-negative will appear blue-purple as it will lose its gentian violet-iodine complex in the decolorization step and appear pink after counterstaining with safranin. The Gram-positive bacteria appear purple due to retention of primary dye and Gram-negative bacteria appear pink due to counter-stain. Also, the smear should be assessed for inflammatory cells, arrangement, and shape of the bacteria, and their uniformity of staining.

Clinical Application

- Gram-stained smear showing pus cells and Gram-positive cocci in clusters suggest staphylococcal infection (Fig. 8.1).
- Gram-stained smear showing pus cells and Gram-positive cocci in pairs surrounded by a clear halo suggest *Streptococcus pneumoniae.*
- Gram-stain smear showing pus cells and Gram-negative intracellular and extracellular cocci in pairs (diplococci) suggest *Neisseria* infection (Fig. 8.2).

Potassium Hydroxide Wet Mount

Potassium hydroxide mounts are used for detection of fungal elements in patient's specimens.

Procedure

- Take a clean glass slide.
- Place the specimen in the center of the slide.
- Put one drop of 10% KOH on the specimen.
- Put a coverslip while avoiding any air bubbles.
- Incubate at room temperature for 30–90 minutes to allow clearing of the specimen.
- Screen under 10X objective of the microscope for the presence of fungal elements.
- Confirm the findings by examining under 40X objective.

Principle and Interpretation

Potassium hydroxide digests the animal cells leaving behind the fungal elements intact. KOH helps in loosening the corneal stromal lamellae and exposing more fungal filaments. Fungal elements can be appreciated as

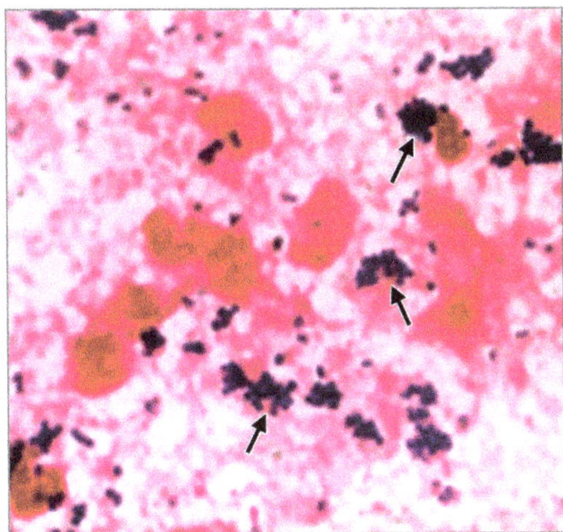

Fig. 8.1: Gram-positive cocci in clusters suggestive of *Staphylococcus* species.

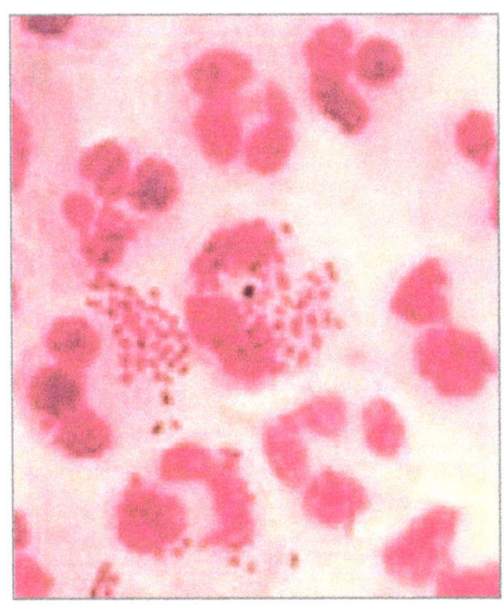

Fig. 8.2: Gram-negative cocci, mostly intracellular.

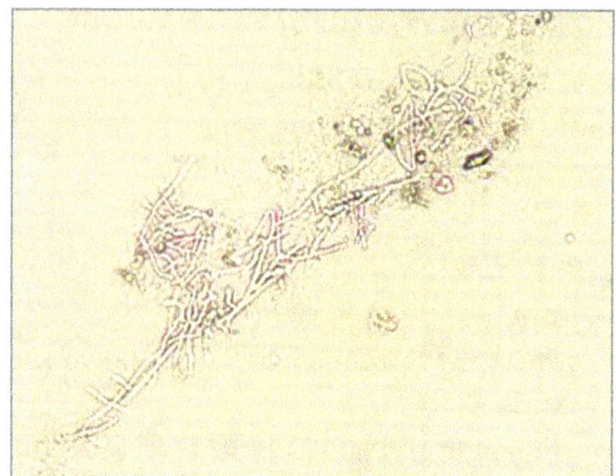

Fig. 8.3: KOH mount showing fungal hyphae.

refractile, septate or aseptate hyphae (Fig. 8.3) yeast cells or conidia with specific morphology. KOH mount also helps to identify *Acanthamoeba.*

Clinical Application

- Septate hyphae with V-shaped acute angle branching is suggestive of infection with *Aspergillus* species.
- Aseptate hyphae with irregular or right-angled branching are suggestive of infection with *Rhizopus/Mucor*.

Figures 8.4A to H depict the characteristics of common fungi implicated in ocular infections.

Ziehl–Neelsen (Acid-fast) Stain

It is a special stain used for the identification of suspected *Mycobacteria, Actinomyces* or *Nocardia.*

Procedure

- Flame the slide to hit fix (as described above).
- Flood the entire slide with carbol fuchsin.
- The slides are then heated slowly with a Bunsen burner until steaming. The steaming is maintained for 5 minutes using low or intermittent heat.
- Wash the slide with water.
- Using 3% acid alcohol, flood the slide and allow to decolorize for 5 minutes.
- Wash the slide with water.
- Flood the slide with methylene blue (counterstain) for 1 minute.
- Wash the slide with water.

Principle and Interpretation

Mycobacteria, few strains of *Nocardia* resist decolorization by a strong acid (hence the name acid fast) after staining with basic carbol fuchsin. These organisms have unique lipid-rich cell walls that resist decolorization. Acid-fast organism appears red against a blue background.

Clinical Application

Mycobacteria are acid-fast, *Nocardia* stain variably, whereas *Actinomyces* are nonacid-fast.

Culture

Culture is the gold standard tool for diagnosing bacterial and fungal infections. Most organisms appear on culture media with distinct characteristics, which helps in easy identification of causative pathogen. The features to be noted while studying the colonies on solid media include shape, size, elevation, margins, surface, edges, color, structure, and consistency.

Culture Media

In ocular microbiology, the commonly used culture media are:

- *Nutrient agar*: It is a type of basic media that support the growth of most nonfastidious bacteria.
- *Blood agar*: It is a type of enriched media, which is used to grow nutritionally exacting (fastidious) bacteria. This

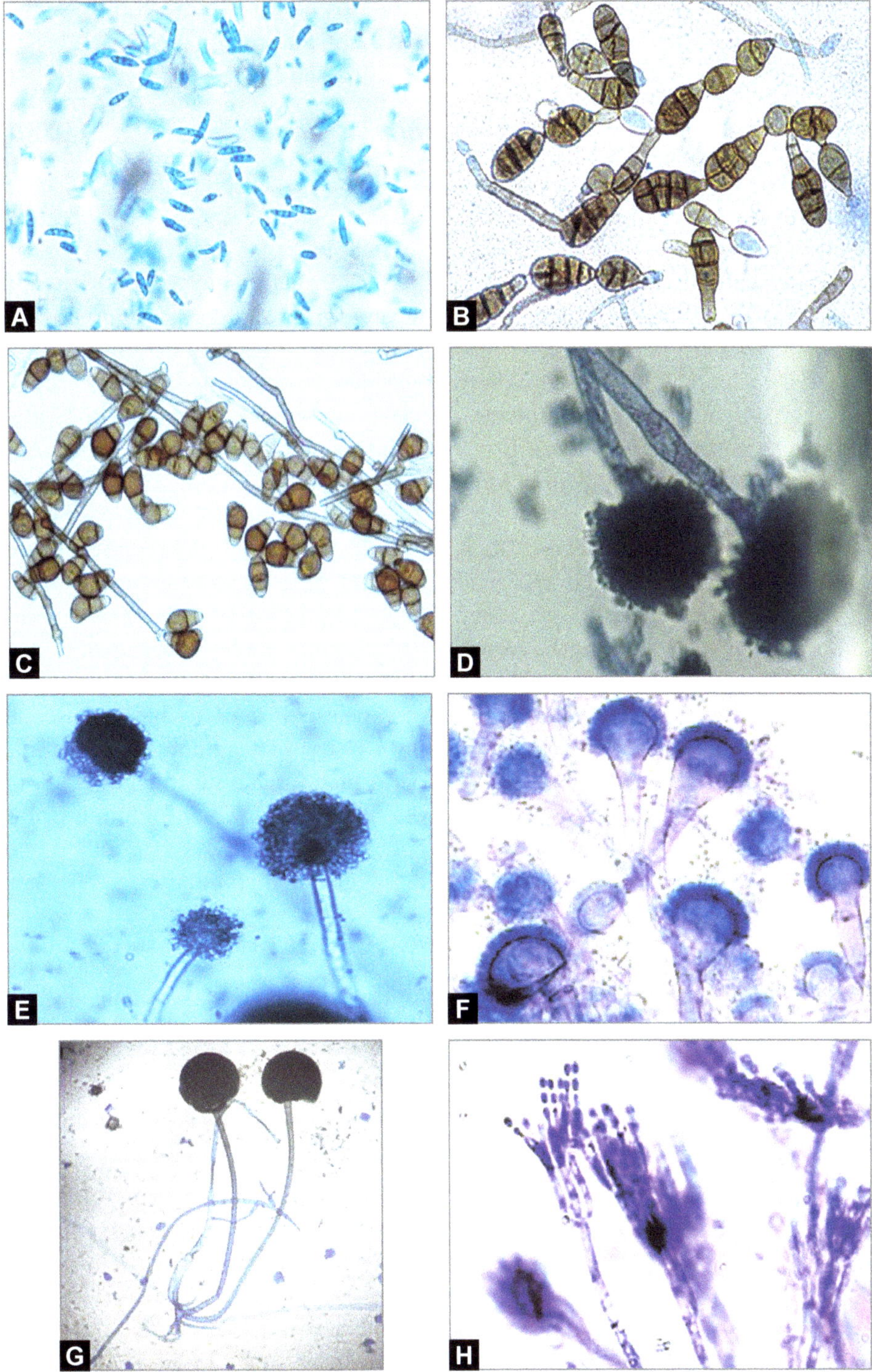

Figs. 8.4A to H: (A) *Fusarium* species (note the sickle-shaped spores); (B) *Alternaria* species (note the vertically and horizontally divided spores); (C) *Curvularia* species; (D) *Aspergillus flavus*; (E) *Aspergillus niger*; (F) *Aspergillus fumigatus*; (G) *Rhizopus* species; (H) *Penicillium* species.

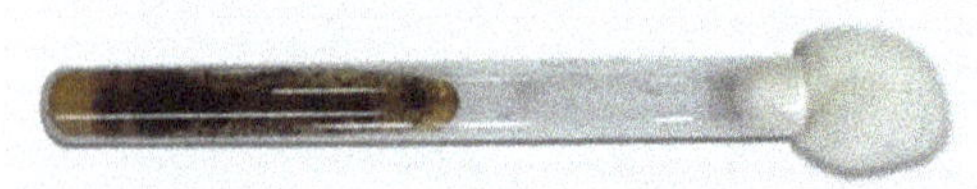

Fig. 8.5: Sabouraud's dextrose agar depicting fungal growth.

contains 5-10% (by volume) blood added to a blood agar base.

- *Chocolate agar*: It is also an enriched media also known as heated blood agar or lysed blood agar.
- *Thioglycollate broth*: It is a liquid medium used for growth of anaerobic organisms.
- *Sabouraud's dextrose agar (SDA)*: It is a nonselective medium for growth of fungi (Fig. 8.5).
- *Lowenstein-Jensen (LJ) medium*: It is a selective medium which is designed to suppress the growth of some microorganisms while allowing the growth of others. LJ medium is used to recover *Mycobacterium tuberculosis* and is made selective by incorporating malachite green.

Culture Techniques[5]

For aerobic bacterial cultures, all media are incubated at 37°C for 48-72 hours. Chocolate agar is incubated in 3-5% CO_2 in a candle jar or CO_2 incubator. For anaerobic bacterial cultures, anaerobic chamber or anaerobic jar with a gas pack is required. Anaerobic cultures are incubated at least for 5 days before discarding. SDA requires a temperature of 25-27°C and a biochemical oxygen demand (BOD) incubator. Fungal cultures are incubated for at least 2 weeks before a specimen is considered negative. The *Mycobacteria* may take as long as 4-6 weeks to grow. *Acanthamoebae* are grown on non-nutrient agar with an overlay of *Escherichia coli* and are incubated at 37°C for 2 weeks. Once the culture shows positive growth, the organisms are subjected to various procedures like microscopy, biochemical tests, subcultures to special media, etc. for identification.

Antimicrobial Susceptibility Testing

The pathogenic microorganisms, especially bacteria, are known to develop resistance to antibiotics or may be insensitive to a particular antibiotic. Thus, susceptibility testing is a must at least for all bacterial pathogens.[6] It helps in determining the most effective drug that can be used for treatment. The two commonly used methods are disck diffusion method and broth dilution.

Disc diffusion method is the most widely used method; it is easy to perform, cost-effective, and reasonably accurate. It consists of using a standard disc of filter paper impregnated with a standard strength of antibiotic under investigation. Dilution method is mostly employed to titrate the therapeutic dose of antibiotic. Susceptibility testing against antifungal drugs can be performed for various fungi by broth or agar dilution methods, where minimum inhibitory concentration (MIC) is determined or by the disc diffusion method.

MOLECULAR METHODS

Molecular methods, especially polymerase chain reaction (PCR), are highly sensitive and specific in diagnosing ocular infections. PCR involves using a pair of priming complementary sequences (oligonucleotide primers), through which multiple copies of a targeted chimeric gene are obtained. The three major steps involved are denaturation, annealing, and elongation. It is particularly useful in diagnosing infections due to organisms which are difficult to isolate by traditional techniques like culture including viruses, microsporidia, chlamydia, etc. or those organisms that take a long time to grow, such as *M. tuberculosis*.

IMMUNODIAGNOSTIC METHODS

These tests are useful for detection of chlamydia antigen by immunofluorescence in conjunctival swabs and that of herpes simplex virus (HSV) in corneal scrapings. Antibody detection is also sometimes helpful in ocular manifestations of systemic diseases like syphilis, toxoplasmosis, etc. The direct immunofluorescence (DIF) assay involves fixing the specimens with methanol on a slide and staining with monoclonal immunoglobulin G (IgG) Ab conjugated with fluorescein according to manufacturer instructions. DIF is more sensitive and more reliable than Giemsa staining for detection of *Chlamydia trachomatis* in the conjunctiva samples of patients with follicular conjunctivitis.[7] Indirect immunofluorescent antibody techniques are a useful tool detection of HSV and have a high sensitivity (97%) and specificity (73%) when compared to HSV cultures.[8]

IN VIVO CONFOCAL MICROSCOPY

It is a noninvasive technique for direct visualization of pathogen throughout the entire depth of the cornea. In vivo confocal microscopy (IVCM) allows for rapid identification of fungi and *Acanthamoeba*. The fungal branching angle detected in IVCM imaging of keratitis can be used to differentiate between fungal species, with a 90° angle reported in *Fusarium* species and 45° in *Aspergillus* species.[9] There is increasing evidence that keratitis caused by *Aspergillus* species may have worse clinical outcomes, higher risk of serious complications such as corneal perforation and respond less well to natamycin therapy compared with *Fusarium* species. Therefore, IVCM is a useful tool to distinguish between the two species early on in the clinical course. It is particularly useful when corneal infiltrates are deep-seated. It can also be used to monitor the patients' response based on the density of organisms before and after the treatment. However, there are limitations in its widespread use as it requires the expensive machine and expertise in confocal microscopy along with excellent patient cooperation. Moreover, it can only be used for cases of keratitis.

Table 8.3: Classification of antifungals.

Class of drug	*Examples*
Antibiotics	Polyenes—amphotericin B, nystatin, natamycin Echinocandins—caspofungin, micafungin Heterocyclic benzofuran—griseofulvin
Antimetabolites	Flucytosine
Azoles	Imidazoles—clotrimazole, econazole, miconazole, ketoconazole Triazoles—fluconazole, itraconazole, voriconazole, posaconazole
Allylamine	Terbinafine

VIVA QUESTIONS

1. Give the intrastromal/intracameral dose of various antifungals used in ophthalmology.

Ans.

- Amphotericin B: 5–7.5 µg/0.1 mL
- Natamycin: 1 µg/0.1 mL
- Voriconazole: 50–100 µg/0.1 mL.

2. Classify various antifungals.

Ans. Refer to Table 8.3.

REFERENCES

1. Klotz SA, Penn CC, Negvesky GJ, et al. Fungal and Parasitic Infections of the Eye. Clin Microbiol Rev. 2000;13:662-85.

2. Armstrong RA. The microbiology of the eye. Ophthalmic Physiol Opt. 2000;20(6):429-41.
3. Ahmed NH, Satapathy G. Primary microscopy as a point of care test in ophthalmology. Ocular Microbiol DOS Times. 2016;22(3):47-50.
4. Gram HC. "Über die isolierte Färbung der Schizomyceten in Schnitt-und Trockenpräparaten" (in German). Fortschritte der Medizin. 1884;2:185-9.
5. Ahmed NH, Satapathy G. Ocular infections: microbiological perspective. Ocular Microbiol DOS Times. 2017;22(4):35-42.
6. CLSI. Performance Standards for Antimicrobial Susceptibility Testing; Twenty-Third Informational Supplement. CLSI document M100-S26. Wayne, PA: Clinical and Laboratory Standards Institute; 2016.
7. Abedinyfar Z, Doustdar F, Amoli FA, et al. Comparison of Direct Immunofluorescence (DIF) Method and Giemsa Staining with PCR Method for Detection of *Chlamydia trachomatis* in Patients with Follicular Conjunctivitis. J Med Microbiol Diagn. 2016;5(4):216-60.
8. Schwab IR, Raju VK, McClung J. Indirect immunofluorescent antibody diagnosis of herpes simplex with upper tarsal and corneal scrapings. Ophthalmology. 1986;93(6):752-6.
9. Chidambaram JD, Prajna NV, Larke N, et al. In vivo confocal microscopy appearance of *Fusarium* and *Aspergillus* species in fungal keratitis. Br J Ophthalmol. 2017;101(8):1119-23.

9 CHAPTER Community Ophthalmology

9.1 BLINDNESS: DEFINITION, BURDEN, PREVENTION, AND REHABILITATION

Vivek Gupta, Pallavi Shukla, Suraj S Senjam, Meenakshi Wadhwani, Praveen Vashist

DEFINITION

Standardized measurement and classification of visual impairment and blindness are vital to ensuring the correct comparison of the burden of them across regions and countries. An initial definition recommended by the 1948 World Health Organization (WHO) Expert Committee on Health Statistics was a central visual acuity (VA) of 6/60 (20/200) or worse with the best correcting lens, or widest diameter of visual field no greater than 20°. The definition has changed over the years and before 2006, the definition endorsed by the WHO under ICD-10 (International Statistical Classification of Diseases and Related Health Problems-10) was based on best-corrected visual acuity (BCVA) of less than 3/60 in better eye or a visual field of under 10°. In 2006, the definition was changed to reflect the importance of refractive errors as a cause of blindness. The standardized definition adopted by WHO since 2006 is as shown in Table 9.1.1.[1] Thus, the current definition of blindness by WHO is—*"presenting visual acuity (PVA) of less than 20/400 (3/60) or a visual field of no greater than 10° in radius around central point of fixation in the better eye".* The term "low vision" was present in ICD-10 before 2006. This term was replaced by category 1 and 2. This was done so since the term "low vision" is commonly used to identify patients who need low vision care and services (as described later in the chapter) and has a different definition.

In India, the National Programme for Control of Blindness used to define blindness as "presenting distance visual acuity less than 20/200 (6/60) in the better eye" or decrease in field of vision to less than 20° around the central point of fixation in the better eye. However, with this definition in place, it was difficult to compare the blindness data of India with the worldwide statistics. As a result, there used to be wide disparity in estimation of blindness and visual impairment as per WHO and National Programme for Control of Blindness (NPCB). Another implication of this definition was that uncorrected refractive error (URE) emerged as an important cause of blindness as per Indian data. This also decreased

Table 9.1.1: Definition of blindness after the 2006 revision of ICD-10.

Category	*Presenting visual acuity (PVA) for distance vision*	
	Worse than	*Equal to or better than*
Category 0, early or mild or no visual impairment (EVI)	-	6/18
Category 1, moderate visual impairment (MVI)	6/18 3/10 (0.3) 20/70	6/60 1/10 (0.1) 20/200
Category 2, severe visual impairment (SVI)	6/60 1/10 (0.1) 20/200	3/60 1/20 (0.05) 20/400
Category 3, blindness: OR visual field 10° or less radius around central point of fixation in the better eye	3/60 1/20 (0.05) 20/400	1/60 1/50 (0.02) 20/1200 or counts finger (CF) at 1 m
Category 4, blindness: OR visual field 10° or less radius around central point of fixation in the better eye	1/60 1/50 (0.02) 20/1200	Light Perception
Category 5, blindness: OR visual field 10° or less radius around central point of fixation in the better eye	No light perception	
Category 9, unspecified or undetermined		

the emphasis on other causes of blindness such as glaucoma and posterior segment diseases.[2] After due considerations, the definition of blindness in India was changed in 2017 as follows—"*presenting distance VA less than 3/60 (20/400) in the better eye or limitation of field of vision less than 10° from center of fixation*".[3]

BURDEN

Globally, around 216.6 million are estimated to be suffering from moderate-severe visual impairment and another 36 million are estimated to be suffering from blindness in 2015. The trends in blindness in India are displayed in Table 9.1.2.

In India, there were 7.2 million (<3/60 vision) blind people in 1990, which have increased to 8.8 million in 2015. India is home to almost a quarter of the total 36 million blind people globally.

Causes of Blindness and Visual Impairment

The major causes of blindness (<3/60 vision) in India as reported by the National Blindness survey of 2001 in population aged 50 years and above are given in Table 9.1.3.

Avoidable blindness includes blindness that is either preventable or treatable—refractive errors, cataract, aphakia, cataract surgical complications, trachoma, corneal opacities, and diabetic retinopathy. Approximately 80–90% of blindness in India is considered avoidable. The profile of blindness has changed and infectious causes such as trachoma which were the most important causes of blindness at the time of independence have decreased in importance. Trachoma is on the verge of elimination with less than 5% prevalence of active trachoma infection in children.

- *Cataract:* Cataract surgical rate (CSR) measures cataract surgeries per million population per year. India has a CSR of

Table 9.1.2: Trends in the prevalence of blindness.

Survey	*Definition*	*50+ years*	*All ages*
ICMR survey 1974	<6/60 in better eye	-	1.38%
WHO-NPCB National Blindness Survey (1986–89) across all ages	<6/60 in better eye	-	1.49%
NPCB National Blindness Survey (1999–2001) in population aged 50 years or more	Presenting vision <6/60 in better eye	8.5%	-
	BCVA <6/60 in better eye	4.3%	1.1%
National Blindness Survey (2006–07) in population aged 50 years or more	Presenting vision < 6/60 in better eye	8.0%	-
	BCVA <6/60 in better eye	5.9%	1.0%

(BCVA: best-corrected visual acuity: ICMR: Indian Council of Medical Research; NPCB: National Programme for Control Blindness: WHO: World Health Organization)

Table 9.1.3: Major causes of blindness.

Cause	*Percent of blindness <6/60*
Cataract	62.6
Refractive errors	19.7
Glaucoma	5.8
Post. Seg. disorders	4.7
Corneal blindness	0.9
Surgical complication	1.2
Others	5

approximately 5,000/million. The cataract surgical coverage (CSC) measures among the persons who are suffering from cataract related blindness, what proportion has been operated and was 82.3% in 2007 for India among persons having vision less than 3/60. *In the 2007 survey, 64% of all cataract surgeries and 82% of surgeries conducted in last 5 years* were with intraocular lens (IOL) implantation. Currently over 6,500,000 cataract surgeries occur annually in India.

- *Refractive errors:* Nearly 11.0% children in schools and 8% children in community suffer from refractive errors. Burden is higher in urban children as compared to rural and in students of private schools as compared to government schools. School vision screening and distribution of free spectacles are the major strategy for control. Presbyopia is also an important condition affecting all persons aged 50+ years.
- *Corneal blindness:* In India, approximately 1–1.2 million are affected by bilateral corneal blindness and another 5–6 million have unilateral corneal involvement. The annual rise is estimated to be 50,000 cases. We need 100,000 keratoplasties and collection of 200,000 corneas per year in India. Setting of eye-collection centers, eye banks, training of surgeons in corneal transplantation and promoting eye donation through public awareness, and hospital-based cornea retrieval program (HCRP) are some key strategies.
- *Glaucoma:* Prevalence of glaucoma ranges from 1% to 4% among 40+ years population in India of which approximately one-third is angle closure glaucoma. An important issue is that over 90% of people with glaucoma remain undiagnosed. Compliance among patients diagnosed with glaucoma is poor. Opportunistic screening in eye clinics is advised as is family-based screening among blood relatives of diagnosed patients. Glaucoma screening is also advised in comprehensive eye camps.
- *Diabetic retinopathy:* India is the diabetic capital of the world and the diabetic

retinopathy is also rising. The prevalence of *diabetic retinopathy* in India is estimated as 16.37% in 40+ year aged population. Risk factors include uncontrolled blood glucose levels, longer duration of disease, concurrent dyslipidemia, being overweight, use of insulin, and presence of comorbid diabetic complications. Annual retinal screening of patients with diabetes is the recommended strategy for early diagnosis, alongside ensuring blood sugar control for prevention.

- *Childhood blindness and retinopathy of prematurity (ROP):* Childhood blindness is estimated to affect 0.8/1,000 children in India. Of this, one-fifth is attributable to corneal scars, one-fifth to pediatric cataract and glaucoma and rest to other causes. ROP is increasing in India due to opening of a large number of private as well as government neonatal intensive care units (NICUs), and increasing survival of prematurely born children (<30 weeks, 1,500 g birth weight). Approximately 10% of childhood blindness in India can be attributed to ROP. Under the Rashtriya Bal Swasthya Karyakram (RBSK), weekly ROP screening of infants by ophthalmologist is recommended in case of (1) low birth weight less than 2,000 g; (2) gestation less than 35 weeks; and (3) infants having risk factors—sepsis, hypotension, apnea, poor weight gain, anemia, and blood transfusion.

PREVENTION

Objective of "prevention" is to prevent development or progression of disease and its complications. It comprises of health promotion, preservation, and restoration.

Primary Prevention

It refers to preventing development of risk factors for blindness. This often includes health education and health promotion interventions. Some primary prevention strategies for prevention of blindness and visual impairment include:

- *Corneal blindness*: Preventing ocular injuries
- *Trachoma*: Facial hygiene and environmental sanitation interventions
- *Uncorrected refractive errors:* Evidence is emerging toward increasing outdoor activity for prevention of myopia
- *Diabetic retinopathy:* Encouraging healthy behaviors that prevent development of diabetes mellitus through lifestyle interventions and environmental modifications will prevent diabetic retinopathy
- *Glaucoma*: Cessation of smoking in high risk groups and observance of the glaucoma awareness week.

Secondary Prevention

It includes early diagnosis and treatment of blinding conditions. This includes screening and case finding interventions. This also includes interventions aimed to improving the access eye care services such as development of vision centers, ensuring availability of refractive services, availability of eye surgeries, etc. Some of secondary prevention strategies for prevention of blindness and visual impairment include:

- *Corneal blindness:* Vitamin A supplementation to prevent keratomalacia, measles vaccination to prevent vitamin A deficiency precipitated by measles infections, improving quality of antenatal care, intranatal practices and essential newborn care to prevent ophthalmia neonatorum, involving local volunteers to ensure immediate referral of ocular injuries, and setting up of eye collection centers, eye banks, and keratoplasty units
- *Trachoma*: Mass drug administration with azithromycin and surgical interventions for trichiasis

- *Uncorrected refractive errors*: School vision screening programs for early detection and presbyopia spectacle dispensing
- *Diabetic retinopathy*: Promoting treatment and ensuring blood sugar control among patients with diabetes, screening programs for diabetic retinopathy, improving cross-referral linkages between diabetes treatment clinic and ophthalmology clinics, and provisioning treatment of diabetic retinopathy
- *Cataract*: Cataract screening camps, ensuring cataract surgeries
- *Glaucoma*: Implementing opportunistic screening, family member screening, screening for glaucoma after cataract surgeries, provisioning antiglaucoma medications, training physicians in awareness, etc.
- *Retinopathy of prematurity*: ROP screening in NICUs.

TERTIARY PREVENTION (REHABILITATION)

It targets minimizing complications of illness and limiting visual disabilities and helping a person to utilize the remaining vision to the fullest through visual rehabilitation. There are multiple components of rehabilitation, which are discussed below.

Low Vision and Rehabilitation

The concept of visual disability has now extended beyond simple anatomical impairments or disease. It is recognized now that multiple other personal, social, and environmental factors are extremely important for an individual's functioning and daily living skills. Under the International Classification of Functioning (ICF), following concepts are used currently:

1. *Impairments:* These are problems in physiological body function of the eye (vision, color vision, stereopsis, etc.) or alterations in anatomical structures of the eye (ulceration, lens opacities, etc.).
2. *Activity limitations:* Due to the impairment of vision, a person may find difficulty in performing various activities. At the same time, with the same type of visual impairment, another person may be still able to perform the same activities.
3. *Participation restrictions:* Due to the impairment, an individual may not be able to participate in various social, vocational, educational, or other types of activities.

Disability includes all these three above mentioned concepts. *Also* use of the term "handicap" is discouraged.

It has been observed that majority of individuals who are visually impaired or blind even after best correction person still have useful residual vision. These are the target group for low vision and rehabilitation activities.[4,5]

The term *"functional low vision"* was introduced in 1989 as "a level of vision that with standard correction hinders an individual in the planning and/or execution of a task, but which permits enhancement of the functional vision through the use of optical or nonoptical devices, environmental modifications, and/or techniques". WHO redefined functional low vision in 2005, as *"VA of less than 6/18 to light perception, or a visual field of less than 10° from the point of fixation, after treatment and refractive correction, in the better eye, which is useful or potentially useful for planning and/or execution of a task"*.

The WHO in 1993 defined *low vision* as "person with low vision is one who has impairment of visual functioning even after treatment and/or standard refractive correction, and has a VA of less than 6/18 to light perception, or a visual field of less than 10° from the point of fixation, but who uses, or is potentially able to use, vision for the planning and/or execution of a task".

Magnitude of low vision: The data on low vision across the globe is extremely lacking. These include people with visual impairment due to causes other than UREs, cataract, and corneal opacities. Roughly, it may be estimated that nearly 20% of visual impairment can account for low vision. As per the 2010 global estimates on blindness and visual impairment, 285 million individuals had visual impairment.[6] It has been estimated that among children less than 15 years of age, 1.4 million need vision rehabilitation interventions.[7] Scenario in India is no better. Functional low vision prevalence of 1.05% was reported in the Andhra Pradesh Eye Disease study (APEDS) which translates to approximately 12 million in India.[8,9]

Visual Disability Certification

In January 2018, updated guidelines have been notified by the Ministry of Social Justice and Empowerment, Government of India for assessing quantum of visual disability for certification purposes. These are based on two criteria, (1) VA and (2) field of vision.

As per the act, a medical authority has been defined and it should include one ophthalmologist. Vision assessment should be done using Snellens chart after best possible correction (medical, surgical, or usual or conventional spectacles). Under the provisions of the act, a temporary certificate can be issued, if condition is likely to worsen while clearly mentioning the period after which reassessment should be done (Table 9.1.4).

Low Vision Rehabilitation

Visual rehabilitation is defined as interventions that help in achieving optimized functioning and reduce disability in individuals with visual disability. The major focus of these interventions is helping person with visual disability to be independent, and help them participate in various activities in their home or community, and to help them live independently.

Table 9.1.4: Guidelines for grading the visual disability under the RPWD Act 2016, based on best corrected visual acuity and fields of vision.

Better eye	*Worse eye best corrected*	*Percent impairment*
6/6–6/18	6/6–6/18	0
	6/24–6/60	10
	Less than 6/60–3/60	20
	Less than 3/60, no Light perception	30
6/24–6/60 or visual field less than 40 up to 20° around center of fixation or hemianopia involving macula	6/24–6/60	40
	Less than 6/60–3/60	50
	Less than 3/60 to no light perception	60
Less than 6/60 to 3/60 or visual field less than 20° up to 10° around center of fixation	Less than 6/60–3/60	70
	Less than 3/60–no light perception	80
Less than 3/60 to 1/60 or visual field less than 10° around center of fixation	Less than 3/60–no light perception	90
Only HMCF, only light perception, no light perception	Only HMCF, only light perception, no light perception	100

(HMCF: hand movements close to face; RPWD: rights of persons with disabilities)

Community-based rehabilitation (CBR) is an important strategy for implementing rehabilitation. It focuses involving the entire community in the rehabilitation process by engaging families, peers, local community groups, social organizations, local self-governments, and other community-based organizations in addition to various governmental organizations. Rehabilitation also requires policy level action on the part of the government to ensure adequate opportunities are available and support is provided to persons needing rehabilitation services. In simple words, visual rehabilitation is a cross-sectoral exercise with much wider scope beyond the eye care sector.

Low vision services include low vision aids and rehabilitative services. Setting up of low vision services involves following six main steps:

1. *Needs assessment:* It is done through retrospective analysis of available hospital data, subspecialty outpatient department (OPD), disability certification data, community-based studies, and surveys of blind school. Sometimes the only data which is available is through nongovernment organizations working for the blind.
2. *Situation analysis*: Assessment of human resource availability, infrastructure and equipment availability need to be done beforehand. Space needs to be identified where these services shall be provided.
3. *Capacity building and training-human resource:* Short-term training on optical, nonoptical, adaptive, orientation and mobility and activity of daily living, home-based care, vocational counseling, and assistance for certification.
4. *Networking with other organizations:* Networking is essential in bringing about a significant change. It requires support of various sectors, community and many departments. The activities should no longer be restricted to clinic-based rehabilitation, but also CBR.
5. *Equipment and assistive devices:* WHO has a standard list for low vision assistive devices. These equipment can be made available locally or with the external support. Government also makes provision of such equipment through scheme of Assistance to Disabled persons for purchase or fitting of aids or appliances (ADIP) scheme. Under this scheme, a separate list for the visually disability is included.[10,11] Multiple types of optical devices are available, which work through principles of enlargement or object, enhancement of contrast, selective fixation, or magnification that can be achieved electronically or optically. Apart from optical devices, there are certain nonoptical aids as well which can be of considerable help for the visually disabled like:
   - *Relative size devices:* These include devices such as large print books, large typewriters, etc. which increase the size of object to be viewed.
   - *Positioning and posture devices:* These devices provide more comfort to the disabled in doing vision related work at length.
   - *Light and illumination modification:* These devices increase illumination, control glare, and restrict certain wavelength to increase clarity.
   - *Writing and communication devices* in the form of typoscopes, writing guide, and signature guide.
   - *Mobility assistive devices:* Canes, smart cane, broad beam lights, and dog guide assist the visually disabled in walking from place to place without seeking assistance from others.

- *Visual substitution devices:* These devices are helpful in making their day-to-day activities easier, e.g. talking clocks, Braille, and Notex.

6. *Monitoring:* Last but not the least is the program monitoring. It must be integral part of the low vision services. It includes efficiency indicators and effectiveness indicators. Efficiency indicators include number of patients registered, number of examined and number prescribed aids, number of patients rehabilitated, etc. Effectiveness indicator includes—quality of life, occupational or educational performance, improvement in activities of daily living (ADLs), etc. The Indian Visual Function Questionnaire (Ind-VFQ) is also used to study and track changes in visual function over time.

Visual rehabilitation is multidisciplinary in activities. It involves a wide range of professionals. Various professional along with their engagements is listed in Table 9.1.5.[12,13]

Community-based Low Vision Rehabilitation Matrix

The CBR matrix developed by the WHO consists of five components—each with five elements. These help in identifying the nature of services that are needed by a specific person and also help in identifying the nature of services that can be offered to a specific person within a CBR program. The matrix also helps clarify the roles of CBR organizations that are not directly related to patients suffering from low vision such

Table 9.1.5: Low vision professionals and their roles.

Professional	*Roles*
Ophthalmologists	• Examination and diagnosis of eye disease • Treatment of eye disease • Medication • Surgery
Optometrist	• Low vision examination • Treatment of refractive error • Eye glasses • Contact lenses • Treatment of low vision • Modification of lighting and contrast
Occupational therapist	• Low vision rehabilitation examination • Low vision rehabilitation • Management of multiple disabilities
Vision rehabilitation therapists or rehabilitation teachers	• Low vision rehabilitation examination • Low vision rehabilitation, braille reading instruction
Orientation and mobility specialist	• Orientation and mobility examination • Orientation and mobility
Teachers of the visually impaired	• Special education of children with low vision and blindness
Low Vision Therapist	• Low vision therapist examination • Low vision therapist
Social worker	• Individual and group counseling, facilitate access to resources, and support services

Flowchart 9.1.1: The community-based rehabilitation (CBR) matrix.

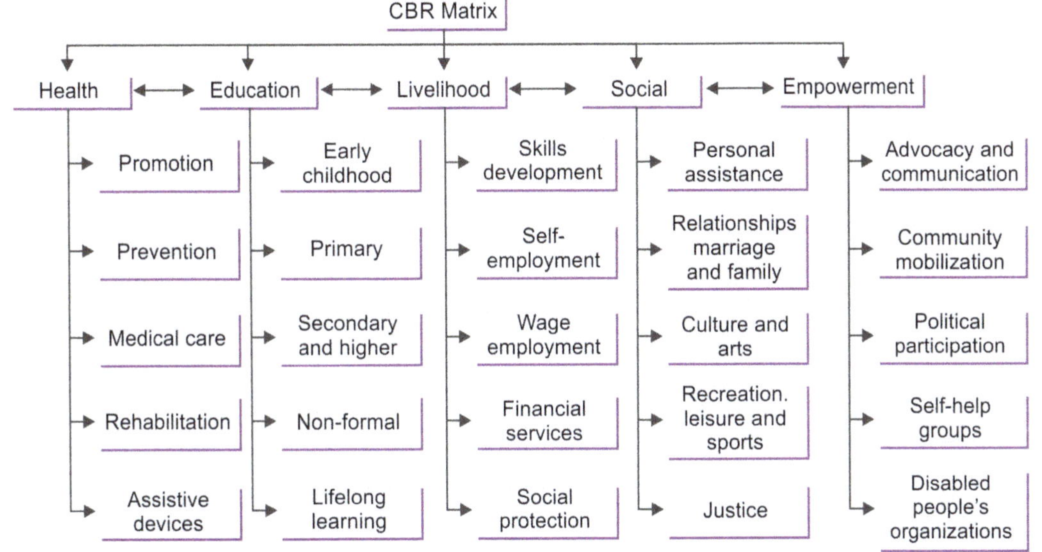

as advocacy and community mobilization (Flowchart 9.1.1).

VISION 2020: THE RIGHT TO SIGHT

Vision 2020: The Right to Sight is a joint global initiative of WHO and IAPB (International Agency for Prevention of Blindness) for elimination of avoidable blindness by 2020. Five priority diseases under Vision 2020 (Global) are—(1) cataract, (2) refractive errors, (3) onchocerciasis, (4) childhood blindness, and (5) trachoma.

A "Vision 2020: The Right to Sight India" initiative has also been launched at the country level. Diseases included under Vision 2020: The Right to Sight India are:

- Cataract
- Refractive Errors and Low Vision
- Childhood Blindness
- Trachoma
- Corneal Blindness
- Diabetic Retinopathy
- Glaucoma

NATIONAL PROGRAMME FOR CONTROL OF BLINDNESS AND VISUAL IMPAIRMENT

The National Programme for Control of Blindness (NPCB) was launched in 1976. The program had set a target of reducing the blindness prevalence from 1.4% to 0.3% by the year 2000. This target was subsequently shifted to 2020. The name of the program has been revised to National Programme for Control of Blindness and Visual Impairment (NPCB&VI) along with the change in definition of blindness in 2016. Under the National Health Policy of 2017, a target of reducing the prevalence of blindness to 0.25/1,000 by 2025 and disease burden by one-third from current levels has been announced. The government of India has also endorsed the Global Action Plan for Universal Eye Health developed by the WHO. The Global Action Plan has set a target of reduction in prevalence of avoidable visual impairment by 25% by the year 2019 (target 2.4%) from the baseline of 2010 (baseline 3.2%).

REFERENCES

1. World Health Organization. List of official ICD-10 updates ratified October 2006. Geneva: WHO; 2006.
2. Vashist P, Senjam SS, Gupta V, et al. Definition of blindness under National Programme for Control of Blindness: Do we need to revise it? Indian J Ophthalmol. 2017;65(2):92-6.
3. Leat SJ, Fryer A, Rumney NJ. Outcome of low vision aid provision: the effectiveness of low vision clinic. Optom Vis Sci. 1994;71(3):199-206.
4. Goodrich G, Bailey I. A history of the field of vision rehabilitation from the perspective of low vision. In: Silverstone B, Lang M, Rosenthal B, Faye E (Eds). The Lighthouse Handbook on Vision Impairment and Vision Rehabilitation. New York: Oxford University Press; 2000. pp. 675-708.
5. Pascolini D, Mariotti SP. Global estimates of visual impairment: 2010. Br J Ophthalmol. 2012;96:614-8.
6. WHO. Vision Impairment and Blindness. [online] Available from: www.who.iny/mediacentre/factsheets/fs282/en/ [Accessed January, 2019].
7. Dandona R, Dandona L. Review of findings of the Andhra Pradesh Eye Disease Study: policy implications for eye care services. Indian J Ophthalmol. 2001;49(4):215-34.
8. WHO. Rehabilitation. [online] Available from: www.who.int/rehabilitation/en/ [Accessed January, 2019].
9. WHO. WHO framework on rehabilitation services: expert meeting. [online] Available from: www.who.int/rehabilitation/expert-meeting-june17/en/ [Accessed January, 2019].
10. ADIP Scheme. National Board of Examination in Rehabilitation. [online] Available from: www.niepmdexaminationsnber.com/documents/niepmd_scheme.pdf [Accessed January, 2019].
11. Whittaker SG, Scheiman M. Low Vision Rehabilitation: A Practical Guide for Occupational Therapists, Second edition. USA: Slack Incorporated Publishers; 2015.
12. WHO. About the community-based rehabilitation (CBR) matrix. [online] Available from: www.who.int/disabilities/cbr/matrix/en/ [Accessed January, 2019].
13. Johnson GJ (Ed). The Epidemiology of eye diseases. London: Imperial College Press; 2012.

9.2 SURVEY METHODS IN OPHTHALMOLOGY

Vivek Gupta, Meenakshi Wadhwani, Praveen Vashist, Suraj S Senjam

INTRODUCTION

Eye health surveys are instrumental tools in ophthalmic epidemiology and community eye health. Survey data have proven indispensable in situation analysis, development planning, program management, and decision-making at all levels. Very often the health systems in developing countries are not adequately developed and the data generated routine reporting mechanisms is not adequate for programmatic planning or evaluations. Ophthalmic surveys fill this gap. The basic premise in any survey is that systematic data collection from an adequate number of participants, who are representative of a larger reference population, can yield valid information about the entire reference population. However, a rigorous methodology and execution with population-based data collection and a sufficiently large sample size are key aspects of a survey. The most common design of ophthalmological surveys is cross-sectional studies. Results of surveys have shaped India's National Programme for Control of Blindness (NPCB) and have provided extremely useful data the world over. Some of the landmark ophthalmic surveys in

India include the National Trachoma Pilot Project Survey, ICMR National Survey of Blindness, Andhra Pradesh Eye Disease Study (APEDs), Aravind Comprehensive Eye Study (ACES), and the National Blindness Surveys of 1989, 2001, and 2007.

USES OF OPHTHALMOLOGICAL SURVEYS

The most common uses of surveys include:

- Assessment of the magnitude of blindness and visual impairment
- Assessment of the major causes of blindness and visual impairment
- Assess trends in magnitude and causes over time and across regions
- Identify the magnitude of treated and untreated visual impairment
- Estimate indicators of healthcare utilization such as cataract surgical coverage
- Assessing barriers to utilization of eye health services
- Generate hypothesis about possible relationships between eye health status and risk factors
- Evaluating the effectiveness of health programs and interventions in reducing blindness and visual impairment.

Survey Approaches

Conventional ophthalmological surveys usually included very detailed data collection about ocular symptoms, vision, and included detailed ophthalmic examination. Conducting extensive eye examination in population-based surveys also decreases participation rates. This makes comprehensive surveys very resource intensive, time intensive, and expensive. Since 1990s, there has been a trend toward developing rapid assessment survey methodologies. Rapid ophthalmological survey methodologies have been developed for cataract, onchocerciasis, and trachoma and now for blindness and visual impairment. The surveys become rapid by leveraging local resources, simplifying sampling methodology, omitting detailed history taking, simplifying ocular examination, and automating data management and analysis. These rapid surveys aim to generate data that satisfies the needs of a program manager for planning and evaluation of ongoing eye care programs. Some of these standard approaches include Rapid Assessment of Cataract Surgical Services (RACSS), Rapid Assessment of Avoidable Blindness (RAAB), Rapid Assessment method for Refractive Errors (RARE), Trachoma Rapid Assessment (TRA), Rapid Assessment of Visual Impairment (RAVI), etc. The RAAB surveys have become especially popular due to their low cost and rapidity and have been extensively conducted all over the world. The 2007 and the 2015 National Blindness Surveys of India are also based on the RAAB methodology.

CONDUCT OF AN EYE HEALTH SURVEY

Objectives

This first step is to clarify the focus and the priority conditions that are the target of the survey. Objectives should be unambiguous and precise and having clarity in objectives makes the entire survey methodology much more focused.

Objectives of the National Blindness Survey of India 2015-2018 include:

- To determine the prevalence of blindness (including avoidable blindness) among the 50+ population
- To identify the major causes of blindness (including avoidable blindness)
- To ascertain the visual outcomes after cataract surgery amongst operated cases

- To estimate the cataract surgical coverage
- To ascertain barriers for uptake of cataract surgery
- To assess the prevalence of diabetes and diabetic retinopathy in the study population
- The proportion of people with known diabetes who have had a previous fundus examination.

Survey Instruments

The survey instruments include not only the eye examination equipment, but also the survey questionnaire or the examination record (proforma). Comprehensive surveys require more extensive equipment depending on the objectives framed. The survey questionnaire and examination records are carefully designed to ensure simplicity in language, avoiding leading and double-barreled questions, and having a proper flow. Responses are restricted to only a certain set of possible values (closed ended) wherever possible. Questionnaires are broken down in logical sections by grouping questions of similar type together. Having a well-designed questionnaire goes a long way toward avoiding information biases in the survey. The equipment needed for trachoma prevalence surveys, are torchlight and corneal loupe. The National Blindness Survey India involves the following survey instruments:

- *Equipment:*
  - Snellen 6 meters single optotypes of 6/12, 6/18, and 6/60
  - One tape or rope of 6 meters (20 feet) with a knot or ring in the middle at 3 m (10 feet)
  - Torch with focused light and spare batteries
  - Direct ophthalmoscope with spare batteries
  - Occluder with pinhole, preferably with multiple holes (of size 0.5–1 mm)
  - *Indirect ophthalmoscope*: For evaluation of diabetic retinopathy.
- Timetable listing all population units and the dates they will be visited by which team
- Maps of the entire survey area with all selected population units marked
- Forms
- The RAAB survey records. Staple exactly as many forms as the total number of persons 50+ to be examined per cluster together to form one bundle for each cluster
- Referral slips for hospital
- Tally sheet of participants enumerated, dilated, examined, referred, and gender
- *Cluster summary form*: Include survey area, the number and the name of the population area, the date of examination, and the name and signature of the team leader
- One set of coding instructions and a set of instructions for examiners
- Map of population unit to be divided in segments
- Basic medicines to treat common minor ailments
- Necessary stationary and bags.

Study Area

The study area refers to the geographical area in which the survey will be conducted and to which the results of the survey can be generalized. This may be the entire country, a state, a district or a village, or a city. This has an important bearing on the sampling methodology since potentially any person living in the survey area is a potential participant of the survey. The selected survey areas should be safe and accessible. Survey should not be done in an area where the safety of field staff cannot be guaranteed. India's National Blindness Surveys are done to represent entire India as the Study Area.

In the trachoma prevalence surveys, the districts were chosen to be representative of former hyperendemic areas of the country.

Study Population

The entire population of the study area often constitutes the study population. Many population groups exist in the study area who would be extremely difficult to include in the survey. These would include for example the incarcerated populations, migratory labor, army personnel, etc. It is required clearly enunciate the target study population for the survey and list out their selection criteria. In the RAAB survey, the study population consists of all individuals aged 50 years or more who are usual residents of the selected study area. Residency has been defined as usual resident of the area over the last 6 months. Any visitors are excluded from the study population. In the trachoma surveys, the entire usual resident population comprises the study population—individuals aged 1–9 years are the study population for active trachoma infection prevalence assessment while older residents are the study population for assessment of trachoma sequelae.

Sample Size

It is vital that a proper sample size estimation is done before survey is initiated. The standard formula used to calculate the sampling method for ophthalmic surveys is:

Sample Size for Prevalence Survey =

$$\frac{Z_{a}^{2} \times p \times (100 - p)}{d^{2}} \times Deff \times \left[\frac{(100 + NR)}{100}\right]$$

The formula includes:

- *Prevalence (p%):* The estimated or assumed or anticipated prevalence of the disease (p) expressed as a % of population affected by the disease. In case, there are multiple ocular disorders under consideration, the prevalence of an important disease with lowest prevalence should be used for calculation in the formula. The formula also includes the term (100-p).
- *Absolute error (d%):* It occurs because of selecting a sample rather than examining the whole population. Sampling error can be reduced but cannot be completely eliminated. Other terms used for this are precision or allowable error. This usually calculated as between 10% and 20% of the anticipated prevalence. As an example, if the anticipated prevalence of blindness is 9.0%, and the investigators feel that true prevalence be within 20% of the anticipated prevalence, then the value of *d* becomes 1.8% (20% of 9.0%). In case, anticipated prevalence is low (<1%), then *d* can be fixed as 0.2–0.5%.
- *Confidence interval or type 1 error rate (Z):* It is usual to work with 5% type-I error rate which corresponds to a *Z* value of 1.96. A *Z* of 1.96 refers to 95% probability that the true population prevalence is within "p – d% to p + d%" range.
- *Design effect (Deff):* It is an adjustment made to adjust for cluster sampling methodology used in ophthalmic surveys. The design effect is high in case we have few clusters each with large participants within each cluster (cluster size) while the design effect decreases as we increase the number of clusters and decrease cluster size. Convention is to use design effect in 1.5–3.0 range. In the RAAB surveys, the design effects recommended are 1.6 for cluster size of 40, 1.7 for cluster size of 50, and 1.8 for cluster size of 60.
- *Nonresponse (NR%):* The sample size needs to be increased because despite all efforts, we will rarely have 100% participation of selected individuals in a survey. A nonresponse rate of 10% is

considered acceptable and the overall sample size needs to be increased accordingly by 10%.

Example Sample Size Calculation

- *Prevalence (p%):* 7.5%
- *Absolute error (d%):* 0.75% (= 10% of p)
- *Confidence interval or type 1 error rate ($Z\alpha$):* 1.96
- *Design effect (Deff):* 1.8 for cluster size of 60
- *Nonresponse (NR%):* 10%.

Sample Size =

$$\frac{1.96^2 \times 7.5 \times (100 - 7.5)}{0.75^2} \times 1.8 \times \left[\frac{(100 + 10)}{10}\right]$$

$$= \frac{2665.11}{0.5625} \times 1.8 \times 1.1$$

$$= 9382$$

In addition, the total population size from which the sample is to be drawn (N) is adjusted for by adding a finite population correction, in case the total population of district is small (convention—less than 100,000). It is important to note that in surveys, the type-II error is not considered since the main purpose of survey is to estimate prevalence. However, type-II error will come into the play, and a different formula will be used for sample size calculation, if the primary objective of the survey is to measure association between a disease and risk factor.

Sampling Methodology

The most common sampling method used in ophthalmic surveys is multistage cluster random sampling. The first stage is sampling and selection of districts in the country. Districts with larger populations have larger probability of selection, making this a *probability proportionate to size (PPS) simple random sample.* The next stage is the selection of clusters within the district. The clusters are villages and urban wards as defined by the census lists. In the National Blindness Survey, the clusters are selected from all over this district, while in the National Trachoma Prevalence Survey, one of the administrative blocks in the district was randomly selected first and then villages were selected within the block. In RAAB surveys, we take a cluster size of 60 participants per cluster, but the total number of participants aged 50 years or more may be in hundreds in each cluster. To facilitate this selection, *compact segment sampling* method is used within the cluster. Compact segment sampling involves dividing the cluster into smaller segments based on a cluster map. Each segment by itself can yield the number of participants that we need to survey. In the National Blindness Survey 2015–2018, a segment of total 400 population (all ages) will yield 60 participants aged 50 years or more, based on results of the Census 2011. Accordingly, with the help of a local volunteer, the selected cluster is divided into segments of 400 population each (6 segments will be made if cluster population is 2,450), each segment is numbered on the map, and one segment is chosen randomly by draw of chits. The survey will start from any randomly selected starting household in the segment, and the team will proceed from house to house till the sample size is achieved. In case, the sample size is not achieved, then next contiguous segment is selected.

Multistage cluster random sampling method reduces the cost, but is less precise compared to the simple random sampling. To adjust for this loss of precision, we include the design effect term when calculating sample size (as described above). This method also facilitates planning for field work because a predetermined number of individuals is interviewed in each unit selected, and staff can be allocated accordingly. This method is still a probability sampling technique since the selection of districts, clusters, and segments was all done using random sampling methods.

In the TRA surveys, nonprobability sampling is used wherein in the district, the areas with worst hygiene and areas most likely to harbor trachoma infections are purposively selected. The results of these nonprobability TRA surveys therefore, must never be generalized to entire districts.

Survey Duration

The cluster size if planned in a manner that one-three complete clusters can be covered by one team, in one day. In the National Blindness Survey 2015-18, three clusters are completed per day by one team. To complete one district having 50 clusters, 9 working days are required with two teams working in parallel. Adding a period of 5 days of presurvey preparations, one day for local training and one day for coordination with the local district administration, 3 days for travel, and one day of postsurvey debriefing, each district requires 20 days of work. Additionally, about 1 week is required subsequently for dual data entry and report generation. Overall, one district is realistically covered per month. In trachoma prevalence surveys, two clusters are being covered per day per team, while in the TRAs, three clusters can be covered by one team per day.

Training and Manual of Operations

A detailed manual of operations is also developed and finalized before the start of the survey. It is important that the study protocol remains constant throughout the survey and having the manual of operations ensures that if at any point of time there is a confusion about what needs to be done, the team can refer to the manual of operations and therefore be guided with the survey methodology. A copy of the manual of operations is given to the survey team for their reference, at all times.

All the staffs enrolled in the survey are trained comprehensively in the survey methodology. This includes both classroom teaching as well as a field pilot. An interobserver variation (IOV) assessment is conducted wherein the same patient is examined by two or more optometrists and two or more ophthalmologists. The findings of the teams are matched against each other and the calculation of kappa coefficient is done and recorded. A low value of kappa coefficient indicates the need for further training and discussion to bring consistency in study implementation while a high kappa value (>0.6) indicates consistency.

Survey Resources and Logistics

Managing logistics for the survey is a very important exercise. Through use of survey logistic checklists, it is ensured that all the requirements for the survey are organized well in time before the team departs for the survey district. Logistic planning also includes planning for the travel of the team from the headquarters to the survey district, identification and planning of accommodation for the team in the survey district, organizing local transport, and organizing food for the team members. If the resources are managed well, it means that the survey team can focus on the real work with minimal disturbances. Financial management is also very important since the expense of the survey can run into several lakhs of rupees.

Approval of State and District

Before starting any survey, proper approval from the State Program Officer (SPO), Chief Medical Officer (CMO), District Health Officers (DHO), and District Program Officers (DPO), is arranged to inform them about the survey activities to be conducted in their areas. The district health authorities are also requested to provide maps, list of Accredited Social Health Activist (ASHA) workers, paramedical staff, cluster details, etc. Law and order can sometimes pose problems and therefore the District Collector (DC) is always informed of the plan. The local community leaders (panchayats) are also involved in the implementation of survey. With the involvement of the district administration and health system, a detailed microplan for conduct of survey is prepared. This plan is also shared with the district health administration so that they can mobilize the health system to assist the survey team.

Survey Execution

Survey in the cluster typically consists of activities spread over 2 days—enumeration activities on day 1 and clinical evaluation and examination on day 2.

Enumeration: Two members of the survey team go to the cluster selected for the survey. Once they reach the cluster, they contend the local lusher worker and do compact segment sampling in the cluster. This involves preparing for cluster map, dividing the cluster into segments and selection of one segment randomly by draw of chits. In the selected segment, a random starting household is identified and enumeration begins. The visited household is informed about the survey that will be done on the next day and the eligible members from the household are requested to be available on the next day for the survey team. In an enumeration sheet, the number of male and female eligible from the household are noted. Using a permanent marker or chalk, a visual marking is done near the gate of the household. The team proceeds from house to house till the required sample size is reached.

Examination: On the next day, one member from the enumeration team of the previous day brings the clinical team to the selected cluster. This person is able to guide the examination team directly to the household where the survey has to begin. In the examination team, two identified members are responsible for taking informed consent and collecting the demographic information in the study proforma. Thereafter, the study optometrists along with field supervisors conduct visual acuity assessments. The participant is then examined by the study ophthalmologists who do lens evaluation, eye examination, and assign the cause of visual impairment or blindness. In case, the patient requires referral to a clinic or hospital, an optometrist and the local health worker accompanying the ophthalmologist counsel the participant and provide a referral card. This optometrist also is responsible for managing all the forms and keeping record of any patients that require evaluation under mydriasis. All the forms that have been filled are checked in the field at completion of a cluster to ensure completeness. After completion of one cluster, the team moves on to the next cluster. The survey investigators and the district medical officer of the CMO also visit the survey team from time to time for supervision and verification of the survey records (Fig. 9.2.1).

ETHICS

The integrity, reliability, and validity of the survey rely heavily on adherence to ethical principles. All the surveys are approved by the institutional ethical board before initiation. Prior to collection of any information, a written informed consent is taken from the participant. The participant information sheet form includes all following points:

- Purpose of the survey
- Procedures involved for the participant in the survey and time involvement required
- Risks and benefits of taking part
- Costs of (or lack of costs of) taking part
- Participation is voluntary

RAPID ASSESSMENT FOR AVOIDABLE BLINDNESS

A. GENERAL INFORMATION

Survey area: ______________ [ ][ ] **Cluster:** [ ][ ][ ] **Year - month:** [ ][ ][ ][ ] - [ ][ ]

Name: ______________ **Sex:** Male: O (1) Female: O (2) **Individual no.:** [ ][ ] **Age (years):** [ ][ ]

Optional 1: [ ][ ]
Optional 2: [ ][ ]

Examination status:

Examined: O (1) (go to B) Refused: O (3) (go to E)
Not available: O (2) (go to E) Not able to communicate: O (4) (go to E)

Always ask: "Did you ever have any problems with your eyes?" Yes: O (1) No: O (2)

If not available - details (availability / tel number / address)

B. VISION

Uses distance glasses: No: O (1) Yes: O (2)
Uses reading glasses: No: O (1) Yes: O (2)

Presenting vision	Right eye	Left eye
Can see 6/12	O (1)	O (1)
Cannot see 6/12 but can see 6/18	O (2)	O (2)
Cannot see 6/18 but can see 6/60	O (3)	O (3)
Cannot see 6/60 but can see 3/60	O (4)	O (4)
Cannot see 3/60 but can see 1/60	O (5)	O (5)
Light perception (PL+)	O (6)	O (6)
No light perception (PL-)	O (7)	O (7)

Pinhole vision	Right eye	Left eye
Can see 6/12	O (1)	O (1)
Cannot see 6/12 but can see 6/18	O (2)	O (2)
Cannot see 6/18 but can see 6/60	O (3)	O (3)
Cannot see 6/60 but can see 3/60	O (4)	O (4)
Cannot see 3/60 but can see 1/60	O (5)	O (5)
Light perception (PL+)	O (6)	O (6)
No light perception (PL-)	O (7)	O (7)

C. LENS EXAMINATION

	Right eye	Left eye
Normal lens / minimal lens opacity:	O (1)	O (1)
Obvious lens opacity:	O (2)	O (2)
Lens absent (aphakia):	O (3)	O (3)
Pseudophakia without PCO:	O (4)	O (4)
Pseudophakia with PCO:	O (5)	O (5)
No view of lens:	O (6)	O (6)

D. MAIN CAUSE OF PRESENTING VA<6/12
(Mark only one cause for each eye)

	Right eye	Left eye	Principal cause in person
Refractive error:	O (1)	O (1)	O (1)
Aphakia, uncorrected:	O (2)	O (2)	O (2)
Cataract, untreated:	O (3)	O (3)	O (3) (F)
Cataract surg. complications:	O (4)	O (4)	O (4)
Trachoma corneal opacity:	O (5)	O (5)	O (5)
Other corneal opacity:	O (6)	O (6)	O (6)
Phthisis:	O (7)	O (7)	O (7)
Onchocerciasis:	O (8)	O (8)	O (8)
Glaucoma:	O (9)	O (9)	O (9)
Diabetic retinopathy:	O (10)	O (10)	O (10)
ARMD:	O (11)	O (11)	O (11)
Other posterior segment:	O (12)	O (12)	O (12)
All globe/CNS abnormalities:	O (13)	O (13)	O (13)
Not examined: can see 6/12	O (14)	O (14)	O (14)

E. HISTORY, IF NOT EXAMINED
(From relative or neighbour)

Believed	Right eye	Left eye
Not blind	O (1)	O (1)
Blind due to cataract	O (2)	O (2)
Blind due to other causes	O (3)	O (3)
Operated for cataract	O (4)	O (4)

F. WHY CATARACT SURGERY WAS NOT DONE
(Mark up to 2 responses, if VA<6/18, not improving with pinhole, with visually impairing lens opacity in one or both eyes)

Need not felt	O (1)
Fear of surgery or poor result	O (2)
Cannot afford operation	O (3)
Treatment denied by provider	O (4)
Unaware that treatment is possible	O (5)
No access to treatment	O (6)
Local reason (optional)	O (7)

G. DETAILS ABOUT CATARACT OPERATION

	Right eye	Left eye
Age at operation (years)	[ ][ ]	[ ][ ]
Place of operation		
Government hospital	O (1)	O (1)
Voluntary / charitable hospital	O (2)	O (2)
Private hospital	O (3)	O (3)
Eye camp / improvised setting	O (4)	O (4)
Traditional setting	O (5)	O (5)
Type of surgery		
Non IOL	O (1)	O (1)
IOL implant	O (2)	O (2)
Couching	O (3)	O (3)
Cost of surgery		
Totally free	O (1)	O (1)
Partially free	O (2)	O (2)
Fully paid	O (3)	O (3)
Cause of VA<6/12 after cataract surgery		
Ocular comorbidity (Selection)	O (1)	O (1)
Operative complications (Surgery)	O (2)	O (2)
Refractive error (Spectacles)	O (3)	O (3)
Longterm complications (Sequelae)	O (4)	O (4)
Does not apply - can see 6/12	O (5)	O (5)

Fig. 9.2.1: Survey form used in the National Blindness Survey 2015–18 (sample front page).

- Participant can say no or withdraw from survey at any time without any danger or risk
- All information collected will be kept confidential to the survey team
- Contact details of investigators.

Additionally, an aim of surveys is to provide services and all possible support to participants identified as having ocular diseases. In RAAB survey, free antibiotic and lubricating drops are provided to all the needy participants of the survey. All participants needing referral are also appropriately guided. Adequate provision of cataract surgery is made with local district authorities and NGOs. In trachoma surveys, azithromycin and epilation forceps are distributed to participants with active infection or trichiasis, respectively.

DATA ENTRY AND ANALYSIS

Data collected during the day are entered into the data entry system on the same day. The data entry system has inbuilt logical consistency checks that flags records with missing or inconsistent data. This helps in minimizing the data entry errors. Furthermore, this also identifies the records in which errors are present and these records are then shared with the survey team in the evening and the discussion takes place over minimizing them. The team is now able to ensure that the errors do not arise in the field. A second data entry is done once the survey team returns from the district to the headquarters. The first and the second data entry is compared, all nonmatched entries are then corrected by taking out the original survey records. By creating a uniform data analysis code in the statistical software, a uniform data analysis is the run on the updated dataset and the results are generated. In the National Blindness Survey 2015–2018, the use of RAAB 6 software has greatly minimized the time for data analysis.

DISSEMINATION AND USE OF RESULTS

The ultimate aim of the survey is to use the results for the prevention of blindness and severe visual impairment in planning interventions. Otherwise, it becomes a redundant academic exercise. The survey should also be used to develop future programs and policies. The results of all the surveys are shared with the NPCB and visual impairment and the concerned SPO. This helps the program managers to develop and implement various programs and interventions to address the issue of blindness and in turn this helps the nation as it strives to achieve elimination of avoidable blindness and visual impairment. Mass Drug Administration with azithromycin and implementation of safe interventions was done in Nicobar Island in 2011 with the aim to eliminate trachoma based the results of the TRA survey done in the island in which a very high burden of active trachoma infection was observed. This led to reduction in burden of active trachoma infection to subthreshold levels in 2016 which was documented through two repeat trachoma prevalence surveys conducted in Car Nicobar.

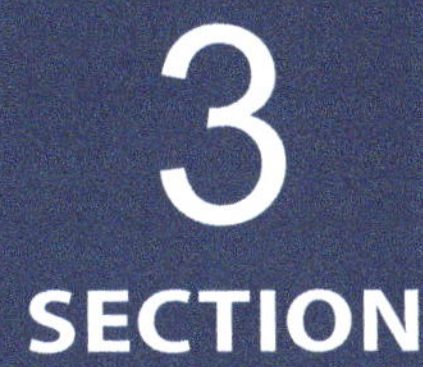

INTERPRETATION OF IMAGES AND REPORTS

10 CHAPTER

Interpretation of Images

Pranita Sahay, Jyoti Shakrawal, Gunjan Saluja, Siddhi Goel

INTERPRETATION OF GOLDMANN VISUAL FIELDS

General Principles

Look for following while interpreting a Goldmann visual field (GVF). The report should be interpreted under following headings:

- Eye involved
- Size of stimulus used. The various size of stimulus used have been summarized in Table 10.1
- The area involved general or local
- *The density of scotoma:*
  - *Absolute*: No visual sensation perceived
  - *Relative*: Depressed visual sensation perceived.
- *The position of field defect:*
  - Central, temporal, nasal, superior, and inferior.
- *Shape*:
  - Sectoral (hemianopia)
  - Non-sectoral (regular or irregular).
- Differential diagnosis of conditions in which the given filed defect is found.

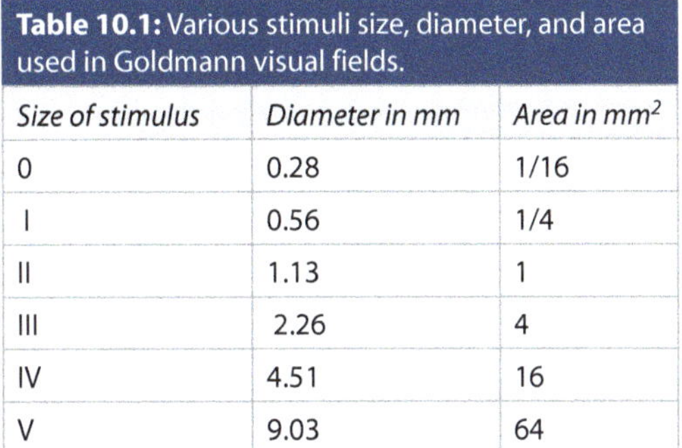

Table 10.1: Various stimuli size, diameter, and area used in Goldmann visual fields.

Size of stimulus	*Diameter in mm*	*Area in mm^2*
0	0.28	1/16
I	0.56	1/4
II	1.13	1
III	2.26	4
IV	4.51	16
V	9.03	64

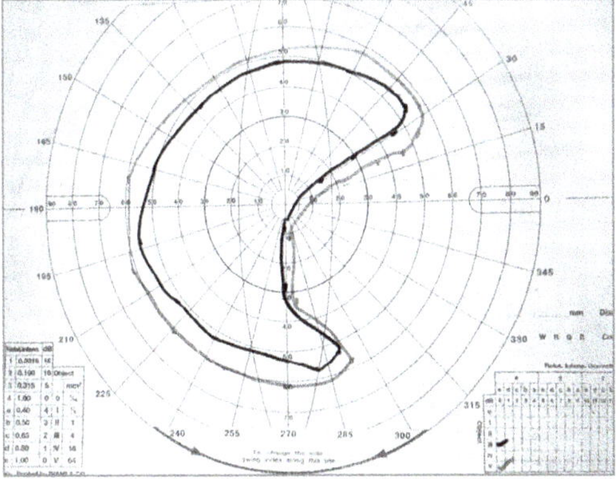

Fig. 10.1: Goldmann visual field (GVF) showing right inferior quadrantanopia.

Specific Examples

- *Example 1 (Fig. 10.1):*
  - The given GVF is of the right eye and has been plotted using a stimulus size of IIIe0 and Ve0.
  - The field shows a depressed response in the inferonasal quadrant suggestive of inferior quadrantanopia.
  - Differential diagnosis of inferior quadrantanopic field defects includes:
    - Neoplasia

- Infarction
- Infections involving occipital lobe.

- *Example 2 (Fig. 10.2):*
  - The given GVF is of the right eye and has been plotted using a stimulus size of I4e0, V4e0, and I3e5.
  - The field shows a dense central scotoma
  - Differential diagnosis of this defect includes:
    - Optic neuritis
    - Hereditary optic neuropathy (bilateral central scotoma will be present)
    - Toxoplasma scar
    - Neurosensory detachment as in central serous choroidopathy

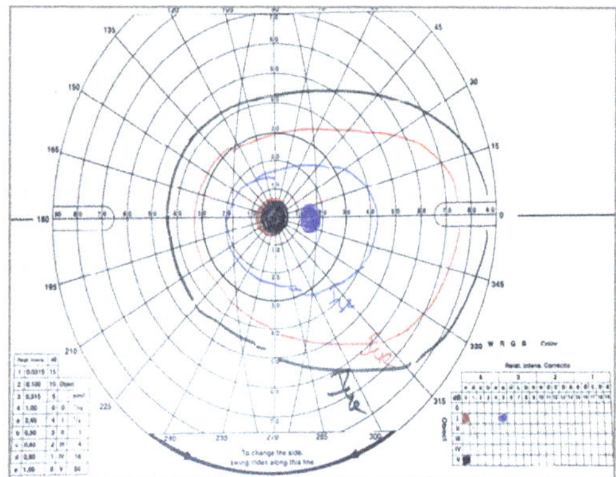

Fig. 10.2: Goldmann visual field showing right central scotoma.

    - Macular edema
    - Macular degeneration.

- *Example 3 (Figs. 10.3A and B):*
  - The given GVF shows a depressed response in the nasal quadrant of the right eye and a depressed response in the temporal quadrant of the left eye.
  - This is suggestive of right eye homonymous hemianopic field defect.
  - *Differential diagnosis of these defects include*:
    - Retrochiasmal lesions
    - Alzheimer's disease
    - Cortical basal ganglion degeneration
    - Mitochondrial encephalomyopathy
    - Neurosyphilis
    - Neuromyelitis optica
    - Posterior cerebral artery occlusion
    - Epilepsy.

- *Example 4 (Fig. 10.4):*
  - The given GVF is of the left eye and has been plotted using a stimulus size of V4e0
  - The field shows a dense scotoma involving the center and area surrounding it, suggestive of centrocecal scotoma
  - *Differential diagnosis of this defect includes*:
    - Optic neuritis

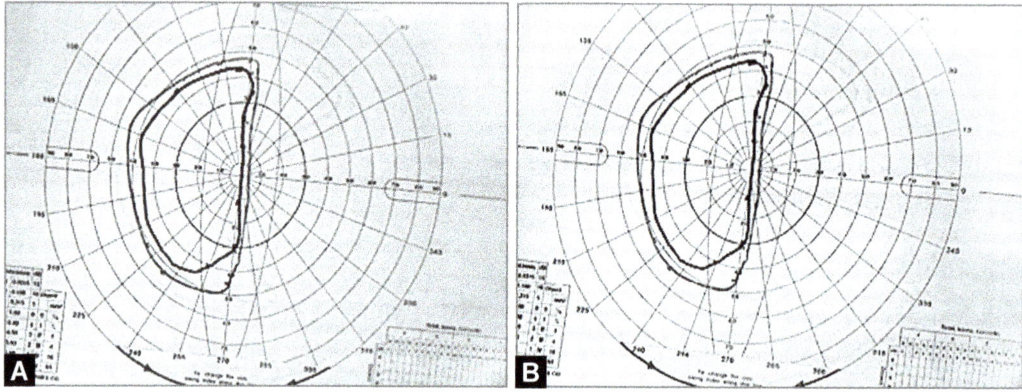

Figs. 10.3A and B: Goldmann visual field showing right homonymous hemianopia.

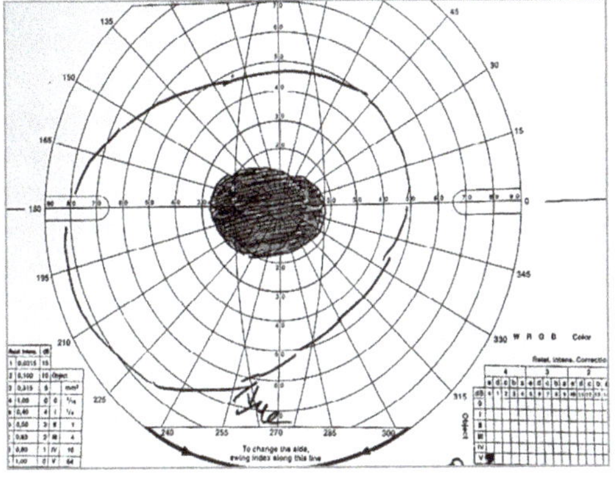

Fig. 10.4: Goldmann visual field showing left centrocecal scotoma.

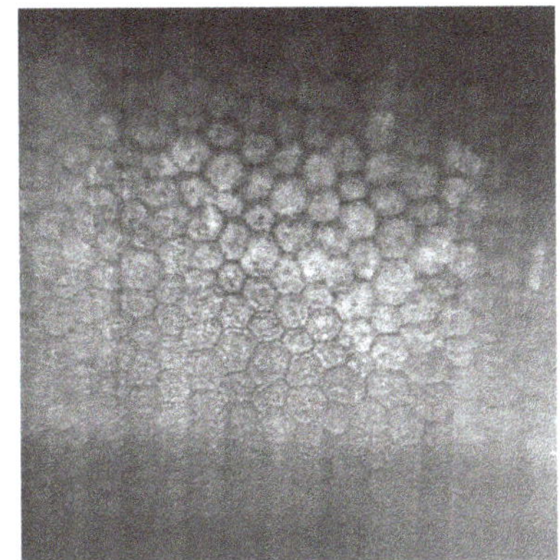

Fig. 10.5: Normal corneal endothelial cell.

- Toxic optic neuropathy
- Stargardt disease.

INTERPRETATION OF SPECULAR MICROSCOPY

General Principles

Look for following while interpreting specular microscope images. The interpretation should be made under the following headings as mentioned below:

- Endothelial cell shape
- Endothelial cell morphology
- Presence of cell dropout or guttae
- Differential diagnosis.

Specific Examples

- *Example 1 (Fig. 10.5):*
    - This is specular microscope image showing:
        - Hexagonal endothelial cells
        - Cells have a bright center and dark border
        - Some variability in the cell size is visible (polymegathism)
        - No cell dropout or guttae.
    - This appears to be a normal scan showing normal endothelial cells.

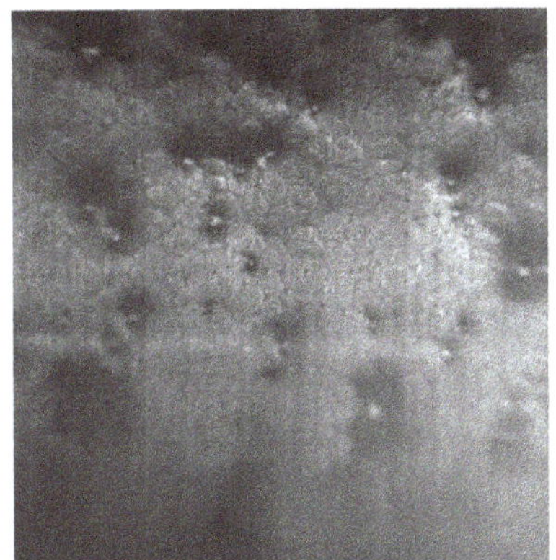

Fig. 10.6: Corneal guttae.

- *Example 2 (Fig. 10.6):*
    - This is a specular microscope image showing:
        - Few hexagonal endothelial cells
        - Corneal guttae are present that are visible as dark areas
        - Few intervening endothelial cells between the corneal guttae have abnormal shape with missing cell boundaries.
    - This image suggests the presence of corneal guttae, which can be seen in various conditions like Fuchs' endothelial corneal dystrophy, glaucoma, uveitis, and old age.

- *Example 3 (Fig. 10.7):* This is a specular microscope image showing:
  - Endothelial cells of variable shape (pleomorphism) and size (polymegathism)
  - The cells have a dark area with a light central spot
  - A light peripheral zone is visible with a dark border.

All the above findings suggest that this is a specular microscopy image of a case with iridocorneal endothelial syndrome. The typical appearance of this endothelial cell is called "iridocorneal-endothelial (ICE) cell."

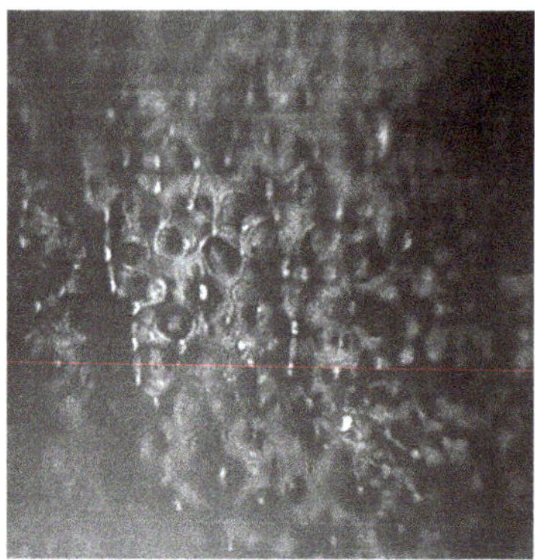

Fig. 10.7: Iridocorneal-endothelial (ICE) cells.

INTERPRETATION OF PENTACAM

General Principles

Look for the following while interpreting a Pentacam map. The interpretation should be made under the following headings as mentioned below. The normal values, as well as screening criteria for diagnosing keratoconus, must be remembered before going through this section (refer the chapter on Pentacam).

- Type of map
- Eye involved
- Age of patient
- K mean
- K_{max}
- Pachymetry apex
- Thinnest pachymetry
- Anterior elevation
- Posterior elevation
- Differential diagnosis.

Specific Examples

- *Example 1 (Fig. 10.8):*
  - This is a Pentacam map showing:

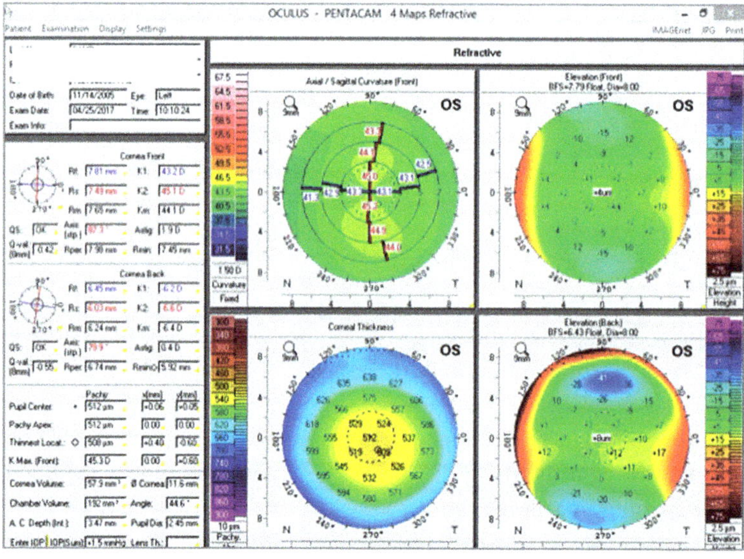

Fig. 10.8: A normal cornea.

- Four maps refractive display
- The left eye
- A 12-year-old patient
- A mean keratometry of 44.1 D
- K_{max} of 45.3 D
- Pachymetry apex of 512 µm
- Thinnest pachymetry of 508 µm
- Anterior elevation 4 µm
- Posterior elevation 12 µm.

◆ This appears to be a normal scan showing with the rule corneal astigmatism.

▪ *Example 2 (Figs. 10.9A and B):*

◆ This is Pentacam map showing:
  - Four maps refractive display
  - Right eye
  - A 12-year-old patient

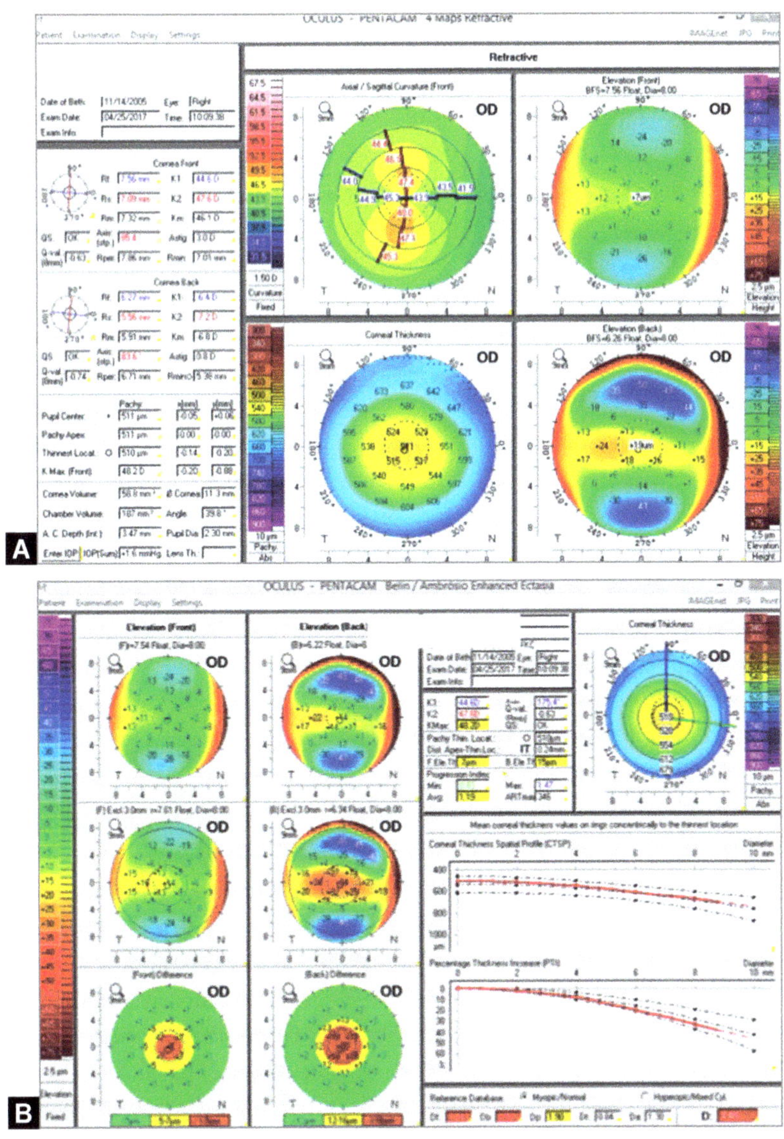

Figs. 10.9A and B: (A) Four maps refractive display of forme fruste keratoconus (FFKC); (B) Belin/Ambrósio enhanced ectasia display showing FFKC.

- A mean keratometry 46.1 D
- K_{max} of 48.2 D
- Pachymetry apex of 511 µm
- Thinnest pachymetry of 510 µm
- Anterior elevation 7 µm
- Posterior elevation 24 µm (abnormal).

◆ This scan shows with the rule corneal astigmatism that appears suspicious for forme fruste keratoconus (FFKC) based on the increased posterior elevation. Hence, I would like to evaluate the Belin/Ambrósio enhanced ectasia display of this patient.

◆ This is a Pentacam map showing:
- Belin/Ambrósio enhanced ectasia display
- The right eye
- A 12-year-old patient
- K_{max} of 48.2 D
- Thinnest pachymetry of 510 µm
- Inferotemporal displacement of the thinnest location by 0.24 mm (normal range)
- Posterior elevation 22 µm (abnormal)
- Posterior elevation on enhanced ectasia map 34 µm (abnormal)
- Both front and back difference map is abnormal (in red)
- Corneal thickness spatial profile is normal
- Percentage thickness increase is abnormal (curve touching the lower border in the 6 mm zone)
- D value is 3.05 (abnormal).

◆ Hence this is a case of FFKC.

- *Example 3 (Figs. 10.10A and B):*

◆ This is Pentacam map showing:
- Four maps refractive display
- The right eye
- A 34-year-old patient
- A mean keratometry 49.1 D
- K_{max} of 54.9 D
- The axial curvature map shows inferior steepening
- Pachymetry apex of 423 µm
- Thinnest pachymetry of 410 µm
- Pachymetry map shows the inferotemporal displacement of the thinnest location on the y-axis by 0.63 mm (suspicious)
- Anterior elevation 33 µm (abnormal)
- Posterior elevation 67 µm (abnormal)

◆ This scan suggests that it is a case of keratoconus as the area of corneal thinning is corresponding with the area of corneal ectasia.

◆ This is a Pentacam map showing:
- Belin/Ambrósio enhanced ectasia display
- The right eye
- A 34-year-old patient
- K_{max} of 54.9 D
- Thinnest pachymetry of 410 µm
- Inferotemporal displacement of the thinnest location by 0.24 mm (normal range)
- Posterior elevation 37 µm (abnormal)
- Posterior elevation on enhanced ectasia map 82 µm (abnormal)
- Both front and back difference map is abnormal (in red)
- Corneal thickness spatial profile is abnormal (curve outside the normal range with a sudden dip at 4 mm zone)
- Percentage thickness increase is abnormal (curve outside the normal range)
- D value is 9.36 (abnormal).

◆ Hence this is a case of keratoconus.

- *Example 4 (Fig. 10.11):*

◆ This is a Pentacam map showing:
- Four maps refractive display
- The left eye

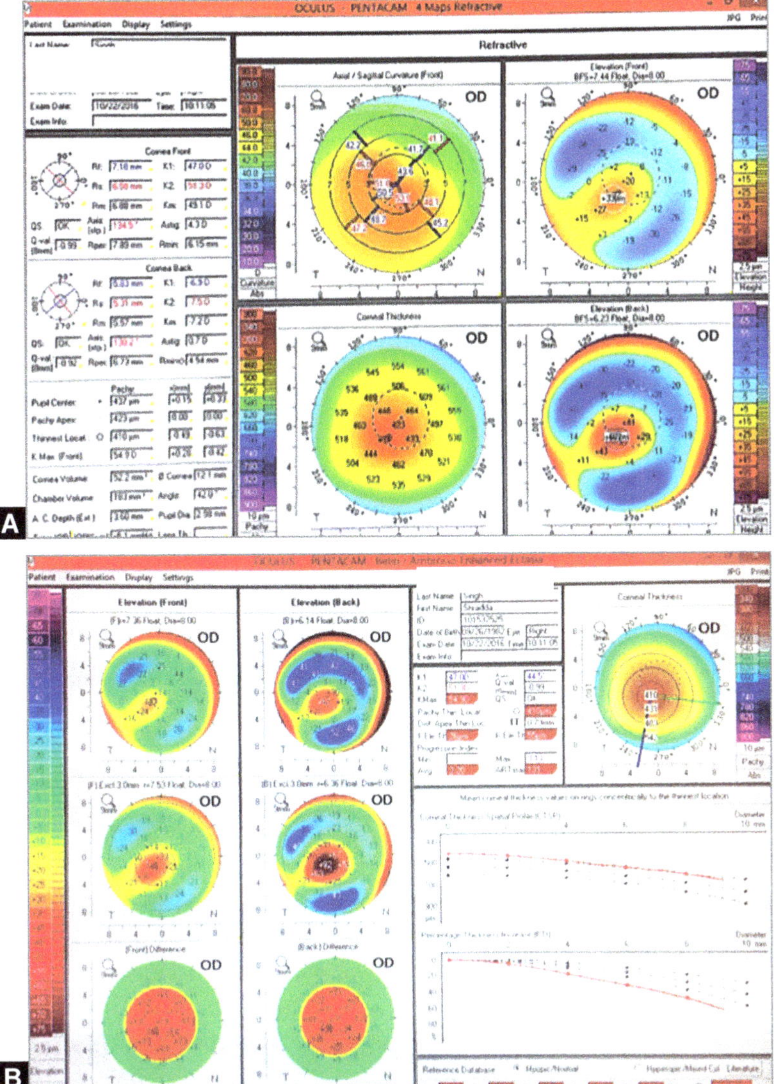

Figs. 10.10A and B: (A) Four maps refractive display; (B) Belin/Ambrósio enhanced ectasia display.

- A 37-year-old patient
- A mean keratometry 43.9 D
- K_{max} of 50.6 D
- The axial curvature map shows superior flat corneal contour with an inferior band of corneal steepening in the pattern of "crab claw" or "kissing doves"
- Pachymetry apex of 495 µm
- Thinnest pachymetry of 480 µm
- Pachymetry map shows inferotemporal displacement of the thinnest location on y-axis by 1.12 mm (suspicious)
- Anterior elevation 43 µm (abnormal)
- Posterior elevation 61 µm (abnormal).

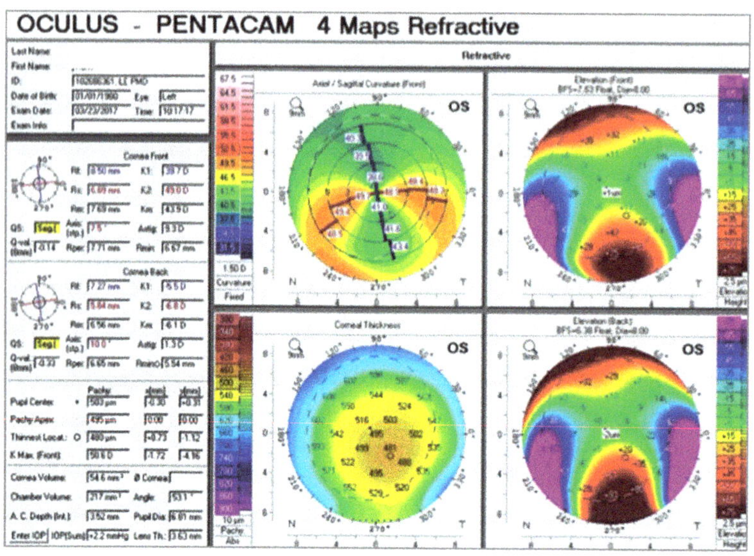

Fig. 10.11: Four maps refractive display showing pellucid marginal corneal degeneration (PMCD).

- This scan suggests a diagnosis of an ectatic corneal disorder, likely pellucid marginal corneal degeneration because the area of maximum corneal ectasia is superior to the area of corneal thinning and the typical "crab claw" appearance on the axial curvature map.

INTERPRETATION OF HUMPHREY VISUAL FIELD

Specific Examples

- *Example 1*—Steps to Interpret (Fig. 10.12A):
  - *Step 1:* This is a single field analysis of right eye of a 61 years old patient.
  - *Step 2:* By using central 30-2, Swedish Interactive Threshold Algorithm (SITA)-fast strategy with appropriate near correction given.
  - *Step 3:* The visual field is reliable.
  - *Step 4:* Total deviation probability plot shows scotoma or defect in the superior half area.
  - *Step 5:* Pattern deviation probability plot also shows a similar defect indicating localized damage, suggestive of superior arcuate going into the periphery.
  - *Step 6:* Global indices are abnormal (Visual field index (VFI) 71%, Mean deviation (MD) –10.83 dB, and Pattern standard deviation (PSD) 15.65 dB).
  - *Step 7:* Glaucoma Hemifield test is outside normal limits.
  - *Step 8:* Anderson's criteria will be met with if these defects are reproducible on consecutive visual fields. Therefore, given visual field shows a superior arcuate scotoma breaking into the periphery, suggestive of glaucomatous damage. Clinical correlation is needed.
- *Example* 2 *(Fig. 10.12B):*
  - *Step 1:* Single field analysis of the right eye of a 56 years old patient.
  - *Step 2:* By using central 30-2, SITA-Fast strategy with appropriate near correction given.

- *Step 3:* The visual field is reliable.
- *Step 4:* Total deviation probability plot shows scotoma or defect in nasal area inferiorly.
- *Step 5:* Pattern deviation probability plot also shows a similar defect indicating localized damage. Global indices are abnormal (VFI 94%, MD 2.75 dB and PAD 7.63 dB).
- *Step 6:* Glaucoma Hemifield test is outside normal limit.
- *Step 7:* Anderson's criteria will be met with if these defects are reproducible on consecutive visual fields. Therefore, given visual field shows an inferior nasal step, suggestive of glaucomatous damage. Clinical correlation is needed.

■ *Example 3 (Fig. 10. 12C):*
- *Step 1:* Single field analysis of the right eye of a 55 years old patient.
- *Step 2:* By using central 30-2, FASTPAC strategy with appropriate near correction.
- *Step 3:* The visual field is reliable.
- *Step 4:* Total deviation probability plot shows superior and inferior arcuate scotoma, breaking into the periphery.
- *Step 5:* Pattern deviation probability plot also shows a similar defect indicating localized damage.
- *Step 6:* Global indices are abnormal (MD-26.15, PSD 7.72).
- *Step 7:* Anderson's criteria will be met with if these defects are reproducible on consecutive visual fields. Therefore, given visual field shows a double arcuate scotoma breaking into the periphery, suggestive of advanced glaucomatous damage. Clinical correlation is needed.

■ *Example 4 (Fig. 10.12 D):*
- *Step 1:* Single field analysis of left eye of a 49 years old patient.
- *Step 2:* By using central 30-2, SITA-Fast strategy with appropriate near correction given.
- *Step 3:* The visual field is reliable.
- *Step 4:* Total deviation probability plot shows generalized depression which is not present in pattern deviation probability plot, suggestive of a nonglaucomatous defect like cataract. Clinical correlation is needed.

■ *Example 5 (Fig. 10.13):*
- *Step 1:* Guided progression analysis (GPA) report of the left eye of a patient named, ...
- *Step 2:* The upper two fields depict the baseline fields of the patient on presentation showing VFI 96%, MD –4.13 dB, and PSD 3.10 dB.
- *Step 3:* Below that is the VFI plot with a steeper slope, showing significant progression based on VFI values. It also shows that this much amount of 3–5 years progression is going to happen in future, if the current trend follows.
- *Step 4:* The rate of progression is –3.0± 0.9%/year.
- *Step 5:* Below that is the current visual field summary showing VFI 73%, MD –13.67 dB, and PSD 6.55 dB. GPA alert shows "likely progression."

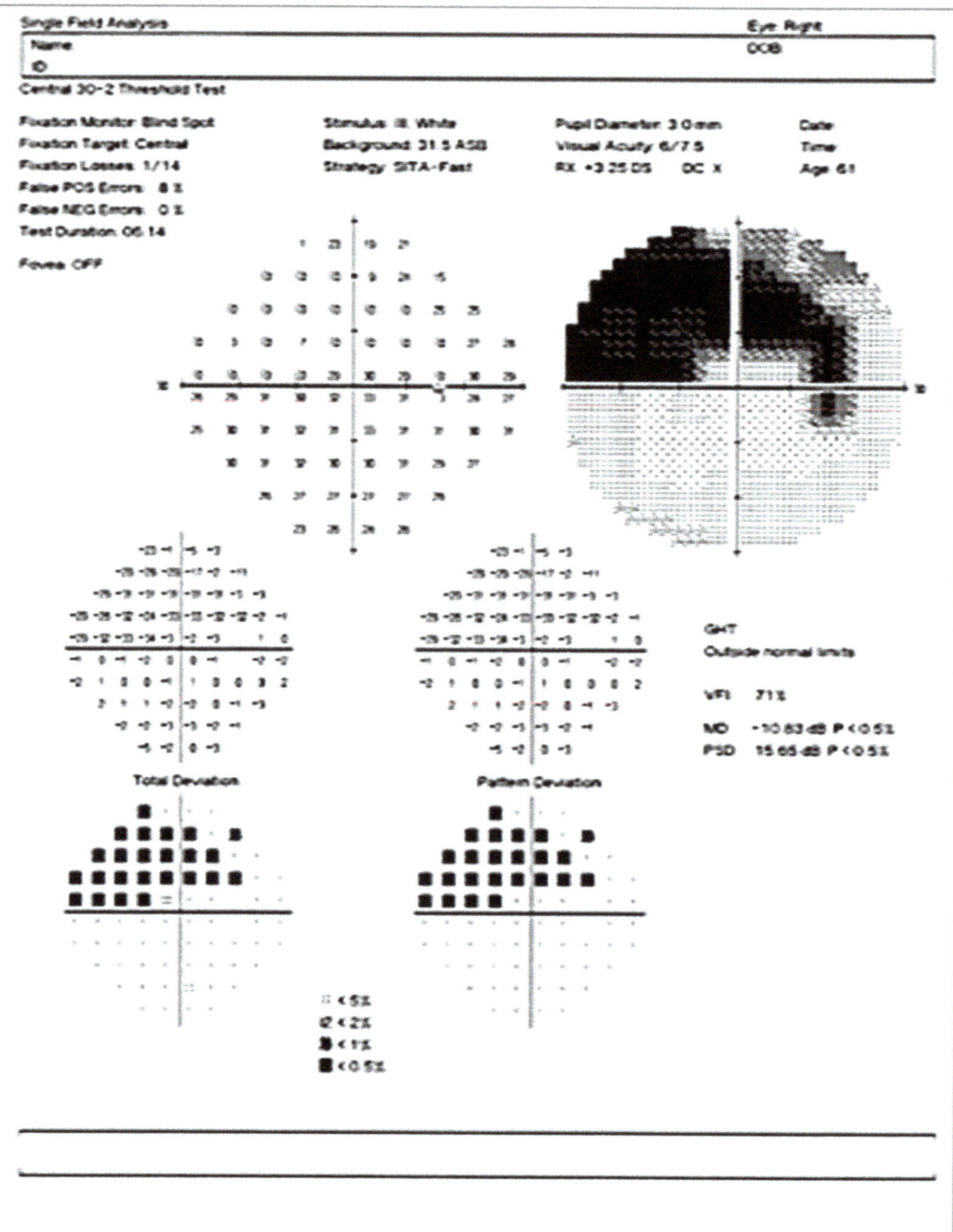

Fig. 10.12A

Single Field Analysis
Eye: Right
Name
DOB
ID
Central 30-2 Threshold Test
Fixation Monitor: Blind Spot
Fixation Target: Central
Fixation Losses: 0/13
False POS Errors: 3 %
False NEG Errors: 0 %
Test Duration: 04:55
Fovea: OFF
Stimulus: III, White
Background: 31.5 ASB
Strategy: SITA-Fast
Pupil Diameter: 3.0 mm
Visual Acuity: 6/6
RX: +3.00 DS DC X
Date
Time
Age: 56
GHT
Outside normal limits
VFI 94%
MD -3.75 dB P < 1%
PSD 7.63 dB P < 0.5%
Total Deviation
Pattern Deviation
< 5%
< 2%
< 1%
< 0.5%

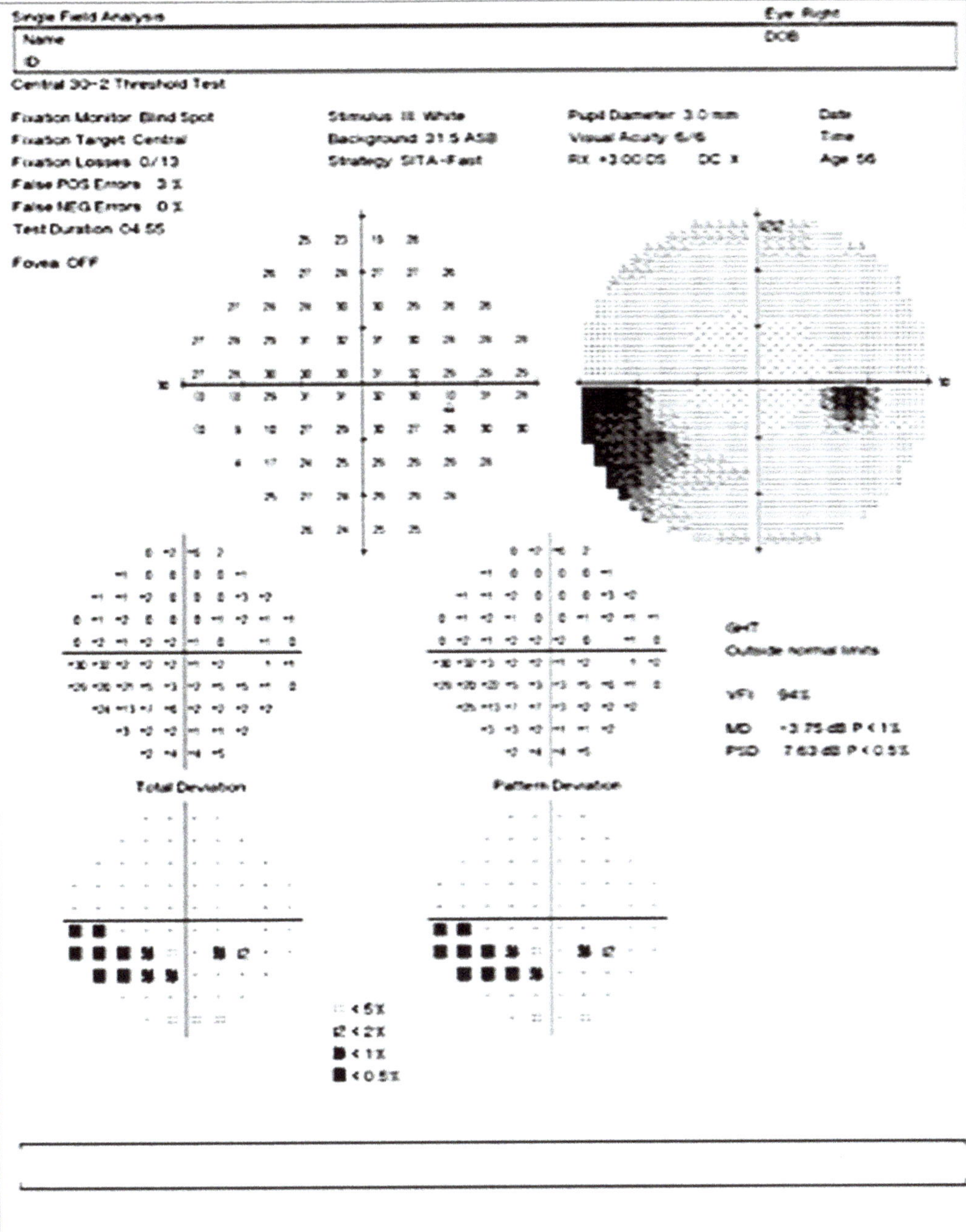

Fig.10.12B

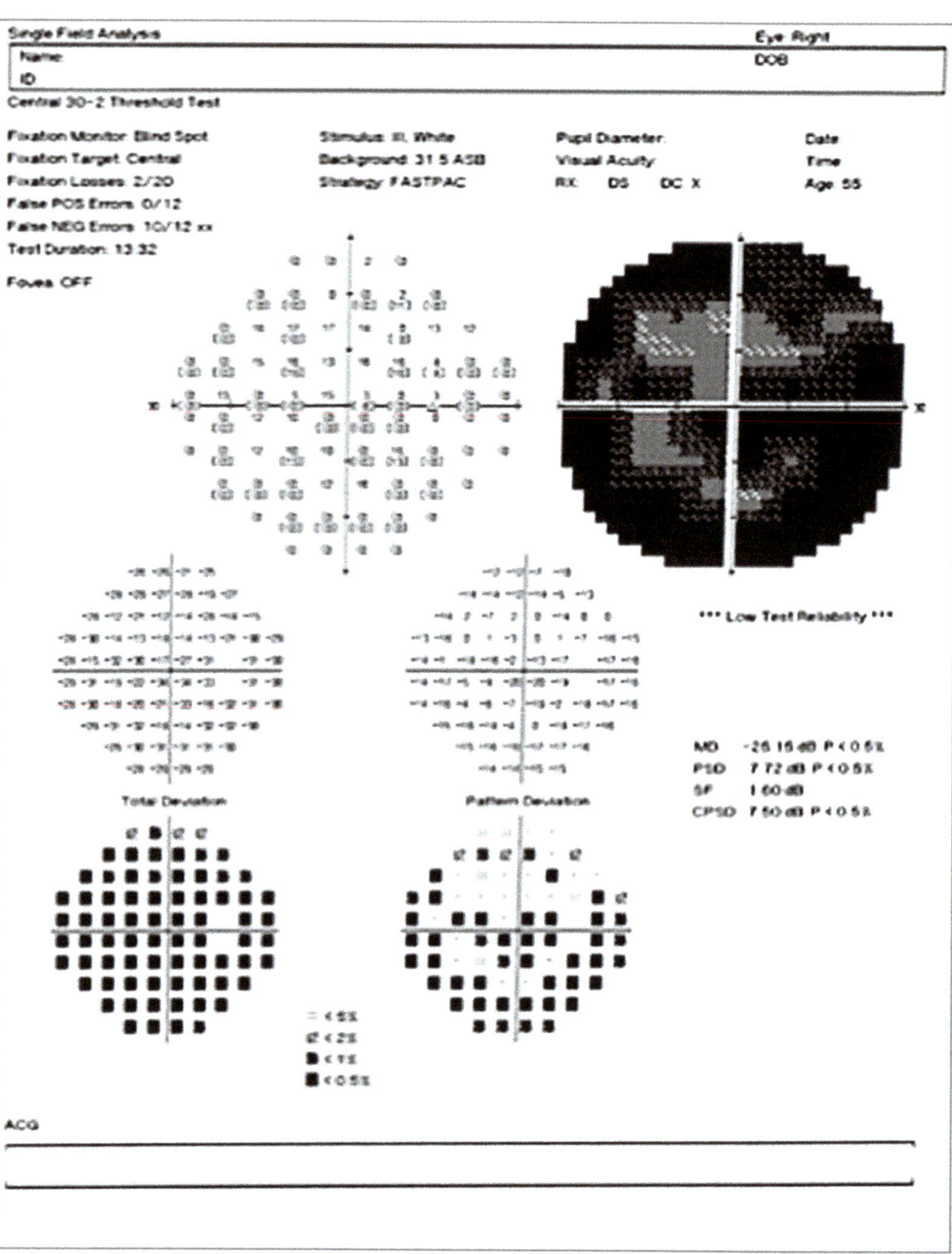

Fig. 10.12C

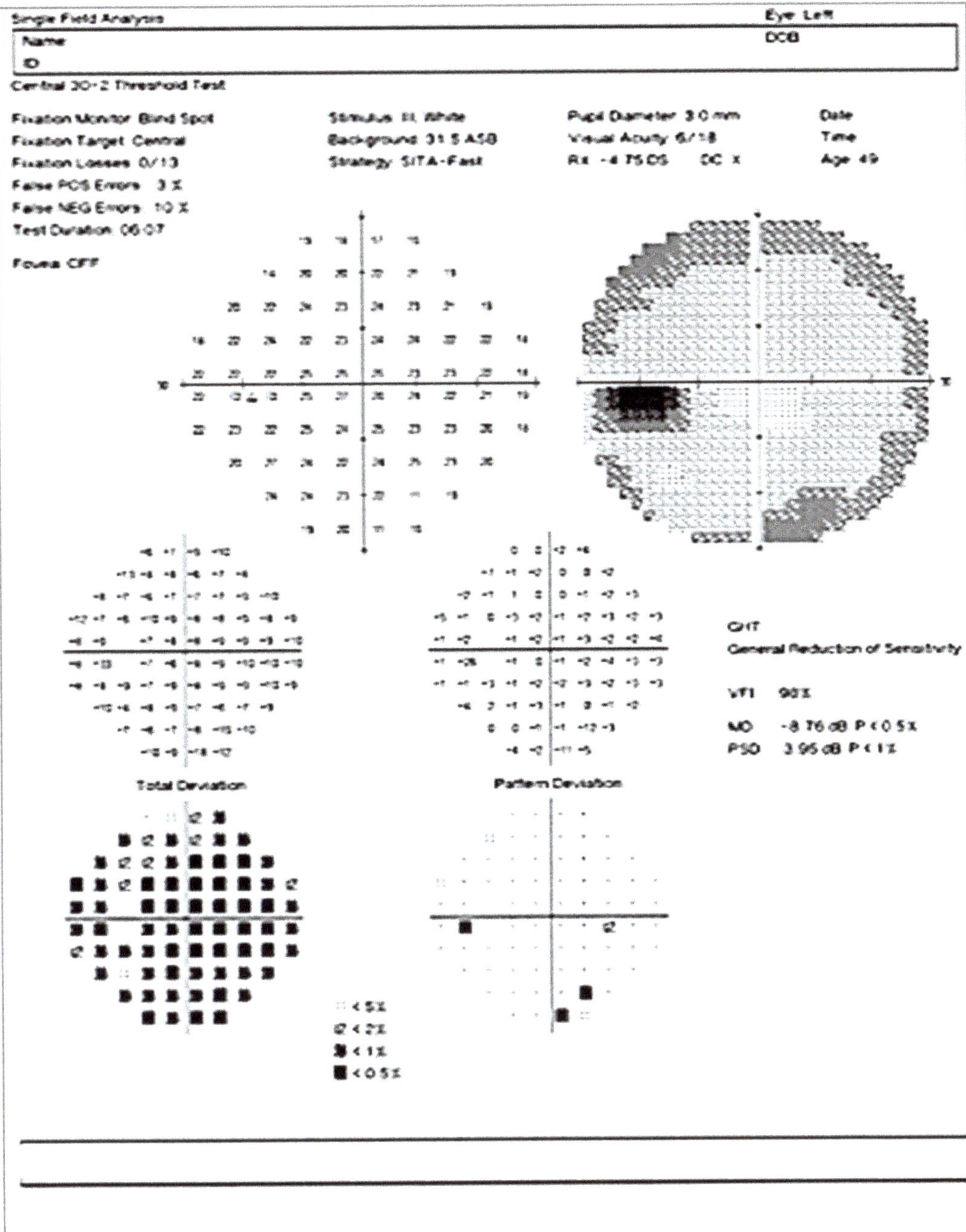

Fig. 10.12D

Figs. 10.12A to D: Humphrey visual field.

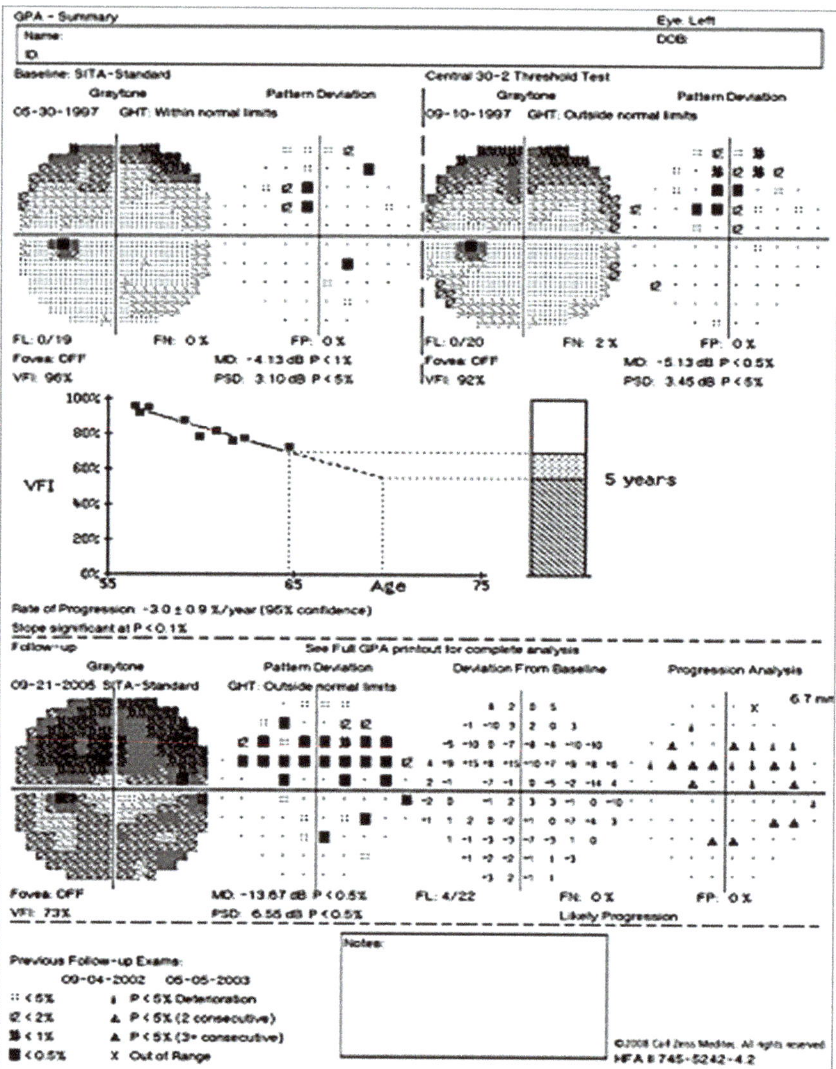

Fig. 10.13: Guided progression analysis.

INTERPRETATION OF ANTERIOR SEGMENT OPTICAL COHERENCE TOMOGRAPHY

Specific Examples

- *Example 1 (Fig. 10.14):* This is an anterior segment optical coherence tomography (ASOCT) image showing Descemet membrane detachment with a corneal thickness of 571 μm.
- *Example 2 (Fig. 10.15):* This is an ASOCT image of a case of operated endothelial keratoplasty. The total corneal thickness is 421 μm, and the thickness of donor corneal lenticule is 56 μm. The patient most likely seems to have undergone an ultrathin Descemet stripping automated endothelial keratoplasty (DSAEK) considering the graft thickness and the smooth interface.
- *Example 3 (Fig. 10.16):* This is an ASOCT image of a case of operated phakic intraocular lens (IOL). The vault, in this case, is 620 μm.

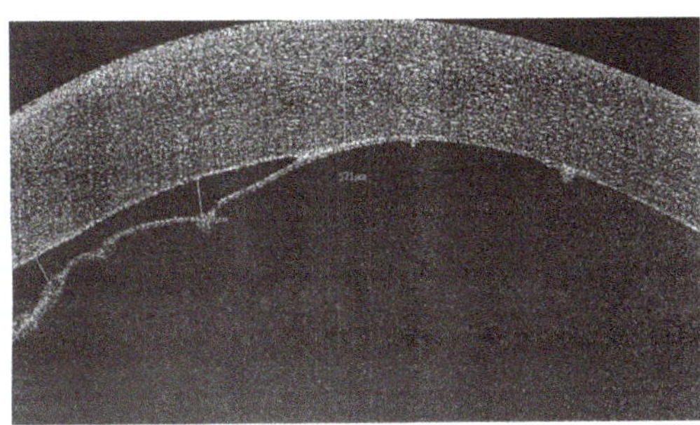

Fig. 10.14: Anterior segment optical coherence tomography (ASOCT) image showing Descemet membrane detachment.

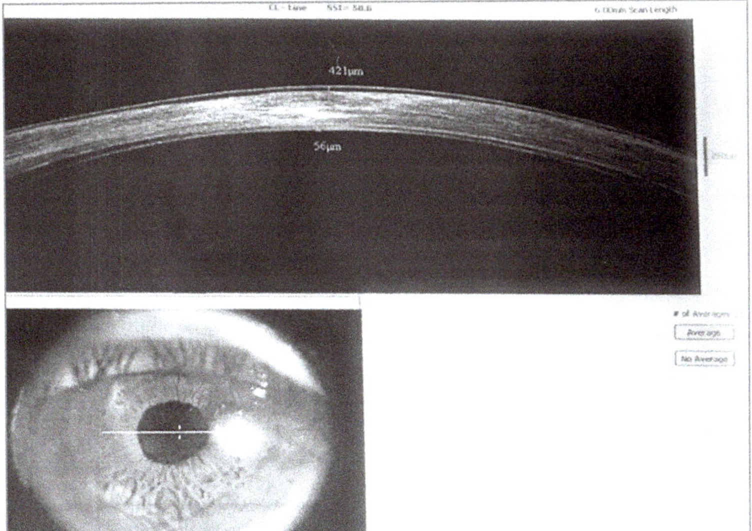

Fig. 10.15: Anterior segment optical coherence tomography image of a case of operated endothelial keratoplasty.

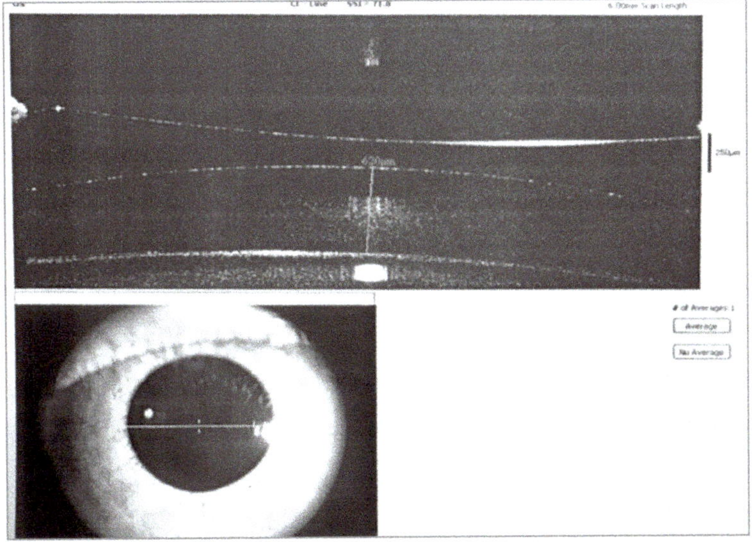

Fig. 10.16: Anterior segment optical coherence tomography image of a case of operated phakic intraocular lens.

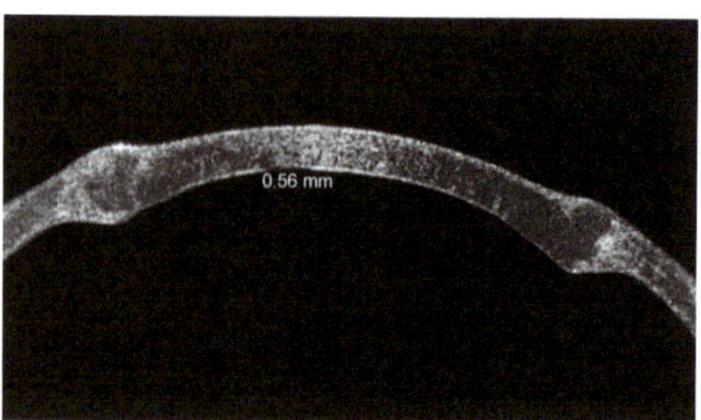

Fig. 10.17: Anterior segment optical coherence tomography image of a case of operated penetrating keratoplasty.

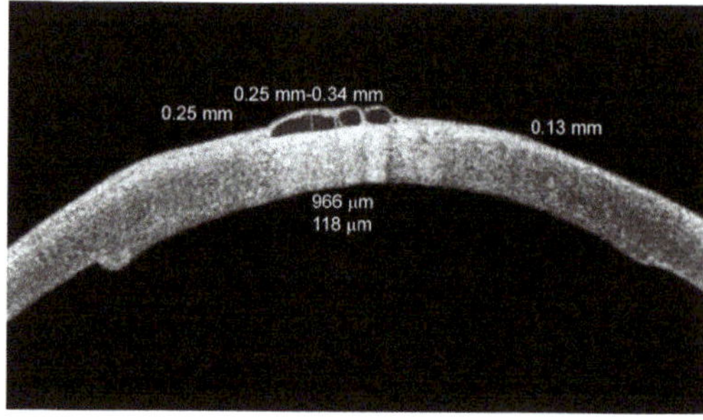

Fig. 10.18: Anterior segment optical coherence tomography image of a case of operated endothelial keratoplasty.

- *Example 4 (Fig. 10.17):* This is an ASOCT image of a case of operated penetrating keratoplasty. The graft thickness is 560 μm. The image shows an irregular contour of the posterior graft-host junction.
- *Example 5 (Fig. 10.18):* This is an ASOCT image of a case of operated endothelial keratoplasty. The total corneal thickness is 966 μm, and the thickness of donor corneal lenticule is 118 μm. Corneal epithelial bullae are visible. On the basis of the presence of epithelial bullae with increased corneal thickness, this appears to be a case of failed endothelial keratoplasty.

INDEX

Page numbers followed by *f* refer to figure, and *t* refer to table.

B

C

D

E

F

G

H

I

J

K

L

M

N

O

P

Q

R

S

T

U

V

W

Y

Z

EU GSPR Authorised Reprsentative
Logos Europe, 9 rue Nicolas Poussin
1700, La Rochelle, France
Phone: +33 (0) 6 67 93 73 78
E-mail: contact@logoseurope.eu

www.ingramcontent.com/pod-product-compliance
Ingram Content Group UK Ltd.
Pitfield, Milton Keynes, MK11 3LW, UK
UKHW050923290726
14058UKWH00011B/683

* 9 7 8 9 3 8 9 1 8 8 6 0 8 *